TABLE OF CONTENTS

Evolve®

YOU'VE JUST PURCHASED

MORE THAN A TEXTBOOK!

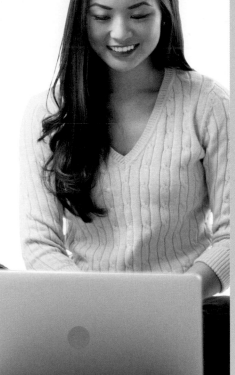

Enhance your learning with Evolve Student Resources.

These online study tools and exercises can help deepen your understanding of textbook content so you can be more prepared for class, perform better on exams, and succeed in your course.

Activate the complete learning experience that comes with each NEW textbook purchase by registering with your scratch-off access code at

http://evolve.elsevier.com/Muscolino/palpation/

If your school uses its own Learning Management System, your resources may be delivered on that platform. Consult with your instructor.

If you rented or purchased a used book and the scratch-off code at right has already been revealed, the code may have been used and cannot be re-used for registration. To purchase a new code to access these valuable study resources, simply follow the link above.

Muscolino
Scratch Gently to Reveal Code

REGISTER TODAY!

ELSEVIER

2019v1.0

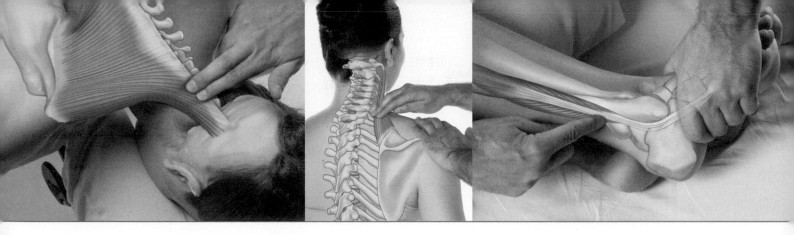

Third Edition

The MUSCLE *and* BONE PALPATION MANUAL

with Trigger Points, Referral Patterns, and Stretching

JOSEPH E. MUSCOLINO, DC

Owner, The Art and Science of Kinesiology and
LearnMuscles.com,
Stamford, Connecticut

ELSEVIER

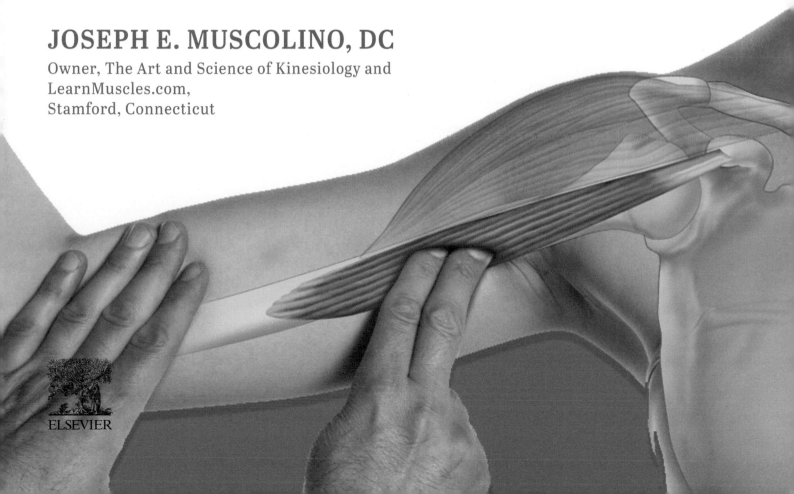

Elsevier
3251 Riverport Lane
St. Louis, Missouri 63043

THE MUSCLE AND BONE PALPATION MANUAL WITH TRIGGER POINTS,
REFERRAL PATTERNS, AND STRETCHING, THIRD EDITION   ISBN: 978-0-323-76136-9

Previous editions copyrighted 2016, 2009

Content Strategist: Melissa Rawe
Senior Content Development Specialist: Sarah Vora and Beck Rist
Publishing Services Manager: Shereen Jameel
Project Manager: Gayathri S
Design Direction: Bridget Hoette

Printed in India

Last digit is the print number: 9   8   7   6   5   4   3   2

Working together
to grow libraries in
developing countries

www.elsevier.com • www.bookaid.org

DEDICATION

This book is dedicated to all of my students, past, present, and future.
I have always felt that both the classroom and life are about learning and growing.
It was a gift to be a part of your lives as we meandered through the intricacies
as well as the bigger picture of anatomy, physiology, kinesiology, palpation, and treatment.
So much of my learning took place in the classroom along with you.

Thank you.

SPECIAL DEDICATION

This book is lovingly dedicated to Diane C. Schwartz.
Her courage, spirit, and passion for life, learning, and love
have always been and always will be an inspiration to me
and everyone's life she touched.

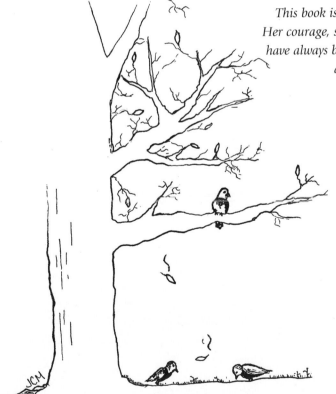

First Edition Contributors and DVD Presenters

Sandra K. Anderson, BA, NCTMB

Leon Chaitow, ND, DO

Judith DeLany, LMT

Neal Delaporta, NCTMB

Mike Dixon, RMT

Sandy Fritz, MS, NCTMB

Beverley Giroud, LMT, NCTMB

Gil Hedley, PhD

Glenn M. Hymel, EdD, LMT

Bob King, LMT, NCTMB

George Kousaleos, BA, LMT, NCTMB

Whitney Lowe, LMT

Bob McAtee, NCTMB, CSCS, CPT

Thomas Myers, LMT, NCTMB, ARP

Fiona Rattray, RMT

Monica J. Reno, LMT, NCTMB

Susan G. Salvo, BEd, LMT, NCTMB

Diana L. Thompson, LMP

Benny Vaughn, LMT, ATC, CSCS, NCTMB

Tracy Walton, MS, LMT

Ruth Werner, LMP, NCTMB

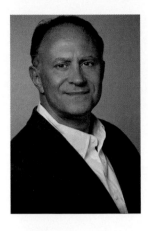

Dr. Joe Muscolino has been teaching neuro-myo-fascio-skeletal and visceral anatomy and physiology, kinesiology, and pathology courses for more than 35 years. He has published the following books with Elsevier: *The Muscular System Manual: The Skeletal Muscles of the Human Body, 5th Edition; Kinesiology: The Skeletal System and Muscle Function, 4th Edition; Musculoskeletal Anatomy Coloring Book, 3rd Edition; Know the Body, along with its companion Workbook;* and *Musculoskeletal Anatomy Flashcards.* He has also published *Manual Therapy for the Low Back and Pelvis: A Clinical Orthopedic Approach* and *Advanced Treatment Techniques for the Manual Therapist: Neck.*

Dr. Muscolino is the author of more than 90 articles on manual and movement therapy published in the *Massage Therapy Journal,* the *Journal of Bodywork and Movement Therapies,* and other journals, both in the United States and overseas. He has also published numerous DVDs for manual and movement therapists, and he has several online learning platforms for both core-curriculum anatomy and physiology as well as continuing education techniques of manual and movement therapies. Dr. Muscolino is also a global lecturer and instructor, running continuing education workshops in the world of manual and movement therapy. Topics include palpation and orthopedic assessment, manual and movement therapy treatment techniques, body mechanics, cadaver labs, and fundamental biomechanics/kinesiology. He also offers a Certification in *Clinical Orthopedic Manual Therapy (COMT).* He is an NCBTMB-approved provider of continuing education, and CEUs are available for Massage Therapists toward Certification renewal.

Dr. Muscolino holds a Bachelor of Arts degree in Biology from the State University of New York (SUNY) at Binghamton, Harpur College. He attained his Doctor of Chiropractic Degree from Western States Chiropractic College in Portland, Oregon, and is licensed in Connecticut, New York, and California. Dr. Joe Muscolino has been in private practice in Connecticut for more than 35 years and incorporates soft tissue work into his chiropractic practice for all his patients.

If you would like further information regarding Dr. Muscolino's Elsevier publications previously listed or if you are an instructor and would like information regarding the many supportive materials available from Elsevier such as PowerPoint slides, test banks of questions, or TEACH Instructor Resources, please visit http://www.us.elsevierhealth.com. If you would like to contact Dr. Muscolino directly, please contact him at his website: www.learnmuscles.com.

Foreword to Second Edition

It was my honor to write the foreword for the first edition of *The Muscle and Bone Palpation Manual* in the summer of 2008. I was most taken with the accessibility of the text and the usability of the format along with beautiful artwork. Now, several years later, I am still impressed by these features, but I am most moved by how this text has grown to meet and anticipate the needs of today's students.

I am frankly envious of massage therapy students who start school today. The array of educational settings is varied, the skillsets to which they are exposed are far more broad than my 125 hours of entry-level education afforded, and most of all, people who enter massage school today have texts and other learning tools developed specifically for them. Such things simply didn't exist back in my day (when we carried our tables to school, uphill, through the snow, barefoot, you get the idea). In those olden days of the early '80s we didn't have books on the musculoskeletal system to help us mount the intimidating learning curve of kinesiology. Moreover, we had barely enough time to develop a rudimentary understanding and appreciation for human function. The ability to use that knowledge to make appropriate clinical decisions was something that developed very much on the fly for many of us—me included.

Many massage therapy students approach the project of learning muscle anatomy with an understandable degree of apprehension. They look at those long lists of muscles with attachments and functions, and feel utterly overwhelmed. The topic seems abstract, the language is unfamiliar, and the goal of truly "getting it" seems out of reach. Gifted educators find ways to make this information jump off the page, but the process is daunting. What a gift to have a text that illustrates these concepts with such thoroughness, clarity, and beauty.

Even better, this updated edition is supplemented with tools for putting those concepts directly into clinical application. Massage therapy education today puts increasing emphasis on the development of strong skill competencies, and *The Muscle and Bone Palpation Manual, 2nd Edition* is well designed to answer that call. The illustrated therapist-assisted stretches, the case studies that conclude each chapter, and the printable client self-care charts reflect this priority. Students will find this text indispensable long after they graduate, because the information here isn't just for beginning a career: it's for a lifelong calling in this field.

The Muscle and Bone Palpation Manual, 2nd Edition continues to identify the needs of massage practitioners and students, and consistently meets them with accessible language,

beautiful art that represents a wide range of bodies, and a sharp focus on how this knowledge can inform the way every massage therapist touches another human being. Meticulous attention to accuracy is obvious on every page. This book can provide tools for massage therapists and students not only to become soft tissue experts but to communicate professionally with other health care providers to obtain the best outcomes for their clients.

I am confident that *The Muscle and Bone Palpation Manual, 2nd Edition* is a tool that can help to launch new generations of therapists ready to improve the quality of life for all their clients. It and texts like it will continue to set the best possible standards in massage education: a goal that supports us all.

Ruth Werner, BCTMB
Waldport, Oregon
May, 2014

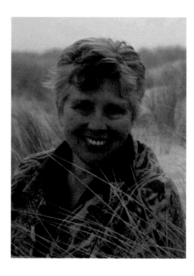

Ruth Werner is an award-winning writer and educator with a passionate interest in the role of massage therapy for people who struggle with health. Her book, *A Massage Therapist's Guide to Pathology*, is in its seventh edition, with Books of Discovery, and is used in massage schools worldwide. She writes columns for *Massage and Bodywork* magazine and *Massage New Zealand* and teaches live and online continuing education workshops all over the world. She is a past president of the Massage Therapy Foundation and an avid volunteer in the field of massage therapy education.

ORGANIZATION

The Muscle and Bone Palpation Manual is organized into four parts.

Part 1 covers assessment techniques. Two chapters are provided that explain the art and science of how to palpate. These chapters simply and clearly explain the guidelines that will help you become an effective and confident palpator. Chapter 3, new to this edition, covers orthopedic assessment testing.

Part 2 covers treatment techniques. There is a chapter that provides an atlas of soft tissue manipulation (massage) strokes and draping methods for massage. Another chapter explains what trigger points are and how they are formed, along with what is likely a treatment method superior to ischemic/sustained compression. There is a chapter that explains how to reason out stretches for the muscles of the body and explains how to perform advanced stretching techniques, such as contract relax (CR) stretching (also known as proprioceptive neuromuscular facilitation [PNF] stretching) and agonist contract (AC) stretching. And given the crucial importance of body mechanics to the student and therapist, there is also a chapter that offers 10 guidelines that will appreciably improve the efficiency with which you work.

Part 3 is composed of three chapters that cover palpation of the bones, bony landmarks, and joints of the body, as well as covering the ligaments of the body. Effective palpation of the bones and bony landmarks of the body is a crucial first step before muscle palpation can be tackled. Effective palpation of the joints is also a necessary skill for assessment of clients. Each chapter in Part 3 also contains a thorough set of anterior, posterior, and lateral illustrations depicting the ligaments of the body.

Part 4 is the masterpiece of the book. It contains 11 chapters that cover palpation of the skeletal muscles of the body. Each chapter presents a tour of the body's muscles in each region. For each muscle, a step-by-step palpation is presented, with the reasoning given for the steps so that the palpation can be understood and reasoned out instead of being memorized. The illustrations are superbly done with the bones and muscles drawn over photographs of real people, offering the most accurate and clear renderings of the muscles and muscle palpations possible. In addition, unique muscle stretch illustrations, for both self-care and therapist-assisted stretches, are given for each and every muscle covered, as well as trigger point and trigger point referral zone information and illustrations for all the muscles.

DISTINCTIVE FEATURES

- An Alternate Palpation Position is given when appropriate, often with an accompanying illustration.
- General muscle information is provided, including attachments, actions, and a drawing of the individual muscle.
- Full-color musculoskeletal drawings depict muscles and bones exactly as they appear when palpated to help locate tissues and landmarks with confidence, explained by detailed palpation steps and supplemented with a photo of the starting position.

- Trigger points, referral patterns, and both self-care and therapist-assisted stretches included for each muscle provide convenient access to guidelines for additional client assessment and treatment.
- Included throughout the chapters are *Detours* to individual muscles that are not featured in a full spread, briefly discussing palpation and trigger point aspects of those muscles.
- Palpation Notes and a *Palpation Key* for each muscle palpation provide more in-depth information to enhance palpation knowledge and provide interesting notes to trigger memory recall.
- Chapters 8, 9, and 10 contain comprehensive coverage of bones and how to palpate bones and their landmarks. These chapters feature four-color line drawings of bone palpation showing the therapist palpating the client's bone, with the bone visible beneath the skin.
- Each chapter begins with a chapter overview, outline, objectives, and key terms.
- A robust Evolve website is available with not only the unique Interactive Muscle Program and other learning tools for students, but also videos that demonstrate and reinforce correct palpation of the muscles of the body. Furthermore, there are video lecture presentations by Dr. Joe Muscolino for the entirety of Chapters 8, 9, and 10.

This text also includes:

- Review Questions allow students to discuss concepts and synthesize chapter information.
- *Deeper Thoughts* questions actively engage students and challenge their reasoning skills.
- Case studies provide students with the opportunity for integrative, clinical reasoning.
- Drawings of therapist-assisted stretches are shown with the client on the table with draping. These stretches alongside existing drawings of self-care stretches provide the user with a comprehensive look at stretching.
- Unique Interactive Muscle Program are available on Evolve. For each major region of the body, a base photograph is presented with the skeleton drawn in. A list of every muscle of that region is given, and the user can choose any combination of muscles and place them onto the illustration. This exciting program allows the user to see muscle attachments and the relationship among the muscles of the region. Any combination of muscles can be chosen!
- An invaluable Self-Care Stretching Customization form for Clients asset on the Evolve website allows you to drag and drop the self-care stretching figures into a template that can be printed and handed to your clients to aid them in their self-care program at home!

EVOLVE RESOURCES FOR THE INSTRUCTOR

In addition to the clear and simple, yet thorough, approach to the content of this book, the accompanying Evolve resources for instructors is complimentary for any school that adopts this book into their curriculum. Instructors can access Power-Point presentations accompanied by complete TEACH lesson plans along with learning objectives, critical reasoning questions, classroom activities, and more. An image bank containing every illustration in the book, a 600-question test bank, answers to Review Questions and Case Studies, bonus video, and more are also available.

EVOLVE RESOURCES FOR THE STUDENT/THERAPIST

Students and therapists who purchase a new book are given free access to the student/therapist resources on Evolve, which include the unique Interactive Muscle Program, exercises, a new Body Systems Quick Guide, a Self-Care Stretching Customization form for Clients asset, and more! And to enhance muscle palpation illustrations and text in Parts 3 and 4 of this book, Evolve also has more than 17 hours of video of Dr. Muscolino demonstrating the bone and muscle palpations of the book. The videos also contain cameo presentations by some

of the most prestigious names in the world of massage therapy education, including Tom Myers, Leon Chaitow, Whitney Lowe, Bob King, Gil Hedley, and many more.

FINAL NOTE

No other book offers as much to you as *The Muscle and Bone Palpation Manual*. It contains the most thorough and clear palpation methods accompanied by the highest-quality illustrations possible, and it includes an accompanying Evolve website that contains a wealth of valuable study aids! Furthermore, it offers a complete set of stretches and trigger point illustrations for the skeletal muscles of the body. With chapters on how to palpate and stretch, orthopedic assessment testing, understanding trigger points, a complete coverage of the ligaments, a compendium of all major massage strokes and draping methods, and a thorough chapter on body mechanics, *The Muscle and Bone Palpation Manual* will easily take the place of three or four books needed in your library.

Joseph E. Muscolino
December 2021

Acknowledgments

The longer I have been writing, the more I have come to realize that a book of this scope does not come to fruition without enormous contributions from many, many people. I am so thankful that this Acknowledgments page offers me the chance to publicly thank everyone who helped create this book.

First, I am indebted to all of my students, past and present, both in the United States and overseas. Few people may realize it, but teaching in front of a group of sharp, motivated students is the best way to learn a subject! Each and every time a student questioned my presentation of content, it helped me to hone how to best say and present it the next time. This has helped me immeasurably as a teacher and as an author!

A number of students specifically helped me by modeling for photos that were the basis for the artwork in Chapters 8 through 10. Thank you so very much. I also must thank Ania Kazimierczuk and Amy Van Buren, massage therapists who helped me create the therapist-assisted stretching figures in this book. As always, I reserve a special thank you for William Courtland, the student who first sparked my interest in writing books. His statement, "You should write a book," many years ago placed me on my current path as an author.

Many years ago, a professor of mine once said that we all stand on the shoulders of those who have come before us. This is so true. I would like to thank the authors of past and present books on musculoskeletal anatomy, physiology, kinesiology, palpation, assessment, and treatment. We all learn from each other and then offer our best to the students, therapists, trainers, and instructors who buy our books.

One of the highlights of this book is the artwork. Indeed, much of the time my writing is more of an addendum to the artwork than the other way around. I am indebted to Jeanne Robertson for her sharp, clean, and clear figures in Parts 1 and 2 of this book. I am also indebted to Ken Vanderstoep of Lightbox Visuals out of Canada who provided the wonderful trigger point and stretching illustrations in Part 4. For the muscle and bone artwork superimposed over photographs of models (also found in Part 4), I cannot thank Frank Forney and Dave Carlson of Colorado and Giovanni Rimasti of Lightbox Visuals enough. Their stunning artwork makes this book shine. A big thank you also goes out to Jodie Bernard of Lightbox Visuals who was fabulous to work with. She was super competent, always available by phone, and fun to work with – a great combination of traits! And a fond thank you to my son, JC, for the illustration that accompanies the Special Dedication on the Dedication page.

For the beautiful photographs that were the basis of most of the artwork for Part 3, as well as the other photographs throughout this book, I thank Yanik Chauvin, another great Canadian, once again. Yanik is a wonderful photographer and a pleasure to work with.

At Elsevier, thank you again to my entire editorial, design, and production team for the First Edition: specifically, Laura Loveall, Ellen Kunkelmann, Linda McKinley, Julia Dummitt, April Falast, Linda Duncan, and Kellie White. And, as always, a huge thank you to Jennifer Watrous, my developmental editor who was my partner throughout the First Edition project; no author could have asked for a better partner! Also, a big thank you to my Elsevier team for the Second Edition: Pat Costigan, Rachel McMullen and Julia Dummitt; and the biggest thank you to Shelly Stringer, my partner throughout the Second Edition. And finally, a big thank you to my Elsevier team for the Third Edition: Melissa Rawe and Gayathri S.

A special thank you to Sandy Fritz and Susan Salvo for writing the principal body of the chapter on massage strokes and draping. This book also contains a great number of cameo presentations on the Evolve website. Thank you to the extraordinary assemblage of massage therapy educators who donated their time to be a part of this project. I am humbled and honored by your participation. I am also honored to have had my good friend, Ruth Werner, write the foreword to the Second Edition of this book.

Thank you also to all the models for the artwork in the book and Evolve website that accompany the book. A special thank you goes to Betsyann Baron for her invaluable assistance in finding many of the models! Thank you to Chuck and his video team at Visionary Production for making the video shoot efficient and fun. Thank you to Steve and Lois at Top Graphics for their fast and excellent work. And a blanket "thank you!" to all the people who worked on this project who I do not know personally. You all share in the success of this book.

Finally, a huge thank you to my entire family, especially my wife and angel, Simona Cipriani. Thank you for your patience, understanding, and support during all the hours that I have spent away from you to create this book. I love you all and look forward to spending more time with you now that this project is finally completed!

And thank you Diane for all the love and support that you gave me and the inspiration that you continue to give me every day of my life!

CHAPTER 1

Introduction to Palpation

Overview

This chapter is an introduction to the general principles of palpation. The two major objectives of palpation, location and assessment of the target structure, are discussed first. General principles that explain how to palpate are then presented. The importance of palpating not only during a client examination but also during treatment is emphasized. The chapter concludes with an exercise that can help develop palpation skills and a recommendation to incorporate the practice of palpatory skills whenever our hands are on a client.

Note: The introductory palpation information covered in this chapter is sufficient to allow the reader to successfully palpate the bones and bony landmarks of the skeleton presented in Chapters 8 to 10. Palpating skeletal landmarks is relatively easy because they are hard tissue surrounded by the many soft tissues of the body; therefore their many features, such as tubercles, shafts, fossas, and condyles, stand out amongst the surrounding tissues. However, muscle palpation can be more nuanced and challenging. For this reason, it is strongly recommended that Chapter 2, The Art and Science of Muscle Palpation, is read before attempting the muscle palpations covered in Chapters 11 to 21. Chapter 2 explores palpation in much greater depth and offers more subtle and sophisticated methods and guidelines that are directly applicable to muscle palpation.

Chapter Outline

What Is Palpation?
Objectives of Palpation: Location and Assessment
How to Palpate
When Do We Palpate?
How to Learn Palpation

Chapter Objectives

After completing this chapter, the student/therapist should be able to perform the following:
1. Define the key terms of this chapter.
2. Discuss how palpation with mindful touch incorporates both the therapist's hands and mind.
3. State and discuss the importance of the two major objectives of palpation.
4. Describe the importance of moving slowly when palpating.
5. Discuss the importance of using appropriate pressure when palpating.
6. Discuss the importance of tissue barrier and how it relates to palpation.
7. Discuss the importance of the quality of palpation.
8. Discuss the importance of palpating not only during the examination of the client, but also when treating the client.
9. Describe one exercise that can be used to improve palpatory skills.
10. Explain the importance of constantly practicing palpation skills.

Key Terms

Appropriate pressure	Palpation	Target structure
Mindful intent	Palpatory literacy	Tissue barrier
Mindful touch	Target muscle	

WHAT IS PALPATION?

Palpation may be defined in many ways. The word *palpation* itself derives from the Latin palpatio, meaning "to touch." However, defining palpation as simply touching is too simplistic, because there is more involved. Inherent in the term palpation is not just touching, but also the act of sensing or perceiving what is being touched. In this sense, palpation involves more than just the fingers and hands. Palpation also involves the mind. Successful palpation requires us to feel with our minds as well as our fingers. When palpating, the therapist should be focused with a mindful intent; in other words, the therapist must be in his/her hands. All of the therapist's correlated knowledge of anatomy must be integrated into the sensations that the therapist's fingers are picking up from the client's body and sending to the brain. The therapist's mind must be open to the sensations that are coming in from the client, yet at the same time interpret these sensations with an informed mind (Figure 1-1). Incorporating mindful intent into examination and treatment sessions creates mindful touch.

BOX 1-1

A therapist may touch and palpate the client with more than just the fingers or hands. Sometimes the forearm, elbow, or even the feet are employed to contact the client. As a rule, this text refers to fingers or hands when referring to the therapist's contact upon the client.

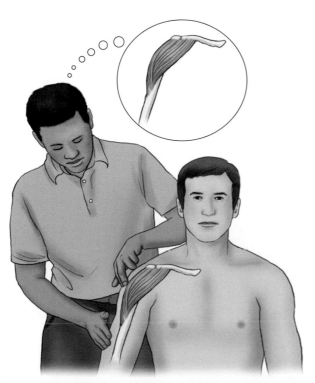

Figure 1-1 Palpation is as much an act of the mind as it is of the palpating fingers. Sensory stimuli entering through the therapist's hands must be correlated with a knowledge base of anatomy.

OBJECTIVES OF PALPATION: LOCATION AND ASSESSMENT

There are two main objectives when palpating. Step one is locating the target structure. Step two is assessing the target structure.

BOX 1-2

The term **target structure** is often used to name the particular structure of the body that the therapist is targeting to palpate. If the target structure is a muscle or muscle group, it is often called the **target muscle.**

The first objective, and indeed perhaps the major objective of the novice manual therapist, is to locate the target structure being palpated. This is no easy feat to achieve. It is one thing to simply touch the tissues of the client. It is an entirely different matter to be able to touch the tissues and discern the target structure from all the adjacent tissues. This requires the therapist to be able to locate all borders of the structure, superiorly, inferiorly, medially, laterally, and even superficially and deep. If the structure is immediately superficial to the skin, this may not be very difficult. Indeed, the olecranon process of the ulna or a well-developed deltoid muscle may be visually obvious and located without even touching the client's body. However, if the target structure is deeper in the client's body, locating the structure may present a great challenge.

BOX 1-3

As a rule, it is always best to first visually inspect the region that is to be palpated before placing your hands on the client. Once palpating hands are placed on the client, they block any visual information that might be present. See Chapter 2, The Art and Science of Muscle Palpation, for more on this idea.

As basic as palpation for the purpose of determining location seems, it is a supremely important first step, because it follows that if a structure cannot be accurately located, it cannot be accurately assessed. Once the target structure is located, then the process of assessment can begin. Assessment requires interpretation of the sensations that the palpating fingers pick up from the target structure. It involves becoming aware of the qualities of the target structure; its size, shape, and other characteristics. Is it soft? Is it swollen? Is it tense or hard? All of these factors must be considered when assessing the health of the target structure.

It is worthy of note that as high-tech diagnostic and assessment equipment continues to be developed in Western medicine, palpating hands remain the primary assessment tool of a manual therapist. Indeed, for a manual therapist, palpation, the act of gathering information through touch, lies at the very heart of assessment. Armed with both an accurate location and an accurate assessment of the health of the target structure through careful palpation, the manual therapist can develop an effective treatment plan that can be confidently carried out.

BOX 1-4

As crucial as palpation is to assessment, it is still only one piece of a successful assessment picture. Visual observation, history, findings from specific orthopedic assessment procedures, and the client's response to treatment approaches must also be considered when developing an accurate client assessment.

HOW TO PALPATE

Move Slowly

Given that palpation is a cooperative effort between the hands and the mind, it is important that the therapist's mind has sufficient time to interpret and make sense of the sensory stimuli that are coming in through the palpating fingers. This requires that palpation is performed slowly. Moving too quickly or frenetically jumping around the client's body does not allow for effective and mindful palpation.

Use Appropriate Pressure

The next question that arises when exploring how to palpate is how much pressure do we use? In other words, what is **appropriate pressure**? Because palpation is an exercise in sensation, it is imperative that the therapist's fingers are sensitive to the client's tissues that underlie them. However, quantifying palpation pressure is difficult. Recommendations for the degree of palpation pressure vary from 5 grams to 4 kilograms of pressure; there is an 800-fold difference between these two figures! One method recommended to gauge light pressure is to press on your eyelids; whatever pressure is comfortable there would then be considered appropriate pressure when palpating lightly. How much pressure is too much when palpating with deep pressure? A good measure of this is to look for blanching of the fingernails of the palpating fingers. If they are blanched, sensitivity is most likely lost.

BOX 1-5

An exercise to see how ineffective too much pressure can be is to press the pad of your thumb forcefully against a hard surface for 5 to 10 seconds. Directly afterward, try to palpate something on a client's body and note how much sensitivity is lost.

Generally, most new therapists use too little pressure, probably because they are afraid of hurting the client. Being unfamiliar with exactly what structures are under the client's skin and where they are located, the therapist fears damaging tissue and hurting the client. An analogy can be made to entering a dark room. Because we cannot see the objects in the room, we fear to enter and explore. However, if we can turn on the light and illuminate the room, we find it easy to move through it with ease. Learning anatomy well is like turning on the light. A stronger knowledge base of the underlying anatomy, along with more hands-on experience, allows for our fear to recede and be replaced with clarity and confidence.

Conversely, there are those therapists who are heavy handed, using too much pressure and being oblivious to the comfort of the client. If a client tightens the target musculature because your palpation pressure is causing pain, then an accurate assessment of the tone of the muscle is not possible. This pressure would be considered to be too much.

BOX 1-6

There are techniques that comfortably enable the use of more palpatory pressure with a client. Generally, if you enter the client's tissues slowly while asking the client to breathe using deep and steady breaths, it is usually possible for the client to remain comfortable while you palpate more deeply. Techniques and guidelines such as these are discussed in more detail in Chapter 2, The Art and Science of Muscle Palpation.

The optimal pressure to use is whatever pressure is appropriate to the circumstance. Some clients are not comfortable with strong pressure because it hurts them; others prefer it. Some clients are not comfortable with very light pressure, because it tickles their skin and/or it feels like a tease because the subcutaneous tissues are not being engaged; others prefer light pressure. The same client may even prefer light pressure in one region of the body, but deeper pressure in another.

Although the health and comfort of the client must be kept foremost in mind, the therapist should remember that the primary purpose of palpation is to locate and assess the structures of the client's body. When pressing into the client's tissues, palpating fingers usually sink in until a **tissue barrier** is felt. A tissue barrier is felt when the client's tissues offer an increased resistance to the pressure of the therapist's fingers. The tissue that is providing the barrier is often the tissue that is important to locate and assess. It is important to not blindly push past this tissue barrier, but rather to match the resistance of this tissue and explore it more fully. Therefore appropriate pressure employed to palpate a client's tissues is usually whatever pressure is necessary to reach and explore the tissue that is providing the tissue barrier.

If a structure is located three layers down, then it may be impossible to palpate it unless deeper pressure is employed. For example, accessing the psoas major muscle within the abdominopelvic cavity requires a good amount of pressure.

This does not mean that the therapist should be rough, but if enough pressure is not used, the muscle cannot be reached and therefore cannot be palpated, located, and assessed. When we are working clinically, if we do not accurately assess the health of a client's structure because it requires deeper pressure that might temporarily be slightly uncomfortable for the client, then we will never be able to assess the client's condition; without an accurate assessment, we cannot treat the client to help them improve and feel better. Having said that, when lighter pressure can be used, it should. For example, if the medial or lateral epicondyle of the humerus is being palpated, there is simply no reason to press with anything more than light pressure, because these structures are located superficially (Figure 1-2). The same may be said for a thin superficial muscle of the body.

Quality of Palpation Touch

There is another aspect of palpation that must be addressed, which is the quality of the palpation touch. The quality of the palpation touch should be comfortable to the client. Generally, palpation is best achieved by the therapist using their fingers. When palpating with fingers, finger pads should ideally be used, not fingertips. Fingertip palpation tends to feel to the client as though he or she is being poked, not palpated. From the point of view of the therapist, finger pad palpation is also more desirable, because the pads of the fingers are much more sensitive than the fingertips and better able to pick up subtle palpatory clues in the client's body.

WHEN DO WE PALPATE?

Always. Whenever we are contacting the client, we should be palpating. This is true not only during the assessment phase of the session, but also during the treatment phase. Too many therapists view palpation and treatment as separate entities that are compartmentalized within a session. A therapist often spends the first part of the session palpating and gathering sensory input for the sake of assessment and evaluation. Using the information gathered during this palpation assessment stage, a treatment plan is determined and

the therapist then spends the rest of the session implementing the treatment plan by outputting pressure into the client's tissues. Rigidly seen in this manner, palpation and treatment might each be viewed as a one-way street: palpation is sensory information in from the client, and treatment is motor pressure out to the client. The problem with this view is that we can also glean valuable assessment information while we are treating.

Treatment should be a two-way street that involves not just motor pressure out to the tissues of the client, but also continued sensory information in from the tissues of the client's body (Figure 1-3). While we are exerting pressure on the client's tissue, we are also sensing the quality of the tissue and its

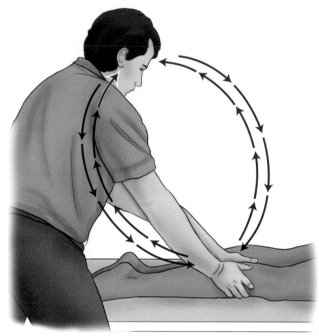

Figure 1-3 This figure illustrates the idea that palpation should be done whenever the therapist contacts the client, even when administering treatment strokes.

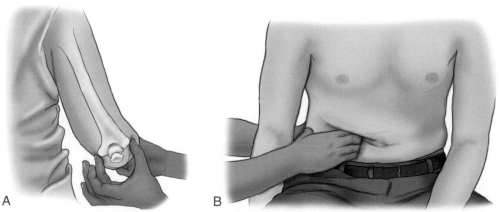

A   B

Figure 1-2 This figure illustrates the idea of using pressure that is appropriate to the structure being palpated. When the medial and lateral epicondyles of the humerus are being palpated, only light pressure is needed (A). However, when the psoas major muscle is palpated, deeper pressure is required (B).

response to our pressure. This new information might guide us to alter or fine-tune our treatment for the client. Thus while we work, we continue to assess, gathering information that guides the pace, depth, or direction of the next strokes. Ideally, no stroke should be carried out in a cookbook manner, performed as if on autopilot. Treatment is a dynamic process. How the middle and end of each stroke are performed should be determined from the response of the client's tissues to that stroke as we perform it. This is the essence of mindful touch, having a fluid interplay between assessment and treatment; assessment informs treatment and treatment informs assessment, creating optimal therapeutic care for the client.

HOW TO LEARN PALPATION

A long-standing exercise to learn palpation is to take a hair and place it under a page of a textbook without seeing where you placed it. With your eyes closed, palpate for the hair until you find it and can trace its shape under the page. Once found, now replace the hair, this time under two pages, and palpate to locate and trace it. Continue to increase the number of pages placed over the hair until you cannot find it. If this exercise is repeated, the number of pages under which you can locate and trace the hair will gradually increase, and your sensitivity will improve.

Even more important than performing palpation exercises with textbooks, it is imperative that palpation is applied directly to the client. When your hands are on your fellow students in school, or on your clients or patients if you are in professional practice, constantly try to feel for the structures about which you have learned in your anatomy, physiology, and kinesiology classes. As your hands are moving on the client's skin, close your eyes so that you block out extraneous sensory stimuli, and try to picture all the subcutaneous structures over which your hands are passing. The better you can picture an underlying structure, the better you will be able to feel it with your palpating hands and your mind. Once felt, you can focus on locating its precise location and assessing its tissue quality.

Given that the foundation of all manual skills rests upon our palpatory ability to read the clues and signs that a client's body offers, the better we hone this skill, the greater **palpatory literacy** we gain. Perfecting our palpatory literacy is a work in progress, an endless journey. The greater we polish and perfect this skill, the greater our therapeutic potential becomes, bringing greater benefit to our clients. However, written chapters can only provide guidelines and a framework for how to palpate. Ultimately, palpation is a kinesthetic skill, and as such can only be learned by kinesthetic means. In other words, "palpation cannot be learned by reading or listening; it can only be learned by palpation."[1]

Review Questions

1. What is meant by the term *palpation?*
2. What does the concept of *mindful intent* involve?
3. What is the term used to describe incorporating mindful intent into the processes of examination and treatment?
4. List the two main objectives during palpation.
5. What problem will arise due to the lack of ability to accurately locate the target structure?
6. What is the importance of the therapist's speed in regard to palpation?
7. Issues of therapist experience and client comfort aside, what best describes an appropriate amount of pressure?
8. What is meant by the term *tissue barrier?*
9. What part of the fingers should be used for palpating? Why?
10. When, during a session, should a therapist palpate the client's body tissues?
11. How may a therapist increase their palpatory literacy?

 Deeper Thoughts

In addition to the example of palpating a hair under layers of textbook pages, in what other ways can a therapist try to increase their sensitivity?

REFERENCE

1. Frymann VM: Palpation, its study in the workshop, *AAO Yearbook:* 16–31, 1963.

CHAPTER 2

The Art and Science of Muscle Palpation

Overview

This chapter expands on the principles of palpation covered in Chapter 1, specifically discussing palpation as it applies to the skeletal muscles of the body. Twenty guidelines are discussed that comprise the art and science of muscle palpation. The two most basic guidelines, described as the *science of muscle palpation*, are knowing the attachments and actions of the target muscle. The additional 18 guidelines describe how to begin and perfect the *art of muscle palpation*. In all, these guidelines can help increase palpatory literacy of the muscles of the body.

Chapter Outline

Introduction
List of Muscle Palpation Guidelines
The Science of Muscle Palpation
Beginning the Art of Muscle Palpation
Perfecting the Art of Muscle Palpation
Conclusion

Chapter Objectives

After completing this chapter, the student/therapist should be able to perform the following:
1. Define the key terms of this chapter.
2. Explain why and demonstrate how knowing the attachments of a muscle is useful for its palpation.
3. Explain why and demonstrate how knowing the actions of a muscle is useful for its palpation.
4. Discuss and give an example of the importance of choosing the best action of a target muscle to isolate its contraction.
5. Discuss and give an example of the idea of using critical reasoning to figure out how to palpate a muscle instead of memorizing its palpation procedure.
6. Discuss the value of and be able to demonstrate how to add resistance to the client's contraction of the target muscle.
7. Explain and give an example of why another joint should not be crossed when adding resistance to the client's contraction of the target muscle.
8. Explain why it is best to look for a target muscle before placing the palpating hand on the client.
9. Explain why it is best to first locate a target muscle in the easiest place possible.
10. Discuss the value of and demonstrate strumming perpendicularly across the belly or tendon of a target muscle.
11. Explain the value of and be able to use baby steps when palpating a muscle.
12. Discuss the importance of alternately contracting and relaxing the target muscle.
13. Explain, give an example of, and demonstrate how knowledge of coupled actions can help palpation of scapular rotator muscles.
14. Explain, give an example of, and demonstrate how to use neural (reciprocal) inhibition to palpate a target muscle.
15. Explain the importance of using appropriate pressure, and give examples of when using light pressure is preferable and when using deep pressure is preferable.
16. Discuss the importance of slow palpation and the client's breathing pattern when palpating deeper muscles.
17. Explain and give an example of using one muscle as a landmark to locate and palpate another muscle.
18. Discuss why it is important to relax and passively slacken a target muscle when palpating its bony attachments.
19. Explain why it can be helpful for therapists to close their eyes when palpating.

20. Explain why it can be helpful for the therapist to construct a mental image of the client's anatomy under the skin.
21. Describe an approach that can be tried to lessen the sensitivity of a client who is ticklish.
22. Explain the importance of having short and smooth fingernails.
23. Discuss the relationship between using the optimal client position for target muscle palpation and treating the client.

Key Terms

Add resistance	Isolated contraction	Science of muscle palpation
Alternately contract and relax	Look before you touch	Stabilization hand
Appropriate pressure	Neural inhibition	Strumming perpendicularly
Art of muscle palpation	Optimal palpation position	Target muscle
Baby steps	Palpation hand	Target structure
Coupled actions	Reciprocal inhibition	Visual observation

INTRODUCTION

As described in Chapter 1, palpation of the client's body involves the location and assessment of a structure termed the target structure. The first step of palpation is to accurately locate the target structure. Once located, the second step is to assess its health. When the target structure is a bone or bony landmark, the process of palpation is relatively easy, because the skeleton is a hard tissue that is surrounded by soft tissues. Therefore bones and bony landmarks stand out. However, when the target structure is a muscle, palpation can be more difficult, because a muscle is a soft tissue that is usually surrounded by other soft tissues; this makes the discernment of one muscle from all the adjacent muscles and other soft tissues more challenging.

Given that massage therapists and many other manual therapists work primarily on myofascial tissues, accurate palpation of the musculature is of the utmost importance; this is especially true when working clinically. The emphasis of this chapter is to learn how to carry out the first step of muscle palpation; that is, to learn how to locate a target muscle. When we speak of palpating a muscle, as a rule we are referring to the location of the muscle. Toward this end, twenty guidelines are offered in this chapter that will help increase palpatory literacy of the musculature of the body. A list of these guidelines is given here; a detailed explanation of each of the guidelines follows. It is recommended that this chapter is read in its entirety before attempting the palpations of the skeletal muscles covered in Chapters 11 to 21.

LIST OF MUSCLE PALPATION GUIDELINES

Each of the following muscle palpation guidelines will be discussed in this chapter. All twenty are summarized in list form here.

1. Know the attachments of the target muscle so that you know where to place your hands.
2. Know the actions of the target muscle. The client will most likely be asked to perform one of them to contract the target muscle so that it can be discerned from the adjacent musculature. (Make sure that the client is not asked to hold the contraction too long or the target muscle may fatigue and the client may become uncomfortable.)
3. Think critically to choose exactly which joint action of the target muscle best isolates its contraction.
4. If necessary, add resistance to the client's contraction of the target muscle. (When resistance is added, do not cross any joints that do not need to be crossed; in other words, be sure to resist only the action of the target muscle that is desired.)
5. Look before placing your palpating hand on the client. (This is especially important with superficial muscles.)
6. First find and palpate the target muscle in the easiest place possible.
7. Strum perpendicularly across the belly or tendon of the target muscle.
8. Once located, follow the course of the target muscle in small successive baby steps.
9. At each baby step of palpation, have the client alternately contract and relax the target muscle, and feel for this tissue texture change as the muscle goes from relaxed and soft, to contracted and hard, to relaxed and soft again.
10. Use knowledge of coupled actions to palpate target muscles that are scapular rotators.
11. To aid palpation of the target muscle, use reciprocal inhibition of another muscle when needed. (When reciprocal inhibition is used, do not have the client contract the target muscle too forcefully, or the other muscle that is being reciprocally inhibited may be recruited anyway.)
12. Use appropriate pressure. Appropriate pressure is neither too heavy nor too light.
13. When using deep palpation pressure, sink slowly into the client's tissues as the client breathes slowly and evenly.
14. Once the palpation of one muscle is known, it can be used as a landmark to locate other muscles.
15. Relax and passively slacken the target muscle when palpating it at its bony attachment.
16. Close your eyes when you palpate to focus your attention on your palpating fingers.
17. Construct a mental picture of the client's anatomy under the skin as you palpate.
18. If the client is ticklish, use firm pressure and have the client place a hand over your palpating hand.
19. Fingernails need to be very short and smooth.

20. Place the client in a position that is optimal for the muscle palpation.

ⓔ Refer to http://evolve.elsevier.com/Muscolino/palpation for a demonstration of how to palpate.

THE SCIENCE OF MUSCLE PALPATION

Guideline #1: Know the Attachments of the Target Muscle

When a target muscle is superficial, it is usually not difficult to palpate. If we know where it is located, we can simply place our hands there and feel for it. Unless there is a great deal of subcutaneous fat in that region of the body, apart from the client's skin and some thin fibrous fascial membranes, we will be directly on the muscle. Therefore the first step of muscle palpation is to know the attachments of the target muscle. For example, if we know that the deltoid attaches from the lateral clavicle, acromion process, and spine of the scapula, to the deltoid tuberosity of the humerus, then we need simply place our palpating hand there to feel it (Figure 2-1).

Guideline #2: Know the Actions of the Target Muscle

Often, even if a target muscle is superficial, it can be difficult to discern the borders of the muscle. If the target muscle is deep to another muscle, it can be that much harder to palpate and discern from superficial and other nearby muscles. To better discern the target muscle from all adjacent musculature and other soft tissues, it is helpful to ask the client to contract the target muscle by doing one or more of its actions. If the target muscle contracts, it will become palpably harder. Assuming that all the adjacent muscles stay relaxed and therefore palpably soft, the difference in tissue texture between the hard target muscle and the soft adjacent muscles will be clear. I like to refer to the contracted muscle as being "the only hard, soft tissue amidst a sea of soft, soft tissues." This will allow an accurate determination of the location of the target muscle. Therefore the second step of muscle palpation is to know the actions of the target muscle (Figure 2-2).

Guidelines #1 and #2 of muscle palpation involve knowing the "science" of the target muscle; in other words, knowing the attachments and actions of the muscle that were learned when the muscles of the body were first learned. Armed with this knowledge, the majority of muscle palpations can be reasoned out instead of memorized. Using the attachments and actions to palpate a target muscle can be thought of as the science of muscle palpation.

BEGINNING THE ART OF MUSCLE PALPATION

Guideline #3: Choose the Best Action of the Target Muscle to Make It Contract

Applying knowledge of the attachments and actions of a target muscle to palpate it is a solid foundation for palpatory literacy. However, effective palpation requires not only that the target muscle contracts, but that an isolated contraction of the target muscle occurs. This means that the target muscle needs to be the only muscle that contracts, and all muscles near the target muscle must remain relaxed. Unfortunately, because adjacent muscles often share the same joint action

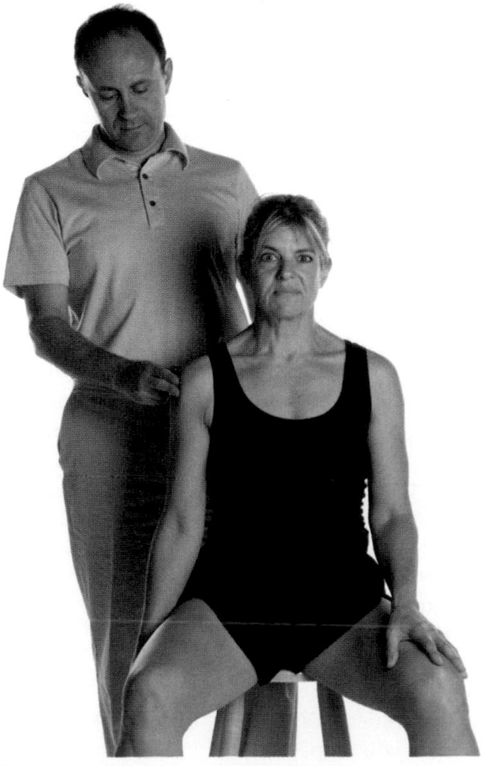

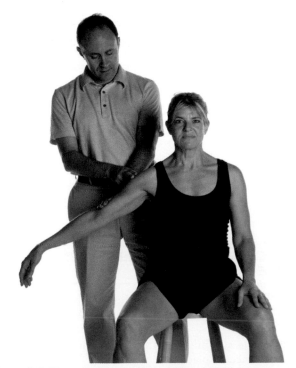

Figure 2-1 The deltoid is a superficial muscle and can be palpated by simply placing our palpating hand on the muscle between its attachments.

Figure 2-2 The precise location of the deltoid is more easily palpated if the deltoid is contracted. In this figure, the client is asked to abduct the arm at the shoulder (glenohumeral) against the force of gravity.

with the target muscle, it is usually not enough to simply place our hands on the location of the target muscle and then choose any one of its actions to contract it. If the action chosen is shared with an adjacent muscle, then it will also contract, making it very difficult to discern the target muscle from the adjacent muscle.

For this reason, knowing which joint action to ask the client to perform is where the therapist needs to be creative and think critically. This is where the art of muscle palpation begins. It requires knowledge of not only of the actions of the target muscle, but also the actions of all adjacent muscles. With this knowledge, the client can be asked to perform the best joint action for the palpation of the target muscle. This joint action will usually be the one that is most different from the joint actions of adjacent muscles.

BOX 2-1

The goal when engaging the target muscle to contract is to have an isolated contraction of the target muscle. This means that the target muscle must be the only muscle that contracts and every other muscle must remain relaxed. Although this is the ideal, it is not always possible to achieve.

BOX 2-2

There are times when the client is not able to perform only the action that is asked for by the therapist; this is especially true with actions of the toes, because we do not usually develop the coordination necessary to isolate certain toe motions. For example, if the target muscle is the extensor digitorum longus (EDL) and the client is asked to engage this muscle by extending toes two through five at the metatarsophalangeal and interphalangeal joints, the client may be unable to extend these toes without also extending the big toe (toe one) at the same time. This poses a problem because extending the big toe will also engage the extensor hallucis longus (EHL) muscle. When this happens, it is tempting to isolate extension of toes two through five by holding down the big toe of the client so that it does not move into extension. However, the goal of engaging the target muscle is for it to be the only muscle that contracts. If the big toe is held down in this scenario, even though the big toe is not moving, the EHL muscle is still contracting; it is simply contracting isometrically instead of concentrically. This will still cause the EHL to contract and harden, making it harder to palpate and discern the EDL. For this reason, any time that a client contracts a muscle that he or she is not supposed to, preventing the client's body part from moving does not help the palpation. It is the *contraction* of any muscle other than the target muscle that is undesirable, not the movement of a client's body part.

For example, if the flexor carpi radialis (FCR) of the wrist flexor group is the target muscle, then asking the client to flex the hand at the wrist joint will engage not only the FCR, but also the other two wrist flexor group muscles, the palmaris longus (PL) and flexor carpi ulnaris (FCU). In this case, to palpate and discern the FCR from the adjacent PL and FCU, the client should be asked to do radial deviation of the hand at the wrist joint instead of flexion of the hand at the wrist joint. This will better isolate the contraction to the FCR. It becomes palpably harder than the relaxed and palpably softer PL and FCU muscles, which facilitates palpating and discerning the FCR (Figure 2-3).

PERFECTING THE ART OF MUSCLE PALPATION

Knowing the attachments and actions of the target muscle are the first two steps of learning the science of muscle palpation. Determining which joint action to ask the client to perform is the beginning of learning the art of muscle palpation. However, perfecting the art of muscle palpation

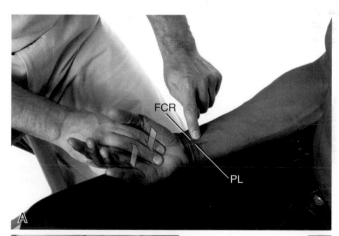

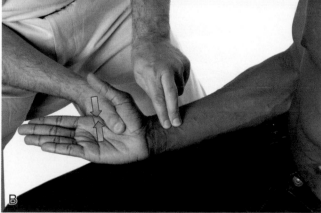

Figure 2-3 The flexor carpi radialis (FCR) muscle is being palpated. If the client is asked to flex the hand at the wrist joint as shown in **A**, the FCR will contract, but so will the adjacent palmaris longus (PL) muscle. However, if the client is asked to radially deviate the hand at the wrist joint as shown in **B**, the contraction is isolated to the FCR while the adjacent PL remains relaxed.

2

involves the knowledge and application of many more guidelines. These additional guidelines are presented in the following pages. A summary list of all twenty muscle palpation guidelines has already been given. It is difficult if not impossible to memorize a list this long; rather these guidelines need to be learned by using them as the palpations of the skeletal muscles of the body are covered in Chapters 11-21 of Part IV of this book. With practice, these guidelines will become familiar and comfortable to you and will enhance the art and science of your muscle palpation technique.

Guideline #4: Add Resistance to the Contraction of the Target Muscle

When a client is asked to do one of the joint actions of the target muscle to make it contract, harden, and stand out, there are times when this contraction is not forceful enough to make it easily palpable. This is especially true if the joint action does not require a large body part to be moved and/or if the body part that is moved is not moved against gravity. When the client's contraction of the target muscle is not forceful enough, it might be necessary for the therapist to add resistance so that the target muscle contracts harder and stands out more. A good example is when the target muscle is the pronator teres and the client is asked to pronate the forearm at the radioulnar joints. Because the forearm is not a very large body part and pronation does not occur against gravity, the pronator teres muscle will contract, but most likely not forcefully enough to make it stand out and be easily palpable. In this case, the therapist can add resistance to the client's contraction by resisting the forearm during pronation. This requires a more forceful contraction of the pronator teres, making it easier to palpate and discern from the adjacent musculature (Figure 2-4).

Resisting a client's target muscle contraction is not a battle between the therapist and client to see who is stronger. The role of the therapist is simply to oppose the force of the

client's muscle contraction, not overpower the client. The degree that the client is asked to contract the target muscle can vary. Ideally, it should be the lightest amount necessary to bring out the target muscle's contraction so that it is palpable. This is especially true if the target muscle is a small muscle that is deep to a larger muscle that has the same action, for example, the piriformis deep to the gluteus maximus. Both of these muscles are lateral rotators of the thigh at the hip joint. As a rule, a gentle lateral rotation contraction engages the smaller deeper piriformis without engaging the larger more superficial gluteus maximus. This allows us to discern the piriformis's contraction without the gluteus maximus contracting and blocking our palpation. Ideally, we want just enough contraction to feel the piriformis "pop," in other words, to feel its contraction, while the gluteus maximus remains relaxed and soft. However, there are also times when a more forceful contraction is needed to feel a target muscle's contraction. A good guideline is to begin with a gentle resistance as you try to palpate the target muscle. If it not successful, then gradually increase the force of the resistance as necessary.

Whenever resistance is added to the contraction of the target muscle by the client, it is extremely important that the therapist does not cross any additional joints with the placement of the stabilization hand. The goal of having a

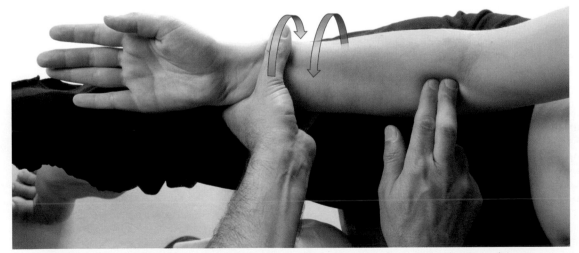

Figure 2-4 To create a more forceful contraction of the pronator teres muscle, the therapist can hold on to the client's distal forearm and resist forearm pronation at the radioulnar joints. Note that the stabilization hand resisting the client's forearm pronation is placed on the distal forearm and does not cross the wrist joint to hold the client's hand.

BOX 2-4

When you ask the client to contract the target muscle or to contract it against your resistance during palpation, remember to give the client a rest every few seconds or so. Holding a sustained isometric contraction can become uncomfortable and painful. It is more comfortable for the client and actually better for our palpation procedure if the client is asked to alternately contract and relax the target muscle instead of holding a sustained isometric contraction. (See Guideline #9 for more on alternately contracting and relaxing the target muscle.)

of the target muscle, because the direction that the client must move to press against your contact is better focused at the joint where resistance is being offered. Continuing with the wrist flexor musculature again as our example, if the client is asked to contract against our resistance with the hand in neutral position at the wrist joint, it is likely that their contraction will originate at the elbow joint instead of the wrist joint, because contraction of elbow joint flexors will also push against our resistance as seen in Figure 2-5, *A*. However, if the client's hand is first slightly flexed, then the angle of the client's force will less likely be generated from the elbow joint, because the line of force of elbow joint flexion

client contract the target muscle during palpation is to limit contraction to the target muscle. This way, it will be the only muscle that is palpably hard and can be discerned from the adjacent relaxed and palpably soft muscles. However, if the therapist's stabilization hand does cross other joints, it is likely that muscles crossing these joints will also contract. This defeats the purpose of having an isolated contraction of the target muscle.

For example, in the case of the pronator teres palpation, when resistance to forearm pronation is added, it is important that the therapist's stabilization hand does not cross the wrist joint and hold the client's hand. If the stabilization hand holds the client's hand, then other muscles that cross the client's wrist joint, such as the muscles of the wrist flexor group that move the hand at the wrist joint, or flexor muscles of the fingers, will likely also contract, making it difficult to discern the pronator teres from these adjacent muscles. Therefore the resistance hand should be placed on the client's forearm (see Figure 2-4). Ideally, placing the resistance hand on the distal end of the forearm affords the best leverage force so that the therapist does not have to work as hard.

Generally, if the therapist is resisting an action of the arm at the shoulder joint, the therapist's stabilization hand should be placed just proximal to the elbow joint and not cross the elbow joint to grasp the client's forearm. If the therapist is resisting an action of the forearm at the elbow joint, the therapist's stabilization hand should be placed on the distal forearm and not cross the wrist joint to grasp the client's hand. If the therapist is resisting an action of the hand at the wrist joint, the therapist's stabilization hand should be placed on the palm of the hand and not cross the metacarpophalangeal joints to grasp the client's fingers. The same reasoning can be applied to the lower extremity and the axial body.

One other aspect of adding resistance is the angle of the client's joint when the resistance is added. As a rule, it is better to first allow the client to slightly move the joint being crossed and then contact the client to add the resistance. For example, if the muscle being palpated is a wrist flexor muscle, make sure that the client's hand is first slightly flexed at the wrist joint and then add resistance to wrist flexion (Figure 2-5). This usually creates a better isolated contraction

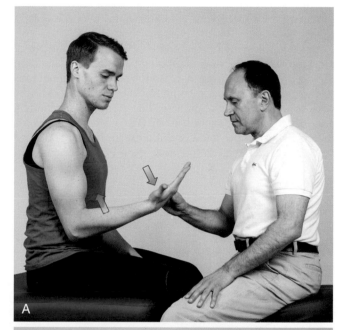

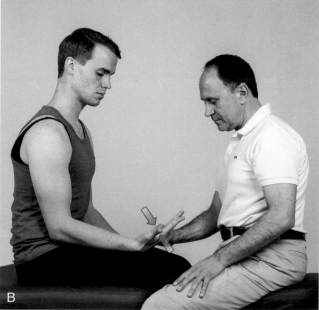

Figure 2-5 Optimizing the angle of the client's wrist joint when offering resistance to flexion is important. **A,** The wrist joint is in neutral position. **B,** The wrist joint is first slightly flexed.

is now different from the line of force of wrist joint flexion as seen in Figure 2-5, *B*.

Guideline #5: Look Before You Palpate

Even though palpation is done via touching, **visual observation** can be a valuable tool for locating a target muscle. This is especially true for muscles that are superficial and whose contours show through the skin. Very often, a target muscle visually screams, "Here I am!" yet the therapist doesn't see it because the palpating hand is in the way. This may be true when the target muscle is relaxed, but is even more likely to be true when the target muscle is contracted (especially if it contracts harder from increased resistance), because when it contracts and hardens, it often pops out visually. For this reason, whenever attempting to palpate a target muscle, look first; then place your palpating hand over the muscle to feel for it.

For example, when palpating the PL and FCR muscles of the wrist flexor group, before placing your palpating hand on the client's anterior forearm, first look for the distal tendons of these two muscles at the anterior distal forearm near the wrist joint. They may be fully visible, aiding you in finding and palpating them (Figure 2-6, *A*). If they are not visible, ask the client to flex the hand at the wrist joint, and add resistance if you would like. Now look again before placing your

palpating hand on the client. When contracted, it is even more likely that these distal tendons will tense and visually pop out, helping you to locate and palpate them (see Figure 2-6, *B*). There are many muscles whose visual information can help with their palpation. For this reason, it is a good rule to always **look before you touch.**

> ## BOX 2-5
>
> It should be noted that the palmaris longus (PL) muscle is often missing, either unilaterally or bilaterally, in many individuals.

Guideline #6: First Find the Target Muscle in the Easiest Place Possible

Once a target muscle has been found, it is much easier to continue to palpate along its course than it is to locate it in the first place. For this reason, a good palpation guideline is to always feel for the target muscle wherever it is easiest to first find. Once located, then you can continue to palpate it toward

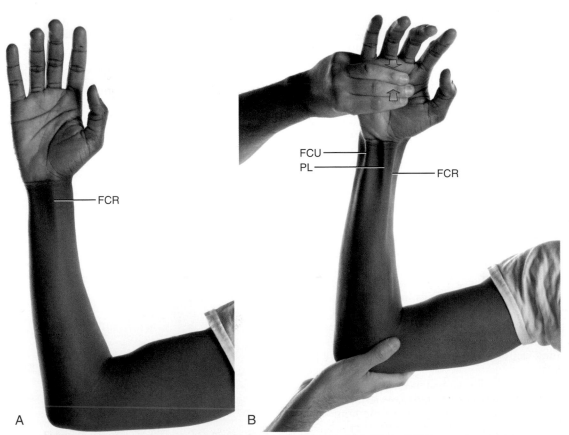

A   B

Figure 2-6 A shows that the distal tendon of the flexor carpi radialis (FCR) muscle might be visible even when it is relaxed. **B** shows that when contracted (in this case, against resistance), its distal tendon tenses and becomes even more visually apparent. Note: The palmaris longus (PL) and flexor carpi ulnaris (FCU) tendons are also visible.

one or both of its attachments. For example, using the FCR as an example, if the distal tendon is visually apparent (see Figure 2-6) then begin your palpation there. Once it is clearly felt, then continue to palpate toward its proximal attachment on the medial epicondyle of the humerus.

Guideline #7: Strum Perpendicularly Across the Target Muscle

When first locating a target muscle or when following a target muscle that has already been found, it is best to strum perpendicularly across its belly or tendon. Strumming perpendicularly across a muscle belly or its tendon is like strumming or twanging a guitar string; you begin on one side of the belly or tendon, then you rise up onto its prominence, and then fall off the other side of it. This change in contour is much more palpably noticeable than if your palpating fingers simply glide longitudinally along the muscle (which offers little change in contour and thus does not help to define the location of the target muscle).

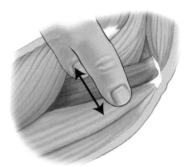

Figure 2-7 The pronator teres is being palpated by strumming perpendicularly across its belly. (Muscolino JE: Kinesiology: the skeletal system and muscle function, 2nd ed., St Louis, 2011, Mosby.)

It is important to note when strumming perpendicularly across a muscle's belly or tendon that the movement of your palpating fingers is not a short vibration motion; rather it must be large enough to begin off one side of the target muscle, rise onto it, go all the way across it, and end off the other side of it. This means that the length of excursion of your strumming motion must be fairly long. Figure 2-7 illustrates the belly of the pronator teres being strummed perpendicularly.

Guideline #8: Use Baby Steps to Follow the Target Muscle

Once a target muscle has been found in the easiest place possible by strumming perpendicular to it, it should then be followed all the way to its attachments. This should be done in baby steps. Using baby steps to follow a muscle means that each successive "feel" of the muscle should be immediately after the previous feel so that no geography of the muscle's contour is skipped. If you feel the target muscle in one spot, then you should not skip a couple of inches down the muscle to feel it again. The farther down you skip, the more likely it is that you will no longer be on the muscle and will lose the course of its palpation. Figure 2-8 illustrates the idea that once a target muscle has been located, baby steps should be used to follow it toward its attachments.

BOX 2-6

When following the course of a target muscle with baby steps, it helps to have a clear picture in mind of the orientation of the muscle so that each baby step of palpation will be in the correct direction and therefore stay on the target muscle.

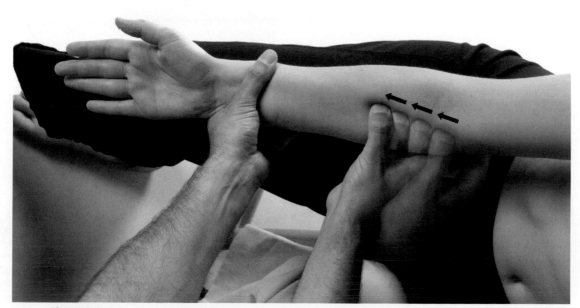

Figure 2-8 The pronator teres muscle is palpated in "baby steps" toward its distal attachment.

Guideline #9: Alternately Contract and Relax the Target Muscle

It has already been stated that it can be uncomfortable for the client to hold a sustained isometric contraction of the target muscle while it is being palpated; therefore it is better for the client to alternately contract and relax it. In addition, having the client alternately contract and relax the target muscle while the therapist follows its course with baby steps aids in successful palpation. At each baby step of the palpation process, if the target muscle alternately contracts and then relaxes, the therapist can feel its *change in texture* from being soft when it is relaxed, to being hard when it is contracted, to being soft when it is relaxed again. This assures the therapist that he or she is still on the target muscle. If the therapist does accidentally veer off the target muscle onto other tissue, it will be evident because the tissue texture change from soft to hard to soft (as the relaxed target muscle contracts and then relaxes again) will not be felt.

When the therapist does veer off course, the palpating fingers should be placed back at the last spot where the target muscle was felt clearly and then make the next baby step in a slightly different direction to relocate the course of the target muscle as the client is asked once again to alternately contract and then relax it.

Guideline #10: When Appropriate, Use Coupled Actions

There are certain instances in which knowledge of coupled actions can help isolate contraction of a target muscle so that its palpation is facilitated. Most of these instances involve rotation of the scapula at the scapulocostal joint because scapular rotation cannot occur on its own; rather the scapula can only rotate when the arm is moved at the shoulder (glenohumeral) joint. For example, if the target muscle to be palpated is the pectoralis minor, even though it has a number of actions that could be used to make it contract, most of these actions would also cause the overlying pectoralis major to contract, which would block palpation of the pectoralis minor. The most effective action that would isolate contraction of the pectoralis minor in the anterior chest is downward rotation of the scapula. However, this rotation will occur only in conjunction with extension and/or adduction of the arm at the glenohumeral joint. Therefore, to create downward rotation of the scapula to engage the pectoralis minor, ask the client to extend

and adduct the arm at the glenohumeral joint. This can be accomplished by having the client first rest the hand in the small of the back; then, to engage the pectoralis minor, have the client move the arm further into extension by moving the hand posteriorly away from the small of the back. This will immediately engage the pectoralis minor, allowing it to be easily palpated through the pectoralis major (Figure 2-9). This same procedure can be used to palpate the rhomboid muscles through the middle trapezius (see Figures 11-15 and 11-16).

Guideline #11: When Appropriate, Use Neural (Reciprocal) Inhibition

Reciprocal inhibition is a neurologic reflex that causes neural inhibition, in other words relaxation, of a muscle whenever an antagonist muscle is actively contracted. This neurologic reflex can be used to great advantage when palpating certain target muscles. For example, if our target muscle is the brachialis and we want to make it contract so that it hardens and is easier to feel, we have no choice but to ask the client to flex the elbow joint, because that is the only

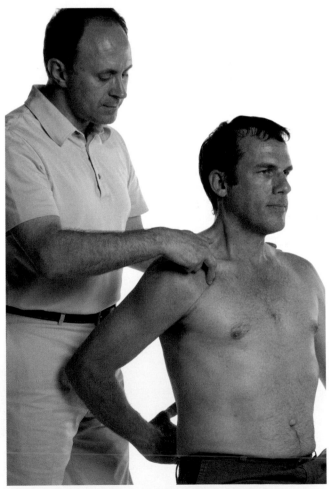

Figure 2-9 When the client moves the hand posteriorly away from the small of the back, extension of the arm occurs. This requires the coupled action of downward rotation of the scapula at the scapulocostal joint, which engages the pectoralis minor muscle so that it can be easily palpated through the pectoralis major muscle.

BOX 2-7

Knowledge of coupled actions can also be used with neural (reciprocal) inhibition to palpate a target muscle. For example, when palpating the levator scapulae, the client's arm is extended and adducted at the shoulder (glenohumeral) joint by placing the hand in the small of the back. This requires the coupled action of downward rotation of the scapula at the scapulocostal joint, which then reciprocally inhibits and relaxes the upper trapezius (because it is an upward rotator of the scapula). With the upper trapezius relaxed, palpation of the levator scapulae through it can now be done. For a fuller explanation of this, see the discussion on reciprocal inhibition in Guideline #11.

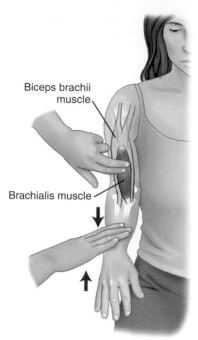

Figure 2-10 The biceps brachii, which is also a supinator of the forearm, is reciprocally inhibited because the forearm is pronated (as it is flexed), facilitating palpation of the brachialis. (Muscolino JE: Kinesiology: the skeletal system and muscle function, 2nd ed., St Louis, 2011, Mosby.)

action of the brachialis. The problem with this is that if the client flexes the forearm at the elbow joint to contract the brachialis, the biceps brachii will also contract. This makes it difficult to palpate the brachialis, because the biceps brachii overlies the brachialis in the anterior arm. Given that it is always the goal of a muscle palpation to have an isolated contraction of the target muscle (in this case, we want only the brachialis to contract), the biceps brachii needs to remain relaxed. Even though the only action of the brachialis (elbow joint flexion) is an action of the biceps brachii, it is possible to achieve this if we can neurally inhibit the biceps brachii by using the principle of reciprocal inhibition (Figure 2-10). To do this, we ask the client to flex the forearm at the elbow joint while the forearm is in a position of full pronation. Because the biceps brachii is also a supinator of the forearm, having the forearm pronated neurally inhibits it from contracting, so it remains relaxed as the brachialis contracts to flex the forearm at the elbow joint. Thus we have achieved the goal of having an isolated contraction of our target muscle, the brachialis.

Another example of using the principle of neural inhibition to isolate the contraction of a target muscle is palpating the scapular attachment of the levator scapulae. If we ask the client to elevate the scapula to contract and palpably harden the levator scapulae, the problem is that the upper trapezius will also contract and harden, making it impossible to feel the levator scapulae at its scapular attachment deep to the upper trapezius. To stop the upper trapezius from contracting, ask the client to place the hand in the small of the back. This position of humeral extension and adduction requires downward rotation of the scapula at the scapulocostal joint. Because the upper trapezius is an upward rotator of

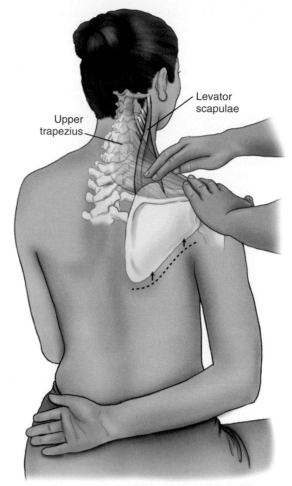

Figure 2-11 The upper trapezius, which is also an upward rotator of the scapula, is neurally inhibited, because the scapula is downwardly rotated (as it is elevated) because of the position of the hand in the small of the back. This facilitates palpation of the levator scapulae.

the scapula, it will be inhibited and stay relaxed. This allows for an isolated contraction of and a successful palpation of the levator scapulae when the client is asked to elevate the scapula (Figure 2-11).

BOX 2-8

The downward rotation of the scapula at the scapulocostal joint when palpating the levator scapulae not only aids palpation of the levator scapulae by reciprocally inhibiting the upper trapezius, but also increases the contraction strength of the levator scapulae, because downward rotation of the scapula is another one of its actions.

There is one important caution when using the principle of neural reciprocal inhibition for a muscle palpation. When the client is asked to contract and engage the target muscle, the force of its contraction must be small. If the contraction is forceful, the client's brain overrides the neural inhibition reflex in an attempt to recruit as many muscles as possible for the joint action. This results in a contraction of the muscle that was supposed to be inhibited and relaxed. Once this other muscle contracts, it will likely block successful palpation of the target muscle. For example, when palpating for the brachialis, if flexion of the forearm at the elbow joint is performed forcefully, the biceps brachii will be recruited, making palpation of the brachialis difficult or impossible. Another example is palpating for the levator scapulae; if elevation of the scapula at the scapulocostal joint is performed forcefully, the upper trapezius will be recruited, making palpation of the levator scapulae at its scapular attachment difficult or impossible.

Guideline #12: Use Appropriate Pressure

The concept of using appropriate pressure has already been discussed in Chapter 1; however, the use of appropriate pressure is so critical to muscle palpation that the key points are repeated here. (For a more complete discussion of palpation pressure, please see Chapter 1.) It is important to not be too heavy handed; sensitivity can be lost with excessive pressure. On the other hand, it is important to not be too light with your pressure either; some muscles are quite deep and require moderate to strong pressure to feel. Generally, when most new students have a difficult time palpating a target muscle, it is because their pressure is too light. Appropriate pressure means applying the optimal palpation pressure for each target muscle palpation.

BOX 2-9

There are occasional times when a deep muscle palpation is facilitated by extremely light pressure. If a muscle is so deep that its borders cannot be felt, then its location must be determined by feeling for the vibrations of its contraction through the tissues. This can only be felt with a very light touch. One example of this approach is palpation of the extensor hallucis longus (EHL) muscle in the leg deep to the tibialis anterior and extensor digitorum longus (EDL) muscles.

Guideline #13: For Deep Palpations, Sink Slowly into the Tissue and Have the Client Breathe

All deep muscle palpations should be done slowly. Although deep pressure can be uncomfortable for many clients, it is often accomplished quite easily if we work with the client as we palpate. This can be accomplished by sinking slowly into the client's tissues and having the client breathe with the palpation process in a slow and rhythmic manner. An excellent example of this is palpating the psoas major in the abdominopelvic cavity. The psoas major must be palpated from the anterior perspective. This requires firm pressure to reach through the abdominal viscera, because the psoas major lies against the spinal column and forms part of the posterior abdominal wall. For the client to remain comfortable, the therapist needs to sink into the client's tissues very slowly as the client breathes slowly and evenly. To begin the palpation, ask the client to take in a moderate

to deep breath; then as the client slowly exhales, slowly sink in toward the psoas major. It is not necessary to reach the psoas major at the end of the client's first exhalation. Instead, ease off slightly with your pressure, and ask the client to take in another moderate-sized breath; then continue to slowly sink in deeper as the client slowly exhales again. This process may need to be repeated a third time to reach the psoas major; a deep muscle can usually be accessed in this manner with two or three breaths by the client. What is most important to remember is that firm deep pressure must be applied slowly.

BOX 2-10

When having a client breathe with your palpation as you sink slowly and deeply in the client's tissues to access a deep muscle, it is important that the client's breath is not quick and shallow. However, the breaths do not need to be very deep either; a very deep breath may push your palpating hands out, especially if you are palpating in the abdominal region. More important than the depth of the breath is its pace. The client's breathing should be slow, rhythmic, and relaxed. This type of breathing on the part of the client is facilitated if you breathe in a similar manner.

Guideline #14: Use Muscles as Landmarks

Once the bones and bony landmarks of the skeleton have been learned, it is common to use a bony landmark to help locate and palpate a target muscle. However, once the palpation of one muscle has been learned, it can also be a useful landmark for locating another adjacent muscle. For example, if palpation of the sternocleidomastoid (SCM) has been learned, then it is a simple matter to palpate the scalene muscles. All that is required is to locate the lateral border of the clavicular head of the SCM and then drop off it immediately laterally, and you will be on the scalene group. This is a much easier way to locate the scalenes than to first try to palpate the anterior tubercles of the transverse processes of the cervical vertebrae. Similarly, the SCM can also be used to locate and palpate the longus colli muscle. First locate the medial border of the sternal head of the SCM and then drop off it just medially, and sink in toward the spinal column. There are countless other examples wherein the knowledge of one muscle's location can help the therapist locate another muscle that might otherwise be more difficult to find.

Guideline #15: Relax and Passively Slacken the Target Muscle When Palpating Its Bony Attachment

It is always desirable to palpate as much of a target muscle as possible; preferably it should be palpated all the way from one bony attachment to its other bony attachment. However, there are times when it is difficult to follow a target muscle all the way to its bony attachment. This is especially true if the client is contracting the target muscle, because this tenses and hardens its tendon, making it difficult to discern from its bony attachment. Ironically, even though contracting the target muscle helps us discern its belly from adjacent soft tissue because the muscle belly becomes hard, contracting the target muscle tenses and hardens the tendon of the muscle too; and that makes it harder to discern the hard tendon from the adjacent hard bony tissue of its attachment. In other words, contracting a target muscle helps to discern it from adjacent soft tissue, but makes it more difficult to discern from adjacent hard tissue. Therefore one guideline that can help the therapist follow a target muscle all the way to its bony attachment is to have the client relax the target muscle and have it passively slackened as the therapist reaches its bony attachment. Examples that use this guideline are palpating the proximal attachment of the rectus femoris muscle on the anterior inferior iliac spine (AIIS) of the pelvis (see Figure 19-30), and palpating the distal attachment of the subscapularis muscle on the lesser tubercle of the humerus (see Figure 11-60).

The concept of slackening soft tissue can also be applied to adjacent muscles and other soft tissues and is helpful when palpating a target muscle that is deep. For example, if we want to palpate the transverse process attachments of the scalenes in the anterior neck, we need to slacken the overlying SCM muscle; this is accomplished by flexing, (ipsilaterally) laterally flexing, and contralaterally rotating the client's neck. We can now gently push our palpating fingers deep to the slackened SCM to access the transverse process attachments of the scalenes. Similarly, to palpate the rib attachment of the scalenes, we need to reach deep to the client's clavicle; this is best achieved if we slacken the tissue of the anterior neck with flexion and (ipsilateral) lateral flexion.

Guideline #16: Close Your Eyes When You Palpate

Although it is important to visually inspect the palpation region when beginning palpation of the target muscle (see Guideline #5), once the visual inspection is done, it is usually not necessary for a therapist to continue looking at the client's body as the palpation procedure continues. In fact, it can be greatly beneficial if the therapist closes his or her eyes when palpating. By closing the eyes, the therapist can block out extraneous sensory stimuli that might otherwise distract from what is being felt in the palpation fingers. Closing the eyes allows the therapist to focus all attention on the palpating fingers, thereby increasing their sensory acuity.

Guideline #17: Construct a Mental Picture of the Client's Anatomy under the Skin as You Palpate

As the therapist's eyes are closed during palpation, it can be further beneficial to picture the target muscle and other adjacent anatomic structures under the client's skin. Creating this mental picture of the client's anatomy under the skin can facilitate correct initial location of the target muscle and facilitate use of baby steps as the target muscle is followed toward its attachments.

Guideline #18: If a Client Is Ticklish, Have the Client Place a Hand over Your Palpating Hand

Unfortunately, when clients are ticklish, it often makes it difficult if not impossible to palpate them, because touching causes them to pull away. This is especially true if we touch the client lightly. Therefore it is usually best to palpate ticklish clients with firm pressure. However, some clients are extremely ticklish whether we touch them lightly or firmly. This can interfere with

palpation assessment and also with treatment. One thing that can be done to help lessen the sensitivity of a ticklish client is to ask the client to place one of his or her hands over the therapist's palpating hand. Ticklishness is a perceived invasion of one's space by another individual; this is why a person cannot tickle himself or herself. Therefore if the client's hand is placed over our palpating hand, the client subconsciously has a sense that he or she is in control of this space and tends to be less ticklish. Using this guideline does not work with everyone in every circumstance, but it is often successful and worth trying.

Guideline #19: Keep Fingernails Short and Smooth

For some muscle palpations, the therapist's fingernails need to be very short (Figure 2-12, A). This is especially true when it comes to deeper palpations; for example, when palpating the subscapularis muscle, quadratus lumborum muscle, or the vertebral attachments of the scalene muscles. Unfortunately, it seems that everyone has a different sense of what *short* means when it comes to the length of fingernails. As a result, some therapists allow their nails to be too long. Consequently they are unable to comfortably palpate some muscles and either cause pain and leave fingernail marks on the client or, just as bad, avoid adequately palpating or working musculature of the client that is in need of treatment because they are afraid of hurting the client with their nails. The exact fingernail length that is necessary varies from one palpation to another. A good way to check for appropriate fingernail length is to place the pads of your palpating hand fingers away from you and try to catch the fingernails of your palpating hand with a fingernail of your other hand (see Figure 2-12, B). If you can, then the fingernails are likely too long. If you cannot, then the length of your fingernails is short enough for deep palpations.

It is just as important that fingernails are smooth (i.e., their edges are not sharp). When filing fingernails, it is important to finish with a fingernail file that buffs and smoothes the edges of the nails. Short nails that are sharp can be just as uncomfortable or painful to the client as long fingernails.

Guideline #20: Use the Optimal Palpation Position

The optimal palpation position is simply the client position that is most effective for the palpation of a particular target muscle. It is important to realize that the optimal position in which to palpate a certain target muscle might not be the position that a client is usually in when that muscle is being treated. Clients are usually treated in the prone or supine position. However, some muscles are optimally palpated with the client side lying, standing, or seated. For example, the pectoralis minor is most often treated with the client supine. However, the optimal client position in which to palpate the pectoralis minor is probably seated. This is because the seated position better allows the client to first place the hand in the small of the back and then move the hand posteriorly away from the small of the back (creating downward rotation of the scapula to engage the pectoralis minor) (see Figure 11-80). For this reason, even though it is usually preferred to not have the client change positions in the middle of a treatment session, if accurate palpation is critical to the assessment and treatment of the client, it might be necessary to do so. To avoid this interruption to the flow of a treatment session, the therapist may choose to do all palpation assessments at the beginning of the session before commencing with treatment.

2

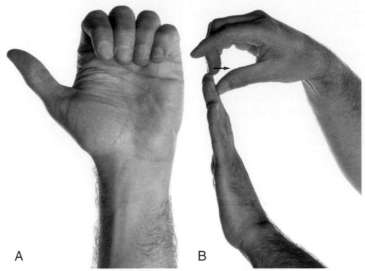

A   B

Figure 2-12 A Shows the proper length for fingernails when palpating and working deeply. An easy way to check that fingernail length is short enough for deeper palpations is seen in **B.** See if you can catch the fingernails of your palpating hand (when the pads are oriented away from you) with a fingernail of your other hand. If you can, that fingernail may be too long.

BOX 2-11

Often the client can be placed in more than one position to palpate a particular target muscle. Although one position might generally be considered optimal for palpation of that target muscle, some therapists may prefer an alternative position. However, even if one client position and palpation procedure is the favorite approach, an alternative position and procedure might work better for certain clients. For this reason, it is always desirable to be creative and flexible when approaching muscle palpation. The more palpation positions and methods you are comfortable with, the more likely it is that you will be successful when working with your clients. For each muscle palpation given in Part IV of this book, alternative client positions are given whenever applicable. Alternative palpation methods are also often presented.

CONCLUSION

Although the science of muscle palpation begins with a solid knowledge of the attachments and actions of the target muscle, turning palpation into an art requires much more. The art of muscle palpation involves weaving the knowledge of the attachments and actions of the target muscle and all adjacent musculature, as well as the many guidelines listed in this chapter, into a cohesive approach that allows the target muscle to be discerned from adjacent tissues. Overall, what are necessary are sensitive hands, critical thinking, and a willingness to be creative.

Review Questions

1. What is the difference between palpating bone and bony landmarks versus palpating soft tissues?
2. What advantages does knowing the attachments of a muscle give a therapist?
3. What is the importance of an isolated contraction of the target muscle?
4. Aside from touch, which of the other senses can be a valuable tool for the palpating therapist?
5. List three of the important details about adding resistance to the contraction of the target muscle.
6. In what way should a target muscle be palpated: longitudinally or perpendicularly? Why?
7. Describe the process of deep palpation.
8. Describe the optimal palpation position. How does this relate to treatment?
9. What is reciprocal inhibition and how can it be used during palpation?
10. When approaching a muscle's bony attachment, what can a therapist do to make palpation potentially easier?

 Deeper Thoughts

Given all of the palpation guidelines in this chapter, which one presents the biggest challenge for you? What steps might you take to overcome this difficulty?

CHAPTER 3

Orthopedic Assessment Testing

Overview

Although the principal focus of this book is to explore palpation assessment, orthopedic assessment testing is another major area of musculoskeletal assessment that all manual and movement therapists/practitioners should be familiar with when performing a physical examination on the client. This chapter begins with the essential components of the physical exam process. It then describes the three major types of general orthopedic assessment testing: active range of motion, passive range of motion, and manual resistance. This chapter then covers the major special orthopedic assessment tests for the body, covering them regionally, beginning with the axial body, then the lower extremity, and finishing with the upper extremity. For each test, three major aspects are addressed: the objective(s) of the test, the mechanics of how it is performed, and the objective and/or subjective results that would determine a positive test. High-quality photographs are also provided to demonstrate how the tests are carried out. Alternate names and additional notes for some of the tests are also included.

Chapter Outline

Introduction
General Orthopedic Assessment Tests
Active Range of Motion (AROM)
Passive Range of Motion (PROM)
Manual Resistance (MR)
Making the Assessment
Perform AROM
Perform PROM
Perform MR to Mover Musculature
Determine Location of Pain with Prom and Perform MR to Antagonist Musculature
Putting It All Together
Special Orthopedic Assessment Tests
Neck
Thoracic Spine
Sacroiliac Joint (SIJ)
Lumbar Spine
Hip Joint/Thigh
Knee Joint
Ankle Joint/Foot
Shoulder Joint
Elbow Joint
Wrist Joint/Hand

Chapter Objectives

After completing this chapter, the student/therapist should be able to perform the following.
1. List the major aspects of the physical examination process.
2. Describe and demonstrate active range of motion testing.
3. Describe and demonstrate passive range of motion testing.
4. Describe and demonstrate manual resistance testing.
5. State the name, objective(s), mechanics, and indications of a positive test result for each of the special orthopedic assessment tests covered in this chapter.

3

Key Terms

Active Range of Motion
Passive Range of Motion
Manual Resistance
Foraminal Compression Test
   (Spurling's Test)
Maximal Foraminal Compression
   Test
Cervical Distraction Test
Cough Test
Valsalva Test/Maneuver
Vertebral Artery Competency Test
Slump Test
Adson's Test
Eden's Test (Military Brace
   Position)
Wright's Test
Brachial Plexus Tension Test
   (BPTT) – Median Nerve
Brachial Plexus Tension Test
   (BPTT) – Ulnar Nerve
Brachial Plexus Tension Test
   (BPTT) – Radial Nerve
Nachlas Test
Yeoman's Test
SIJ Compression Tests
Gaenslen's Test
Patrick FABER Test

Active Straight Leg Raise (ASLR)
   Test
Passive Straight Leg Raise
   (PSLR) Test
Lumbar Extension for Facet
   Syndrome
One Leg Lumbar Extension Test
Bowstring Test
Thomas Test
Piriformis Syndrome Test
Pace Abduction Test
Ober's Test
Noble Compression Test
Anterior Draw Test
Posterior Drawer Test
Medial Collateral Ligament Test
Lateral Collateral Ligament Test
Apley's Compression Test
Apley's Distraction Test
Patellofemoral Syndrome
   (Clarke's) Test
Patellofemoral Mobility Test
Metatarsal Head Assessment
Achilles Tendon Pinch Test
Morton's (Compression/Squeeze)
   Test
Interdigital Squeeze Test

Dorsiflexion Eversion Test
Tinel's Sign at the Ankle
Ankle Anterior Drawer
Talar Tilt Test
Apley's Scratch Test
Drop-Arm Test
Empty Can Test
Hawkins-Kennedy Impingement
   Test
Subacromial Bursitis Abduction
   ROM Test
Speed's Test
Cross Over Test
Radial Tunnel Syndrome/Posterior
   Interosseus Nerve (PIN)
   Syndrome Assessment
Phalen's Test
Prayer Test
Tinel's Sign at the Wrist
Tethered Median Nerve Stress
   Test
Finklestein's Test
Froment's Sign
Pinch Grip Test

INTRODUCTION

The primary focus of this book is palpation assessment. Indeed, palpation is the principal assessment tool for the manual therapist. However, orthopedic assessment testing should accompany palpation during the physical exam process. Palpation and orthopedic assessment are the two principal components of an accurate and thorough physical examination.

This chapter offers a critical-thinking exploration of general orthopedic assessment testing as well as the major special orthopedic assessment tests that the manual therapist should employ in their practice.

General Orthopedic Assessment Tests
a. Active Range of Motion (AROM) – positive for muscle strain, ligament sprain, and muscle spasm
b. Passive Range of Motion (PROM) – positive for ligament sprain and muscle spasm
c. Manual Resistance (MR) – positive for muscle strain and muscle spasm

GENERAL ORTHOPEDIC ASSESSMENT TESTS

There is a saying in the world of medicine: "Never treat without a diagnosis." This concept could be slightly modified for the world of clinical orthopedic manual therapy (COMT): "Never treat without an accurate assessment." The essence of COMT is that treatment is not oriented toward general

wellness but is performed to remedy a specific myofascial complaint. This requires an accurate assessment.

There are many special orthopedic assessment tests that can be learned, and it is certainly good to know as many of them as possible; indeed, the major ones are explored in this chapter. However, a majority of clients who present for clinical orthopedic work have hypertonicity and strains of musculature and/or ligament complex (ligament/joint capsule/fascial) sprains, and can be assessed with three key orthopedic tests described as "general orthopedic assessment tests." These three tests are: active range of motion (AROM), passive range of motion (PROM), and manual resistance (MR).

AROM is done by asking the client to actively move the target joint through a range of motion by contracting the musculature of that joint (Fig. 3-1). With PROM, the client remains relaxed as the therapist brings the client's joint through the range of motion (Fig. 3-2). MR is performed by asking the client to attempt to move the joint through a range of motion but adding resistance with the hand so that the client cannot succeed in moving the joint (Fig. 3-3). In each case, the test assesses a certain tissue of the body by placing a physical stress on it. If the tissue is healthy, no pain/discomfort will be experienced, and the test is negative. If the tissue is unhealthy, the client will experience pain/discomfort, and the test is positive. Understanding which tissues are stressed with each assessment test allows the therapist to critically reason and accurately determine the client's condition. This allows for more efficient and effective treatment. Note: Each client's sensitivity to pain and when they report pain varies, therefore it should be kept in mind that orthopedic assessment tests are not always 100% accurate.

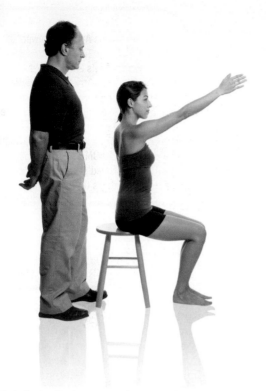

Figure 3-1 Active flexion range of motion of the glenohumeral joint.

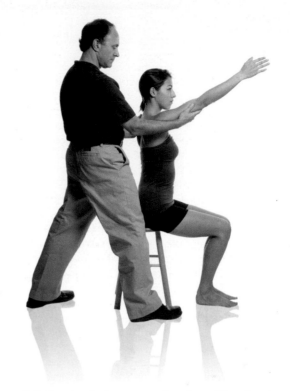

Figure 3-2 Passive flexion range of motion of the glenohumeral joint.

Active Range of Motion (AROM)

AROM stresses/assesses the client's mover musculature by requiring it to concentrically contract; if the mover musculature is strained, spasmed, or injured in any way, pain will be felt. It also requires the joint to move through a range of motion; this stresses/assesses the ligament complex by moving and stretching it. So, if the ligament complex is sprained or injured, it will cause pain. And it stresses/ assesses the antagonist musculature because it causes it to be lengthened/stretched as the joint moves through its range of motion. So, if the antagonist musculature is strained/ spasmed/injured, it will cause pain. Therefore AROM will show positive if the client has a mover muscle strain, a ligament complex sprain, and/or an antagonist muscle strain. For this reason, AROM is a screening test that is performed first. If it is negative, the client has no strain or sprain, and theoretically the other two assessment tests do not need to be performed. However, if it is positive, we know that the client either has a strain, a sprain, or both. PROM and MR are then performed to determine exactly which condition(s) the client has (Box 3-1).

Passive Range of Motion (PROM)

The mover musculature remains relaxed during PROM, therefore it is not assessed. However, because the joint moves through a range of motion, the ligament complex is stressed; therefore sprained ligaments will show as positive. Similarly, joint motion causes the antagonist musculature to be stretched; therefore if it is strained, it will show as painful.

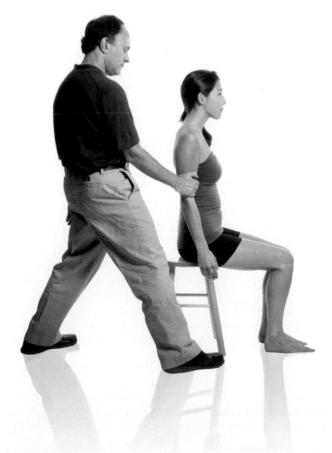

Figure 3-3 Manual resistance to flexion range of motion of the glenohumeral joint.

BOX 3-1

Joint Surfaces

When a joint is moved, if the bony joint surfaces are unhealthy (for example, degenerative joint disease, also known as osteoarthrosis/osteoarthritis), pain will be present, and the assessment test will be deemed positive. The health of the bony joint must be considered when making the assessment. A pathologic joint surface will show positive with AROM and PROM but usually not MR (because the joint surface is not moved); in this regard, it is similar to the presentation of a sprain. Differentiating between the bony joint surface and the ligament complex is challenging but can be done. Making this discernment is accomplished by keeping in mind that ligament sprains usually exhibit pain when they are stretched, whereas joint surfaces exhibit pain when they are compressed. Therefore, if we add compression to the joint, it will show positive for the joint surface and not the ligament complex, whereas if we stretch the soft tissue on one side of the joint, it will show positive for the ligament complex and not the joint surface. For example, if we right laterally flex the cervical spine, this compresses the right facet joints and stretches the left facet joint ligament complex. If the right facet joint is unhealthy, the client will experience pain on the right side, whereas if the client has a ligamentous sprain on the left, the client will experience pain on the left side.

BOX 3-2

Manual Resistance

MR is meant to stress and assess only the musculature being asked to contract, not other tissues. Therefore for MR assessment to be accurate, it is extremely important for resistance to be sufficiently strong so that the joint is not allowed to move. If the joint does move, then ligaments and the antagonist musculature will be stretched, and therefore also stressed and assessed, making a clear assessment of the contracting musculature more difficult to determine.

Manual Resistance (MR)

MR stresses/assesses the mover musculature because it is required to isometrically contract. However, neither the ligament complex nor the antagonist musculature is stressed/assessed because the joint does not move (Box 3.2).

MAKING THE ASSESSMENT

Making an accurate assessment is like assembling the pieces of a puzzle. Each test result gives us a piece. The key is to understand what each test does so that we can critically think through and reason what each result means. In effect, we are detectives who place these pieces into the puzzle to determine our client's condition. Following are the conclusions that can be reached from performing these assessment tests. Figure 3-4 places this information into flow chart form.

Perform AROM

If AROM is negative, the client does not have a strain or a sprain because all tissues were stressed/assessed, and no pain was reported.

If AROM is positive, we know that the client either has a strain of mover musculature, a sprain of the ligament complex, a strain of antagonist musculature, or a combination of these conditions because all these tissues were stressed and therefore assessed. We now need to perform PROM to discern between these conditions.

Perform PROM

If PROM is negative, then the client does not have a ligament sprain or an antagonist musculature strain, because this test stresses these tissues, and they were not painful. If the client does not have a ligament sprain or antagonist strain, the client must have only a strain of the mover musculature.

If PROM is positive, then we know that the client has either a sprain of the ligament complex and/or a strain of the antagonist musculature because these tissues were stretched and assessed. It must be kept in mind that the client may also have a mover strain as well.

Perform MR to Mover Musculature

To determine whether they do also have a strain of the mover musculature, perform MR to the mover musculature. This causes it to contract, thereby stressing and assessing it. If it is negative, they do not have a mover strain. If it is positive, they also have a mover strain; now we need to determine whether the positive PROM was due to a ligament sprain, an antagonist strain, or both.

Dertermine Location of Pain with Prom and Perform MR to Antagonist Musculature

To discern between a ligament sprain and antagonist strain (or to determine whether both are present), two things can be done. First, determine the location of pain during PROM. Was it on the same side of the joint as motion occurred, the opposite side, or both?

- If the pain was on both sides of the joint, the client has a ligament sprain and an antagonist strain.
- If the pain is located only on the same side of the joint, they have a ligament sprain and not an antagonist strain. Now perform MR to the antagonist musculature. It should be negative, confirming that the client does not have an antagonist strain.
- If the pain is located only on the other side of the joint in the antagonist musculature, the client has an antagonist strain and does not have a ligament sprain. Now perform MR to the antagonist musculature. It should be positive, confirming that the client does have an antagonist strain.

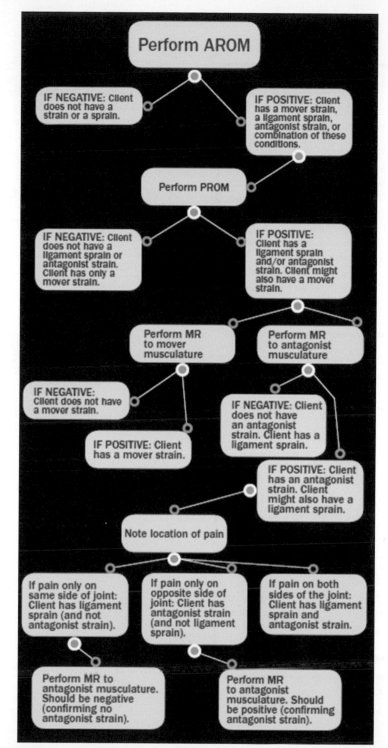

Figure 3-4 Flow chart rubric for analysis of AROM, PROM, and MR results. (Used with permission from: Muscolino JE: Body mechanics: orthopedic assessment of strains and sprains, *Massage Ther J.* Summer:74-80, 2012)

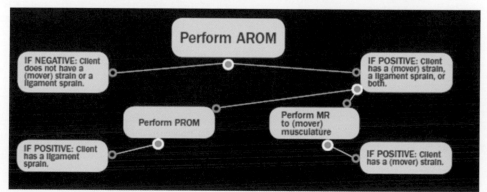

Figure 3-5 Flow chart rubric for analysis of AROM, PROM, and MR without consideration of the antagonist musculature. (Used with permission from: Muscolino JE: Body mechanics: orthopedic assessment of strains and sprains, *Massage Ther J.* Summer:74-80, 2012)

BOX 3-3

A Simpler Approach

Discussions of AROM, PROM, and MR often do not include consideration of the antagonist musculature. This simpler method of assessment can potentially lead to errors because strains of the antagonist musculature will be missed and can be blamed on ligament sprains. Therefore this method of assessment might not be as accurate, but it is much simpler. AROM stresses/assesses (mover) musculature and the ligament complex; PROM stresses/assesses the ligament complex only; and MR stresses/assesses (mover) musculature only. Therefore positive AROM tells us that the client has a strain and/or a sprain. Positive PROM then tells us if they have a sprain, and positive MR tells us if they have a strain (Fig. 3-5).

BOX 3-4

Contractile and Noncontractile Tissues

The terms contractile tissue and noncontractile tissue are often used when describing the soft tissues of the body. Classically, it has been stated that musculature is contractile, and the ligament complex is noncontractile. However, it is now understood that fascia can contract due to the development and presence of myofibroblastic cells. But this new understanding of fascial contraction does not affect our assessment using AROM, PROM, and MR assessment tests because fascial contraction is not voluntary, therefore we do not engage fascial contraction during AROM and MR. Fascial contraction is mediated through local tissue factors instead of the nervous system and is very slow to engage, requiring many minutes, whereas muscular contraction via the nervous system is instantaneous.

Putting it All Together

Even though AROM, PROM, and MR assessment tests for mover and antagonist musculature and the ligament complex are simple and straightforward, there are times when the combinations of positive and negative results for these tests can be a bit complicated. However, if we understand what is being stressed and assessed in each test and reason through the results, we can form an accurate and complete assessment of muscular strains and ligaments sprains with which our clients present. This will allow for thorough and effective clinical orthopedic manual therapy (Boxes 3-3 and 3-4).

SPECIAL ORTHOPEDIC ASSESSMENT TESTS

Neck

Foraminal Compression Test (Spurling's Test)
- Objective: Space-Occupying Lesion (to compress spinal nerves in the intervertebral foramina [IVFs])
- Mechanics: Press down on head
- Positive: Referral into the upper extremity

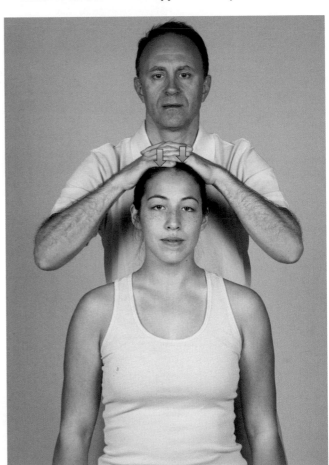

Maximal Foraminal Compression Test
- Objective: Space-Occupying Lesion
- Mechanics: Same as Foraminal Compression with client's head/neck in rotation and lateral flexion to same side
- Positive: Referral into the upper extremity

Cervical Distraction Test
- Objective: To decompress spinal nerves in the IVFs for Space-Occupying Lesions
- Mechanics: Traction head
- Positive: Decrease in referral symptoms into the upper extremity

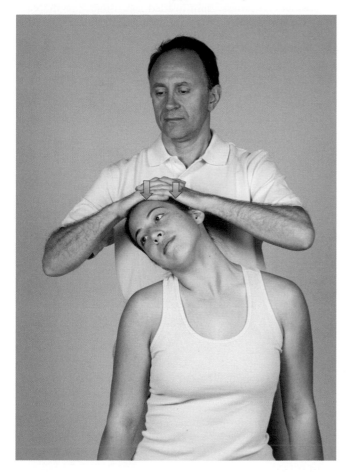

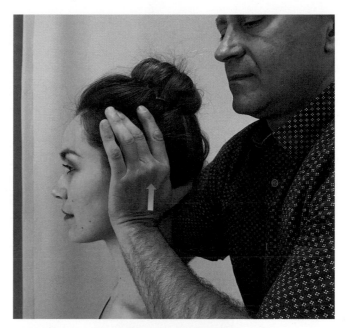

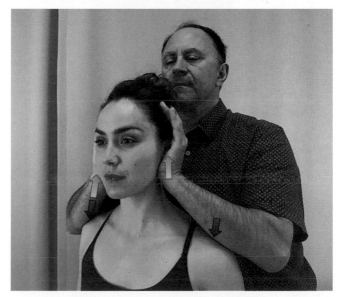

Cough Test
- Objective: Space-Occupying Lesions (entire spine)
- Mechanics: Strong cough to increase intrathecal pressure against the spinal nerves
- Positive: Referral into the upper (or lower) extremity

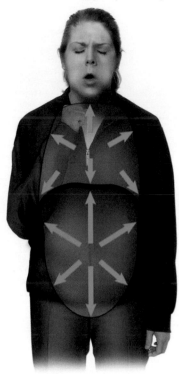

Valsalva Test/Maneuver
- Objective: Space-Occupying Lesions (entire spine)
- Mechanics: Client bears down as if at stool in the bathroom to increase intrathecal pressure against the spinal nerves
- Positive: Referral into the upper (or lower) extremity

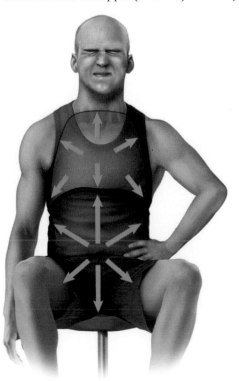

Vertebral Artery Competency Test
- Objective: To check for the competency of the Vertebral Arteries
- Mechanics: Rotation to one side with lateral flexion to the opposite side, and extension
- Positive: Dizziness, light-headedness, ringing in the ears, nausea, nystagmus (…neural symptoms)

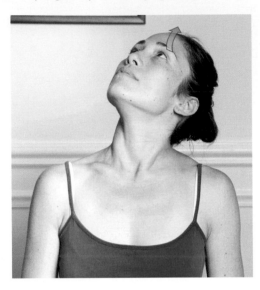

Thoracic Spine
Slump Test
- Objective: To tauten neural tissue against a Space-Occupying Lesion (entire spinal cord and sciatic nerve)
- Mechanics: Hands clasped behind back; flexion of head/neck; flexion of trunk; flexion of thigh at hip joint; extension of leg at knee joint; dorsiflexion of foot at ankle joint; therapist can augment head/neck flexion or foot dorsiflexion
- Positive: Referral into the upper or lower extremities

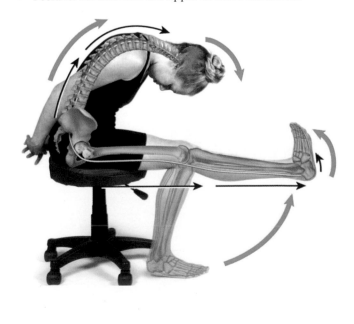

Adson's Test

- Objective: Thoracic Outlet Syndrome (TOS) – Anterior Scalene Syndrome
- Mechanics: Neck rotation to one side with contralateral lateral flexion and extension; monitor radial pulse
- Positive: Decrease in the strength of the pulse (and/or increase in referral symptoms)
- Note: *Halstead Test* (lower photo) is similar but with opposite-side rotation.

Eden's Test (Military Brace Position)

- Objective: TOS – Costoclavicular Syndrome
- Mechanics: Client pushes chest out and pulls shoulder girdles back into retraction, as if in front of commanding officer; monitor radial pulse
- Positive: Decrease in the strength of the pulse (and/or increase in referral symptoms)

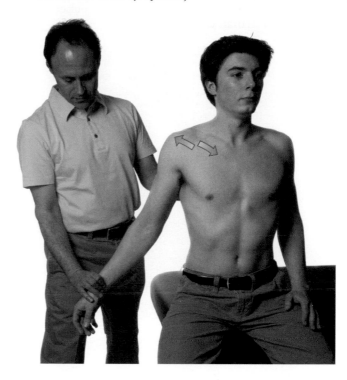

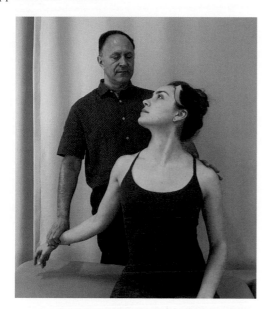

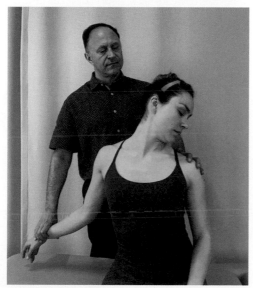

3

Wright's Test

- Objective: TOS – Pectoralis Minor Syndrome
- Mechanics: Version 1 (upper photo): Bring arm into abduction (approximately 145 degrees) and extension (i.e., horizontal extension); monitor radial pulse
- Mechanics: Version 2 (lower photo): Bring client's hand over head; monitor radial pulse
- Positive: Decrease in the strength of the pulse (and/or increase in referral symptoms)

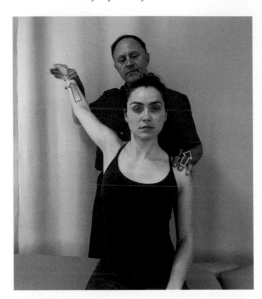

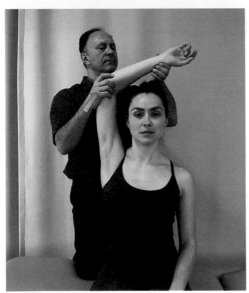

BPTT (Brachial Plexus Tension Test) – Median Nerve

- Objective: Median Nerve Compression
- Mechanics: Stretch median nerve long with contralateral lateral flexion of head/neck; depression of shoulder girdle; abduction of arm; elbow joint extension; forearm supination; wrist extension; finger extension
- Positive: Referral into median nerve distribution

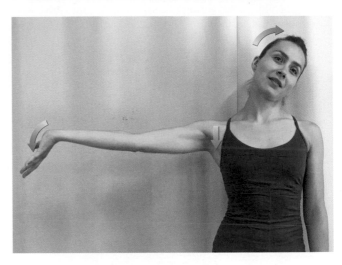

BPTT – Ulnar Nerve

- Objective: Ulnar Nerve Compression
- Mechanics: Stretch ulnar nerve long with contralateral lateral flexion of head/neck; depression of shoulder girdle; abduction of arm; elbow joint flexion; forearm pronation; wrist extension; finger extension
- Positive: Referral into ulnar nerve distribution

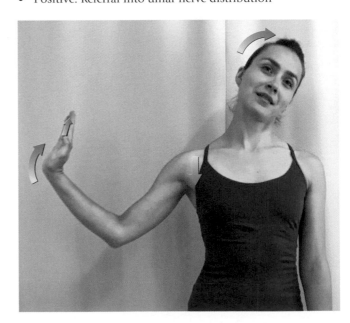

BPTT – Radial Nerve
- Objective: Radial Nerve Compression
- Mechanics: Stretch radial nerve long with contralateral lateral flexion of head/neck; depression of shoulder girdle; abduction of arm; elbow joint extension; forearm pronation; wrist flexion; finger flexion
- Positive: Referral into radial nerve distribution

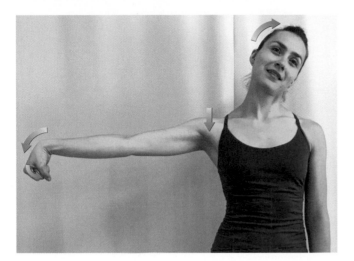

Sacroiliac Joint (SIJ)
Nachlas Test
- Objective: SIJ Sprain/Inflammation
- Mechanics: Bring client's heel to buttock
- Positive: Pain at either SIJ (or lumbosacral [LS] joint)
- Note: Also known as *Prone Knee Bend Test*.

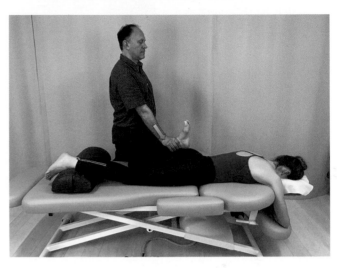

Yeoman's Test
- Objective: SIJ Sprain/Inflammation
- Mechanics: Bring client's thigh into extension while stabilizing ipsilateral PSIS
- Positive: Pain at either SIJ (or LS joint)

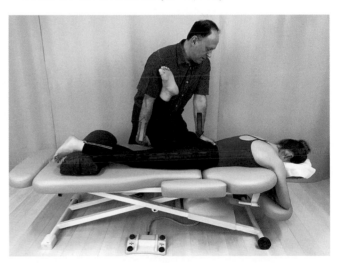

3

Medley of SIJ Compression Tests
- Objective: SIJ Sprain/Inflammation
- Mechanics: Test 1 (both photos below): Client prone with compression on PSIS

- Mechanics: Test 2 (both photos below): Client side-lying with compression on iliac crest
- Note: A cushion can be used (lower photo)

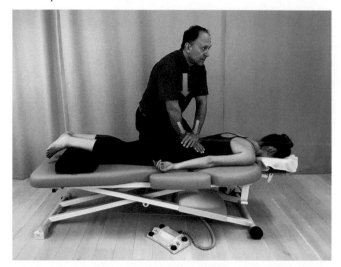

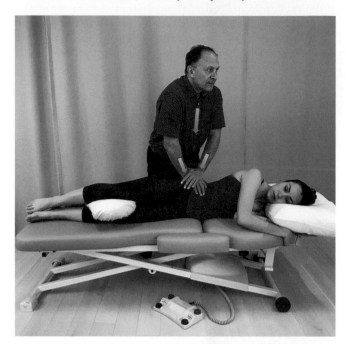

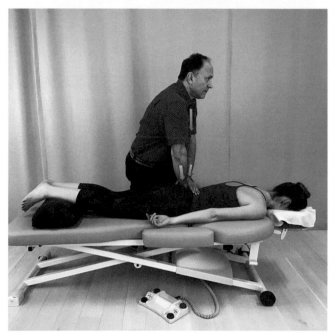

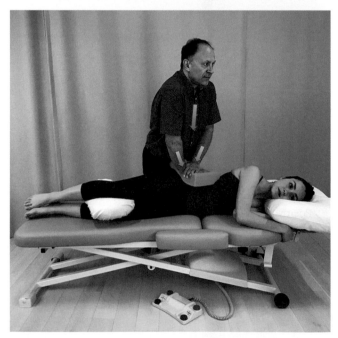

- Mechanics: Test 3 (both photos below): Client supine with compression on ASISs bilaterally

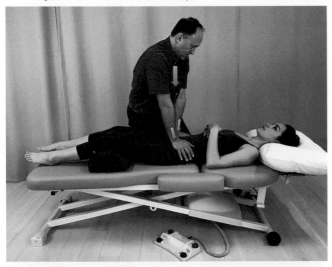

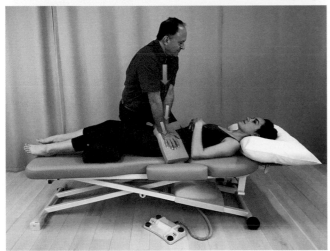

- Mechanics: Test 4: Client supine with thigh flexed to 90 degrees and compression of femur into acetabulum
- Positive: Pain at the SIJ

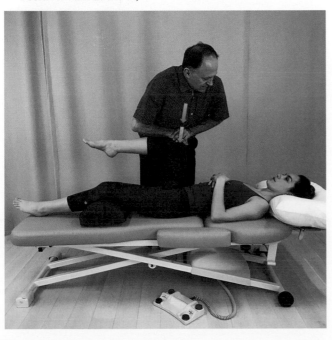

Gaenslen's Test
- Objective: SIJ Sprain/Inflammation
- Mechanics: Client supine with thigh off table into extension; stabilize at contralateral ASIS
- Positive: Pain at either SIJ (or LS joint)
- Note: Original Gaenslen's test was performed side-lying.

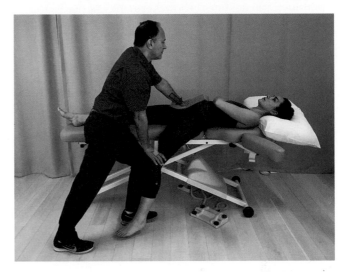

Patrick FABER Test
- Objective: SIJ Sprain/Inflammation (and/or Hip Joint Capsule Sprain and/or Adductor/Medial Rotator Musculature Tightness)
- Mechanics: Place client's thigh into Flexion, Abduction, and External Rotation; knee joint flexion with ankle/foot on opposite distal anterior thigh; pressure applied on client's knee downward toward the floor; opposite ASIS stabilized
    - Positive: Pain at SIJ (and/or hip joint capsule and/or adductors/medial rotators)
    - Note: Effectively a "Figure-4" position.
    - Note: FABER stands for Flexion, ABduction, External Rotation

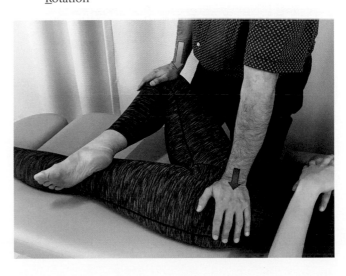

3

Lumbar Spine
Active Straight Leg Raise (ASLR) Test
- Objective: Space-Occupying Lesion, Lumbar/SIJ Strain and/or Sprain (and/or Muscle Spasm)
- Mechanics: Thigh flexion with knee joint extension (ankle joint dorsiflexion can be added)
- Positive: Referral into the lower extremity (space occupying lesion) or pain in the lumbar spine/SIJ (strain and/or sprain and/or muscle spasm)

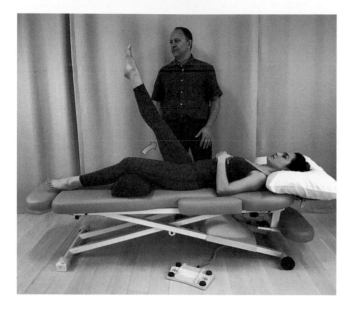

Passive Straight Leg Raise (PSLR) Test
- Objective: Space-Occupying Lesion, Lumbar/SIJ Sprain (and/or Muscle Spasm)
- Mechanics: Thigh flexion with knee joint extension (ankle joint dorsiflexion can be added)
- Positive: Referral into the lower extremity (space occupying lesion) or pain in the lumbar spine/SIJ (sprain and/or muscle spasm)

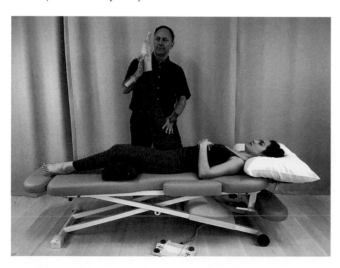

Manual Resistance (MR)
- Objective: Lumbar/SIJ Strain
- Mechanics: Isometric contraction of thigh flexors
- Positive: Pain in the lumbar spine/SIJ

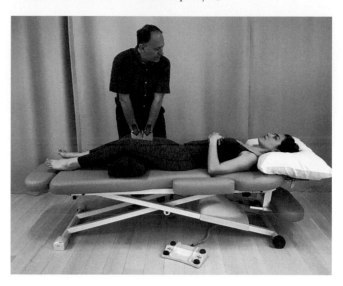

Cough Test
Valsalva Test/Maneuver
Slump Test

Lumbar Extension for Facet Syndrome
- Objective: Facet Syndrome
- Mechanics: Extension of the lumbar spine to approximate and load the facet joints
- Positive: Pain in the lumbar spine

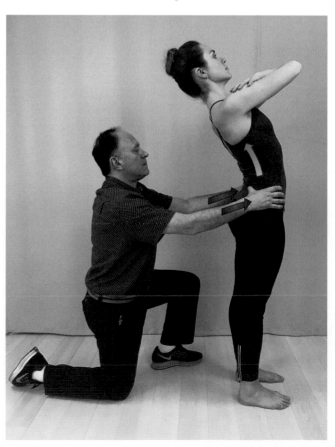

One-Leg Lumbar Extension Test
- Objective: Spondylolysis (pars fracture)/Spondylolisthesis (slippage)/(and Facet Syndrome)
- Mechanics: Stand on one leg and then extend the lumbar spine
- Positive: Pain in the lumbar spine
- Note: Repeat for the other side.

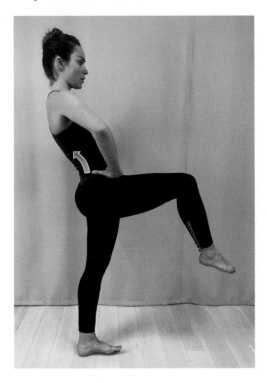

Bowstring Test
- Objective: Sciatica (to discern from tight hamstrings)
- Mechanics: Perform passive SLR and then back off from tension by flexing the knee joint until there is no pain, and then push into the popliteal region
- Positive: Referral into the lower extremity
- Note: Lower extremity referral pain likely indicates sciatica because the hamstrings are slackened.

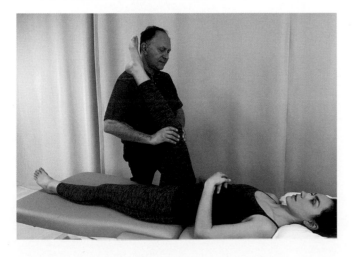

Hip Joint/Thigh
Thomas Test (Modified)
- Objective: Hip Flexor Tightness (perhaps psoas major)
- Mechanics: Supine at end of table and one thigh grasped to chest; note the level of the other thigh
  - Positive: Level of thigh is above table/horizontal (lower photo)
  - Note: Which hip flexor is restricting thigh extension?
  - Note: The original Thomas Test was performed with client's entire body supine on table.

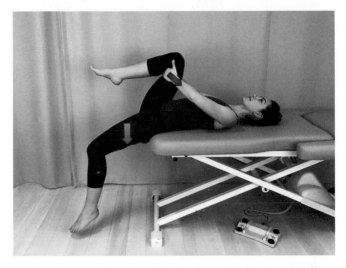

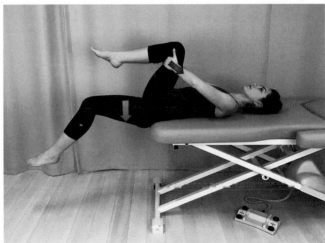

3

Piriformis Syndrome Test
- Objective: Piriformis Syndrome
- Mechanics: Horizontally adduct the thigh at the hip joint
- Positive: Referral pain/symptoms into the lower extremity
- Note: Also known as FAIR test (Flexion, Adduction, Internal Rotation – but there may little or no internal rotation).

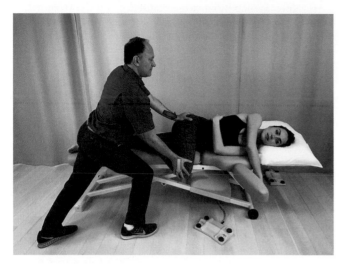

Pace Abduction Test
- Objective: Piriformis Syndrome, SIJ Sprain
- Mechanics: Client seated; resist horizontal abduction of thighs at the hip joints (bilaterally)
- Positive: Referral pain/symptoms into the lower extremity for piriformis syndrome; pain at the SIJ for SIJ sprain

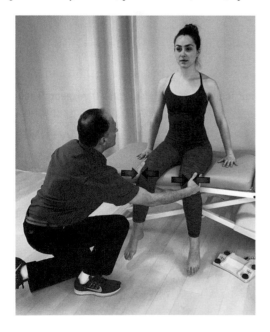

Patrick FABER Test

Ober's Test
- Objective: Hip Abductor/ITB (TFL/Gluteus Maximus) tightness
- Mechanics: Client side-lying with thigh in extension off back of table
- Positive: Level of thigh above horizontal
- Note: The original Ober's Test had the knee joint flexed to 90 degrees.

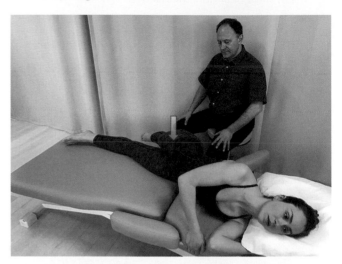

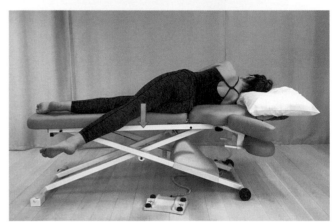

Noble Compression Test

- Objective: Iliotibial Band (ITB) Friction Syndrome
- Mechanics: Client supine with hip flexed and knee joint extended; therapist presses into ITB immediately proximal to lateral femoral epicondyle; slowly flex the leg
  - Positive: Pain at approximately 30 degrees of flexion
  - Note: The ITB lies anterior to the lateral epicondyle when the knee joint is in full extension; at approximately 30 degrees of flexion, the ITB passes over the epicondyle (causing friction) to move to its posterior side.

Knee Joint

Anterior Draw Test

- Objective: Anterior Cruciate Ligament Tear
- Mechanics: Client seated with hip and knee flexed; therapist sits on client's foot; grasps posterior proximal leg and draws the tibia anteriorly
  - Positive: Excessive anterior translation of the tibia
  - Note: *Lachman Test* (lower photo) is an alternative position to rule out/discern from tight hamstrings (client supine with knee in full extension or partial flexion; stabilize distal anterior thigh, grasp the posterior proximal leg and draw the tibia anteriorly).

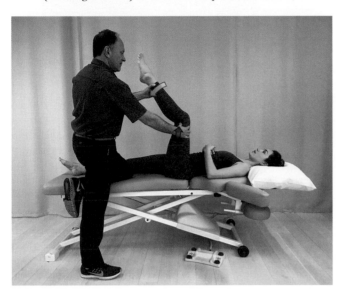

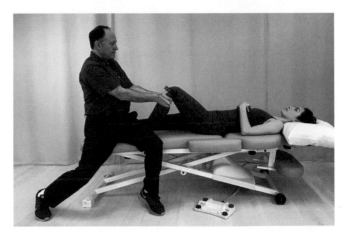

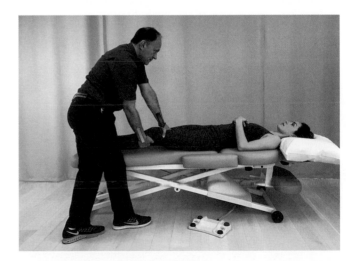

3

Posterior Drawer Test
- Objective: Posterior Cruciate Ligament Tear
- Mechanics: Client seated with hip and knee flexed; therapist sits on client's foot; pushes proximal leg/tibia posteriorly
- Positive: Excessive posterior translation of the tibia

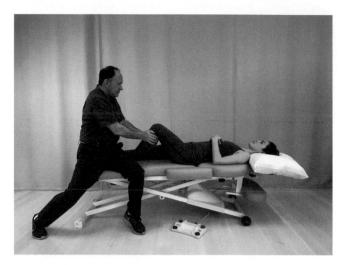

Medial Collateral Ligament Test
- Objective: Medial (Tibial) Collateral Ligament Tear
- Mechanics: Client supine; knee joint in approximately 10 to 15 degrees of flexion; apply genu valgum force (stabilize distal lateral thigh as the distal medial leg is pulled laterally)
- Positive: (Excessive) genu valgum movement

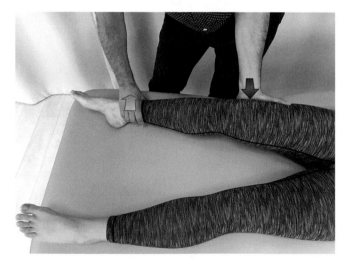

Lateral Collateral Ligament Test
- Objective: Lateral (Fibular) Collateral Ligament Tear
- Mechanics: Client supine; knee joint in approximately 10 to 15 degrees of flexion; apply genu varum force (stabilize distal medial thigh as the distal lateral leg is pulled medially)
- Positive: (Excessive) genu varum movement
- Note: A small bolster can be used under the knee to support the knee joint in slight flexion.
- Note: This test can be performed contralaterally as seen below.

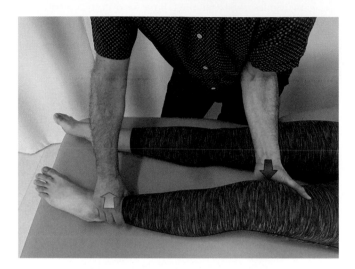

Apley's Compression Test

- Objective: Meniscus Tear (and possibly Ligament Sprain)
- Mechanics: Client prone with knee joint flexed to 90 degrees; apply downward compression force and rotate the leg at the knee joint
- Positive: Pain in the knee joint
- Note: Flexing the leg to approximately 135 degrees preferentially stresses the posterior menisci
- Note: Compression alone does not greatly stress the ligaments; leg rotation increases the stress to the ligaments. (Leg rotation also increases stress to the menisci.)

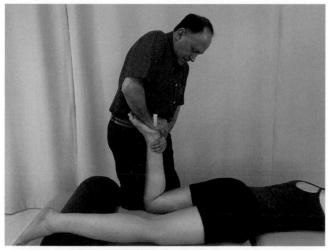

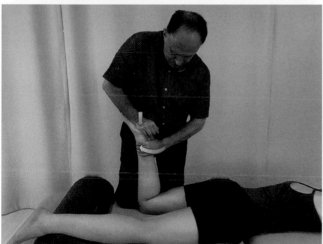

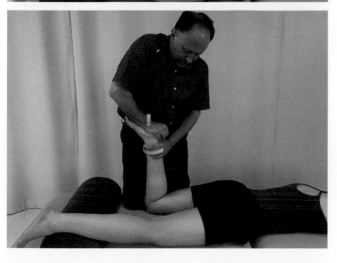

Apley's Distraction Test

- Objective: Ligament Sprain
- Mechanics: Same position as Apley's Compression Test but distal posterior thigh is stabilized and the tibia is tractioned away from the knee joint
- Positive: Pain in the knee joint

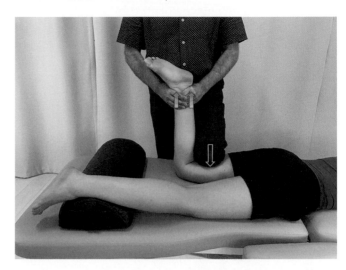

Patellofemoral Syndrome (Clarke's) Test

- Objective: Patellofemoral Syndrome (Chondromalacia Patella)
- Mechanics: Client supine; thumb web around superior/proximal pole of patella; client contracts quadriceps femoris
- Positive: Pain and/or crepitus in knee joint
- Note: Caution: Must be done in gradually increasing degrees of resistance; once pain/crepitus is felt, do not perform further repetitions.

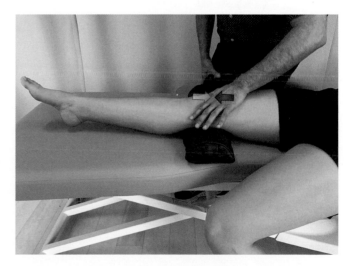

3

Patellofemoral Mobility Test
- Objective: Patellofemoral Syndrome (Chondromalacia Patella) and Restriction of Patellar Motion
- Mechanics: Client supine; apply pressure on patella from lateral to medial and medial to lateral
- Positive: Pain and/or crepitus (patellofemoral syndrome) or restriction of motion (less than ¼ to ½ of patellar width in medial direction indicates tautness of lateral retinacular fibers/vastus lateralis)
- Note: Move the patella lateral to medial to lateral, etc.

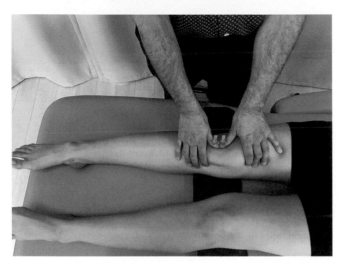

Ankle Joint/Foot
Metatarsal Head Assessment
- Objective: Morton's Foot
- Mechanics: Flex the toes at the MTP and IP joints
- Positive: Visualization of the second metatarsal projecting further distally than the metatarsal of the big toe (lower photo)
- Note: Simple visualization of the length of the second toe relative to the great toe (upper photo) may not be indicative of actual metatarsal length, and therefore Mortons' Foot.

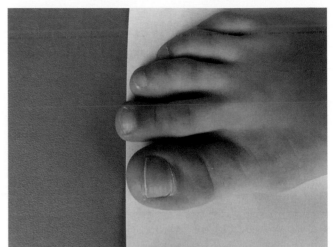

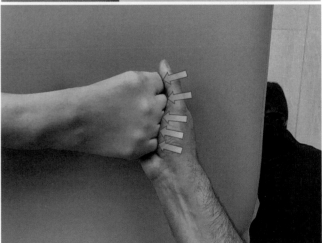

Achilles Tendon Pinch Test

- Objective: Achilles Tendinitis
- Mechanics: Therapist pinches the Achilles tendon making sure to press only on tendon and not the bursa deep/anterior to it (to discern tendinitis from bursitis)
- Positive: Pain in the Achilles tendon

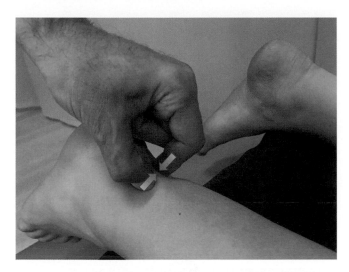

Morton's (Compression/Squeeze) Test

- Objective: Morton's Neuroma
- Mechanics: Compress metatarsal heads together
- Positive: Pain between the metatarsals (usually #3-#4)
- Note: Be sure to compress metatarsals directly into each other and not simply increase the transverse arch (placing thumbs on dorsal surface of foot can be helpful for this).

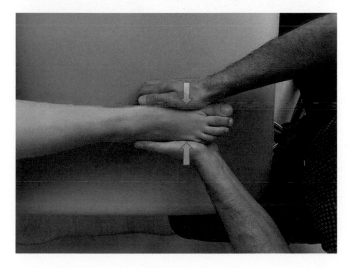

Interdigital Squeeze Test

- Objective: Morton's Neuroma
- Mechanics: Compress/squeeze intermetatarsal space between the metatarsal heads (especially #3-#4)
- Positive: Pain in the intermetatarsal (heads) space

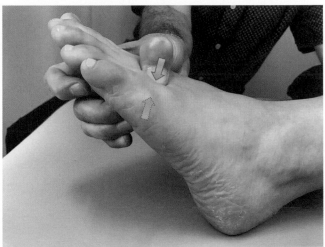

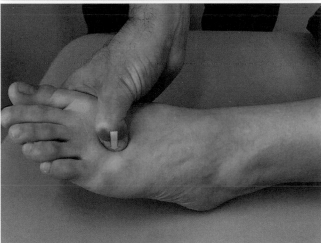

Dorsiflexion Eversion Test

- Objective: Tarsal Tunnel Syndrome (Tibial Nerve Compression)
- Mechanics: Therapist pushes the client's foot into dorsiflexion and eversion with the toes held in full extension, which maximally stretches the tibial nerve in the tarsal tunnel on the posterior side of the medial malleolus
- Positive: Neural symptoms (e.g., sharp shooting pain, tingling) in the medial ankle and/or plantar foot

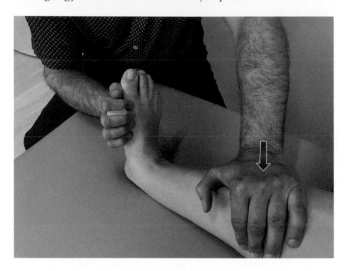

Tinel's Sign at the Ankle

- Objective: Tarsal Tunnel Syndrome
- Mechanics: Therapist taps directly over the tibial nerve in the tarsal tunnel
- Positive: Neural symptoms (e.g., sharp shooting pain, tingling) in the medial ankle and/or plantar foot

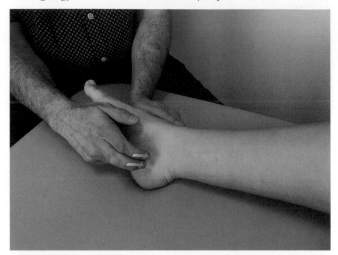

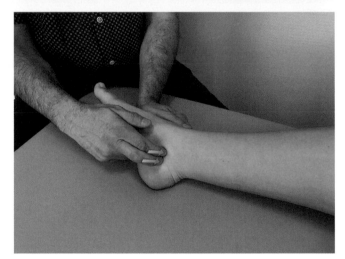

Ankle Anterior Drawer
- Objective: Anterior Talofibular Ligament Sprain
- Mechanics: Client seated with leg off end of table; therapist stabilizes the anterior distal leg and, grasping the posterior calcaneus, draws the calcaneus anteriorly
- Positive: Excessive movement
- Note: The anterior talofibular ligament resists anterior draw/translation of the talus at the talocrural/ankle joint.

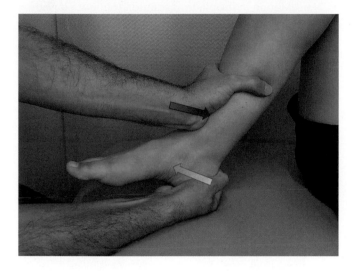

Talar Tilt Test
- Objective: Calcaneofibular Ligament Sprain
- Mechanics: Client side-lying; therapist inverts the foot at the subtalar joint (two different contacts to achieve this are shown below)
- Positive: Excessive movement
- Note: The calcaneofibular ligament resists pure inversion.

3

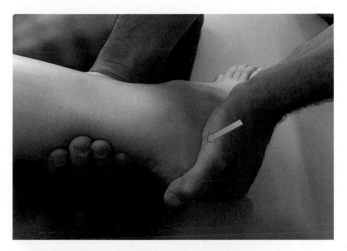

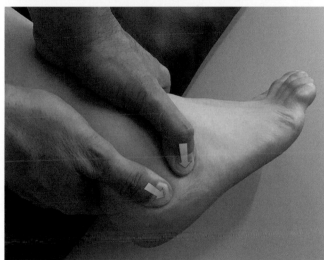

3

Shoulder Joint

Apley's Scratch Test

- Objective: Glenohumeral (GH) Joint ROM/Frozen Shoulder
- Mechanics: Upper: Abduction and lateral rotation
- Mechanics: Lower: Adduction and medial rotation
- Positive: Limited ROM
- Note: Positive Upper indicates decreased abduction/lateral rotation, which indicates tight adductors/medial rotators (more common).
- Note: Positive Lower indicates decreased adduction/medial rotation, which indicates tight abductors/lateral rotators.
- Note: Perform bilaterally.

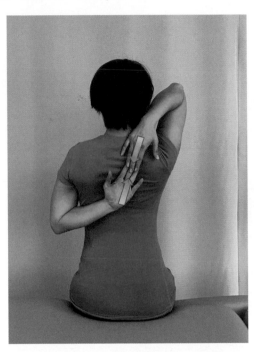

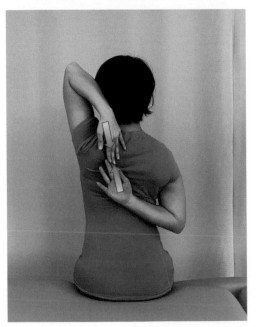

Drop-Arm Test

- Objective: Supraspinatus Tear (Impingement/Tendinitis)
- Mechanics: Client raises the arm to 90 degrees of abduction, then holds arm in this position, then slowly lowers the arm back down
- Positive: Pain at supraspinatus and/or inability to move smoothly and/or client "drops" the arm (because of neurologic inhibition)
- Note: Motion in the plane of scaption (oblique plane of abduction with approximately 30 degrees toward flexion in the sagittal plane) might be more effective.
- Note: Therapist may add resistance (as pictured). With resistance, Drop–Arm Test becomes similar to Empty Can Test; the difference is that Empty Can Test involves GH joint medial rotation to increase impingement.
- Note: Drop-Arm Test without resistance is usually positive only if the supraspinatus tear is moderate to severe.

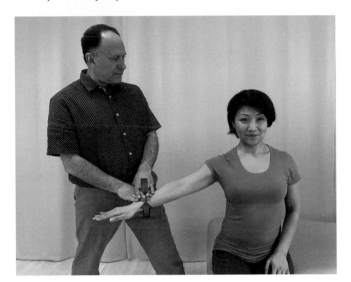

Empty Can Test

- Objective: Shoulder Impingement (especially Supraspinatus Distal Tendon impingement)
- Mechanics: Client actively brings arm to approximately 90 degrees of abduction with approximately 30 degrees of flexion (scaption); client then medially rotates the arm ("empty the can"); Part 2: Therapist adds moderate to strong resistance downward toward floor
- Positive: Pain at shoulder joint
- Note: If pain is only felt during the resistance phase of the test, impingement of the supraspinatus tendon is more likely indicated.
- Note: This test is often performed bilaterally (as seen below) for comparison to other side.

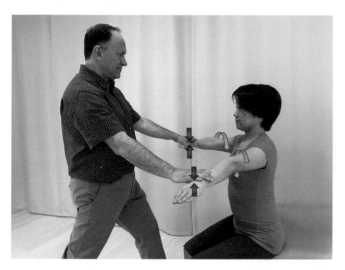

Hawkins-Kennedy Impingement Test

- Objective: Shoulder Impingement Syndrome
- Mechanics: Client's GH and elbow joints are passively flexed to 90 degrees; the therapist then passively medially rotates the arm at the GH joint (approximating greater tubercle with acromion process)
- Positive: Pain at the GH joint
- Note: Tissues impinged may be the supraspinatus distal tendon, subacromial bursa, long head of biceps brachii, coracohumeral ligament.

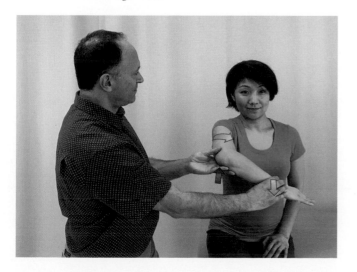

Subacromial Bursitis Abduction ROM Test

- Objective: Shoulder Impingement Syndrome/Subacromial Bursitis (Impingement)
- Mechanics: Client actively abducts the arm at the GH joint starting at anatomic position and ending above 135 degrees; having the arm in medial rotation during the abduction arc of motion increases the sensitivity of this test
- Positive: Pain during abduction which subsides above approximately 135 degrees
- Note: At approximately 135 degrees of abduction, the subacromial bursa slips deep to the acromion and is no longer impinged/compressed between head of humerus and acromion.

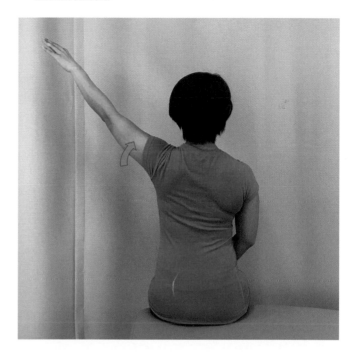

3

3

Speed's Test

- Objective: Biceps Brachii Pathology (Tendinitis/ Tenosynovitis/Tear)
- Mechanics: Client is in a position of 90 degrees of GH joint flexion, full elbow joint extension, and full forearm supination; therapist then adds downward resistance as the client attempts to hold this position
- Positive: Pain in biceps brachii
- Note: Some GH abduction (pictured) in addition to flexion will increase the stress to the biceps brachii long head.
- Note: Alternate mechanics are to have the client create an eccentric contraction of the biceps brachii by therapist resisting the client's arm as it lowers.

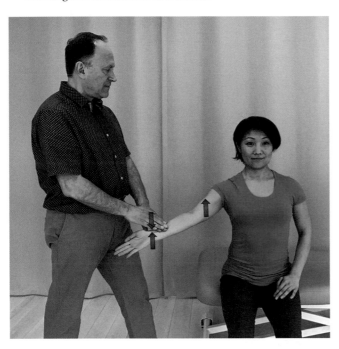

Cross Over Test

- Objective: Acromioclavicular (AC) Joint/Ligament Sprain and/or Coracoclavicular (CC) Ligament Sprain
- Mechanics: Passively bring the client's arm into full horizontal flexion/adduction (with the elbow joint flexed)
  - Positive: Pain at the AC joint/ligament and/or CC ligament
  - Note: Full horizontal flexion/adduction pushes the distal/lateral end of the clavicle against the acromion and places a tension stress on the AC and CC ligaments to prevent accessory (excessive) motion.

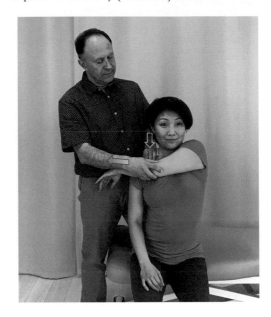

Elbow Joint

Radial Tunnel Syndrome / Posterior Interosseus Nerve (PIN) Syndrome Assessment

- Objective: Radial Tunnel Syndrome – PIN Syndrome (Compression) Assessment
- Mechanics: Version 1 (below): Palpation: Palpate the supinator, distal to lateral epicondyle

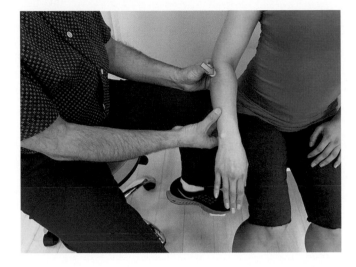

- Mechanics: Version 2 (below): MR to supinator contraction

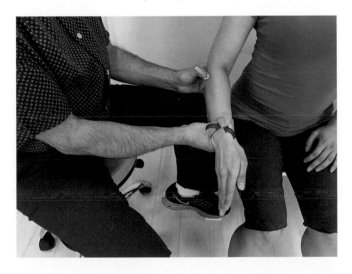

- Mechanics: Version 3 (below): Stretch the supinator by fully pronating the forearm.

- Positive (for all versions): Paresthesia near lateral epicondyle and/or distal into the anterolateral forearm
- Note: The PIN, a branch of the radial nerve (which is composed mostly of motor fibers but also contains some sensory fibers that may cause the paresthesia), runs between the two heads of the supinator muscle, and may be entrapped deep to a band of fibrous tissue called the *Arcade of Frohse* and/or compressed due to muscle hypertonicity/myofascial trigger points.
- Note: BPTT – Radial Nerve Test may also show positive for this condition.
- Note: Radial Tunnel Syndrome/PIN Syndrome must be differentially assessed from tennis elbow.

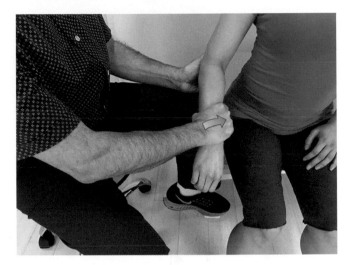

Wrist Joint/Hand

Phalen's Test

- Objective: Carpal Tunnel Syndrome
- Mechanics: Client approximates hands in full (90 degrees) of flexion for approximately 30+ seconds (compresses carpal tunnel contents)
- Positive: Referral into the median nerve distribution in the hand

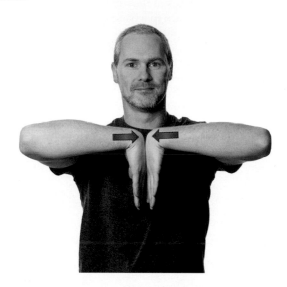

Prayer Test

- Objective: Carpal Tunnel Syndrome
- Mechanics: Client approximates hands in full (90 degrees) of extension for approximately 30+ seconds (compresses carpal tunnel contents)
- Positive: Referral into the median nerve distribution in the hand

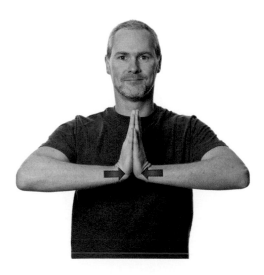

Tinel's Sign at the Wrist

- Objective: Carpal Tunnel Syndrome
- Mechanics: Therapist taps over the median nerve in the carpal tunnel
- Positive: Referral into the median nerve distribution in the hand

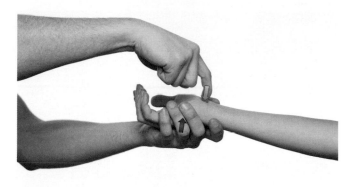

Tethered Median Nerve Stress Test

- Objective: Carpal Tunnel Syndrome
- Mechanics: The client's hand and index finger are passively brought into full extension and held for approximately 30+ seconds
- Positive: Referral into the median nerve distribution in the hand
- Note: For this test to be specific for median nerve compression in the carpal tunnel, the client's elbow joint should be flexed to relieve any tension in the median nerve proximal to the carpal tunnel.

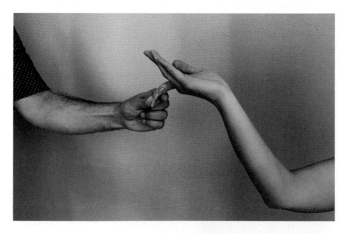

Finklestein's Test

- Objective: deQuervain's Syndrome
- Mechanics: Client flexes thumb under other fingers and then ulnar deviates the hand at the wrist joint
- Positive: Pain at or near the styloid process of the radius
- Note: This test stretches the abductor pollicis longus and extensor pollicis brevis.
- Note: deQuervain's syndrome is also known as deQuervain's stenosing tenosynovitis/deQuervain's disease.

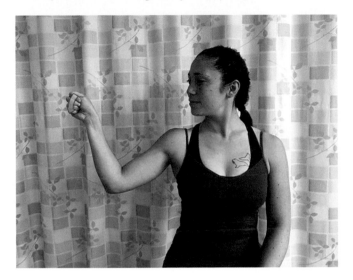

Froment's Sign

- Objective: Guyon's Canal Syndrome (Ulnar Nerve Compression)
- Mechanics: Therapist attempts to pull piece of paper held by client between thumb and base (proximal phalanx) of the index finger
- Positive: Client unable to hold onto piece of paper
- Note: This test challenges the adductor pollicis, which is innervated by the ulnar nerve.
- Note: Positive could be due to ulnar nerve compression other than in Guyon's Canal.

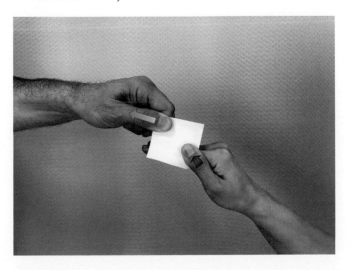

Pinch Grip Test

- Objective: Pronator Teres Syndrome/Anterior Interosseus Nerve (AIN) Syndrome
- Mechanics: Client pinches/grips the distal phalanges of the thumb and index finger against each other
- Positive: Inability to prevent the distal interphalangeal (DIP) joint of the index finger from hyperextending
- Note: The AIN, a branch of the median nerve (which branches off from the median nerve between the two heads of the pronator teres), innervates the flexor digitorum profundus, which flexes the DIP joint.
- Note: Positive could be due to median nerve compression other than at the pronator teres.

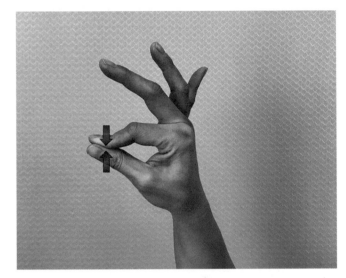

Review Questions

1. What are the three general orthopedic assessment tests?
2. What structures are assessed for with active range of motion testing?
3. What structures are assessed for with passive range of motion testing?
4. What structures are assessed for with manual resistance testing?
5. What is the objective of foraminal compression testing?
6. Describe the mechanics for performing cervical distraction testing.
7. What pulse is monitored during the assessment tests for thoracic outlet syndrome?
8. What orthopedic assessment tests can be used to assess carpal tunnel syndrome?
9. What are the three brachial plexus tension tests?
10. What joint do Nachlas and Yeoman's tests assess?
11. What are the client positions for the medley of SIJ assessment tests?
12. Describe the position for assessment of facet syndrome of the lumbar spine.
13. Thomas test assesses for tightness in what functional group of muscles?
14. What test assesses for tightness of hip abduction musculature?
15. Name two tests that assess for injury to cruciate ligaments of the knee.
16. What is the objective of Apley's compression test?
17. What test assesses for Morton's neuroma in the foot?
18. What orthopedic test assesses for frozen shoulder?
19. Empty can test assesses for the presence of what condition?
20. What orthopedic test assesses for deQuervain's syndrome?

Deeper Thoughts

If a client presents stating that they have pain in the "low back region" of the body, what is the order of components of the physical examination that you would employ? Further, how would you employ the three general orthopedic assessment tests to discern between muscular strain, ligamentous sprain, and muscle tightness? And what special orthopedic assessment tests might you employ to rule in and/or rule out myofascioskeletal conditions that might contribute to the client's pain pattern?

CHAPTER 4

Draping and Basic Massage Strokes

*Sandy Fritz, Susan Salvo
and Joseph E. Muscolino*

Overview

This chapter covers two topics: draping and massage strokes. The first half of the chapter begins by discussing principles of draping. A compendium of draping techniques is then given that describes and illustrates how to drape each of the major body parts. The second half of the chapter discusses massage strokes. The fundamental characteristics of touch that underlie all massage strokes are discussed first. The major massage strokes are then defined and described with illustrations.

Chapter Outline

Draping
Draping Methods
Compendium of Draping Techniques
Massage Strokes
Characteristics of Touch
Compendium of Massage Strokes

Chapter Objectives

After completing this chapter, the student/therapist should be able to perform the following:
1. Define the key terms of this chapter.
2. Explain the purposes and principles of draping.
3. Describe the two major draping methods.
4. Describe how to drape each major body part.
5. List and describe the seven characteristics of touch.
6. List and describe the six major types of massage strokes.

Key Terms

Compression	Effleurage	Percussion
Contoured draping	Flat draping	Petrissage
Depth of pressure	Frequency	Rhythm
Direction	Friction	Speed
Drag	Gliding	Tapotement
Draping	Kneading	Vibration
Duration	Oscillation	

DRAPING

Introduction to Draping

Draping is essentially covering the body with cloth, and it allows the client to be undressed while receiving massage. Draping serves two major purposes: (1) to maintain the client's privacy and sense of security, and (2) to provide warmth. The most frequently used draping materials are sheets and towels.

Principles of Draping

Many different draping methods exist; however, the following principles consistently apply:

- All reusable draping material must be freshly laundered for each client. Disposable linens must be fresh for each client and then disposed of properly.
- Only the area being massaged is undraped. In most circumstances, after moving the draping material to expose the area to be massaged, the draping material stays where it is placed.
- Always use a bottom drape (usually a sheet) under the client.
- Draping may be secured by tucking it underneath the client's body.
- If placing the drape in position feels invasive to the client, especially if tucking the drape under or around a body part, have the client assist in placement of the drape to preserve the client's modesty.
- Draping methods should keep the client covered in all positions, including the seated position.
- The genital area is never undraped.
- The breast area of women is not undraped during routine wellness massage. Specific breast massage under the supervision of a licensed physician may require special draping procedures.

DRAPING METHODS

The two basic types of draping are flat draping and contoured draping.

Flat Draping Methods

With flat draping, a top drape, usually a sheet, is placed over the client. The top drape, and sometimes the bottom drape, is moved in various ways to cover and uncover the area to be massaged.

Contoured Draping

Contoured draping can be done with two towels or with a sheet and a towel (a pillow case may substitute for a towel). These drapes are wrapped and shaped around the client. This type of draping is very effective for securely covering and shielding the genital region and buttocks. For women, a separate chest drape (usually a towel or pillowcase) can be used to drape the breast area when accessing the abdomen.

Alternative to Draping

As an alternative to draping, the client can wear a swimsuit or shorts and a loose shirt. A bottom drape (sheet) is placed over the table or mat. A top drape is available if the client becomes chilled during massage.

COMPENDIUM OF DRAPING TECHNIQUES

Table 4-1 demonstrates a compendium of draping techniques. A description and illustration of how to drape each major body part are given.

TABLE 4-1 Draping Techniques		
Position	**Description**	
Prone back	The client is in the prone position and the top sheet is folded over to expose the back (Figure 4-1).	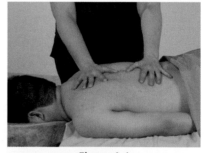 **Figure 4-1**
Prone buttock and lower extremity	The buttock and lower extremity in the prone position are undraped by folding the top sheet up and around to the inside of the lower extremity and secured under the lower extremity to be massaged. The flat sheet on the bottom can be folded up for additional coverage to maintain warmth (Figure 4-2).	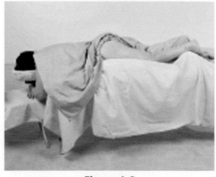 **Figure 4-2**

TABLE 4-1 Draping Techniques—cont'd

Position	Description	
Prone upper extremity	The top flat sheet is folded back on a diagonal to access the upper extremity in the prone position (Figure 4-3).
Figure 4-3
Supine lower extremity	In the supine position the lower extremity is undraped by folding the top sheet up and over and then wrapping it around the inside of the lower extremity (Figure 4-4, *A*). A variation to secure the groin area is to contour the top sheet through the thighs and up and under the buttocks (Figure 4-4, *B*).	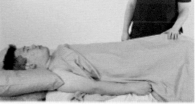
Figure 4-4
Supine upper extremity	The upper extremity in the supine position is exposed by lifting it up and out from under the top sheet and then placing on top of the sheet (Figure 4-5).	**Figure 4-5**
Supine abdomen	The abdominal area is exposed on the female client who is in the supine position. The therapist uses a towel or pillowcase (king size may be preferable) folded horizontally as a bikini top. The top drape over the lower body in this image stops at the anterior superior iliac spines (Figure 4-6).	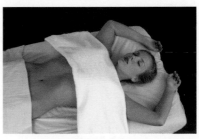
Figure 4-6

Continued

TABLE 4-1 Draping Techniques—cont'd

Position	Description
Supine neck and shoulder	The top sheet is folded down just below the clavicles to expose the inferior attachments of the sternocleidomastoid muscles and to keep the female breasts draped. Note: In this image, the therapist is taking advantage of this draping technique to address trigger points in these muscles while supporting the base of the skull with the opposite hand (Figure 4-7). 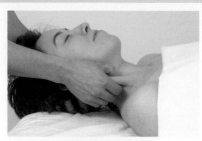 **Figure 4-7**
Side lying back	To expose the back of a side lying female client, the therapist uses contoured draping. To keep the sheet in place and cover the female breasts, the therapist incorporates a towel folded horizontally to anchor the top edge of the sheet. A cushion or rolled-up towel is placed under the head to maintain the spine in neutral alignment. The client may also be given a pillow to place in front of the trunk and "hug." This provides further security and privacy (Figure 4-8). 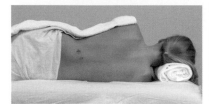 **Figure 4-8**
Side lying upper extremity	To access the upper extremity of a side lying female client, pull the upper extremity from under the sheet, and then arrange the sheet to cover the breasts. The exposed upper extremity can be placed on a draped cushion for client comfort. Note that the neck is placed on a cushion to maintain the spine in a neutral alignment (Figure 4-9). 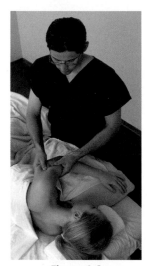 **Figure 4-9**
Side lying lower extremity (that is away from the table)	To access the lower extremity that is away from the table of a side lying client, undrape the area, gather the fabric, and then tuck the sheet around the upper part of the thigh. Be sure the knee joint is flexed approximately 90 degrees. The undraped lower extremity can be placed on a draped cushion for client comfort (Figure 4-10). 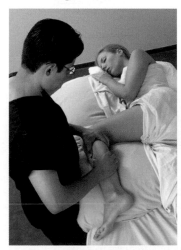 **Figure 4-10**

TABLE 4-1 Draping Techniques—cont'd	
Position	**Description**
Side lying lower extremity (that is closer to the table)	To access the lower extremity that is next to the table of a side lying client, undrape the area, gather the fabric, and then tuck the sheet around the upper part of the thigh. The knee joint is slightly flexed. A rolled-up towel can be placed under the ankle for client comfort. Note that the other lower extremity remains draped and supported by a draped cushion (Figure 4-11).

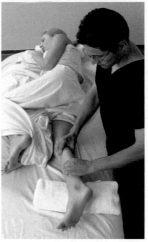

Figure 4-11

MASSAGE STROKES

Introduction to Massage Strokes

Massage application involves touching the body to manipulate soft tissues, influence body fluid movement, and stimulate neuroendocrine responses. During a massage session, many different strokes are often employed. However, more fundamental than the strokes themselves are the characteristics of the touch of the strokes. Following is the classification of massage by pioneer Gertrude Beard, as well as current trends in therapeutic massage.

The touch of a massage stroke can be characterized by the following seven characteristics: depth of pressure, drag, direction, speed, rhythm, frequency, and duration. Each of these seven characteristics is described. Following their description, a compendium of the major treatment strokes employed in massage therapy is presented with a brief description and illustration of each stroke.

CHARACTERISTICS OF TOUCH

Depth of Pressure

Depth of pressure, or the compressive force of massage, can be light, moderate, or deep.

Most areas of the body consist of four major tissue layers. These layers are the skin, superficial fascia, layers of musculature, and various fascial sheaths. Soft tissue dysfunction can develop in any or all of these layers. When dysfunction is present more superficially, the depth of pressure necessary is usually light. When dysfunction is present in deeper layers, deeper pressure is usually necessary. Pressure should be delivered through each successive layer, reaching deeper layers without damage and discomfort to superficial tissues. As a rule, the deeper the pressure, the broader the base of contact required on the body's surface, and the more slowly the therapist should sink into the client's tissues. To treat any soft tissue dysfunction, such as a trigger point or spasm, the therapist applies the proper level of pressure to reach the location of the dysfunction. It should be noted that pressure, by virtue of compressing tissues, also alters the circulation of fluids within the body.

Drag

Drag describes the amount of pull (stretch) on the tissue. Drag is a component of connective tissue massage wherein one layer of tissue is dragged/pulled along an adjacent layer, helping to break up patterns of adhesions. Drag is also used during palpation assessment of various soft tissue dysfunctions to identify areas of ease and bind within the tissues. *Ease* occurs when tissue moves freely and easily; *bind* occurs when tissue feel stuck, leathery, or thick.

Direction

Direction can move out from the center of the body (centrifugal) or in from the extremities toward the center of the body (centripetal). Furthermore, direction can proceed longitudinally, along a muscle following the direction of its fibers; transversely, across the direction of the fibers; or circularly. Direction is a factor in broadening and lengthening tissues containing soft tissue dysfunctions or in the methods that influence blood and lymphatic fluid movement.

Speed

Speed is the rate that massage methods are applied. The speed of a stroke can be fast, slow, or variable, depending upon the demands of the tissues being addressed and the state of the client (faster and more energizing in situations where stimulation is called for, slower and more rhythmic where calming influences are needed).

Rhythm

Rhythm refers to the regularity of technique application. If the method is applied at regular intervals, it is considered even, or rhythmic. If the method is disjointed or irregular, it is considered uneven, or arrhythmic. Rhythmic stroking tends to be more calming, especially if applied slowly and with mild to moderate pressure. Arrhythmic strokes, especially arrhythmic jostling and shaking, tend to be more stimulating.

Frequency

Frequency is the number of times that a treatment method is repeated in a given time frame. This aspect relates to how many repetitions of a stroke, such as a compression or gliding stroke, are performed. In general, the massage practitioner repeats each stroke three to five times before moving or switching to a different one. Although every application of a stroke is therapeutic, the therapist should also be assessing the health of the client's tissues as they are treated with the strokes. If the final stroke indicates remaining dysfunction, then the frequency can be increased and more strokes performed on that tissue.

Duration

Duration has two aspects. It can mean the length of time the session lasts or the length of time that a particular stroke or other treatment application, such as a stretch, is used in the same location. Typically, duration of a specific stroke application is approximately 30 to 60 seconds. Certain treatment protocols may call for less or more time.

COMPENDIUM OF MASSAGE STROKES

Following is a description of the six major types of massage therapy strokes: gliding, kneading, friction, compression, percussion, and vibration.

Gliding

A gliding stroke (historically known as effleurage) is a long, broad stroke that is usually applied along the direction of the muscle fibers. It can also be applied across the muscle fibers; when this is done, it is often called *stroking*.

In this example of gliding (Figure 4-12), the therapist starts at the top of the client's back and applies pressure using the palms of her hands on both sides of the spinous processes until she arrives at the sacrum. The hands then separate and slide back toward the top of the back using just the weight of the hands. Contact with the client's skin is maintained when moving from pushing to pulling and between repetitions.

In Figure 4-13, the client is supine with her head and neck rotated to one side. Pressure is applied with the fist from the occiput to the acromion process and then back to the occiput. While on the cervical vertebrae, the pressure is focused over the laminar groove. While on the top of the shoulder, the pressure is focused on the thickest portion of the upper trapezius.

Kneading

A kneading stroke (historically known as petrissage) lifts the tissue, and then the full hand is used to squeeze the tissue as it rolls out of the hand, while the other hand prepares to lift additional tissue and repeat the process. Skin rolling is a variation of a kneading stroke.

The therapist positions herself between the supine client's head and shoulder; this helps keep her wrist joint as straight as

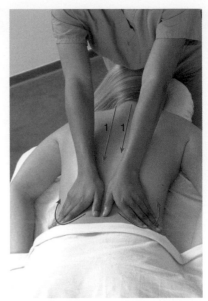

Figure 4-12 Gliding example #1: Long stroke gliding along the back.

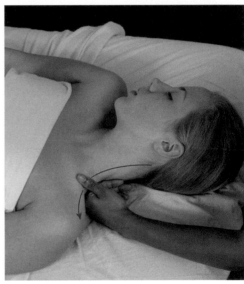

Figure 4-13 Gliding example #2: Gliding along the neck and shoulder.

possible. The upper trapezius is compressed, lifted, and then released (Figure 4-14).

In Figure 4-15, the client is lying supine while the therapist kneads the client's left thigh. The hands move in opposite directions; one hand applying a force forward while the other is pulling back. The tissue under the therapist's hands is compressed, twisted, and squeezed. The hands cross each other midstroke.

Compression

A compression stroke directs pressure downward into the tissues at a 90-degree angle to the contour of the surface of the body part being worked (Figure 4-16). A compression stroke spreads or displaces surface layers of tissues. It is often applied with a "pumping" action in which the pressure is gradually increased as the compression is applied.

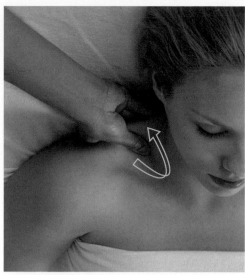

Figure 4-14 Kneading stroke example #1: One-handed kneading of the upper trapezius.

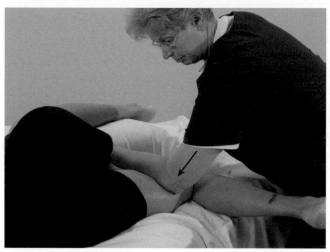

Figure 4-17 Compression stroke example #2: Forearm compression to the medial thigh.

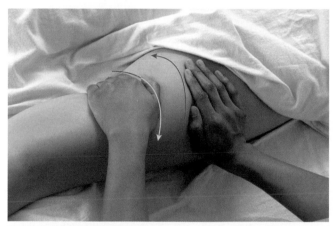

Figure 4-15 Kneading stroke example #2: Two-handed kneading of the anterior thigh.

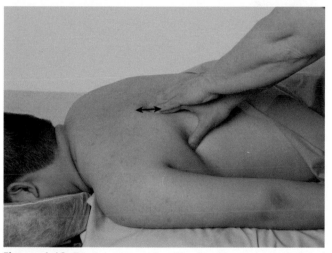

Figure 4-18 Friction example #1: Double-supported hand contact, friction to the back.

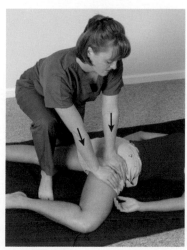

Figure 4-16 Compression stroke example #1: Two-handed compression of the gluteal region.

Compression can be applied with two hands moving simultaneously. In this example, the clothed client lies prone on a draped floor mat; her right hip joint is laterally rotated to shorten the targeted muscles. The therapist positions herself above the client so that she can use her body weight. She places her hands onto the gluteal musculature and leans in, applying rhythmic compression strokes to broaden the muscles.

In Figure 4-17, compression is applied down into the musculature of the medial thigh at a 90-degree angle. The therapist leans forward and uses forearm compression into the musculature.

Friction

A **friction** stroke moves tissue under the skin. The movement is produced by beginning with a specific and moderate-to-deep compression. The surface tissues are moved back and forth across the fibers of deeper tissues for transverse or cross-fiber friction; or the tissues are moved in a circle to produce circular friction.

In Figure 4-18, the therapist braces (double supports) her finger pads and applies friction to the tissues near the medial border of the scapula.

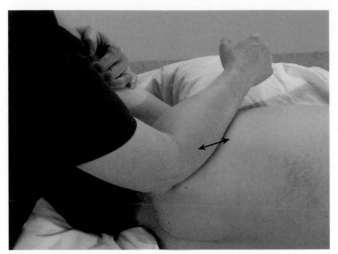

Figure 4-19 Friction example #2: Forearm contact, friction to the back.

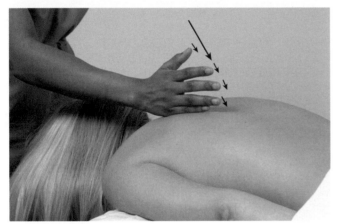

Figure 4-20 Percussion stroke example #1: Hacking the upper back.

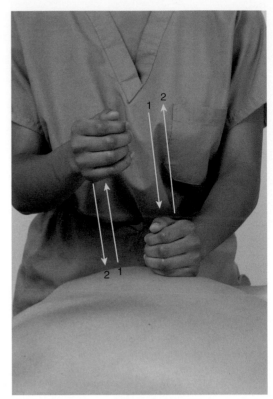

Figure 4-21 Percussion stroke example #2: Loose-fist percussion of the upper back.

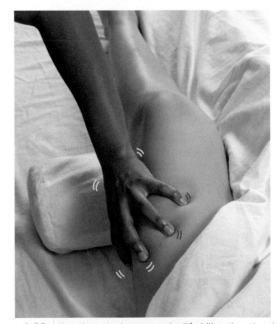

Figure 4-22 Vibration stroke example #1: Vibrating the thigh.

In Figure 4-19, friction is being applied with a broader but still focused contact; the therapist is using the ulnar side of her forearm. The client is in a side-lying position and friction is being applied to the latissimus dorsi muscle.

Percussion

A **percussion** stroke (historically called **tapotement**) is a controlled flailing of the arms or forearms as the wrists snap back and forth and the hands strike the client's tissues. Various methods include slapping, tapping, hacking, pounding, and beating. Percussion can also be classified as **oscillation** movements.

In Figure 4-20, the ulnar surface of one hand is seen striking the client's upper back. The fingers are slightly spread while lifted. On contact, the momentum of the stroke causes each finger to contact the one above it, creating a slight vibratory effect. Two hands can be used instead of one.

In Figure 4-21, the therapist is standing to the side of a prone client and using the ulnar sides of both loosely closed fists to pound the client's upper back. The knuckles of a loosely closed fist can also be used to percuss the back.

Vibration

A **vibration** stroke begins with compression. After the depth of pressure has been achieved, the hand trembles/vibrates and

transmits the action to the surrounding tissues. Shaking is a larger, more abrupt movement and is usually applied to the limbs of the client. Vibration can also be classified as oscillation movements.

In Figure 4-22, the client is lying supine and a draped bolster is placed under the knee joint. Repetitive vibratory shaking movements are used to relax the thigh muscles. The therapist uses the entire palmar surface of her hand to slightly compress

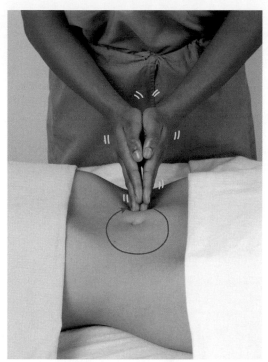

Figure 4-23 Vibration stroke example #2: Abdominal vibration.

Photos in this chapter are from Salvo S: Massage therapy: principles and practice, ed 3, St Louis, 2008, Saunders, and Fritz S: Mosby fundamentals of therapeutic massage, ed 4, St Louis, 2009, Mosby.

Review Questions

1. What are the major purposes of draping?
2. Briefly describe the two basic types of draping.
3. Adjusting the depth of pressure during a session is used to address what four major tissue layers?
4. *Ease* and *bind* are terms used when describing what massage stroke characteristic? What do these terms mean in that context?
5. In what five directions may a stroke be performed?
6. How can the speed of massage strokes affect the client?
7. What is the term for the number of times that a treatment method is repeated in a given time frame?
8. List and describe the two aspects of duration.
9. List the six major types of massage strokes.
10. Describe a kneading stroke.
11. Describe a compression stroke.

and lift the client's tissue before beginning the vibratory shaking motions.

In Figure 4-23, the client is lying supine and the therapist is standing to her side. To access the abdomen, a sheet drapes her lower body and a pillowcase folded horizontally drapes the breast region. Vibratory movements are begun in the therapist's arms and are transmitted to the client's tissues via the tips of the last three fingers. Vibration to the abdomen may help stimulate intestinal peristalsis.

 Deeper Thoughts

While performing a massage, what aspects of the interplay between draping and stroke choice are most challenging? What ways can you think of to overcome these issues?

CHAPTER 5

Anatomy, Physiology, and Treatment of Trigger Points

Overview

This chapter defines a trigger point (TrP) and then covers the foundational anatomy, physiology, and pathology of myofascial TrPs. To understand the mechanism of how TrPs develop, sarcomere structure and the sliding filament mechanism are reviewed. Then the two major hypotheses, the *energy crisis hypothesis* and *dysfunctional endplate hypothesis*, for TrP genesis are discussed, including their fusion into what is called the *integrated trigger point hypothesis*. The relationship of the *pain–spasm–pain cycle* and the *contraction–ischemia cycle* are also related to the genesis of a TrP. Then the relationships between central and attachment TrPs, and key TrPs and satellite TrPs are examined, as well as the general factors that create TrPs. The effects of TrPs are discussed, including the concept and proposed mechanisms for how a TrP refers pain. The chapter concludes with an exploration of how TrPs can be located in clinical practice and a discussion of the major methods used by manual and movement therapists to treat TrPs, including the relative efficacy of the methods of sustained compression compared with deep-stroking massage. Note: Common patterns of TrPs in individual muscles with the typical corresponding referral zone(s) are given in Part IV of this book.

Chapter Outline

What Is a Trigger Point?
Sarcomere Structure
Sliding Filament Mechanism
Genesis of Trigger Point: Energy Crisis Hypothesis
Central Trigger Points: Linking the Energy Crisis and Dysfunctional Endplate Hypotheses to Form the
    Integrated Trigger Point Hypothesis
Central Trigger Points, Taut Bands, and Attachment Trigger Points
General Factors That Create Trigger Points
Effects of a Trigger Point
Key Trigger Points Creating Satellite Trigger Points
Trigger Point Referral Patterns
Locating and Treating Trigger Points

Chapter Objectives

After completing this chapter, the student/therapist should be able to perform the following:

1. Define the key terms of this chapter.
2. List the different types of TrPs.
3. Discuss the similarities and differences between active and latent TrPs.
4. Describe the structure of a sarcomere, and explain how the sliding filament mechanism works.
5. Discuss the relationship between the sliding filament mechanism, the energy crisis hypothesis, and the genesis of a TrP.
6. Describe how the pain–spasm–pain, contraction–ischemia, and pain–spasm–ischemia cycles relate to the genesis of a TrP.
7. Describe the dysfunctional endplate hypothesis.
8. Describe the relationship among the energy crisis, the dysfunctional endplate, and the integrated TrP hypotheses.
9. Discuss the relationship between central and attachment TrPs, including the role of enthesopathy.
10. List and discuss the general factors that tend to create TrPs.
11. Describe the effects of a TrP.
12. Discuss the relationship between a key TrP and a satellite TrP.
13. Discuss the two types of TrP referral patterns and the proposed mechanisms for how TrPs refer pain.

14. Discuss the methods and principles involved in locating a client's TrPs.
15. Discuss the various methods of TrP treatment, including the proposed mechanism for their validity and the possible benefit of one method versus the other.

Key Terms

Active TrP
Adaptively shorten
Attachment TrP
Central TrP
Contraction–ischemia cycle
Contracture
Convergence–projection theory
Cord spillover theory
Deep-stroking massage
Dysfunctional endplate hypothesis
Energy crisis hypothesis
Enthesopathy

Essential referral zone
Integrated TrP hypothesis
Ischemia
Ischemic compression
Key TrP
Latent TrP
Motor point
Myofascial TrP
Pain–spasm–ischemia cycle
Pain–spasm–pain cycle
Pincer grip
Primary referral zone
Sarcomere

Satellite TrP
Sclerotogenous referred pain
Secondary referral zone
Shortened active insufficiency
Sliding filament mechanism
Spillover referral zone
Stripping massage
Sustained compression
Taut band
Trigger point (TrP)
TrP pressure release
Twitch response
Visceral referred pain

WHAT IS A TRIGGER POINT?

A trigger point (TrP) is a focal area of hyperirritability that is locally sensitive to pressure and can refer symptoms (usually pain) to other areas of the body. TrPs are reported to exist in most every soft tissue of the body, including muscle, muscular fascia, periosteum, ligament, and skin. The term myofascial TrP is used to describe TrPs that exist within skeletal muscle tissue or skeletal muscular fascia (usually the tendon or aponeurosis of a muscle). This text will restrict its discussion to myofascial TrPs, which are the most common type of TrPs found in the body.

BOX 5-1

For simplicity of verbiage, unless the context is made otherwise clear, the term *TrP* will be used throughout this text to refer to a myofascial TrP.

Put simply, a skeletal muscle TrP is what the lay public refers to as a tight and painful muscle knot. More specifically, a skeletal muscle tissue TrP is a hyperirritable focal area of muscle hypertonicity (tightness) located within a taut band of skeletal muscle tissue. Furthermore, as with all TrPs, it is locally sensitive to palpatory pressure and can potentially refer pain or other symptoms to distant areas of the body.

All TrPs can be divided into two classifications, active TrPs and latent TrPs. Although the definitions are not fully consistent, it is generally agreed that latent TrPs do not cause local or referred pain unless they are first compressed, whereas active TrPs may produce local or referred pain even when they are not compressed. A latent TrP is essentially at a less severe stage than is an active TrP; if left untreated, a latent TrP often develops into an active TrP.

Furthermore, myofascial TrPs are often divided into central TrPs and attachment TrPs. As their names imply, central TrPs are located in the center of a muscle (or more accurately, in the center of muscle fibers), and attachment TrPs are located at the attachment sites of a muscle.

BOX 5-2

If every muscle fiber of a muscle begins at one attachment of the muscle and ends at the other attachment of the muscle, then the center of a muscle would be the center of all its fibers. However, not all muscles have their fibers architecturally designed this way. For example, pennate muscles by definition do not have their fibers run from attachment to attachment. Furthermore, even fusiform muscles do not always have all their fibers run the entire length of a muscle. For this reason, the center of a muscle is not always synonymous with the center of its fibers.

Effective clinical treatment of clients who present with myofascial pain syndromes requires an understanding of both why TrPs form in the first place and what the essential mechanism of a TrP is. This understanding is not possible unless sarcomere structure and the sliding filament mechanism of muscle contraction are first understood. For this reason, it is necessary to review these topics before continuing on with a discussion of TrPs.

SARCOMERE STRUCTURE

A muscle is an organ that is made up of thousands of muscle fibers. Each muscle fiber is made up of thousands of myofibrils that run the length of the muscle fiber, and each myofibril is composed of thousands of sarcomeres laid end-to-end (as well as side-to-side).

A sarcomere is bordered at each end by a Z-line. Within a sarcomere, there are two types of filaments, actin and myosin. The thin actin filaments are located on both sides of the sarcomere and are attached to the two Z-lines; the thick myosin filament is located at the center of the sarcomere. Furthermore, the myosin filament has projections called *heads* that can reach out and attach themselves to the actin filaments (Figure 5-1). Also important to note is that the sarcoplasmic reticulum of a muscle fiber has stored calcium ions within it.

BOX 5-3

The term *muscle fiber* is synonymous with the term *muscle cell.*

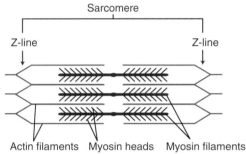

Figure 5-1 A sarcomere is bounded on both sides by Z-lines. The thin actin filaments attach to the Z-lines. The thick myosin filament is located in the center and contains projections called *heads*. (From Muscolino JE: Kinesiology: the skeletal system and muscle function, enhanced edition, St Louis, 2007, Mosby.)

When a muscle contracts, it does so because it has been ordered to contract by the nervous system. Given that a sarcomere is the basic structural unit and the basic functional unit of a muscle, to understand muscle contraction, it is necessary to first understand sarcomere function and its initiation by the nervous system. The process that describes sarcomere function is called the *sliding filament mechanism.*

SLIDING FILAMENT MECHANISM

Following are the steps of the sliding filament mechanism:
1. When we will a contraction of a muscle, a message commanding this to occur originates in our brain. This message travels as an electrical impulse within our central nervous system.
2. This electrical impulse then travels out to the periphery in a motor neuron (nerve cell) of a peripheral nerve to go to the skeletal muscle. Where the motor neuron meets each individual muscle fiber is called the motor point and is usually located at approximately the midpoint (i.e., center) of the muscle fiber.
3. When the impulse gets to the end of the motor neuron, the motor neuron secretes its neurotransmitter (acetylcholine) into the synaptic cleft at the neuromuscular junction (Figure 5-2).
4. These neurotransmitters float across the synaptic cleft and bind to the motor endplate of the muscle fiber.
5. The binding of these neurotransmitters onto the motor endplate causes an electrical impulse on the muscle fiber that travels along the muscle fiber's outer cell membrane. This electrical impulse is transmitted into the interior of the muscle fiber by the transverse tubules (T tubules) (Figure 5-3).

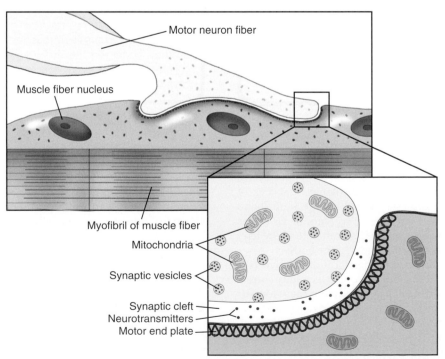

Figure 5-2 Neuromuscular junction. (Note: The *inset box* provides an enlargement.) (From Muscolino JE: Kinesiology: the skeletal system and muscle function, enhanced edition, St Louis, 2007, Mosby.)

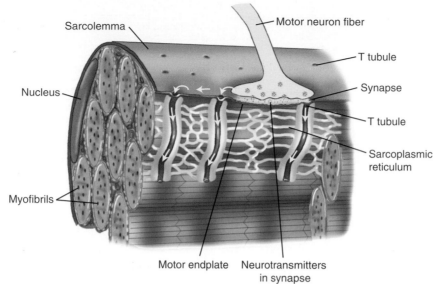

Figure 5-3 Binding of the neurotransmitters onto the motor endplate of the muscle fiber's membrane initiates an electrical impulse that travels along the outer membrane (sarcolemma) of the entire muscle fiber. This electrical impulse is then transmitted into the interior of the muscle fiber by the transverse tubules (T tubules) of the muscle fiber. (From Muscolino JE: Kinesiology: the skeletal system and muscle function, enhanced edition, St Louis, 2007, Mosby.)

6. When this electrical impulse reaches the interior, it causes the sarcoplasmic reticulum of the muscle fiber to release stored calcium ions into the sarcoplasm (the cytoplasm of the muscle fiber).
7. These calcium ions then bind onto the actin filaments, causing a structural change that exposes the binding sites of actin filaments to the myosin heads.
8. Heads of the myosin filaments attach onto the binding sites of the actin filaments, creating myosin-actin cross-bridges.
9. These cross-bridges then bend, pulling the actin filaments in toward the center of the sarcomere (Figure 5-4).

BOX 5-4

The steps listed here illustrate the sliding filament mechanism when the sarcomere (i.e., the entire muscle) is able to contract and shorten (concentrically contract). This only occurs if the force of the muscle's contraction is great enough to overcome whatever resistance force there is to shortening. Alternately, a muscle can contract and stay the same length (isometrically contract) or can contract and lengthen (eccentrically contract). Regardless of the type of contraction, the defining characteristic of a muscle contraction is the presence of the myosin-actin cross-bridges and the pulling force that they create.

10. If no adenosine triphosphate (ATP) molecules are present, these cross-bridges will stay in place (hence the contraction is maintained) and no further sliding of the filaments will occur.
11. When ATP is present, the following sequence occurs: the cross-bridges between the myosin and actin filaments break

because of the expenditure of energy by ATP molecules, and the myosin heads attach to the next binding sites on the actin filaments, forming new cross-bridges. These new cross-bridges bend and pull the actin filaments further in toward the center of the sarcomere.
12. This process in Step 11 will repeat as long as ATP molecules are present to initiate the breakage, and calcium ions are present to keep the binding sites on the actin filaments exposed so that the next cross-bridges can be formed, which then pull the actin filaments further in toward the center of the sarcomere.
13. In this manner, sarcomeres of the innervated muscle fibers will contract to 100% of their ability.
14. When the nervous system message for contraction is no longer sent, neurotransmitters are no longer released into the synapse. The neurotransmitters that were present are either broken down or reabsorbed by the motor neuron.

BOX 5-5

An adenosine triphosphate (ATP) molecule can be likened to a battery because it stores energy in its bonds. Within a muscle fiber, its energy is used to provide the energy that is needed to both break myosin-actin cross-bridges and also reabsorb calcium ions back into the sarcoplasmic reticulum.

15. Without the presence of neurotransmitters in the synapse, no impulse is sent into the interior of the muscle fiber, and calcium ions are no longer released from the sarcoplasmic reticulum.

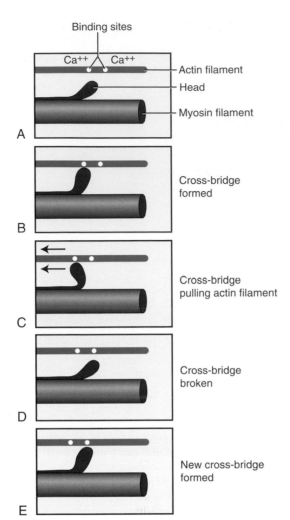

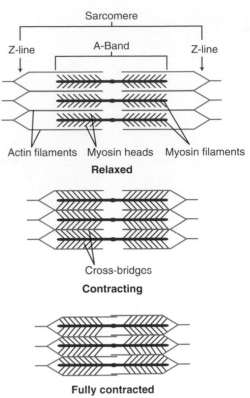

Figure 5-5 Illustration of how the sliding filament mechanism results in a change in length of a sarcomere. (From Muscolino JE: Kinesiology: the skeletal system and muscle function, enhanced edition, St Louis, 2007, Mosby.)

Figure 5-4 Steps of the sliding filament mechanism. **A,** Binding sites are exposed because of the presence of calcium ions (Ca++) that have been released by the sarcoplasmic reticulum. **B,** The myosin head forms a cross-bridge by attaching to one of the actin's binding sites. **C,** The myosin head bends, pulling the actin filament toward the center of the sarcomere. **D,** The myosin cross-bridge breaks. **E,** The process begins again when the myosin head attaches to another actin binding site. (From Muscolino JE: Kinesiology: the skeletal system and muscle function, enhanced edition, St Louis, 2007, Mosby.)

16. Calcium ions that were present in the sarcoplasm are reabsorbed by the sarcoplasmic reticulum by the expenditure of energy by ATP molecules.
17. Without the presence of calcium ions in the sarcoplasm, binding sites on actin filaments are no longer exposed, so it is no longer possible for new myosin-actin cross-bridges to form. Assuming that the old cross-bridges are released (because of the presence of ATP; see Step 11), the muscle contraction ceases.
18. The entire point of this process is that if actin filaments slide along the myosin filament toward the center of the sarcomere, then the Z-lines to which the actin filaments are attached are pulled in toward the center of the sarcomere, and the sarcomere shortens (Figure 5-5).

19. When the sarcomeres of a myofibril shorten, the myofibril shortens, pulling at its attachment ends.
20. When the myofibrils of a muscle fiber shorten, the muscle fiber shortens.
21. When enough muscle fibers shorten, the muscle shortens, moving its two attachments closer to each other.

GENESIS OF TRIGGER POINT: ENERGY CRISIS HYPOTHESIS

Once normal muscle contraction is understood, it is not difficult to understand how a TrP can form. The most prominent theory for TrP genesis is called the energy crisis hypothesis. To understand the energy crisis hypothesis, it is necessary to understand the role that ATP molecules have within the sliding filament mechanism. ATP molecules provide the energy necessary to run the functions of a cell, including the sliding filament mechanism. Specifically, there are two steps within the sliding filament mechanism that require the input of energy from ATP molecules: ATP molecules are necessary to break the myosin-actin cross-bridges (see Step 11 earlier), and they are necessary for reabsorption of calcium ions by the sarcoplasmic reticulum when the sarcomere contraction is complete (see Step 16 earlier). If for any reason ATP molecules are not present during Step 11, the myosin-actin cross-bridges will not break and the affected sarcomeres will not be able to relax, thus forming a TrP. Furthermore, if ATP molecules are not present during Step 16, the calcium ions cannot be reabsorbed into the sarcoplasmic reticulum. As long as calcium ions are present, active sites on actin molecules remain exposed and myosin-actin cross-bridges remain, continuing the contraction, thus forming a TrP.

Essentially, the energy crisis hypothesis is so named because if the sliding filament mechanism is deprived of ATP molecules, there is a crisis due to insufficient energy, and the sarcomere contraction continues, resulting in the formation of a TrP. The underlying cause of the lack of ATP molecules is ischemia (loss of arterial blood flow) to the region of sarcomeres affected due to the tightness of the muscle itself. When a muscle contracts, it becomes palpably harder and has the ability to constrict the blood vessels within it, restricting blood flow. A muscle contraction that is approximately 30% to 50% of its maximum is sufficient to close off arterial vessels located within it. When arterial blood vessels are closed off in this manner, the local muscle tissue loses its blood supply, resulting in a loss of nutrients, including those needed to generate ATP molecules. Furthermore, this loss of ATP molecules occurs during a time of increased metabolic demand by the muscle, because its contraction requires ATP each time a cross-bridge breaks to then reform on a different active site of the actin filament. This initiates a vicious cycle called the contraction–ischemia cycle: muscle contraction causes ischemia, thereby creating a deficiency of ATP; without ATP, the muscle tissue cannot relax and therefore stays contracted; its contraction then continues to cut off the arterial blood supply furthering the ischemia, and so on (Figure 5-6, A). It is for this reason that once TrPs form, they tend to persist unless therapeutic intervention occurs.

Another exacerbating factor is that the venous vessels are also closed off due to the muscle contraction (spasm). Because it is the job of the venous vessels to remove waste products of metabolism, when veins are closed off, the waste products of metabolism remain in the tissues. Unfortunately these metabolic waste products are acidic and irritate the local muscle tissue, resulting in pain in the region, hence the tenderness that TrPs display. Ironically, the pain produced by these waste products tends to cause more spasming due to the pain–spasm–pain cycle (see Figure 5-6, B), which only increases the ischemia. Hence, we have a pain–spasm–ischemia cycle, with TrPs that become entrenched in the muscle tissue.

With an understanding of the energy crisis hypothesis, we see that all that it takes to begin the process of TrP formation is for a part of a muscle to forcefully contract long enough to cause an *energy crisis* in the local muscle tissue. Given this, it is easy to see why TrPs are so prevalent in the body. In fact, it might be asked why TrPs do not form even more often than they do. The answer seems to be that the local muscle contraction must persist long enough to cause sufficient ischemia to create the energy crisis. Most of the time, we contract our muscles intermittently with periods of rest in between; these periods of rest allow a new flow of nutrients that can then be used for the production of ATP molecules in the muscle tissue. However, postural muscles very often contract isometrically for long periods of time without rest, such that ischemia and the resultant depletion of ATP is sufficient to create a TrP. This is one reason that TrPs are so often found in postural muscles; prominent examples include the trapezius and sternocleidomastoid.

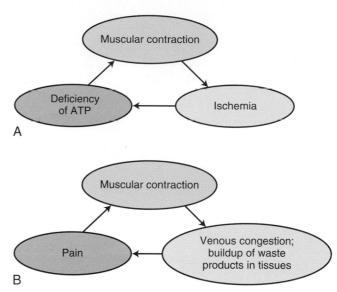

Figure 5-6 The contraction–ischemia and pain–spasm–pain cycles are illustrated. **A** shows the contraction–ischemia cycle. **B** shows the pain–spasm–pain cycle.

Furthermore, irritation or injury to a region of a muscle is another factor often implicated in the formation of a TrP. When a region of a muscle is injured, highly irritating chemicals are released, which directly increases the sensitivity and tenderness of the area and also cause local swelling. This local swelling can press on nerves, causing more pain. It can also compress arterial blood vessels, causing ischemia. Furthermore, the pain caused by the irritating chemicals and the pressure from the swelling can initiate the pain–spasm–pain cycle.

Hence, TrPs tend to form within regions of a muscle that have contracted for long periods without rest, or within regions that have been irritated or injured. It is important to realize that once formed, a TrP is a local phenomenon. It does not continue because a person is directing the TrP to contract from the central nervous system; it is perpetuated because of the local factors in the muscle tissue at the TrP itself.

BOX 5-6

The fact that a TrP is a local phenomenon is an important distinction, because when an entire muscle or a globally large portion of a muscle is tight, it is due to the pattern for tightness that is being directed from the gamma motor system of the central nervous system via muscle spindle reflex mediation. Therefore a globally tight muscle is tight because of central nervous system activity, whereas a TrP is a local phenomenon of muscle tightness. Some sources like to make this distinction by stating that a globally tight muscle occurs because of an excess of contraction, whereas a TrP occurs because of contracture. In this sense, the term *contracture* is used to emphasize that the mechanism of a TrP is not mediated and controlled by the central nervous system, whereas *contraction* denotes that the control is by the central nervous system.

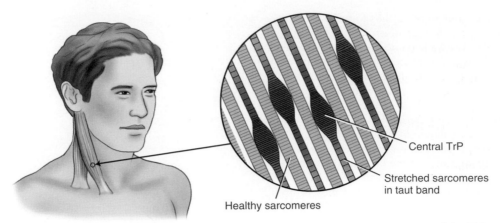

Figure 5-7 A central trigger point (TrP) located within a taut band. The sarcomeres of the TrPs can be seen to be shortened. This results in a pulling along the myofibrils in which the TrPs are located, causing a stretching of the remaining sarcomeres of the myofibrils. (Reprinted with permission by New Harbinger Publications, Inc. Modified from Davies C: The trigger point therapy workbook: your self-treatment guide for pain relief, ed 2, Oakland, CA, 2004, New Harbinger. www.newharbinger.com)

CENTRAL TRIGGER POINTS: LINKING THE ENERGY CRISIS AND DYSFUNCTIONAL ENDPLATE HYPOTHESES TO FORM THE INTEGRATED TRIGGER POINT HYPOTHESIS

Interestingly, even though TrPs can form anywhere within a muscle, they most often form at the motor point of the muscle, usually located at the center of the muscle, where the motor neurons synapse with the muscle fibers. The proposed theory to explain why TrPs so often form at motor points is called the dysfunctional endplate hypothesis. This hypothesis posits that when a motor neuron continually carries the message for contraction to a muscle fiber, it becomes dysfunctional and secretes excessive amounts of acetylcholine into the synapse, causing the muscle fiber's motor endplate to produce excessive numbers of action potentials. This results in a sustained partial depolarization of the motor endplate, which then increases the local metabolic demand for ATP by the muscle fiber. This increased ATP usage by the motor endplate of the muscle fiber membrane further depletes the ATP available in the region of the motor endplate, which increases the energy crisis for the sarcomeres located closest to the motor endplate. Therefore, the dysfunctional endplate hypothesis is, in effect, another mechanism that contributes to the *energy crisis* of TrP genesis. Therefore sarcomeres located most closely to the motor endplate tend to form TrPs more easily than sarcomeres located in other regions of the muscle. Linking the energy crisis hypothesis with the dysfunctional endplate hypothesis is called the integrated TrP hypothesis. Because motor points of a muscle are usually located at the center of muscle fibers, most TrPs formed are central TrPs.

CENTRAL TRIGGER POINTS, TAUT BANDS, AND ATTACHMENT TRIGGER POINTS

Once a central TrP has been created, its sarcomeres contract and shorten, pulling in toward their centers. This creates a constant pull upon the rest of the sarcomeres of the affected myofibril. This pull stretches these sarcomeres, creating a *taut band* of muscle tissue (Figure 5-7). For this reason, central TrPs are usually found within a taut band.

If the pulling force of the central TrP is sufficiently strong, the adjacent sarcomeres of the affected myofibril that lengthen will not be able to dissipate the entire pulling force of the central TrP, and its pull will be transferred to the ends of the myofibrils at their attachment into bone. Unfortunately, this pulling force irritates the ends of the myofibrils at or near the actual attachment into bone. The term enthesopathy is used to describe the condition that results from this constant irritation to the muscle's attachments and can either cause a TrP to form in the sarcomeres of the skeletal muscle tissue near the attachment or cause a TrP to form within the muscle's tendon or the bone's periosteum at the muscle's attachment site. Whether formed within the skeletal tissue or its related fascial tissue, this TrP created by the enthesopathy due to the pull of the central TrP is called an *attachment TrP*. Hence, once central TrPs have formed, they create a taut band that tends to create an enthesopathy, which in turn can create an attachment TrP.

GENERAL FACTORS THAT CREATE TRIGGER POINTS

As stated, via the energy crisis hypothesis, TrPs tend to develop when a muscle is contracted for an excessive length of time. There are a number of factors that tend to create this scenario. Following is a list of these common factors that can lead to the formation of TrPs:

1. Excessive muscle contraction: Certainly this is the prime factor for TrP genesis. A muscle that contracts for an extended period, especially a long-held isometric contraction, tends to close off the blood supply to the muscle tissue, resulting in ischemia and the formation of TrPs via the energy crisis hypothesis. Further, the pulling force of a muscle contraction causes tension within the muscle tissue. If the contraction is excessive (too forceful

or held for too long), it can cause injury to the muscle tissue, which can be a further factor in TrP genesis (see Factor #2).

2. Irritation/injury/trauma: Whenever a muscle is physically irritated or injured, irritating chemicals are released into the local muscle tissue. These chemicals can create swelling in the muscle tissue, which compresses blood vessels, resulting in ischemia, thereby initiating TrP formation. These chemicals can also cause local pain and tenderness that can initiate the pain–spasm–pain and contraction–ischemia cycles, which can further lead to TrP formation.

3. Perceived pain: Any pain perceived to be in a muscle, even if the pain is referred from elsewhere in the body, can result in the tightening of that muscle via the pain–spasm–pain cycle. This tightening predisposes the muscle to TrP formation.

4. Muscle splinting: If there is any pain or damage to an adjacent tissue, especially a nearby joint, muscles in that region of the body tend to tighten up as a protective mechanism to splint the region. Splinting the region decreases motion; therefore the likelihood of further injury is lessened. However, this splinting contraction of the muscle favors the formation of TrPs.

5. Prolonged shortening: Whenever a muscle remains in a shortened state for a prolonged period, it will tend to adaptively shorten. An adaptively shortened muscle tends to tighten (i.e., increased contraction), and this increased tension favors the development of TrPs.

6. Prolonged stretching: Even though stretching any soft tissue, including muscle, is theoretically good, if a muscle is excessively stretched and or stretched too quickly, the muscle spindle reflex will be initiated, causing the muscle to tighten. This will then predispose the muscle to the development of TrPs. Further, as with excessive muscle contraction, stretching also places a tension force into the muscle tissue. If the stretching force is excessive, it can cause injury to the muscle tissue, which can be a further factor in TrP genesis (see Factor #2).

EFFECTS OF A TRIGGER POINT

The most obvious effect of having a TrP within a muscle is that the TrP is locally painful and may have a referral pattern of pain. Beyond that, TrPs tend to be located within taut bands that are also usually tender and painful upon palpation.

However, when a muscle harbors a TrP, there are other consequences that might affect the entire muscle. Given that a TrP creates a taut band in which it is located, the taut band of muscle tissue resists stretching, and if stretching is attempted, pain likely results. For this reason, a muscle with a TrP located within it very often results in decreased range of motion of the joint(s) crossed by that muscle. Furthermore, if a muscle is not stretched and is allowed to stay in a shortened state, the muscle tends to adapt to that shortened state. This adaptation can be both functional and structural. Functionally, the muscle can adaptively shorten because the nervous system, fearing possible pain or muscle tearing, tends to avoid motions of the body that would stretch that muscle. Structurally, the muscle can adaptively shorten

because fibrous adhesions tend to accumulate within the muscle, further decreasing its ability to lengthen and stretch. In addition, because of a principle known as the *length tension relationship curve*, muscles that are excessively tight and shortened become weaker.

BOX 5-7

The phenomenon of a tight and shortened muscle becoming weaker is known as **shortened active insufficiency**. When a sarcomere shortens, its actin filaments overlap, covering up and making inaccessible some of the active binding sites needed for myosin-actin cross-bridges to form. If fewer cross-bridges form, the strength of the contraction will be diminished, resulting in a weaker muscle.

Hence, when a muscle contains one or more TrPs, besides local or referred pain, muscle-wide effects often occur. Muscles harboring TrPs tend to become tighter and weaker. Of course, when one muscle becomes functionally impaired, stresses occur within the body as other muscles try to compensate for this dysfunctional muscle. For this reason, it is often said that the presence of a first TrP, often called a **key TrP**, can cause the creation of other TrPs, called **satellite TrPs**.

BOX 5-8

Perhaps the easiest way to understand why adaptive shortening of a muscle occurs is to look at the example of hip joint flexor muscles. When we sit for prolonged periods of time, our hip flexors are shortened and slackened because sitting places our thigh into 90 degrees of flexion at the hip joint. The problem is that if in this position we want to further flex a thigh at the hip joint, the hip flexor muscles would not be immediately responsive to cause motion when they contract, because any contraction would have to first take out the slack that is present in the muscles. For this reason, the gamma motor system of the brain adaptively shortens these muscles by increasing their tension to match the shortened length that they are in when sitting. They are now no shorter than they were before, but the increased tension has removed the slack. If they are now ordered to contract, they are more responsive and are able to more quickly create further flexion of the thigh at the hip joint. For this reason, whenever we maintain postures for prolonged periods of time wherein a muscle or muscle group is shortened and slackened, the baseline resting tone of these muscles gradually adapts to adjust to that shortened state.

5

It is this increased tension in the adaptively shortened muscle that predisposes it to the formation of TrPs. A further factor is that if a muscle is always held in a shortened state and is never stretched out, fascial adhesions build up within and around the muscle. In time, these adhesions make it that much more difficult for the muscle to lengthen and stretch out.

KEY TRIGGER POINTS CREATING SATELLITE TRIGGER POINTS

Once a key TrP has formed, it is common for its presence to create satellite TrPs, either in the same muscle or within other muscles of the body.

1. Central and attachment TrPs: Key central TrPs often create satellite attachment TrPs within the same taut band of muscle tissue. As previously explained, the attachment TrP is caused by the enthesopathy (irritation) created by the pull of the central TrP's taut band.
2. Functional muscular mover group: Key TrPs within one muscle often create satellite TrPs in other muscles of the same functional group of movers. Given that a TrP often makes the muscle it is located in painful as well as tighter and weaker, the body tends to compensate by using other muscles that share the same joint action to engage and work instead. In time, these other muscles may be overworked and therefore become painful and contracted, and in turn develop satellite TrPs.
3. Antagonist muscles: Key TrPs within one muscle often create satellite TrPs in muscles of the antagonist group of muscles. Given that a muscle with TrPs tends to be tight, antagonist muscles often must increase their contraction to even the pull across their shared joint so that the tight muscle with TrPs does not asymmetrically pull upon the joint, creating an asymmetric posture of the bones (and therefore body parts) at that joint.
4. Referral zones of pain: Key TrPs often cause satellite TrPs to form within the musculature located within the referral pain zone. Even though pain within the referral zone of a key TrP is not indicative of trauma or damage to the tissue of the referral zone, the nervous system interprets this pain as if the referral zone is experiencing trauma or damage. As a result, the pain–spasm–pain cycle may kick in, creating tightness of the musculature of the referral zone, which predisposes TrP formation in this area.

TRIGGER POINT REFERRAL PATTERNS

Perhaps the most enigmatic aspect of a TrP is its referral pattern. Each muscular TrP, when tight enough or sufficiently compressed, tends to have a characteristic pattern of pain referral that may be felt locally or distant from the TrP itself. Usually the pain refers to what is known as the primary referral zone (also known as the essential referral zone). However, when more severe, a TrP may refer pain into what is called the secondary referral zone (also known as the spillover referral zone) in addition to the primary referral zone. In this textbook,

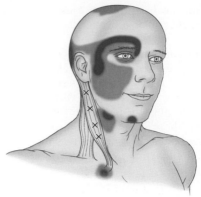

Figure 5-8 Four TrPs, indicated by the Xs, are illustrated within the sternal head of the sternocleidomastoid (SCM) muscle. The primary (essential) referral zones of pain are indicated by the *areas of dark red*. When more severe, SCM sternal head TrPs may also refer pain into secondary (spillover) referral zones, indicated by the *areas of light red*.

the primary zone is indicated by a *dark red color* and the secondary zone is indicated by a *lighter red color* (Figure 5-8). It should be emphasized that even though typical TrP locations and referral patterns are mapped out for most muscles of the body, this does not mean that TrPs can only occur where shown in the illustrations in this book, or that the referral zones must always follow the patterns shown here. Although usual TrP locations and referral patterns are known, TrPs can occur anywhere within a muscle, and their referral patterns are not necessarily restricted to the patterns shown here.

TrP referral patterns of pain do not simply follow the course of a peripheral nerve as if the TrP entrapped a nerve and caused projection of pain along its course (similar to how a lumbar disc herniation can compress the sciatic nerve and cause pain along the course of the sciatic nerve). Rather, TrP referral is more similar to the type of referred pain that a heart attack is well known to cause. Only in the case of a TrP, instead of an internal visceral organ referring pain to the skin of the body (to the shoulder and chest region in the case of a heart attack), a TrP in a muscle usually refers pain to another region of the muscle, or just as commonly, to an entirely different muscle of the body.

BOX 5-9

TrPs most often refer pain; however, they sometimes refer other symptoms, such as numbness or tingling.

The prevailing theory for how myofascial TrPs refer pain is called the convergence–projection theory. According to this theory, the sensory neurons that detect sensation and pain in one muscle converge with the sensory neurons that come from another muscle of the body (Figure 5-9). For example, if the sensory neurons from muscles A and B converge in the spinal cord, then when pain occurs due to a TrP in muscle A, these signals travel within sensory neurons that enter the spinal cord and converge with the sensory neurons that come from muscle B. When these signals of pain reach the brain along the

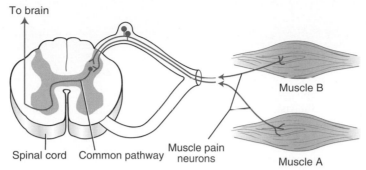

Figure 5-9 The convergence–projection theory for TrP referral. The convergence–projection theory posits that sensory pain neurons from different muscles converge in the spinal cord onto a common pathway that carries that information up to the brain, allowing the brain to mislocalize the source of the pain. (Modified from Mense S, Simons DG, Russell IJ: Muscle pain: understanding its nature, diagnosis, and treatment, Baltimore, 2000, Lippincott, Williams & Wilkins.)

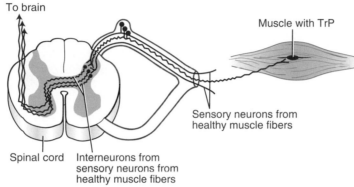

Figure 5-10 The cord spillover theory for trigger point (TrP) referral. The spillover theory posits that when strong pain signals enter the cord from the sensory neurons of a muscle with a TrP, the electrical activity can "spill over" and cause activity within adjacent interneurons that are part of the pathways of other muscles that do not have pain-producing TrPs.

common pathway from muscles A and B, the brain has no way of knowing if the pain originated in muscle A or muscle B. As a result, the pain may be projected (or it could be said to be mislocalized) to muscle B. In this way, the brain can perceive the pain that is caused by a TrP located in muscle A as coming from muscle B, even if there is no TrP located in muscle B.

If this theory were the only theory responsible for explaining TrP referral, then it would mean that all TrP referral pain patterns and the TrPs that caused them must be innervated by the same sensory neurons. This does not seem likely given the widespread referral patterns of some TrPs. Another proposed theory to explain the phenomenon of TrP referral patterns is called the cord spillover theory. It states that when excessive pain signals enter the spinal cord from a strongly active TrP, there is a "spillover" of these electrical signals in the cord from the sensory neurons coming from the muscle housing the TrP to interneurons that come from other muscles that do not have TrPs (Figure 5-10). This spillover causes these other interneurons to carry signals of pain to the brain, telling the brain that these other muscles have pain, even though they contain no pain-producing lesions. In effect, the pain has been referred from the muscle housing the TrP to other muscles that do not have TrPs.

In all likelihood, both theories are probably true and combine to form the most common typical TrP referral patterns of pain that have been mapped. It is important to emphasize that TrP referral patterns do not always follow the most commonly mapped referral patterns that are shown in this and other

BOX 5-10

There is one other explanation that is sometime offered to explain how TrP referral patterns occur. Similar to **sclerotogenous referred pain** (from ligaments and joint capsules) and **visceral referred pain** (from internal visceral organs), it appears that many TrP (myotogenous) referral pain patterns occur within aspects of the body that share the same embryologic origin as the location of the TrP itself. In other words, the location of the TrP and the location of the referral zone were derived from the same embryologic segment. Therefore it is proposed that given the common embryologic origins, the brain may have some mapping that continues to link these areas that may now be spread apart geographically within the body. Thus a TrP in one area of the body may refer pain to another, once embryologically related, area.

books. Figure 5-11 divides the body into regions and then lists which muscles' trigger point referral symptoms are felt in each region. For specific illustrations of the primary and secondary trigger point referral patterns for each individual muscle of the body, please see part IV of the book.

5

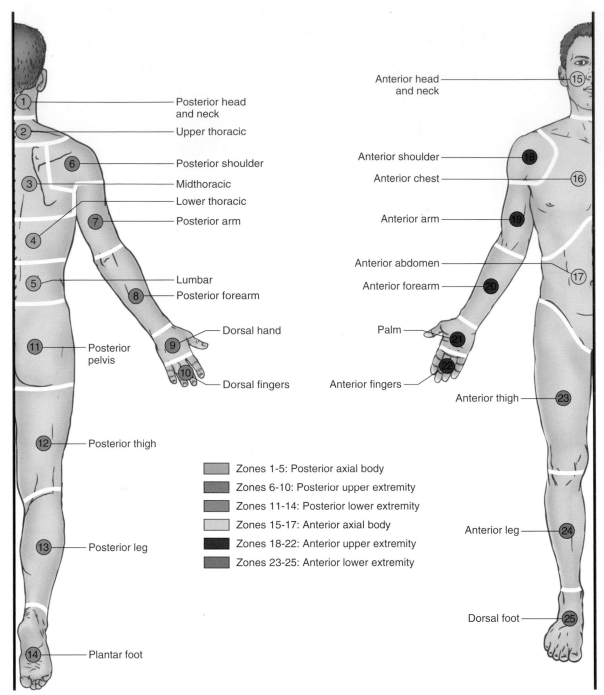

Posterior head and neck
Upper thoracic
Posterior shoulder
Midthoracic
Lower thoracic
Posterior arm
Lumbar
Posterior forearm
Dorsal hand
Posterior pelvis
Dorsal fingers
Posterior thigh
Posterior leg
Plantar foot

Anterior head and neck
Anterior shoulder
Anterior chest
Anterior arm
Anterior abdomen
Anterior forearm
Palm
Anterior fingers
Anterior thigh
Anterior leg
Dorsal foot

Zones 1-5: Posterior axial body
Zones 6-10: Posterior upper extremity
Zones 11-14: Posterior lower extremity
Zones 15-17: Anterior axial body
Zones 18-22: Anterior upper extremity
Zones 23-25: Anterior lower extremity

Figure 5-11 Trigger point referral zones.

Posterior axial body

Zone 1: Digastric, Levator scapulae, Longissimus, Multifidus (cervical), Occipitofrontalis, Rotatores (cervical), Semispinalis thoracis, Semispinalis capitis, Splenius capitis, Suboccipitals, Temporalis, Trapezius (lower), Trapezius (middle), Trapezius (upper)

Zone 2: Levator scapulae, Rotatores (cervical), Semispinalis thoracis, Splenius cervicis, Trapezius (upper)

Zone 3: Erector spinae (iliocostalis), Infraspinatus, Latissimus dorsi, Levator scapulae, Multifidus (thoracic), Rhomboids, Scalenes, Semispinalis thoracis, Serratus anterior, Serratus posterior superior, Transversospinalis (multifidus and rotatores), Trapezius (middle)

Zone 4: Erector spinae (iliocostalis), Iliopsoas, Latissimus dorsi, Rectus abdominis, Serratus anterior, Serratus posterior inferior, Transversospinalis (multifidus and rotatores)

Zone 5: Erector spinae (iliocostalis), Erector spinae (longissimus), Iliopsoas, Serratus posterior inferior, Transversospinalis (multifidus and rotatores)

Posterior upper extremity

Zone 6: Deltoid (middle), Deltoid (posterior), Infraspinatus, Levator scapulae, Semispinalis thoracis, Serratus posterior superior, Subscapularis, Supraspinatus, Teres major, Teres minor, Trapezius (lower), Trapezius (middle), Trapezius (upper), Triceps brachii (long and lateral head)

Zone 7: Brachioradialis, Coracobrachialis, Extensor carpi radialis longus, Extensor digitorum, Scalenes, Supraspinatus, Triceps brachii (long and lateral head)

Zone 8: Anconeus, Coracobrachialis, Extensor carpi ulnaris, Serratus posterior superior, Subclavius, Subscapularis, Supinator, Triceps brachii (long and lateral head)

Zone 9: Adductor pollicis, Brachialis, Brachioradialis, Coracobrachialis, Extensor carpi radialis brevis, Extensor carpi ulnaris, Extensor indicis, Scalenes, Serratus posterior superior, Supinator

Zone 10: Abductor digiti minimi manus, Dorsal interossei manus, Extensor digiti minimi, Extensor digitorum, Lumbricals manus, Palmar interossei, Scalenes

Posterior lower extremity

Zone 11: Erector spinae (iliocostalis), Erector spinae (longissimus), Gluteus maximus, Gluteus medius, Gluteus minimus, Iliopsoas, Piriformis, Quadratus lumborum, Rectus abdominis, Semimembranosus, Semitendinosus, Soleus, Transversospinalis (multifidus and rotatores), Vastus lateralis

Zone 12: Biceps femoris, Gastrocnemius, medial and lateral heads, Gluteus minimus, Plantaris, Popliteus, Quadratus lumborum, Semimembranosus, Semitendinosus, Vastus lateralis

Zone 13: Biceps femoris, Gastrocnemius, medial and lateral heads, Gluteus minimus, Plantaris, Popliteus, Soleus, Tibialis posterior, Vastus lateralis

Zone 14: Abductor and flexor digiti minimi pedis, Abductor hallucis, Adductor hallucis, Adductor longus, Flexor digitorum brevis, Flexor digitorum longus, Flexor hallucis longus, Gastrocnemius (medial head), Interossei pedis, Quadratus plantae, Soleus, Tibialis posterior

Anterior axial body

Zone 15: Buccinator, Digastric, Lateral pterygoid, Levator labii superioris, Masseter, Medial pterygoid, Occipitofrontalis, Orbicularis oculi, Platysma, Semispinalis capitis, Splenius capitis, Splenius cervicis, Sternocleidomastoid sternal and clavicular heads, Suboccipitals, Temporalis, Trapezius (upper), Zygomaticus major

Zone 16: Abdominal obliques (internal and external), Diaphragm, Intercostal muscles, Pectoralis major (sternocostal head), Scalenes, Sternocleidomastoid (sternal head), Subclavius, Transversus abdominis

Zone 17: Abdominal obliques (internal and external), Rectus abdominis, Transversus abdominis

Anterior upper extremity

Zone 18: Biceps brachii, Coracobrachialis, Deltoid (anterior), Deltoid (middle), Diaphragm, Infraspinatus, Pectoralis major (clavicular head), Pectoralis minor, Scalenes, Supraspinatus

Zone 19: Biceps brachii, Infraspinatus, Pectoralis major (sternocostal head), Scalenes, Subclavius, Supinator, Triceps brachii (medial head)

Zone 20: Opponens pollicis, Pectoralis major (sternocostal head), Pronator teres

Zone 21: Adductor pollicis, Flexor carpi radialis, Flexor carpi ulnaris, Flexor pollicis longus, Opponens pollicis, Palmaris longus

Zone 22: Flexor digitorum profundus, Flexor digitorum superficialis

Anterior lower extremity

Zone 23: Abdominal obliques (internal and external), Adductor longus, Adductor magnus, Gracilis, Iliopsoas, Pectineus, Rectus femoris, Sartorius, Tensor fasciae latae, Vastus intermedius, Vastus medialis

Zone 24: Rectus femoris, Vastus medialis

Zone 25: Extensor digitorum longus, Extensor hallucis longus, Extensors digitorum and hallucis brevis, Fibularis longus and brevis, Fibularis tertius, Flexor hallucis brevis, Interossei pedis, Tibialis anterior

Figure 5-11, cont'd

LOCATING AND TREATING TRIGGER POINTS

To treat a TrP, it must first be found. Although TrPs can be located anywhere within a muscle, they tend to occur in certain spots within certain muscles. Generally, TrPs are located at the center of a muscle fiber. If all muscles were fusiform with all their fibers running the full length of the muscle, then all central TrPs would be located at the center of the muscle. Unfortunately this is not always true. Pennate muscles and fusiform muscles that do not have fibers running the full length of the muscle can have their central TrPs in locations other than dead center within the muscle. For this reason, it is helpful to know the fiber architecture of each muscle. In lieu of knowing this, there are commonly mapped-out TrP locations for each muscle of the body. These are shown in Muscle Palpation Tours located in Chapters 11 to 21 of Part IV of this book.

BOX 5-11

Not all roundish nodules palpated within the client's soft tissues are TrPs. Be careful to discern TrPs from lipomas and lymph nodes. Lipomas are benign soft tissue tumors that generally feel soft and have the consistency of a gel caplet inserted under the skin; they may or may not be tender to compression. Lymph nodes/glands may mimic the feeling of a TrP if they are swollen, as they will be if the client has an active infection in that region of the body; swollen lymph nodes usually are tender to compression, but are usually not as hard as TrPs. However, long-standing swollen lymph nodes may calcify over time and eventually feel similar to a TrP on palpation. In addition to assessing palpatory quality, another way to distinguish a TrP from a lipoma or lymph node is to check for the presence of pain referral upon compression. Although not all TrPs refer pain to a distant site, many TrPs do. Lipomas and lymph nodes, however, do not refer pain when compressed.

Once your palpating fingers are in the correct location for a TrP, you should palpate for what likely feels like a small hard knot or marble embedded within the muscle tissue. Often, these TrPs are located within a taut band of fibers that can be strummed or twanged by running your fingers across (perpendicular to) them. Very often, if the taut band is sufficiently taut, a twitch response occurs in which the taut band involuntarily contracts when strummed. Of course, both TrPs and their associated taut bands are usually tender to palpation. Regarding methods of muscle palpation necessary to identify the location of a TrP, see Chapter 2, The Art and Science of Muscle Palpation.

Understanding the genesis of central and attachment TrPs and the mechanism of an actual TrP allows us to reason through the best treatment approach for clients with myofascial TrP syndromes.

For years, the recommended approach for treating TrPs has been the technique known as ischemic compression. Ischemic compression involves the application of deep pressure directly on the client's TrP and holding the pressure for a sustained length of time (approximately 10 seconds or more). The premise of ischemic compression (as its name implies) was to create ischemia in the TrP; then when the therapist removed the pressure, a surge of blood would rush in to the TrP. The problem with ischemic compression, besides the fact that it tended to be an extremely uncomfortable treatment for most clients due to the deep pressure that was recommended, is that given the fact that a TrP is already ischemic, why would therapy be aimed at creating ischemia? This has already been acknowledged by many authorities on TrPs. As a result, ischemic compression technique has been modified and renamed, and is now termed sustained compression or TrP pressure release. However, regardless of the new names, the essence of holding sustained compression upon the TrP is essentially unchanged. (The only substantive change is that less pressure is recommended, making it less painful for the client.) The value to ischemic compression or any sustained compression or TrP pressure release technique is usually stated to create a surge of new blood into the TrP when the pressure is released. Using that logic, it would seem that a better treatment approach could be devised for working with TrPs.

Toward this end, the technique of deep-stroking massage (also known as stripping massage) has been recommended by many of the authorities on TrP theory and practice. David Simons states, "This method is probably the most effective way to inactivate central TrPs when using a direct manual approach, and it can be used to treat TrPs without producing excessive joint movement. The rationale is clear."[1] It is also the preferred method espoused in *The Trigger Point Therapy Workbook* by Clair and Amber Davies.[2]

Deep-stroking massage is done with short strokes that use moderately (but not excessively) deep pressure directly over the TrP. The deep stroking can be done in any direction, but at least some of the strokes should be done along the direction of the taut band containing the TrP. Approximately 30 to 60 short deep strokes should be done consecutively at a pace of 1 to 2 seconds per stroke, totaling a treatment session of approximately 1 minute per TrP.

BOX 5-12

The TrP treatment methods discussed in this chapter are hands-on myofascial approaches. Two other common methods used for the treatment of a TrP are spray and stretch, and TrP injections. Spray and stretch is done by applying a vapocoolant spray to the region of the TrP and then immediately stretching the muscle containing the TrP. TrP injections are injections of either saline solution, a local anesthetic, or steroid (prednisone) directly into the TrP; this treatment is usually performed only by a licensed physician. Certainly other treatment options exist, including stretching, acupuncture, and physical therapy. Of these, stretching is certainly an option for most manual and movement therapists; and given that a TrP is, in effect, a tightening of a small region of a muscle; it stands to reason that stretching would be beneficial. There are many techniques that can be used when stretching a muscle. For a discussion of these techniques, see Chapter 6.

It can also be beneficial to continue the deep stroking along the taut band to the attachment of the muscle. The purpose of deep stroking is twofold. The primary purpose, as stated, is to create a flushing of blood into the TrP with each release of the pressure. This is the major advantage of doing deep-stroking massage 30 to 60 times in a row compared with two to three sustained pressures as recommended in the past. Given that the therapeutic aspect of this technique occurs with each release as new blood flushes in, more strokes mean more releases, which result in a better circulation of blood into the TrP. Given that the pathologic mechanism that creates a TrP is ischemia, the new circulation of blood allows nutrients to enter the TrP so that ATP molecules can be formed, eliminating the "energy crisis."

When done along the direction of the taut band, deep-stroking massage also has the advantage of helping to stretch the shortened sarcomeres within the TrP, breaking the myosin-actin cross-bridges with mechanical force. It is also recommended that the manual treatment be performed with the muscle on stretch to further aid in the stretching of shortened sarcomeres.

BOX 5-13

By the energy crisis hypothesis, any TrP treatment technique whose method depends upon mechanically deforming a TrP to break its cross-bridges would seem to be ultimately ineffective. If the local ischemia is not eliminated, then even if every myosin-actin cross-bridge of the TrP were broken, without the presence of the ATP molecules to reabsorb the calcium ions back into the sarcoplasmic reticulum, the continued presence of the calcium ions in the sarcoplasm would keep the active sites of the actin filaments exposed and new cross-bridges would immediately form, perpetuating the TrP.

If a TrP is long standing, the chance of fibrous adhesion formation increases. The microstretching of deep-stroking massage, especially if performed along the length of the muscle fibers and with the muscle on stretch, helps to break up these patterns of adhesions before they form more fully and become structurally entrenched. In addition, most types of deep tissue work have the advantage of helping to flush out toxins that have accumulated because of the venous congestion present in TrPs.

A special note regarding attachments TrPs: When central and attachment TrPs both exist within a muscle, the recommended course is to treat the central TrPs first. Given that attachment TrPs are usually caused by the pulling of the taut bands created by the central TrPs, if a central TrP is cleared up, its attachment TrP may clear up on its own. However, it is

---

BOX 5-14

Although most TrPs are treated with a flat pressure applied by the therapist's fingers, thumb, hand, or elbow, there are times when a **pincer grip** is recommended. A pincer grip involves grabbing the TrP between the thumb and another finger (usually the index or middle finger) and pinching or squeezing the TrP between them. This method is often employed when it is not desirable to transmit flat pressure deep to the TrP. For example, when working a TrP in the sternocleidomastoid muscle, flat pressure is often contraindicated because of the presence of the carotid artery immediately deep to portions of the muscle; in this region, a pincer grip can be safely used. A pincer grip also offers the ability to increase pressure on the TrP because it is trapped between the two treating fingers. The disadvantage is that pincer grip work is often less comfortable for the client.

---

entirely possible for an attachment TrP in muscle tissue, once created, to now have its own vicious cycle of ischemia causing contraction, causing further ischemia, and so on. Furthermore, once this cycle has begun, the pain present as a result of the attachment TrP can trigger further contraction via the pain–spasm–pain cycle; and of course the pooling of toxins from venous congestion also tend to perpetuate the presence of the TrP based on their irritating nature. For all of these reasons, even though it is probably wisest and most efficient to first treat central TrPs, if central TrP treatment does not result in the easy dissolution of attachment TrPs, then it is advisable to directly treat the attachments TrPs as well.

BOX 5-15

The reasoning used for treating central TrPs before attachment TrPs can be applied to the treatment of any key TrP before treating its satellite TrP(s). Given that it is the presence of a key TrP that creates the satellite TrP, beginning with treatment of key TrPs may obviate the need to treat the satellite TrPs. The challenge is knowing which TrPs are key TrPs and which ones are their satellite TrPs. Of course, even if it is determined which TrPs are key and which are satellite (e.g., central TrPs are often key and attachment TrPs are usually satellite), once formed, a satellite TrP may create its own vicious ischemic cycle and may not disappear unless treated directly.

5

Review Questions

1. How is a TrP defined? What are the two classifications of TrPs?
2. Describe the organizational composition of a muscle.
3. To what degree, represented by a percentage, will sarcomeres of innervated muscle fibers contract?
4. What role does ATP play in muscle contraction?
5. In the energy crisis hypothesis, what is the underlying cause of the lack of ATP?
6. What is the relationship between length and frequency of muscular contraction and the formation of TrPs?
7. Explain the relationship between the energy crisis hypothesis and the dysfunctional endplate hypothesis.
8. What are four general factors that create TrPs?
9. Briefly describe the cord spillover theory.
10. What is the preferred technique for treating TrPs, and how it is done?

 Deeper Thoughts

Given that TrPs can be found anywhere in a muscle, and key TrPs can give rise to satellite TrPs, how is a therapist to know which is which? Is there any pattern to this spiderweb? Where would you begin treatment of a client with multiple TrPs?

REFERENCES

1. Simons DG, Travell JG, Simons LS: *Myofascial pain and dysfunction: the trigger point manual*, ed 2, vol 1. Baltimore, 1999, Lippincott Williams & Wilkins. 41.
2. Davies C: *The trigger point therapy workbook: your self-treatment guide for pain relief*, ed 3, Oakland, CA, 2001, New Harbinger.

Stretching

INTRODUCTION

Stretching is a powerful therapeutic tool that is available to manual therapists and athletic trainers to improve the health of their clients. Although few people disagree about the benefits of stretching, there is a great deal of disagreement about how stretching should be done. There are many possible choices. Stretching can be performed statically or dynamically. Three repetitions (reps) can be done, each one held approximately 10 to 20 seconds, or ten reps can be performed, each one held for approximately 2 to 3 seconds. A technique called *pin and stretching* can be done, or stretches that use neurologic reflexes to facilitate the stretch, such as contract relax (CR) and agonist contract (AC) stretching, can be performed. There are also choices regarding when stretching is best done; stretching can be done before or after strengthening exercise.

To best understand stretching so that we can apply it clinically for the optimal health of our clients, let's first look at the fundamental basis of stretching by posing and answering the following five questions: What is stretching? Why is stretching done? How do we figure out how to stretch muscles? How forcefully should we stretch? When should stretching be done? Then we can examine the types of stretching techniques that are available to the client and therapist/trainer.

1. What Is Stretching?

Simply defined, stretching is a method of physical bodywork that lengthens and elongates soft tissues. These soft tissues may be muscles and their tendons (collectively called *myofascial units*), ligaments, joint capsules, and/or other fascial planes of tissue. When performing a stretch upon our client, we use the term target tissue to describe the tissue that we intend to stretch (or target muscle when we specifically want to stretch a muscle or muscle group). To create a stretch, the client's body is moved into a position that creates a line of tension that pulls on the target tissues, placing a stretch upon them (Figure 6-1). If the stretch is effective, the tissues are lengthened.

2. Why Is Stretching Done?

Stretching is done because soft tissues may increase in tension and become shortened and contracted. Shortened and contracted soft tissues resist lengthening and limit mobility of the joints that they cross. The specific joint motion that is limited will be the motion of a body part (at the joint) that is in the opposite direction from the location of the tight tissues. For example, if the tight tissue is located on the posterior side of the joint, anterior motion of a body part at that joint will be limited, and if the tight tissue is located on the anterior side of the joint, posterior motion of a body part at that joint will be limited (Figure 6-2).

As stated, a shortened and contracted tissue can be described as having greater tension. Two types of tissue tension exist, passive tension and active tension. All soft tissues can exhibit increased passive tension. Passive tension results from increased fascial adhesions that build up over time.

Additionally, muscles may exhibit increased active tension. Active tension results when a muscle's contractile elements (actin and myosin filaments) contract via the sliding filament mechanism, creating a pulling force toward the center of the

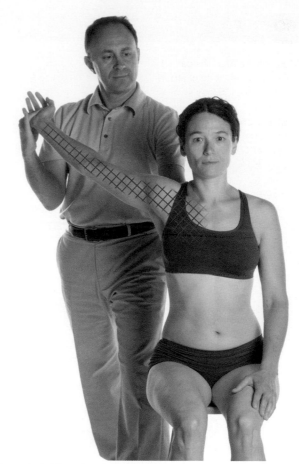

Figure 6-1 The client's right upper extremity is stretched. The line of tension created by this stretch is indicated by *hatch marks*. A stretch is exerted upon all tissues along the line of tension of the stretch.

muscle. Whether a soft tissue has increased passive or active tension, this increased tension makes the tissue more resistant to lengthening. Therefore stretching is done to lengthen and elongate these tissues, hopefully restoring full range of motion and flexibility of the body.

BOX 6-1

The tension of a tissue can be described as its resistance to stretch.

---

3. How Do We Figure Out How to Stretch Muscles?

If our target tissue to be stretched is a muscle, the question is how do we figure out what position the client's body must be put in to achieve an effective stretch of the target muscle or muscle group? Certainly there are many excellent books available for learning specific muscle stretches. Indeed, specific stretches for each of the muscles and muscle groups covered in Part IV of this book are given. However, better than relying on a book or other authority to give us stretching routines that must be memorized, it is preferable to be able to figure out the stretches that our clients need.

BOX 6-2

Muscles have classically been considered to be the only tissue that can exhibit active tension. However, recent research has shown that fibrous connective tissues often contain cells called myofibroblasts, which evolve from fibroblasts normally found in the fibrous connective tissues. Myofibroblasts contain contractile proteins that can actively contract. Although not present in the same numbers that muscle tissue contains, connective tissue myofibroblasts may be present in sufficient number to be biomechanically significant when assessing the tension of that connective tissue.

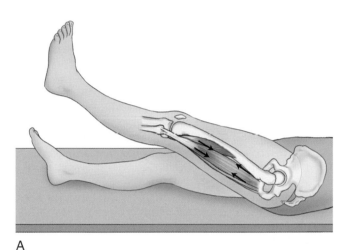

A

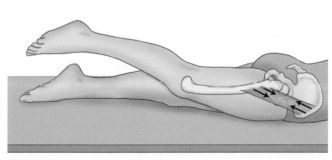

B

Figure 6-2 When tissues located on one side of a joint are tight, motion of a body part at the joint to the opposite side will be limited. **A** shows decreased hip joint flexion due to taut tissues, tight hamstrings, at the posterior side of the hip joint. If anterior hip joint tissues (especially hip joint flexor muscles, such as the tensor fasciae latae [TFL] seen in this illustration) are tight, a decrease in hip joint extension occurs—as seen in **B.**

Figuring out a stretch for a muscle is actually quite easy. Simply recall the actions that were learned for the target muscle, and then do the opposite of one or more of its actions. Because the actions of a muscle are what the muscle does when it shortens, then stretching and lengthening the muscle would be achieved by having the client do the opposite of the muscle's actions. Essentially, if a muscle flexes a joint, then extension of that joint would stretch it; if the muscle abducts a joint, then adduction of that joint would stretch it; if a muscle medially rotates a joint, then lateral rotation of that joint would stretch it. If a muscle has more than one action, then the optimal stretch would consider all its actions.

BOX 6-3

"The Shortest Rope"

Placing a stretch force upon a functional group of muscles, such as the flexors of the thigh at the hip joint, does not actually stretch all the muscles in that group. In reality, only one of the muscles within the group is stretched. To understand this, an analogy called "the shortest rope" can be used. If I am holding five ropes, with lengths of 10 inches, 20 inches, 30 inches, 40 inches, and 50 inches respectively, with the ends of all five ropes in one hand and the other ends of all five ropes in my other hand, and I pull my hands apart, lengthening the ropes, I will stretch the ropes until the shortest one stops the stretch. Therefore, only the shortest rope is actually stretched; no stretch force is placed on the other ropes because the shortest rope stopped the stretch before they could be sufficiently lengthened to stretch them. For example, applying this concept to hip joint extension to stretch the hip flexor functional group, if the hip joint is extended, the excursion of extension continues until the tightest muscle (in other words, the shortest hip flexor muscle) stops the stretch.

For example, if the target muscle that is being stretched is the right upper trapezius, given that its actions are extension, right lateral flexion, and left rotation of the neck and head at the spinal joints, then stretching the right upper trapezius would require either flexion, left lateral flexion, and/or right rotation of the head and neck at the spinal joints.

When a muscle has many actions, it is not always necessary to do the opposite of all of them; however, at times it might be desired or needed. If the right upper trapezius is tight enough, simply doing flexion in the sagittal plane might be sufficient to stretch it. However, if further stretch is needed, then left lateral flexion in the frontal plane and/or right rotation in the transverse plane could be added as shown in Figure 6-3. Considering the action of the target muscle in each of the cardinal planes in which it can cause motion is called multiplane stretching.

Even if not every plane of action is used for the stretch, being aware of all the muscle's actions is still important; otherwise, a mistake might be made with the stretch. For example, if the right upper trapezius is being stretched by flexing and left laterally flexing the client's head and neck, it is important to not let the client's head and neck rotate to the left, because this will allow the right upper trapezius to be slackened in the

6

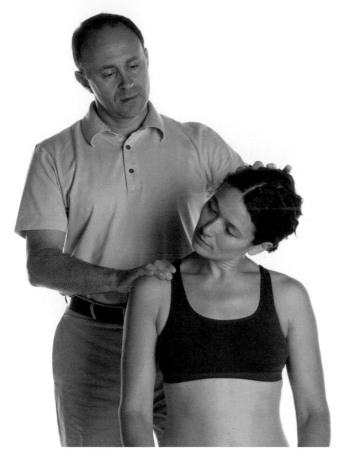

Figure 6-3 The right upper trapezius is stretched in all three planes. The client's head and neck are flexed in the sagittal plane, left laterally flexed in the frontal plane, and right rotated in the transverse plane.

transverse plane and the tension of the stretch will be lost. Furthermore, considering what the actions of the target muscle are at its other attachment is also important, because if this other attachment is allowed to move, the stretch tension could be lost. The right upper trapezius also elevates the right scapula at the scapulocostal joint (as well as retracting and upwardly rotating it). Therefore, it is important to make sure that the right scapula is stabilized and not allowed to elevate during the stretch. Stabilization of the other end of the target muscle is extremely important and often the more challenging aspect of performing a stretch.

Isolating a stretch so that a specific target muscle is stretched can be very challenging. When a stretch is performed, a stretch is placed upon an entire functional group of muscles. For example, if a client's thigh is stretched into extension at the hip joint in the sagittal plane, a stretch will be placed upon the entire functional group of sagittal plane hip joint flexors. To isolate one of the hip flexors usually requires fine-tuning the stretch to achieve the desired result. If the stretch is done into extension in the sagittal plane and adduction in the frontal plane, then all hip flexor muscles that are also frontal plane adductors will be slackened and relaxed by the adduction, and the stretch will be focused on those hip flexor muscles that are also abductors, such as the tensor fasciae latae (TFL), the sartorius, and the anterior fibers of the gluteus medius and minimus.

BOX 6-4

The functional group of flexors of the hip joint includes the tensor fasciae latae (TFL), anterior fibers of the gluteus medius and minimus, sartorius, rectus femoris, iliacus, psoas major, pectineus, adductor longus, gracilis, and adductor brevis.

If medial rotation of the thigh at the hip joint in the transverse plane is also added to the stretch so that the thigh is now being extended in the sagittal plane, adducted in the frontal plane, and medially rotated in the transverse plane, then all hip flexors and abductors that are also transverse plane medial rotators will be slackened and relaxed by medial rotation, and the stretch will now be focused on muscles that do flexion, abduction, and lateral rotation of the thigh at the hip joint. In this case, the sartorius is the principal target muscle to be stretched, because it is the only hip flexor and abductor muscle that also laterally rotates the thigh at the hip joint (the iliopsoas will also be stretched because it is a flexor and lateral rotator at the hip joint, and some sources state that it can also abduct). Of course, given that the sartorius is also a flexor of the leg at the knee joint, it is imperative that the knee joint is extended during the stretch, or the sartorius would be slackened by a flexed knee joint and the effectiveness of the stretch would be lost.

Had lateral rotation of the thigh at the hip joint been added as the third transverse plane component instead of medial rotation, then the sartorius, being a lateral rotator, would have been slackened and the TFL and anterior fibers of the gluteus medius and minimus, being medial rotators, would have been stretched instead. To then isolate the stretch to just the TFL or just the anterior fibers of the gluteus medius or minimus is difficult if not impossible, because these muscles all share the same hip joint actions in all three planes and therefore are stretched by the same joint position.

Therefore, whenever a client's body part is moved into a stretch in one direction, in other words in one plane, the entire functional group of muscles located on the other side of the joint has a stretch force placed upon it. To then fine-tune and isolate the stretch, to one or only a few of the muscles of this functional group, considering the action of the target muscle in each of the cardinal planes in which it can cause motion is necessary. Optimizing a stretch might also involve adding a stretch to another joint if the target muscle crosses more than one joint (i.e., is a multi-joint muscle).

Figuring out exactly how to fine-tune a stretch to isolate a target muscle depends upon a solid foundational knowledge of the joint actions of the muscles involved. Once this knowledge is attained, applying it can eliminate the need for memorizing tens or hundreds of stretches. In the place of memorization comes an ability to critically reason through the steps necessary to figure out whatever stretches are needed for the proper treatment of our clients!

BOX 6-5

If the target tissue to be stretched is not a muscle but rather a ligament, joint capsule, or other fascial tissue of the region, its stretch can still be reasoned out instead of memorized. One way to do this is to think of the ligament or the region of the joint capsule as though it were a muscle; figure out what its action would be if it were a muscle, and then do the action that is antagonistic to that action. Even simpler, move the client's body part at the joint in the direction that is away from the side of the joint where the ligament or region of the joint capsule is located. For example, if the target tissue is a ligament located anteriorly at the glenohumeral joint, then simply move the client's arm posteriorly at the glenohumeral joint to stretch it. Doing this will work for most ligaments and capsular joint fibers, except for the ones that are arranged horizontally in the transverse plane. To stretch these, a transverse plane rotation motion is needed.

4. How Forcefully Should We Stretch?

Stretching should never hurt. If stretching causes pain, the target muscles or muscles in the vicinity of the target tissues will likely tighten in response to the pain via the pain–spasm–pain cycle. Furthermore, if the target muscle is either stretched too quickly or too forcefully, the muscle spindle reflex may be engaged, resulting in a tightening of the target muscle. Given that a stretch should relax and lengthen tissue, stretching that causes musculature to tighten defeats the purpose of the stretch.

For this reason, a stretch should never be done too quickly; stretching should always be done slowly and rhythmically. Furthermore, the therapist should be prudent and judicious regarding how far a client is stretched. The therapist should stretch the client until tissue tension is reached, and then slightly more force should be added. a stretch should never cause pain; theoretically, a stretch can be done as hard as possible, but always without pain. When in doubt, it is best to be conservative regarding the speed and forcefulness of a stretch. It is wiser to gently and slowly stretch a client over a number of sessions, gradually increasing the assertiveness of the stretch, to safely achieve the goal of loosening the target tissues. It may take more sessions, but a positive outcome is essentially guaranteed. Imprudent stretching may not only set back the progress of the client's treatment program but may also cause soft tissue damage and injury that is difficult to reverse.

5. When Should Stretching Be Done?

Stretching should be done when the target tissues are most receptive to being stretched; this is when they are already warmed up. Not only do cold tissues resist stretching, resulting in little benefit, they are also more likely to be injured when stretched. For this reason, if stretching is linked to a physical exercise workout, the stretching should be done after the workout when the tissues are warmed up, not before the workout when the tissues are cold. This general principle is true if the type of stretching is the classic form, called *static stretching*. If dynamic stretching is done instead, then it is safe and appropriate to stretch before an exercise regimen when the tissues are cold, because dynamic stretching is a method of warming the tissues in addition to stretching them. For more on static versus dynamic stretching, see the next section.

BOX 6-6

Clients often describe a stretch as being painful but go on to say that the pain feels good. For this reason, a distinction should be made between what is often described by the client as **good pain** and true pain (or what might be called *bad pain*). Good pain is often the way that a client describes the sensation of the stretch; therefore causing good pain as a result of a stretch is fine. However, if a stretch causes true pain—in other words, the client winces and resists or fights the stretch—then the intensity of the stretch must be lessened. Otherwise, not only will the stretch be ineffective, but the client is likely to be injured. A stretch should never be forced.

If the client wants to stretch but does not have the opportunity to first engage in physical exercise to warm the target tissues, then the client may warm the tissues by applying moist heat. There are a number of ways to do this. Taking a hot shower or bath, using a whirlpool, or placing a moist heating pad or hydrocollator pack upon the target tissues are all effective ways to warm target tissues before stretching them. Of all these choices, perhaps the most effective one is taking a hot shower, because it not only warms the tissues, but also the pressure of the water hitting the skin physically creates a massage that can help to relax the musculature of the region.

BOX 6-7

Warming/heating the soft tissues of the body facilitates stretching them in two ways: first, heat is a central nervous depressant helping the musculature relax; second, fascia is more easily stretched when warm.

BASIC STRETCHING TECHNIQUES: STATIC STRETCHING VERSUS DYNAMIC STRETCHING

Classically, stretching has been what is called static stretching, meaning that the position of the stretch is attained and then held statically for a period of time. The length of time recommended

6

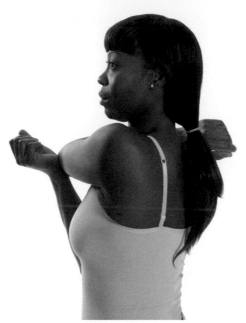

Figure 6-4 A client is performing a stretch of her left arm and scapular region. This (or any) stretch can be performed statically or dynamically. (From Muscolino JE: Stretch your way to better health, Massage Ther J 45[3]:167-171, 2006. Photo by Yanik Chauvin.)

to statically hold a stretch has traditionally been between 10 and 30 seconds, and three reps have usually been recommended. However, the wisdom of this "classic" technique of stretching has recently been questioned. The alternative to static stretching is called **dynamic stretching,** and it is sometimes also known as **mobilization.** Dynamic stretching, as its name implies, is more dynamic. Instead of holding the position of stretch statically for a prolonged period of time, the end-position of the stretch is held for only a few seconds and then released. This is then repeated many times, usually for approximately ten reps (Figure 6-4). Because dynamic stretching involves more movement of the client's body, it is not only a stretch, but also an effective means of warming up the region.

Another factor to consider is whether the stretch is performed actively or passively. An **active stretch** is defined by the client actively contracting the muscles of the joint being moved to bring the joint into stretch. A **passive stretch** occurs when the muscles of the joint being stretched are relaxed. Most often, passive stretching is performed by a therapist/trainer. However, a client can perform a passive stretch without the assistance of another person. Figure 6-5, *A,* demonstrates an active stretch of the client's neck. Figure 6-5, *B,* shows the same stretch performed passively with the assistance of a therapist. And Figure 6-5, *C,* shows the same stretch performed passively by the client without the assistance of a therapist. Typically, static stretching is performed passively and dynamic stretching is performed actively, but this need not be the case.

Regardless of whether a stretch is performed statically or dynamically, or actively or passively, the idea is that whenever a joint is moved in a certain direction, the tissues on the other side of the joint are stretched. Following the example of Figure 6-2, if the hip joint is flexed (whether by the usual action of flexion of the thigh at the hip joint, or the reverse action of anterior tilt of the pelvis at the hip joint), then the tissues on the other side of the joint, the hip joint extensor muscles

and other posterior soft tissues, will be stretched. Similarly, if the hip joint is extended (whether by extending the thigh at the hip joint or posteriorly tilting the pelvis at the hip joint), the hip joint flexor muscles and other anterior tissues, will be stretched.

By this concept, any joint motion of the body stretches some of the tissues of that joint. Of course, it is important when doing dynamic stretching that the joint motions are done in a careful, prudent, and graded manner, gradually increasing the intensity of the motions. For this reason, dynamic stretching begins with small ranges of motion carried out with little or no resistance. It then gradually builds up to full ranges of motion. If dynamic stretching is done before a physical workout, then the ranges of motion that are performed should be the same ranges of motion that will be asked of the body during the physical workout. And if the exercise entails some form of added resistance, then the added resistance of the exercise should gradually be added to the dynamic stretching after the full ranges of motion of the joints are done.

For example, before playing tennis, one would go through the motions of forehand, backhand, and serving strokes without a racquet in hand, beginning with small swings and building up to full range of motion swings. Then the same order of motions would be repeated, but this time with the added resistance of having the tennis racquet in hand (but not actually hitting a ball), starting with small swings and gradually working up to full range of motion swings. Finally, the person adds the full resistance of hitting the tennis ball while playing on the court, again, starting with gentle, short swings and gradually building up to full range of motion and powerful swings (Figure 6-6). The advantage of active dynamic stretching done in this manner as an exercise warm-up is that not only is circulation increased, the tissues warmed up, the joints lubricated and brought through their ranges of motion, and the neural pathways that will be used during the exercise routine engaged, but with each motion that is done, soft tissues on the other side of the joint are stretched. Even though dynamic stretching is the ideal method to employ before engaging in physical exercise, it can certainly be done at any time.

Given the benefits of dynamic stretching, is there still a place for classic static stretching? Yes. As explained earlier, static stretching is beneficial if the tissues are first warmed up. This means that static stretching can be very effective after an exercise routine is done, or if the tissues are first warmed up by the application of moist heat or soft tissue manipulation. Many sources also recommend performing a statically held stretch position after first performing a number of short-held dynamic repetitions.

BOX 6-8

Some sources state that static stretching done before strengthening exercise is actually deleterious to the performance of the exercise. Their reasoning is that when muscles are stretched, they are neurologically inhibited from contracting and consequently less able to contract quickly when needed to protect a joint from a possible sprain or strain during strenuous exercise.

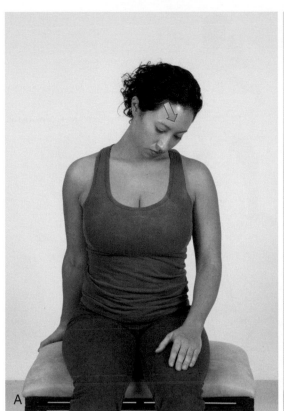

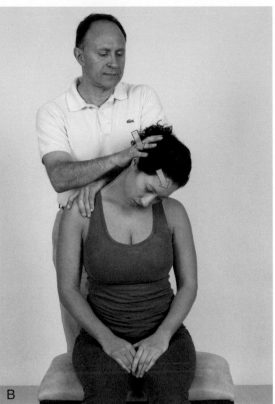

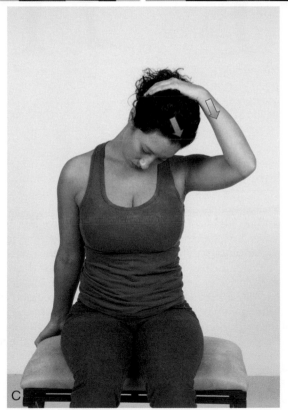

Figure 6-5 Active and passive stretching of the client's neck. **A,** The stretch performed actively. **B,** The stretch performed passively with the assistance of a therapist. **C,** The stretch performed passively by the client without the assistance of a therapist.

6

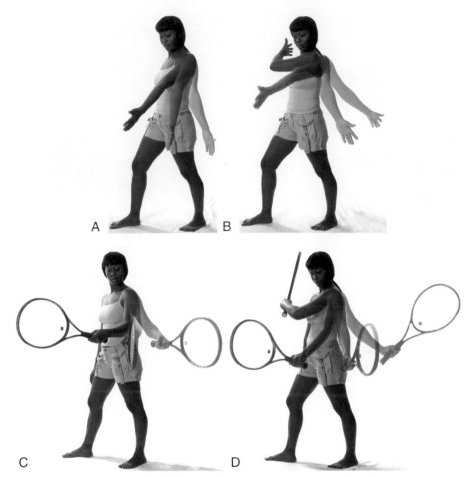

Figure 6-6 Illustration showing the beginning stages of dynamic stretching for a forehand stroke in tennis. In **A,** a short forehand swing is done without holding a racquet. In **B,** a full range of motion swing is done without the racquet. The person then progresses to holding a racquet to provide greater resistance, first with a short swing as seen in **C,** and then with a full range of motion swing as seen in **D.** (From Muscolino JE: Stretch your way to better health, Massage Ther J 45[3]:167-171, 2006. Photos by Yanik Chauvin.)

PIN AND STRETCH TECHNIQUE

Beyond the choice of performing a stretch statically or dynamically, there are other stretching options. One of these options is pin and stretch technique. **Pin and stretch** technique is a stretching technique in which the therapist pins (stabilizes) one part of the client's body and then stretches the tissues up to that pinned spot.

The purpose of the pin and stretch is to direct a stretch to a more specific region of the client's body. It can even be used to direct the stretch to a specific aspect of the target muscle being stretched. As stated previously, when a body part is moved to create a stretch, a line of tension is created. Everything along the line of tension is stretched. However, if we want only a certain region of the soft tissues along that line of tension to be stretched, then we can specifically direct the stretch to that region by using the pin and stretch technique.

For example, if a side-lying stretch is done on a client as demonstrated in Figure 6-7, *A,* the entire lateral side of the client's body from the therapist's right hand on the client's distal thigh to the therapist's left hand on the client's upper trunk is stretched. The problem with allowing the line of tension of a stretch to spread over such a large region of the client's body

is that if one region of soft tissue of the client's body within that line of tension is very tight, it might stop the stretch from being felt in another area of the line of tension that we are specifically targeting to stretch.

To focus the line of tension and direct the stretch to our target tissues, we can use the pin and stretch technique. If the therapist pins the client's lower rib cage, as seen in Figure 6-7, *B,* the stretch is no longer felt in the client's lateral thoracic region; instead it is specifically directed to the client's lateral pelvis and lateral lumbar region. If the therapist instead pins the client's iliac crest, as seen in Figure 6-7, *C,* the stretch is no longer felt in the client's lateral lumbar region and is now directed to only the lateral musculature and other soft tissues of the client's thigh. In effect, the pin and stretch technique pins and stabilizes a part of the client's body, thereby focusing and directing the force of the line of tension of the stretch to the specific target tissue(s).

Continuing with this example, if the target tissues are the gluteus medius and quadratus lumborum (as well as other muscles of the lateral pelvis and lateral lumber region), pinning the client at the lower rib cage, as seen in Figure 6-7, *B,* is the ideal approach. If the target tissue is limited to the gluteus medius (and other muscles/soft tissues of the lateral pelvis), the ideal location to pin the client during this side-lying

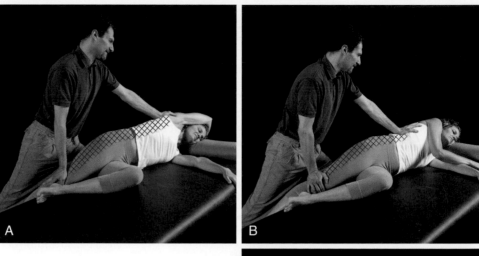

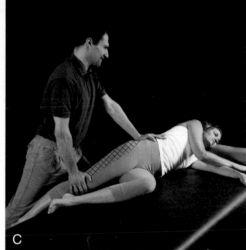

Figure 6-7 A shows a side-lying stretch of a client. When done in this manner, the line of tension of the stretch is very broad, ranging from the therapist's right hand on the client's distal thigh to the therapist's left hand on the client's upper trunk. **B** and **C** demonstrate application of the pin and stretch technique to narrow the focus of the stretch. Note: *Hatch marks* indicate the area that is stretched in all three figures. (Modified from Muscolino JE: Stretching the hip, Massage Ther J 46[4]:167-171, 2007. Photos by Yanik Chauvin.)

stretch is at the iliac crest, as seen in Figure 6-7, *C*. In fact, if desired, the pin could even be placed partway down the gluteus medius (perhaps halfway between the iliac crest and the greater trochanter), thereby focusing the stretch to the distal aspect of the gluteus medius. As can be seen, pin and stretch is a powerful technique that allows for much greater specificity when stretching a client.

ADVANCED STRETCHING TECHNIQUES: NEURAL INHIBITION STRETCHING

Two advanced stretching techniques that are extremely effective are the contract relax (CR) stretching technique and the agonist contract (AC) stretching technique. Both of these advanced stretching techniques are similar in that they employ a neurologic reflex to facilitate the stretching of the target musculature; therefore they are termed neural inhibition stretches. The CR technique has classically been stated to employ the neurologic reflex called the Golgi tendon organ (GTO) reflex. The AC technique uses the neurologic reflex called *reciprocal inhibition*.

CR stretching is perhaps better known as proprioceptive neuromuscular facilitation (PNF) stretching; it is also known as postisometric relaxation (PIR) stretching.

BOX 6-9

Regarding the contract relax (CR) stretching technique, the name *contract relax* is used because the target muscle is first *contracted*, and then it is *relaxed*. The name *proprioceptive neuromuscular facilitation* is used because a *proprioceptive neurologic* reflex (classically considered to be the GTO reflex) is used to *facilitate* the stretch of the target muscle. The name *postisometric relaxation* is used because after (i.e., *post*) an *isometric* contraction, the target muscle is *relaxed* (classically ascribed to the GTO reflex). In each case, the name describes how the stretch is done.

CR stretching is done by first having the client isometrically contract the target muscle with mild to moderate force (usually stated to be approximately 25-40% of the client's maximum force) against resistance provided by the therapist; then the therapist stretches the target muscle by lengthening it immediately afterward. The isometric contraction is usually held for approximately 5 to 10 seconds, and this procedure is usually repeated three or four times. Generally, the client is either asked to breathe out or hold in her breath while isometrically contracting against resistance, and then relax and either exhale or continue exhaling while the target muscle is being stretched.

BOX 6-10

Even though the contraction of a CR stretch is usually isometric, it can be done concentrically. In other words, when the client contracts against the resistance of the therapist, the therapist can allow the client to slightly shorten the muscle and move the joint. What is important is that the muscle generates tension to trigger the GTO reflex, adding to the effectiveness of the stretch.

BOX 6-11

There are two choices for the client's breathing protocol when doing a CR stretch. The client can either hold in the breath when contracting the target muscle against the resistance of the therapist, or the client can exhale when contracting the target muscle (think *e*xertion on *e*xhale) against the therapist's resistance. Although contracting when exhaling is probably slightly preferred, if CR stretching is combined with AC stretching to perform contract relax agonist contract (CRAC) stretching, then it is logistically easier for the client to hold in the breath when contracting the target muscle.

The muscle group that is usually used to demonstrate CR stretching is the hamstring group; however this method of stretching can be used for any muscle of the body (Figure 6-8). The classically stated basis for CR stretching is the GTO reflex and works as follows: If the target muscle is forcefully contracted, the GTO reflex is engaged and results in inhibition of the target muscle (i.e., the muscle is inhibited or stopped from contracting). This is a protective reflex that prevents the forceful contraction from tearing the muscle and/or its tendon. As therapists, we can use this protective reflex to facilitate stretching our client's musculature, because muscles that are neurologically inhibited are more easily stretched. Note: There is some disagreement as to whether the operative reflex for CR stretching is the GTO reflex.

BOX 6-12

It is customary for each rep of a CR stretch to begin where the previous rep ended. However, it is possible and sometimes desirable to take the client off stretch to some degree before beginning the next rep. Given that the proposed mechanism of CR stretching is the GTO reflex, what is most important is that the client is able to generate a forceful enough contraction to stimulate this reflex. Sometimes this is not possible if the client is trying to contract when the target muscle is stretched extremely long.

Like CR stretching, AC stretching also uses a neurologic reflex to "facilitate" the stretch of the target muscle; however, instead of the GTO reflex, AC stretching uses reciprocal inhibition. Reciprocal inhibition is a neurologic reflex that creates a more efficient joint action by preventing two muscles that have antagonistic actions from contracting at the same time. When a muscle is contracted, muscles that have antagonistic actions to the contracted muscle are inhibited from contracting (i.e., they are relaxed). Neurologically inhibited muscles are more easily stretched. For example, if the brachialis contracts to flex the forearm at the elbow joint, reciprocal inhibition inhibits the triceps brachii from contracting and creating a force of elbow joint extension (that would oppose the action of elbow joint flexion by the brachialis).

To use reciprocal inhibition when stretching a client, have the client do a joint action that is antagonistic to the joint action of the target muscle. This inhibits the target muscle, allowing for a greater stretch to be done at the end of this active movement (Figure 6-9). Generally, the position of stretch is only held for 1 to 3 seconds; this procedure is repeated approximately ten times. The client is usually asked to breathe in before the movement, and then exhale during the movement. It should be noted that AC stretching technique is also often referred to as *PNF stretching*.

BOX 6-13

Regarding the agonist contract (AC) stretching technique, the name *agonist contract* is used because the *agonist* (mover) of a joint action is *contracted*, causing the antagonist (the target muscle that is to be stretched) on the other side of the joint to be relaxed (by reciprocal inhibition).

BOX 6-14

Agonist contract (AC) stretching that uses the neurologic reflex of reciprocal inhibition is the basis for Aaron Mattes' active isolated stretching (AIS) technique.

The two methods of CR and AC stretching can be powerful additions to your repertoire of stretching techniques and may greatly benefit your clients. In fact, these two methods may be performed sequentially on the client, beginning with CR stretching followed by AC stretching; this protocol is called contract relax agonist contract (CRAC) stretching (Figure 6-10). CRAC stretching begins with the client isometrically contracting the target muscle against the therapist's resistance for approximately 5 to 8 seconds while holding in the breath (see Figure 6-10, *A*); this is the CR aspect of the stretch. Next, the client actively contracts the antagonist muscles of the target muscle by moving the joint toward a stretch of the target muscle while breathing

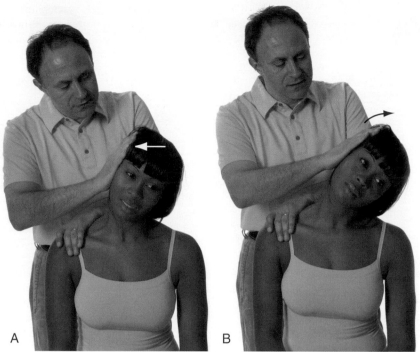

Figure 6-8 Contract relax (CR) stretching of the right lateral flexor musculature of the neck and head is shown. In **A,** the client is isometrically contracting the right lateral flexor musculature against resistance provided by the therapist. In **B,** the therapist is now stretching the right lateral flexor musculature by moving the client's neck and head into left lateral flexion. (From Muscolino JE: Stretch your way to better health, Massage Ther J 45[3]:167-171, 2006. Photos by Yanik Chauvin.)

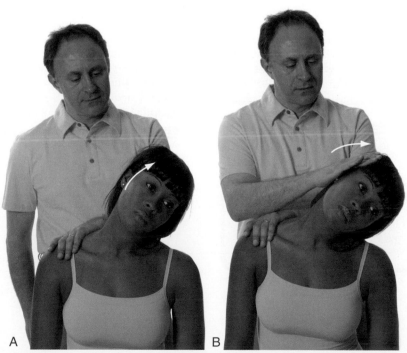

Figure 6-9 Agonist contract (AC) stretching for the right lateral flexor musculature of the neck is shown. **A** shows the client actively performing left lateral flexion of the neck. **B** shows that at the end of range of motion of left lateral flexion, the therapist then stretches the client's neck further into left lateral flexion. (Modified from Muscolino JE: Stretch your way to better health, Massage Ther J 45[3]:167-171, 2006. Photos by Yanik Chauvin.)

6

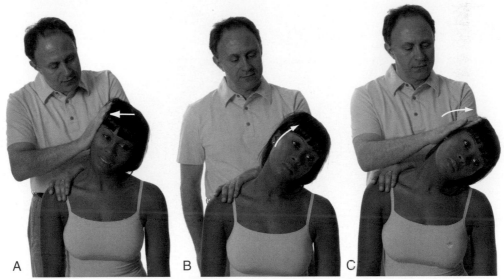

A   B   C

Figure 6-10 Contract relax agonist contract (CRAC) stretching is demonstrated for the right lateral flexion musculature of the neck. When these two stretching methods are both done, contract relax (CR) is usually done first, and then agonist contract (AC) is performed immediately afterward. **A** shows CR stretching technique with the client isometrically contracting the right lateral flexion musculature of her neck against the resistance of the therapist. **B** shows the client actively moving her neck into left lateral flexion. In **C,** the therapist now stretches the client's neck further into left lateral flexion. (Modified from Muscolino JE: Stretch your way to better health, Massage Ther J 45[3]:167-171, 2006. Photos by Yanik Chauvin.)

out (see Figure 6-10, *B*); this is the AC aspect of the stretch. Then the client relaxes and the therapist moves the client into a further stretch of the target muscle while the client continues to breathe out (see Figure 6-10, *C*). The client then breathes in as they are passively brought back to the beginning position of the stretch so they are ready for the next repetition. It is typical to perform anywhere from three to ten reps. Combining CR with AC stretching can create an even greater stretch for the client's target musculature.

BOX 6-15

To simplify the difference between CR and AC stretching, know that with CR stretching, the client actively isometrically contracts the target muscle and then the therapist stretches it immediately afterward; however with AC stretching, the client actively moves his or her body into the stretch of the target muscle and then the therapist further stretches the target muscle immediately afterward.

CONCLUSION

Stretching can be a very powerful treatment option. There are many choices when it comes to choosing the most effective stretching technique. Basic stretching techniques involve the choice between static and dynamic stretching, performed actively or passively. The best choice likely depends upon the unique circumstances of each client. Beyond the choice of static versus dynamic stretching, other stretching options exist, such as pin and stretch, and advanced neural inhibition stretches: CR, AC, and CRAC stretching techniques.

Review Questions

1. What are the soft tissues that can be elongated by stretching?
2. List and define the two types of tissue tension.
3. In simple terms, describe the basic manner in which a stretch is performed.
4. Describe the concept of multiplane stretching.
5. What negative effect might occur if a stretch is performed too quickly or too forcefully?
6. In what ways might a client warm up tissues for the purpose of stretching without first engaging in physical activity? Please give several examples.
7. Describe the procedure for static stretching.
8. Describe the procedure for dynamic stretching.
9. Describe the purpose of, and an advantage to, the pin and stretch technique.
10. What are the names and mechanisms of the two neural inhibition stretches?
11. What is the protocol for combining both contract relax (CR) and agonist contract (AC) stretching?

6

 Deeper Thoughts

Given the many different approaches to stretching discussed in this chapter, how might a therapist determine which method to use on a client? Is there anything you can think of that would lead you to choose one technique over another for a given situation? Think of an occasion in your own life where you were either shown a stretch or were stretched by a professional that was intended to help you. Was it adequate? Did it accomplish the intended goal? Do you think another technique covered in this chapter would have achieved better results? Why or why not?

CHAPTER 7

Body Mechanics for the Manual Therapist*

Overview

This chapter offers a set of ten guidelines designed to create healthy body mechanics when delivering massage or other forms of manual or movement therapy. These guidelines help us to maximize our efficiency while working by showing and explaining how to use the laws of physics to work for us instead of having them work against us. These ten guidelines are divided into three major categories: (1) equipment, (2) positioning the body, and (3) performing the massage stroke.

The section on equipment discusses the importance of the height and width of the table, as well as the quality and quantity of the lotion used. Our discussion on positioning the body addresses how to properly bend the body, align the feet, align the head, and stack the joints of the upper extremity. And the section on performing the massage stroke explains the importance of generating force from the larger proximal muscles of the body instead of the smaller distal ones, how to determine the optimal direction for the line of force, and the advantages of using a larger contact whenever possible as well as bracing/double-supporting the contact. The purpose of these guidelines is to help the manual therapist to work smarter instead of working harder.

Chapter Outline

Introduction
Category 1: Equipment
Category 2: Positioning the Body
Category 3: Performing the Massage Stroke
Summary

Chapter Objectives

After completing this chapter, the student/therapist should be able to perform the following:
1. Define the key terms of this chapter.
2. Explain the importance of table height and table width to the efficient delivery of force.
3. Discuss using internal versus external forces when generating pressure.
4. Explain the importance of the lotion to the delivery of force.
5. Compare and contrast the relative merits of the stoop and squat bends.
6. Discuss the concept of core alignment to the delivery of force.
7. Discuss the relationship between foot position and delivery of force.
8. List and discuss the three positions of the feet.
9. Discuss the importance of the posture of the neck and head.
10. Explain the importance of stacking the joints when performing massage.
11. Discuss the importance of proximal versus distal generation of force.
12. Discuss the importance of the direction of force of a massage stroke.
13. Discuss the importance of using larger versus smaller contacts on the client.
14. Explain why double-supporting the contact is helpful.

*This chapter is modified from Muscolino JE: Work smarter, not harder: body mechanics for massage therapists, *Massage Ther J* Winter:2-16, 2006. Photos by Yanik Chauvin.

Key Terms

Body mechanics	Head position	Slide
Brace	Internal force	Squat bend
Closed-packed position	Joint compression forces	Squat bend with the trunk
Contact	Line of force	inclined forward
Core alignment	Longitudinal stance	Squat bend with the trunk
Direction of force	Lotion	vertically positioned
Distal generation of force	Open-packed position	Stacked joints
Double-support	Pressure	Stoop bend
Drag	Proximal generation of force	Transverse stance
External force	Sagittal plane stance	Weight
Frontal plane stance	Self-support	

INTRODUCTION

Regardless of the technique employed, the essence of all forms of manual therapy is the delivery of pressure—in other words, force—into the tissues of our clients. The efficiency with which we achieve this is crucial, not only to the quality of therapeutic care that we give our clients, but also to our own health and longevity in the field. To examine the efficiency with which our body works, we must study the mechanics of our body; therefore this field is called body mechanics.

Understanding and applying the fundamentals of good body mechanics is simple. We need to apply the laws of physics to our body. The same laws of physics that rule all physical matter, including the moon and stars, governs the forces that our body generates and to which our body is subjected. If we work with these laws of physics, we can generate greater forces with less fatigue, effortlessly working on our clients, and subject our body to less force. But if we work against the laws of physics, generating the force necessary to do our work will be more fatiguing, and our body will be subjected to greater forces that may injure us.

Unfortunately, the study of body mechanics is often given insufficient attention in the world of manual therapy. As a result, many new graduates and established therapists alike are often ill-equipped to do deep tissue work without *muscling* the massage via excessive effort. Instead of working smarter, they work harder, resulting in a high number of injuries. Many of these injuries force otherwise able and successful therapists to prematurely leave the field. Furthermore, many therapists leave the field not because of overt injuries, but because of the physical burnout that occurs from the physicality of doing soft tissue manipulation on a regular basis. Performing soft tissue manipulation can be hard work, especially when done with poor technique! The use of good body mechanics does not eliminate physical stress to the body, but it does minimize it, allowing for a longer and more successful career as a manual therapist.

The goal of this chapter is to offer a set of ten guidelines designed to create healthy body mechanics. Using good body mechanics is important all the time; however, it is crucial when performing deep tissue work, which requires a greater production and delivery of pressure. For this reason, these guidelines are especially recommended to manual therapists who deliver deep pressure on a regular basis. Although this chapter does not address all aspects and facets of body mechanics for manual therapists, it does provide a number of essential basics. As much as following rules and guidelines is important, keep in mind that manual therapy is not only a science, it is also an art. Therefore the following guidelines need to be incorporated into the particular style of the therapist.

CATEGORY 1: EQUIPMENT

Guideline #1: Lower Table Height

Table height is probably the number one factor determining the efficiency of the therapist's force delivery. The proper height of the table is determined by a combination of factors, including the following:

- Height of the therapist
- Size of the client
- Positioning of the client on the table (supine, prone, or side lying)
- Contact being used

When it comes to the production and delivery of force with less effort, if we are working on the "top" of the client's body (the surface that faces the ceiling), the table must be low. Setting the table low allows the therapist to use his/her body weight to create force. Weight is merely a measure of the force that gravity exerts upon mass; given that gravity is an external force that never tires, why not take advantage of it?

When a therapist generates force to work on a client, that force can be created in two ways, internally within the body by muscles, or externally from gravity. Creation of internal force by musculature requires effort on our part and can be fatiguing. However, the creation of force by gravity requires no effort. If the goal is to create force with the minimum effort possible, it is desirable to use gravity as much as possible. However, gravity does not work horizontally or diagonally; it only works vertically downward. Therefore it only works if the therapist's body weight is literally above the client. This requires the client to be placed below the therapist; hence the necessity of low table height. Of course, the contact that the therapist employs makes a big difference. If we are using thumb or finger pads, the table must be at its lowest height. If, instead, we are using the palm, it can be set higher. And if we are using the elbow or forearm, then the table can be set even higher.

BOX 7-1

Although there is not one exact proper height of a table, as a rule for deep work when using the thumb or finger pads as the contact, the top of the table should be no higher than the bottom of the therapist's patella (knee joint).

7

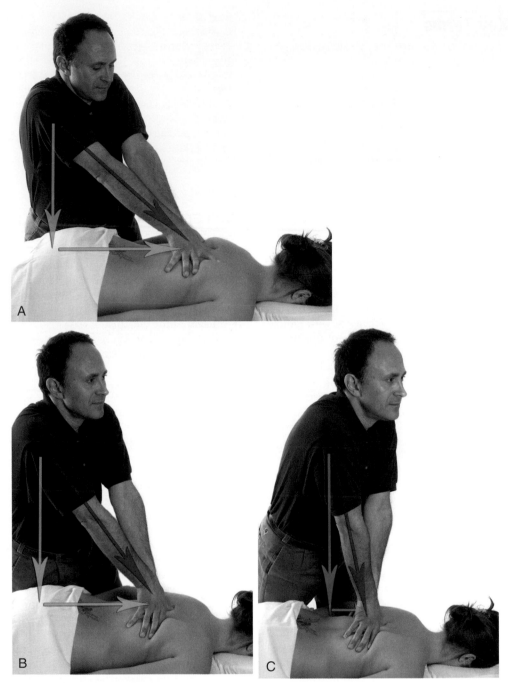

Figure 7-1 Illustration of a therapist working on the "top" surface of a client with the table set at three different heights. In each photo, the *blue arrow* represents the force through the therapist's upper extremity into the client, and the *green vertical arrow* represents the component of that force that is due to gravity (the *green horizontal arrow* represents the force of body weight of the therapist that is lost because it is not purely vertical). Note that the vertical component vector is least when the table is set high **(A)**, and it is greatest when the table is set low **(C)**.

With the client located below the therapist, the therapist does not need to expend much effort; rather it is only necessary to *lean into* the client, letting the therapist's body weight generate forceful deep pressure (Figure 7-1). Given that the greatest weight of the body is located in the core (i.e., the trunk and pelvis) of the body, it is the trunk and pelvis that must be positioned above the client when the therapist leans in.

When generating deep pressure by leaning into the client, it is important for the therapist to maintain a position of **self-support.** This means that even though the therapist is leaning into the client, if the client moved or the therapist needed to remove the pressure from the client, the therapist could quickly stop leaning on the client and regain balance and be able to support his or her body again. Working from a position of self-support maintains the therapist's control and balance, increasing the effectiveness of the session as well as the client's comfort. This self-support can be maintained via a strong and stable stance of the lower extremities. (This is discussed more fully in Guideline #5.)

BOX 7-2

To test the principle of table height at home, place a bathroom scale on a chair or massage table at various heights. At each height, simply lean into the scale and read the force that you are generating on the scale (Figure 7-2). If the scale is low enough that you are directly above it, note how much pressure you can effortlessly generate by passively leaning into the scale. Try to create the same reading on the scale through muscular effort when the scale is located on a higher surface. The difference in effort required is the difference in work that the therapist must do. Multiply this by how many minutes or hours the therapist works per week/month/year, and the cumulative effect of a table set too high can be appreciated.

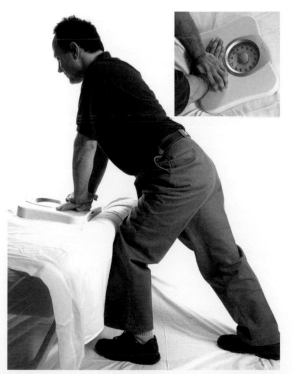

Figure 7-2 Demonstration of an easy method using an ordinary bathroom scale to determine how much effort is necessary at different heights to generate force in a client's body.

In addition to the height of the table, the table width must also be considered. The wider the table, the more difficult it is for the therapist to position body weight over the client; if the client is located at the center of the table, the client is farther away from the therapist. For this reason, a narrow table is more desirable when it comes to using body weight. However, a narrower table might be less comfortable, especially for larger clients. A solution is to use a contour table wherein the width of the table varies to match the contour of the client's body, wide for the client's shoulders, but narrow near the waist so the therapist can be closer to the client. An alternative solution is to use a table with armrests that swing out of the way when closer access is desired. A contour table with armrests would be ideal.

Electric Lift Table. When working with a table set lower, there is another factor to consider. A low table height is ideal when deep pressure is desired and/or thumb/finger pads are the contact being used. However, it is actually easier to work with a higher table height when light pressure is being applied; it requires less effort for lighter pressure if you stand straighter and apply pressure into the client with strokes that are more horizontally oriented. A higher table height is also optimal when we are using the elbow/forearm as the contact. If the table is set low in these scenarios, you either must bend to reach lower or must widen the stance of the lower extremities to bring the upper body down to the height of the client. Between these two choices, widening the stance is preferable; however, it requires greater effort than simply standing upright. For this reason, ideal table height varies during a treatment session based upon the work that is being done and the contact being employed. The solution to this dilemma is to use an electric lift table. Although electric lift tables are viewed as extravagant by many in the manual therapy profession, in my opinion, they are a necessity. Being able to change the height of the table during a session by merely pressing on a foot pedal enables deeper pressure to be delivered with less effort on a low table, and allows you to stand straighter when doing lighter work with the table set higher. It also allows you to alternate between contacts with ease. This allows for better sessions therapeutically for the client and healthier and less fatiguing sessions for the therapist. In the long run, the benefits of an electric lift table far outweigh the increased cost of the initial purchase.

Guideline #2: Use Less Lotion

For beginning therapists, the type and amount of lotion used is often part of the problem. The two competing properties of a lotion are slide and drag. Slide allows the therapist to slide/glide along the client's skin without excessive friction or drag. Drag creates friction, which facilitates translation of the therapist's pressure into the client's tissues. Generally, the more slide that a lotion possesses, the less drag it possesses, and vice versa. When employing deeper pressure, choosing a lotion that offers sufficient drag is important. It is also important to not use too much of the lotion, because the slide factor will increase and the therapist's pressure will translate into slipping and sliding *along* the client's skin instead of delivering pressure *into* the client's tissues. The general guideline for lotion is to use the least amount necessary for the client's comfort. Any amount greater than this decreases the efficiency of pressure delivery into the client. Although it varies from one product to another, generally, oil-based lotions tend to create

7

more slide and are not as efficient as water-based lotions for generating deeper pressure.

CATEGORY 2: POSITIONING THE BODY

Guideline #3: Bend Properly

Although the ideal body posture for delivering deep pressure with maximal efficiency is for you to be positioned directly above the client and delivering the force directly downward, this body posture is not usually possible to attain without some bending. The manner in which the therapist bends is extremely important, because bending tends to create postural imbalances that require effort to maintain and places stress upon the therapist's body. Bending postures can be divided into two general categories: the stoop bend and the squat bend.

Stoop Bend. The stoop bend, which involves flexing the trunk at the spinal joints to bring the body over the client,

is less healthy for the therapist. This is because it unbalances the therapist's body by moving the center of weight of the trunk from being balanced directly over the pelvis to being unsupported (Figure 7-3, *A*). In this position, the only reason that the therapist's trunk does not fall into full flexion is that the spinal extensor musculature must contract isometrically to maintain the partially flexed and imbalanced trunk posture. Furthermore, a stooped posture of spinal flexion places the spinal joints in their open-packed position. The open-packed position of a joint is its least stable position; therefore greater muscular contraction is necessary to stabilize the joints. The result is greater effort on the part of the spinal extensor musculature to maintain the stooped posture.

Squat Bend. A better alternative is the squat bend, which is achieved by flexing the hip and knee joints instead of the spinal joints. In a squat bend, the spine stays erect in its closed-packed position, which is its most stable position. This requires less stabilization contraction effort by the spinal extensor musculature and is healthier for the spine.

BOX 7-3

To Shrug or Not to Shrug?

It seems universally accepted that when doing massage therapy, it is bad body mechanics to work with our shoulders up at our ears—in other words, the scapulae elevated at the scapulocostal joints—giving what could be called "shrugged shoulders." I must admit that I accepted this sacred cow of body mechanics for many years. After all, we always tell our clients that they should relax and let their shoulders drop. And who doesn't have tight muscles of scapular elevation (upper trapezius, levator scapulae, and rhomboids), which are most likely due to our stress patterns of holding our shoulders up in an uptight posture? Therefore it seems perfectly reasonable that when we see massage therapy students or practicing therapists with their shoulders up at their ears while working on their clients, we instinctively tell them to relax and let their shoulders down.

But recently, I started noticing that my shoulders were often up high when working on patients/clients. This puzzled me because I felt relaxed while doing these massages. Yet, I told myself that shrugged shoulders could not be right, so I brought them down and continued with the massage. However, I soon found myself with my shoulders elevated again. So, a doubt began to enter my mind, but remained in the shadows. Once in a while I would think about it for a minute or two, but I never actually came out and said to anyone that shrugged shoulders could be okay. It was when I was demonstrating proper body posture/mechanics while teaching a deep tissue workshop in Tucson, Arizona, that a particularly astute participant pinned me down with the question, "Is working with elevated shoulders always bad?" I was a bit shocked to hear myself answer, "No." It was the first time I ever said that out loud. It seemed heretical, and I am sure that a number of readers right now are shaking their heads and wondering how I could be saying this.

What I realized at that moment is that working with shrugged shoulders is not necessarily right or wrong. It depends on why our shoulders are up there. Most of the

time, it is likely that our shoulders are shrugged because our table is set too high (see Guideline #1), and we are trying in vain to get over our client. In this scenario, we actively contract our scapular elevators to raise our shoulders. Staying like this for more than a moment or two will certainly lead to tight and painful muscles of scapular elevation. In this circumstance, working with shrugged shoulders is definitely bad. However, when the table is set low and we are directly over the client, if we simply lean into the client and relax our scapular muscles, then our shoulders will naturally be pushed up toward our ears.

As a law of physics states, "For every action, there is an equal and opposite reaction." If we are pressing down on our client, our client is pressing back up on us, pushing our shoulders up. In this scenario, if we do not want our shoulders to rise in the air, then we would have to exert muscular effort to hold them down, whereas letting them elevate would be the more relaxed and effortless posture to assume, and (dare I say it…?) good body mechanics!

The one potential drawback to allowing the shoulders to passively rise is that the shoulder girdle is slightly less rigid, and as such, a small amount of pressure and control might be lost when transmitting force from the core through the shoulder girdle to the client. However, I believe this loss is negligible and, depending upon the circumstance, would likely be outweighed by the benefit of having relaxed musculature. Furthermore, having a relaxed shoulder girdle creates a more fluid base from which to work, decreasing the possibility that the client may sense rigidity in our technique.

When working on your clients, examine your own shoulder posture (having a mirror in the massage room is an excellent way to monitor your posture). If your shoulders are up high, feel whether you are actively working to keep them up there or whether you are relaxed. If you are working hard to hold them up there, then I recommend that you lower your table and relax your shoulders. However, if they are comfortably relaxed up there, then maybe there is nothing wrong with letting them be there!

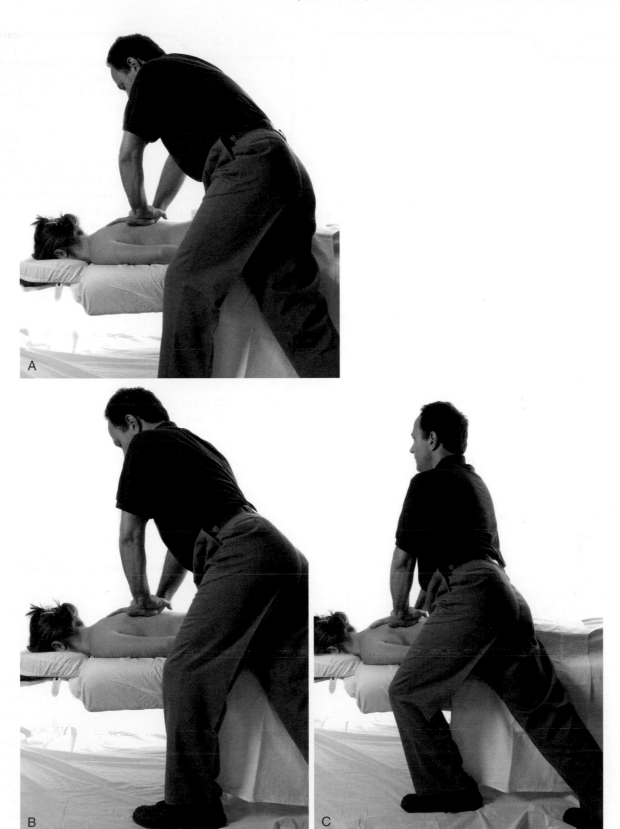

Figure 7-3 A shows the stoop bend, in which the therapist bends by flexing the spinal joints of the trunk. Of the three methods of bending, the stoop bend is least healthy for the therapist's spine. **B** shows the squat bend with the trunk inclined forward, and **C** shows the squat bend with the trunk vertical. The squat bend with the trunk vertical is biomechanically the least stressful on the therapist's spine and should generally be used when bending over a client.

BOX 7-4

In addition to flexion of the hip joints and knee joints, the squat bend also requires the ankle joints to dorsiflex (the dorsum of the legs move toward the dorsum of the feet).

BOX 7-5

The closed-packed position of a joint is the position in which it is most stable. This is usually a combination of the joint surfaces having maximal contact and the ligaments and joint capsules being most taut.

BOX 7-6

It is interesting that even though most everyone knows that it is healthier for our back if we bend with our knees, so many people do not follow this advice and instead fall into a stoop bend. There must be a reason for this. As it turns out, although the squat bend is healthier for the back, it requires more energy expenditure than the stoop bend. Furthermore, even though the squat bend is healthier for the back, it does place a greater stress on the knee joints. All things being equal, it is usually more important to protect the spinal joints. However, when applying these bending guidelines to each therapist's needs, the stress upon the knee joints must be factored in. If a therapist has unhealthy knee joints, a stoop bend may be the lesser of two evils.

There are two squat bend methods:

1. Squat bend with the trunk inclined forward
2. Squat bend with the trunk maintaining its vertical posture

Between these two, maintaining a vertically positioned trunk is preferable, because a squat bend with the trunk inclined forward still places the trunk in an imbalanced posture in which its center of weight is unsupported (see Figure 7-3, *B*). This requires spinal extensor musculature contraction to prevent the trunk from falling into flexion, as well as hip joint extensor musculature contraction to maintain the flexed anterior tilt posture of the pelvis at the hip joints.

The squat bend with the trunk vertically positioned maintains the trunk in a balanced posture, such that its center of weight is aligned and supported over the pelvis (see Figure 7-3, *C*). This eliminates the need for spinal extensor musculature contraction to keep the trunk from falling into flexion and hip joint extensor musculature to maintain pelvic posture.

The key to creating a vertical squat bend instead of an inclined squat bend is the degree of knee joint flexion. As the hip joints are flexed to achieve the squat bend position, the pelvis anteriorly tilts, inclining the trunk forward. However, the more the knee joints are flexed as the hip joints are flexed, the easier it is to keep the trunk vertical. This is "bending with the knees" as we often hear. Hence, a squat bend with the trunk vertically aligned maintains the spine in its most stable closed-packed posture, and maintains the trunk in a balanced and supported posture over the lower body. This allows the therapist to work and deliver pressure efficiently while maintaining a healthy spine. It is often not possible for the therapist to have a perfectly vertical posture to the back when doing massage, but the closer to vertical, the healthier it is for the spine and spinal muscles.

Guideline #4: Align the Core

It has been stated that the key to delivering a strong force is for the therapist to use the weight of the core as much as possible. The importance of core (i.e., trunk and pelvis) positioning was discussed in Guideline #1. However, the orientation and alignment of the core, not just the position, are also critically important to efficiently delivering pressure. As a rule, for body weight to be behind the pressure that is being delivered to the client, your trunk and pelvis must face the same direction as that of the pressure being applied. An easy way to determine your core alignment is to look at your navel. Whatever direction your navel is facing, your core is facing. It is often recommended that the therapist picture a laser beam emanating from their navel. That laser beam should be as parallel and close as possible to the line of the stroke being delivered into the client's body. If the laser beam is in line with the stroke, then the core is aligned with the stroke.

BOX 7-7

Some therapists prefer to look at where their anterior superior iliac spines (ASISs) are facing instead of where their navel is facing to determine the alignment of their core.

For example, if the force of a soft tissue stroke is being applied across the client's body, then your navel should be facing across the client's body in the identical direction. If, on the other hand, the force of the soft tissue stroke is being applied longitudinally along the length of the client's body, then your navel should be similarly oriented. Figure 7-4 demonstrates a few examples of proper orientation and alignment of the core. In these examples, note the change in orientation and alignment of the therapist's core to match the direction of force delivery. Furthermore, note that when working from a seated position, the therapist's elbow is tucked in front of the core of his body. This is best accomplished by adducting and laterally rotating the arm at the glenohumeral joint. This naturally brings the elbow in front of the core, where it can be tucked (close to

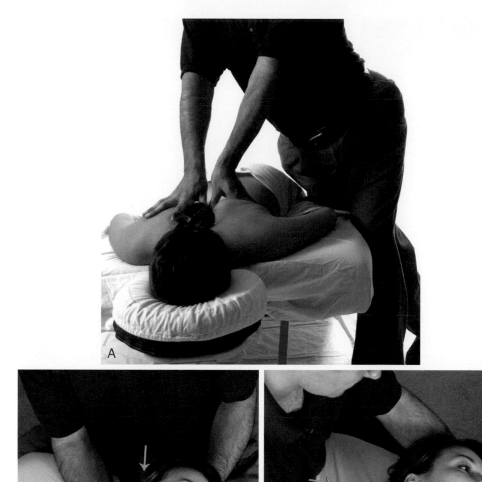

7

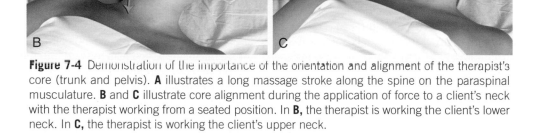

Figure 7-4 Demonstration of the importance of the orientation and alignment of the therapist's core (trunk and pelvis). **A** illustrates a long massage stroke along the spine on the paraspinal musculature. **B** and **C** illustrate core alignment during the application of force to a client's neck with the therapist working from a seated position. In **B,** the therapist is working the client's lower neck. In **C,** the therapist is working the client's upper neck.

being) inside the anterior superior iliac spine (ASIS). When the therapist now leans in with his core, his body weight is transmitted right through his forearm and hand into the client.

Note: When aligning the core of the body longitudinally up the table as seen in Figure 7-4, *A*, it is important to rotate the pelvis from the hip joints and not to rotate the spine. The positioning of your feet is also important and is addressed in the next guideline.

Guideline #5: Position the Feet
Thus far, much has been said about the importance of the positioning, orientation, and alignment of your core. However, there is an old adage in sports that says, "It's all in the

BOX 7-8

Aligning the core along the direction of force is largely a matter of proper positioning of the feet. This is discussed in more detail in Guideline #5.

7

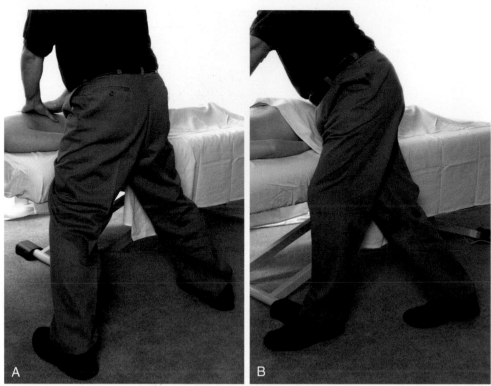

Figure 7-5 The two positions of the therapist's feet relative to the table, and therefore the client's body, when doing bodywork. **A,** The transverse stance. **B,** The longitudinal stance.

footwork." This is no less true when doing bodywork. Your footwork is crucially important, for both aligning and positioning the core and also for pushing off to generate pressure. To achieve all these things, let's look at the placement of the feet. Generally, the direction that the feet are facing is the direction that the core is facing. Therefore, if it is desired to change the orientation of the core, the easiest way to accomplish this is to change the orientation of the feet. Furthermore, if the feet are not positioned correctly, it is not possible to generate force from a lower extremity by plantar flexing a foot against the ground, as well as extending from the knee and hip joints, to push our body weight into the client.

Positioning of the feet can be divided into two general categories—transverse stance and longitudinal stance. Squaring off the feet perpendicular to the length of the table is called the transverse stance, and orienting the feet parallel to the length of the table is called the longitudinal stance. The transverse stance is effective for delivering pressure transversely across the client's body, because it orients your core in that direction (Figure 7-5, *A*); however, it is ineffective when working longitudinally up the client's body, because the core is not facing that direction. On the other hand, the longitudinal stance is effective for delivering pressure longitudinally along the client's body, because it orients your core to face that way (see Figure 7-5, *B*); however, it is ineffective when working transversely across the client's body, because the core is not facing that direction.

Further discussion is warranted regarding the precise orientation of your feet relative to each other. The positioning of the feet relative to each other can generally be divided into the frontal plane stance and the sagittal plane stance. In the frontal plane stance, they are located next to each other in the frontal plane, and may be close together or far apart. In the sagittal plane stance, as its name implies, one foot is farther anterior than the other in the sagittal plane.

An inherent weakness with the frontal plane position of the feet (Figure 7-6, *A*) is that the base of support created by the feet is not very long in the sagittal plane from anterior to posterior. This makes it difficult to maintain balance of the upper body over the feet with movements of the pelvis and trunk in the sagittal plane as you lean forward into the client. For example, if you try to lean into the client by bringing the pelvis and trunk forward (bending at the hip joints), your body weight is projected anterior to the base of the feet and is not supported and balanced. If you compensate for the anterior weight shift of the trunk by shifting the weight of the pelvis posteriorly in an effort to counterbalance the body, then your overall body weight shifts posteriorly and is no longer sufficiently anterior to be over the client's body. In this position, body weight cannot be used effectively to generate force.

Similarly, the therapist is unbalanced and unsupported in this position if the core of the body is propelled forward by pushing off from the feet. The sagittal plane position of the feet is superior in this regard, because the rear foot can be used to push off the ground and project the therapist's body weight forward, while the therapist's body weight is still balanced and supported over the front foot. Hence, the sagittal plane position of the feet provides a stance allowing for balance of the body between the rear foot and front foot. This is especially valuable when performing strokes of any length. It should be added though that if the width of the stance in the sagittal plane becomes too wide, it actually decreases the ease of

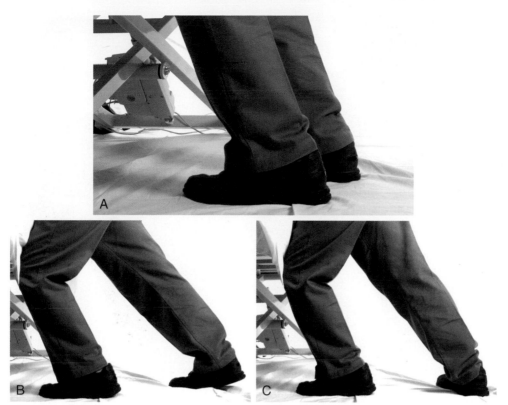

Figure 7-6 Illustration of three positions of the therapist's feet. **A,** The feet are positioned in the frontal plane. **B** and **C,** The feet are positioned in the sagittal plane with one foot in front and one in back. In **B,** the two feet are approximately parallel. In **C,** the rear foot is pointed nearly perpendicular to the front foot.

shifting the balance of our body weight from one foot to the other. For this reason, it is important to also pay attention to the width of the sagittal plane stance.

When positioning oneself in the sagittal plane stance, there are then two choices for the orientation of the rear foot: it can be approximately parallel with or approximately perpendicular to the front foot. Between these two choices, having the rear foot facing approximately the same direction as the front foot (see Figure 7-6, B) is the superior position, because it places the powerful sagittally oriented ankle joint plantar flexor musculature (soleus, gastrocnemius, tibialis posterior, flexors digitorum and hallucis longus, and fibularis longus and brevis), knee joint extensor musculature (quadriceps femoris), and hip joint extensor musculature (hamstrings, adductor magnus, and posterior gluteals) in line with the direction of the stroke. When generating pressure into the client by pushing off with the rear foot of the sagittal plane stance, it is important to generate pressure from all three joints of the lower extremity: the ankle, knee, and hip joints, not just the ankle joint.

The position in Figure 7-6, C, wherein the rear foot is oriented perpendicular to the front foot (and indeed the entire body), loses the orientation of the powerful sagittally-oriented musculature just mentioned and also places the two lower extremities at odds with each other during force generation, because they face in different directions.

There is one final aspect of feet placement that should be addressed. There is no rule that states the feet must be planted at the beginning of a stroke and stay in that planted position for the entire stroke; the feet can be moved. With a short stroke

BOX 7-9

An advantage to having the two feet oriented in opposite directions, such as in Figure 7-6,C, is that it allows the therapist to easily change the direction that the body is facing. Being able to change the direction of the body is extremely important in martial arts; this is why this position is so often employed there. However, for delivering pressure during bodywork, this advantage does not outweigh the disadvantage of losing the strength possible when the feet are oriented in the same direction.

or compression applied to one location, there is little or no need to move the feet. However, with a longer stroke, if the feet are not moved, you will have to reach out horizontally farther away from the initial base of support of the feet. Support and balance will be lost, the trunk cannot be maintained vertically, and therefore body weight can no longer be used as effectively to generate force downward with gravity. To prevent this, especially during longer strokes, it is important to move the feet.

Guideline #6: Position the Head

An often overlooked aspect of body mechanics is the head position of the therapist, or more specifically, the position of

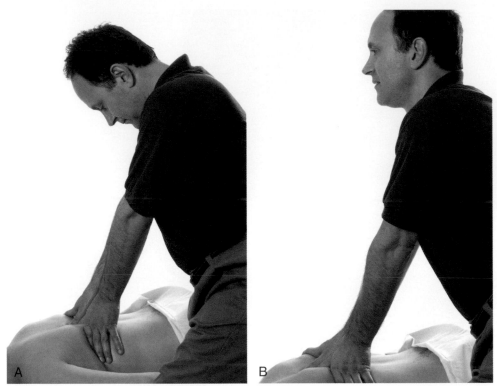

Figure 7-7 Two postures of the therapist's head during bodywork. **A,** The therapist is flexing the neck and head to look at the client as the stroke is being performed. **B,** The therapist is holding the head in a more balanced posture over the trunk.

the therapist's neck and head. The position of the neck and head has little to do with the direct generation and delivery of force while performing a massage. Therefore it makes sense that the therapist should hold the neck and head in whatever position is least stressful for the tissues of the body. The healthiest posture is to hold the head over the trunk so that the center of weight of the head is balanced over the trunk. This position requires little or no muscular effort by neck muscles to support it. Unfortunately, many therapists have a habit of flexing the neck and head at the spinal joints to look down at their client while they work. This unbalances the posture of the head such that its center of weight is no longer over the trunk and instead is over thin air. Therefore it should fall into flexion until the chin hits the chest. The only reason that this does not occur is because the extensor musculature of the neck isometrically contracts to keep the head from falling anteriorly into flexion. Over time, this leads to pain and spasm in the posterior neck musculature. If it is necessary for you to look at the client during a stroke, then this posture is necessary and correct to assume. However, most of the time there is little or no need for it; you even can close your eyes and visualize the structure of the client under your hands. So it is a good reminder for you to occasionally focus on the posture of your neck and head to be sure they are in a posture that is as easy and relaxed as possible (Figure 7-7).

It should be added that it is not possible to place the head in a balanced position over the trunk of the body if the trunk is not vertical or at least near vertical in position. In other words, if we stoop bend or if we squat bend with our trunk inclined forward, it is not possible to position the head over the trunk. This is another disadvantage of these trunk positions. Feet positioning also plays into this scenario. The wider

the stance of the feet in the sagittal plane, the more inclined our trunk position tends to become. This is another reason that we should try to avoid unnecessarily wide sagittal plane positioning of the feet.

When it is not possible to balance the head over the trunk because the trunk is not sufficiently vertical, we have two choices. We can contract our posterior extensor musculature to hold the imbalanced posture of the head. As stated, this can lead to overuse and eventual injury to the musculature. Or we can let our head relax into flexion, allowing the chin to approximate the chest. This relieves the posterior extensor musculature of the neck from having to work to maintain the imbalanced posture of the head, but it also places our neck into a flexion posture that, if done too often, will gradually stretch out the posterior passive ligaments and other fascial tissues. Weakening these fascial structures will eventually increase the workload of the extensor musculature because they will have lost the assistance of the passive tension of the fascia.

Guideline #7: Stack the Joints
Whether the force behind the stroke is created by muscular effort on your part or is due to using body weight, this force must be transmitted through your upper extremity joints (elbow, wrist, fingers, thumb). For this force to travel through the upper extremity joints without loss of strength, it is important that the joints are stacked. Stacked joints are extended and placed in a straight line as seen in Figure 7-8, *A*. This is usually best accomplished by adducting and laterally rotating the arms at the glenohumeral joints, bringing the elbows in front of the core of the body. In this manner, you can deliver pressure for the stroke in a straight line from the core of the body through the stacked joints of the upper extremity to the contact on the client.

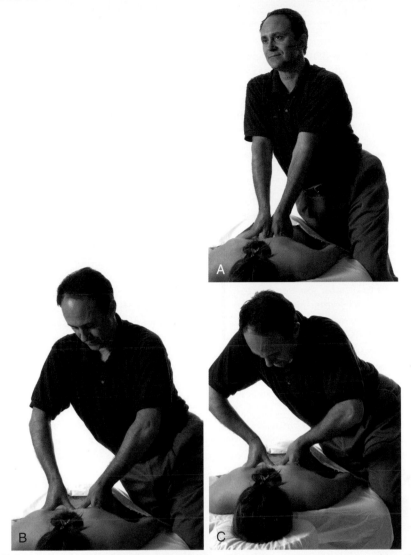

Figure 7-8 Demonstration of force delivery through a therapist's upper extremities that are stacked and not stacked. **A** shows a therapist who has the elbow, wrist, and thumb joints of the upper extremities fully stacked. **B** shows the therapist with the elbow joints unstacked (i.e., flexed). **C,** Collapsing at unstacked upper extremity joints reduces the force delivered into the client.

If you do this as you lean and/or push into the client by pushing off with the back foot, there is little or no loss of strength, and less muscular effort is necessary. However, when your upper extremity joints are not stacked (i.e., they are flexed), the force generated that must pass through them will probably be lost to the client, because the joints of the upper extremity tend to collapse further into flexion. Thus the force that was supposed to be delivered into the client's tissues is lost in creating movement of the therapist's body at the shoulder, elbow, wrist, and finger or thumb joints (see Figures 7-8, B-C). Further, the unwanted motion that occurs at the joint might produce a torque force that will, over time, likely cause arthritic degenerative changes at the joint. This is especially true of the thumb joints.

Note: It is not necessary to bring the elbows all the way to the center of the trunk. This could actually be injurious to the elbow region because a (cubitus valgus–abduction posture of the fore-arm relative to the arm) torque will occur at the elbow, placing greater stress upon the soft tissues around the medial epicondylar region to stabilize the elbow joint. Simply adducting and laterally rotating the glenohumeral joint sufficient to place the (upper) arm in front of the lateral aspect of the trunk/core is sufficient.

It is possible to transmit force through unstacked, flexed upper extremity joints without loss of strength. However, it requires greater effort because muscles around the unstacked joints must be isometrically contracted to stabilize the joints, preventing them from collapsing. For example, if the elbows are bent (flexed) as the stroke is being performed, then the triceps brachii musculature must engage to stabilize the elbow joint from falling into further flexion. Over time, this can become fatiguing for the triceps brachii. This results in greater effort and is less efficient for the therapist, so should be avoided when possible.

CATEGORY 3: PERFORMING THE MASSAGE STROKE

Guideline #8: Generate Force Proximally

It has been stated that use of body weight via the external force of gravity is recommended whenever possible because it requires little or no effort. However, when it is necessary for you to use internal muscular effort to generate the therapeutic force for the treatment technique, there is a choice of which muscles to use.

BOX 7-10

Even perfectly stacked joints do not eliminate all effort and stress to the body. Although markedly less than with unstacked joints, there is still some contraction effort on the part of the musculature to stabilize the stacked joints. Furthermore, because all of the therapist's force is efficiently transmitted through the joints, stacked joints are subjected to greater joint compression forces than are unstacked joints. However, by keeping the joints straight in line with the force being transmitted, all force from your trunk is transmitted without loss of strength to the client.

When choosing between small and large muscles, it is always advantageous for you to generate the force using larger muscles of the body. A smaller muscle cannot generate the same maximal force that a larger muscle can. Furthermore, to the degree that a smaller muscle does generate the same force as a larger muscle, it requires a much greater effort to achieve this.

Looking at the muscles of the upper extremity from distal to proximal, it is evident that smaller muscles are located more distally and larger muscles are located more proximally. For example, the intrinsic finger joint muscles within the hand are smaller than the wrist joint muscles within the forearm, which are smaller than the elbow joint muscles within the arm, which are smaller than the shoulder joint muscles within the trunk. For this reason, whenever possible, it is recommended that a proximal generation of force from the trunk is done instead of a distal generation of force from the upper extremities.

In addition to the larger proximal core muscles of the trunk, large muscle groups of the lower extremities can also be engaged to create great force with little effort. By placing the feet appropriately, the therapist can push off the ground using powerful ankle joint plantar flexors and knee and hip joint extensors to generate strength of force that can be delivered into the client. (See Guideline #5 for more information about proper positioning of your feet.) Furthermore, just as the core of the body should be behind (in other words, in line with the force of the stroke that is transmitted through the upper extremities), the lower extremities should be oriented in the same line. The line of force through the therapist's body should travel in one straight line from the feet to the core and through the upper extremities into the client's body.

BOX 7-11

Putting a number of the these guidelines together, it can be seen that the most efficient delivery of pressure into the client is a straight (stacked) line of force that travels unbroken from the therapist's lower extremities and core, into their upper extremities, and then into the client. This is true when generating force to press into the client. However, having a stacked line of force is just as important and efficient when the therapist is pulling on the client instead. Although pulling strokes are generally not employed as often as compression strokes, they are extremely valuable in certain instances and should be applied with the same efficiency of body mechanics.

Guideline #9: Direct Force Perpendicular to the Contour of the Client's Body

When we discussed table height in Guideline #1, it was emphasized that the most efficient way to use gravity is to direct the force vertically downward into the "top" surface of the client. However, we are not always working the top surface of the client's body; sometimes we are working into the side surface of the client. And when we are working the top surface of the client, the contour of the surface we are working is not always horizontally flat. Therefore, although a vertically downward application of force is the most efficient way to use gravity, it is not always the most efficient direction to transmit force into the client's body.

For example, when a client is prone, the client's back has contours created by the curves of the spinal column. Taking these contours into account, the therapist must change the direction of force so that it is perpendicular to the contour of the client's body at the point of contact. This means that the therapist is not always pressing directly vertically downward; rather the therapist might have to direct the force diagonally so that it is perpendicular to the client's body surface. And if the side surface of the client's body is being worked when the client is prone or supine, then it is optimal for the therapist's line of force to be horizontal; in this case, there is no assistance from gravity with the force generation of the stroke. For these cases, it is important to realize that the most powerful and efficient delivery of force into the client's body is the force that is applied perpendicular to the contour of the body surface being worked. Any deviation from perpendicular involves some loss of strength and efficiency, because some of the force is transmitted into sliding along the tissue instead of pressing into it.

BOX 7-12

Trigonometric formulas (sine, cosine, and tangent) can be used to determine the exact amount of force that is lost when a massage stroke is not delivered perpendicular to the surface of the client's body.

To illustrate this idea, Figure 7-9 shows three different applications of force for a therapist working on a client's back. Note that in each case, the force is applied perpendicular to the contour of the region of the back that is being worked. If you try this in your practice, I believe that you will intuitively find it to be the easiest way to generate pressure with the least effort. A necessary addendum to this concept is that if a long stroke is being done—for example, one that covers the length of the spine—the contours encountered during that stroke vary. For maximal efficiency, it is necessary for the therapist to adjust to these contours by changing the direction that pressure is applied; this necessitates changing the orientation of the core and likely also necessitates changing the position of the feet.

Applying this concept to working along the side-wall of the client's body, generating force into the client's tissue perpendicular to the side-wall would require the therapist to orient the upper extremities horizontally. This obviates the possibility of utilizing gravity and body weight; therefore, force must be generated solely from musculature. In these cases, it is wise to generate the force from the large muscles of the lower extremity. This is best accomplished by using a wide sagittal stance in positioning the feet.

Guideline #10: Choose a Larger Contact Surface When Possible and Brace It

When deep pressure is being delivered, it must be transmitted into the client through whatever body part the therapist uses to contact the client. If the thumb or finger pads are used as the contact, the danger is that over time, continually transmitting deep pressure through the hands will damage these relatively small joints. To protect the therapist's hands against injury, it is important for the contact surface of the hand to be as large as possible. For example, working with the palm of the hand instead of the fingers or thumb allows for deeper pressure to be given with less chance of injury to the therapist. Working with the elbow or forearm allows for an even larger more powerful contact to be used.

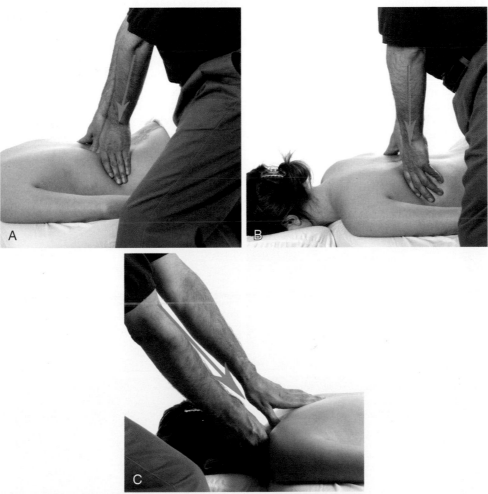

Figure 7-9 Illustration of three applications of force perpendicular to the contour of the body surface that is being worked. **A,** The thoracolumbar region is worked by applying the force diagonally in a cephalad direction (toward the head). **B,** The midthoracic region is worked by applying force vertically downward. **C,** The upper thoracic region is worked by applying the force diagonally in a caudal direction (toward the lower body).

The disadvantage to using a larger contact instead of the fingers or thumb is that larger contacts tend to be less sensitive, making it more difficult for the therapist to assess both the quality of the client's tissues and the response of the client tissues to the pressure of the treatment as the massage is performed. The appropriate contact at any point during the massage can only be determined by the therapist. If you like to use fingers or thumbs a lot, I recommend that you alternate between these contacts as often as possible. This distributes the stress load around the hand, giving each muscle, fascial tissue, and joint a chance to rest. Another good strategy to employ is to begin working an area by using smaller contacts so that assessment will be optimal. Then continue working the area with a larger contact. If desired, the final stroke or two can be done again with a smaller contact to reassess how the client's tissues have responded to the treatment rendered.

In addition to choosing a larger hand contact, it is important to brace or double-support the contact. This means that the two hands are working on the client together instead of separately. One hand should be placed somewhat over the other so that the contact hand on the client is stabilized and reinforced by the other hand (Figure 7-10). Another benefit of bracing/double-supporting the contact is that it strengthens the therapist's contact, allowing for a stronger and more efficient delivery of force into the client. Protecting the contact area of the hand is particularly needed when working with smaller contacts, such as the fingers or thumbs. Although double-supporting the contact means that less surface area of the client can be covered during a stroke, the benefits when doing deep tissue work more than compensate for this. Figure 7-10 illustrates four braced contacts of the therapist's hands upon the client.

BOX 7-13

For a therapist with a hyperextendable interphalangeal joint of the thumb, bracing the thumb is critically important to prevent it from collapsing into hyperextension.

SUMMARY

No matter what technique and style of delivery we have, manual therapy is hard work and physically stresses the body; this reality cannot be avoided. However, if we learn to work more efficiently, we can decrease these stresses. The proposed guidelines of this chapter are meant to help increase the efficiency of our work and thereby minimize the stress to our body. As you practice them, keep in mind that any change made in body mechanics will most likely feel awkward at first, simply because it is different. With time, applying these guidelines should become more comfortable. It is also important to realize that there are times when the application of one guideline somewhat contradicts the application of another guideline. These guidelines are ideals, and it is not always possible to achieve every one of them one hundred percent of the time. In these cases, it is best to find the optimal balance of the competing guidelines.

Although they are not comprehensive of all aspects of body mechanics for manual therapists, these ten guidelines are a

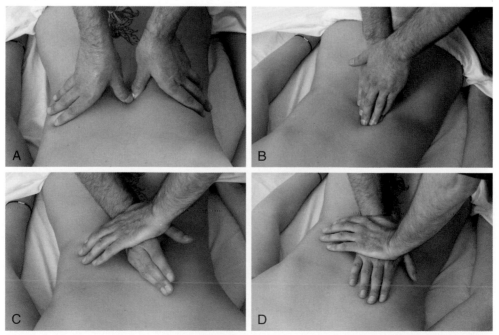

Figure 7-10 Four examples of a braced contact of a therapist's hands upon a client. **A,** Bracing the thumb. **B,** Bracing the fingers. **C,** Bracing the ulnar side of the hand. **D,** Bracing the palm of the hand.

solid foundation to build upon. Note that even though these guidelines were presented and discussed separately in this chapter, it is only by seamlessly weaving them into a cohesive whole that a fluid and efficient style for the delivery of bodywork can be achieved. Furthermore, by increasing the efficiency and decreasing the effort of our work, the quality of our work will likely improve as well. Increasing efficiency is learning to work smarter instead of working harder.

Review Questions

1. What two methods are there for generating force to work on a client?
2. What is the importance of proper table height? What factors contribute to determining proper table height?
3. What are the benefits of an electric lift table over a standard massage table?
4. List and describe the two competing properties of a lotion.
5. Describe the body mechanics to creating a proper vertical squat bend.
6. How is alignment of the core accomplished?
7. What is the advantage of a sagittal stance in which the rear foot is parallel with the front foot as opposed to a sagittal stance in which the rear foot is perpendicular to the front foot?
8. What is the effect of an inclined trunk position on the head and neck of the therapist?
9. How would a therapist position the upper extremities to best transmit force into the client?
10. What is the general rule concerning the choice of contact surfaces?
11. Describe the necessary direction of force for optimal delivery.

Deeper Thoughts

This chapter provided guidelines for optimal use of equipment, position, and performance. Are there other concerns that would come into play while trying to apply these guidelines? Is there any difference if the therapist is working not on a table, but with a massage chair or a shiatsu mat? Are there other pieces of equipment or accessories that would aid in keeping proper body mechanics though a massage?

CHAPTER 8

Upper Extremity Bone Palpation and Ligaments

Overview

Chapter 8 is one of three chapters of Part III of this book that addresses palpation of the skeleton. This chapter is a palpation tour of the bones, bony landmarks, and joints of the upper extremity. The tour begins with the shoulder girdle; then addresses the arm, forearm, and wrist region; and concludes with the hand. Although any one bone or bony landmark can be independently palpated, this chapter is set up sequentially to flow from one landmark to another, so it is recommended that the order presented here is followed. Muscle attachments for each of the palpated structures are also given. Even though specific palpations for these muscles are covered in Part IV of this book, now would also be a good time to palpate and explore these muscle attachments. The ligaments of the upper extremity are presented at the end of this chapter.

Chapter 9 presents the ligaments of the axial body and the palpation of the bones, bony landmarks, and joints of the axial body. Chapter 10 presents the ligaments of the lower extremity and the palpation of the bones, bony landmarks, and joints of the lower extremity.

Chapter Outline

The bones, bony landmarks, and joints of the following regions are covered:
Section 1: Shoulder Girdle
Section 2: Arm and Forearm
Section 3: Radial Side of the Wrist (Scaphoid and Trapezium)
Section 4: Central Carpal Bones of the Wrist (Capitate, Lunate, and Trapezoid)
Section 5: Ulnar Side of the Wrist (Triquetrum and Hamate)
Section 6: Anterior Wrist
Section 7: Hand
Section 8: Ligaments of the Upper Extremity

Chapter Objectives

After completing this chapter, the student/therapist should be able to perform the following:
1. Define the key terms of this chapter.
2. Palpate each of the bones, bony landmarks, and joints of this chapter, which are listed as key terms.
3. State the muscle or muscles that attach to each of the bony landmarks of this chapter.
4. Describe the location of each of the ligaments of the upper extremity.

Key Terms

Acromioclavicular (AC) joint
Acromion process of the scapula
Anatomic snuffbox
Bicipital groove of the humerus
Capitate
Clavicle
Coracoid process of the scapula
Deltoid tuberosity of the humerus
Distal interphalangeal (DIP) joint
Dorsal tubercle of the radius
Greater tubercle of the humerus
Hamate
Hook of the hamate
Humeral shaft

Inferior angle of the scapula
Infraspinous fossa of the scapula
Infraglenoid tubercle of the scapula
Interphalangeal (IP) joint
Lateral border of the scapula
Lateral epicondyle of the humerus
Lateral supracondylar ridge of the humerus
Lesser tubercle of the humerus
Lister's tubercle of the radius
Lunate
Medial border of the scapula

Medial epicondyle of the humerus
Medial supracondylar ridge of the humerus
Metacarpal base
Metacarpal head
Metacarpal shaft
Metacarpals
Metacarpophalangeal (MCP) joint
Olecranon fossa of the humerus
Olecranon process of the ulna
Phalangeal base
Phalangeal head
Phalangeal shaft
Phalanges (singular:phalanx)

Pisiform	Spine of the scapula	Supraspinous fossa of the scapula
Proximal interphalangeal (PIP) joint	Sternoclavicular (SC) joint	Trapezium
Radial head	Styloid process of the radius	Trapezoid
Radial shaft	Styloid process of the ulna	Triquetrum
Root of the spine of the scapula	Subscapular fossa of the scapula	Tubercle of the scaphoid
Saddle joint of the thumb	Superior angle of the scapula	Tubercle of the trapezium
Scaphoid	Superior border of the scapula	Ulnar shaft

ℯ Go to http://evolve.elsevier.com/Muscolino/palpation for identification of bony landmark exercises.

SECTION 1: SHOULDER GIRDLE

Anteromedial View of the Shoulder Girdle (Figure 8-1)

Sternoclavicular Joint. Start palpating the anterior shoulder girdle by first locating the suprasternal notch of the manubrium of the sternum; then press laterally, feeling for the **sternoclavicular (SC) joint** between the sternum and the medial (proximal) end of the clavicle (Figure 8-2). To better palpate the SC joint, ask the client to actively move his or her arm in various ranges of motion while palpating the SC joint.

Clavicle. From the SC joint, slide along the shaft of the **clavicle** from medial to lateral (proximal to distal) to feel its entire length (Figure 8-3). Notice that the medial shaft of the clavicle is convex anteriorly and the lateral end of the clavicle is concave anteriorly.

PLEASE NOTE: The sternocleidomastoid and upper trapezius muscles attach to the superior aspect of the clavicle. The pectoralis major, anterior deltoid, and subclavius muscles attach to the inferior aspect of the clavicle.

Coracoid Process of the Scapula. From the concavity at the lateral (distal) end of the clavicle, drop inferiorly off the clavicle to find the **coracoid process of the scapula** (Figure 8-4). The coracoid process is located deep to the pectoralis major muscle.

When palpating the coracoid process, notice that its apex (tip) points laterally. If it is difficult to locate the coracoid process in this manner, then try to palpate it by first locating its apex. To do this, drop down from the far lateral end of the clavicle onto the head of the humerus and then press medially to find the apex of the coracoid process.

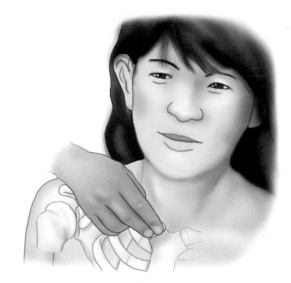

Anteromedial view
Figure 8-2 Sternoclavicular (SC) joint.

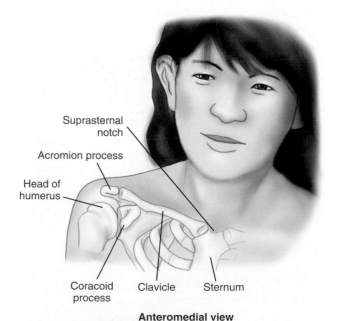

Suprasternal notch
Acromion process
Head of humerus
Coracoid process   Clavicle   Sternum

Anteromedial view
Figure 8-1 Anteromedial view of the shoulder girdle.

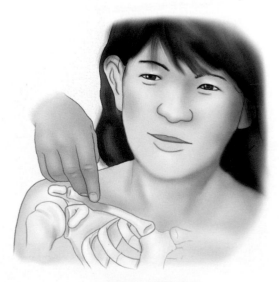

Anteromedial view
Figure 8-3 Clavicle.

8

PLEASE NOTE: Three muscles attach to the coracoid process: the short head of the biceps brachii, coracobrachialis, and the pectoralis minor.

Acromion Process of the Scapula. After palpating the coracoid process of the scapula, move back to the clavicle and continue palpating the clavicle laterally (distally) once again until you reach the **acromion process of the scapula** (Figure 8-5). The acromion process of the scapula is at the far lateral end (i.e., the tip of the shoulder).

PLEASE NOTE: The upper trapezius and deltoid muscles attach to the acromion process of the scapula. The distal tendon of the supraspinatus runs deep (inferior) to the acromion process to attach to the greater tubercle on the head of the humerus.

Acromioclavicular Joint. To best feel the **acromioclavicular (AC) joint**, palpate pressing medially from the acromion of the scapula toward the clavicle until you feel the AC joint

(Figure 8-6). This is usually the easiest way to feel this joint line, because the lateral end of the clavicle sticks up slightly superiorly above the acromion process.

Posterolateral View of the Scapula (Figure 8-7)

Acromion Process and Spine of the Scapula. The **spine of the scapula** is the posterior continuation of the acromion process. To locate the spine of the scapula, begin on the acromion process (Figure 8-8, **A**). Palpate along the acromion process posteriorly onto the spine of the scapula (see Figure 8-8, **B**). The spine of the scapula can be palpated all the way to the medial border of the scapula. The spine of the scapula can be best palpated if you strum it perpendicularly by moving your palpating fingers up and down across it as you work your way posteriorly.

PLEASE NOTE: The posterior deltoid and trapezius muscles attach to the spine of the scapula. The rhomboid minor muscle attaches to the root of the spine of the scapula.

Supraspinous Fossa. To palpate the **supraspinous fossa of the scapula**, locate the spine of the scapula and drop just off it superiorly (Figure 8-9). Palpate along the superior border of the spine of the scapula within the supraspinous fossa.

PLEASE NOTE: The supraspinous fossa is covered by the upper trapezius and the supraspinatus muscles. The supraspinatus muscle attaches to the supraspinous fossa.

Infraspinous Fossa of the Scapula. To palpate the **infraspinous fossa of the scapula**, locate the spine of the scapula and drop just off it inferiorly (Figure 8-10). The infraspinous fossa is larger than the supraspinous fossa.

PLEASE NOTE: The infraspinatus muscle attaches to the infraspinous fossa. The posterior deltoid overlies much of the infraspinous fossa.

Medial Border of the Scapula (at the Root of the Spine of the Scapula). Continue palpating along the spine of the scapula until you reach the **medial border of the scapula** (Figure 8-11). Where the spine of the scapula ends at the medial border is called the **root of the spine of the scapula**. Having the client protract and retract the scapula (at the scapulocostal joint) is

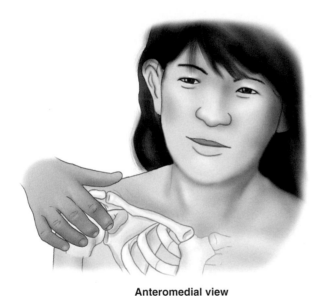

Anteromedial view

Figure 8-4 Coracoid process of the scapula.

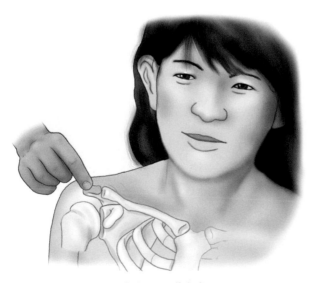

Anteromedial view

Figure 8-5 Acromion process of the scapula.

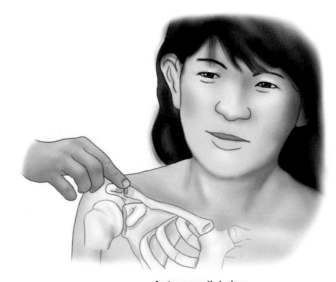

Anteromedial view

Figure 8-6 Acromioclavicular (AC) joint.

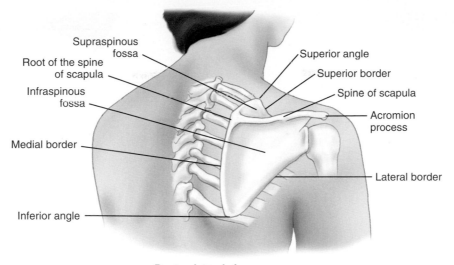

Posterolateral view

Figure 8-7 Posterolateral view of the scapula.

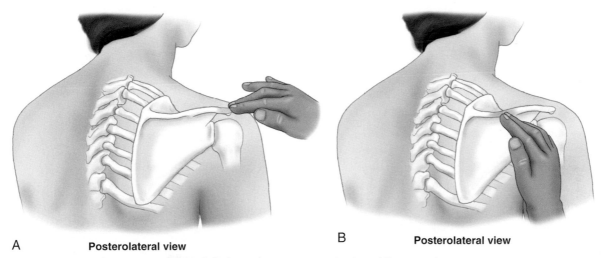

A **Posterolateral view**   B **Posterolateral view**

Figure 8-8 Acromion process and spine of the scapula.

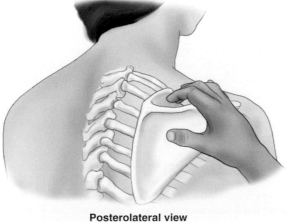

Posterolateral view
Figure 8-9 Supraspinous fossa.

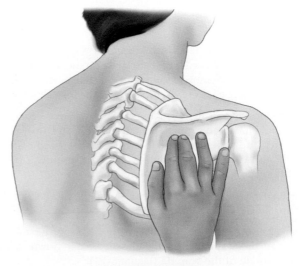

Posterolateral view
Figure 8-10 Infraspinous fossa of the scapula.

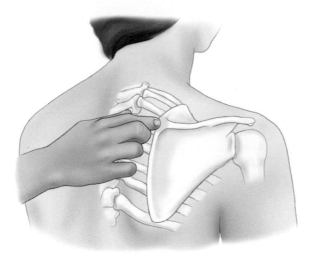

Posterolateral view

Figure 8-11 Medial border of the scapula (at the root of the spine of the scapula).

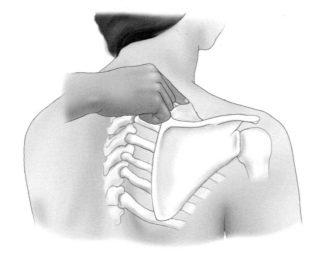

Posterolateral view

Figure 8-12 Superior angle of the scapula.

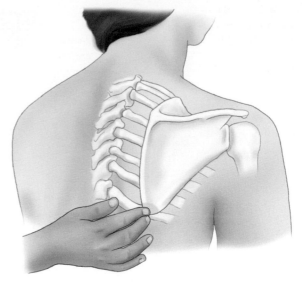

Posterolateral view

Figure 8-13 Inferior angle of the scapula.

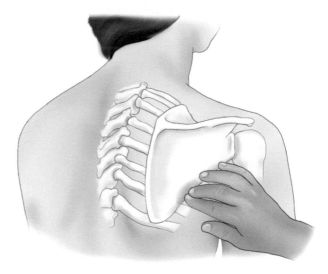

Posterolateral view

Figure 8-14 Lateral border of the scapula.

helpful to bring out the medial border of the scapula. Passively retracting the client's scapula makes it much easier to locate the medial border.

PLEASE NOTE: The levator scapulae and rhomboid muscles attach to the medial border of the scapula on the posterior side. The serratus anterior muscle attaches to the medial border on the anterior side. The trapezius overlies most of the medial border.

Superior Angle of the Scapula. Once the medial border of the scapula has been located, palpate along it superiorly until you reach the **superior angle of the scapula** (Figure 8-12). Having the client elevate and depress the scapula can be helpful as you palpate for its superior angle.

PLEASE NOTE: The levator scapulae muscle attaches to the superior angle of the scapula.

Inferior Angle of the Scapula. Palpate along the medial border of the scapula from the superior angle down to the **inferior angle of the scapula** (Figure 8-13).

PLEASE NOTE: The latissimus dorsi and teres major muscles attach onto or near the inferior angle of the scapula.

Lateral Border of the Scapula. Once you are at the inferior angle of the scapula, continue palpating superiorly along the **lateral border of the scapula** (Figure 8-14). Feeling the lateral border is easiest if your pressure is directed medially. The lateral border of the scapula can usually be palpated all the way to the **infraglenoid tubercle of the scapula**, just inferior to the glenoid fossa of the scapula. To confirm that you are on the infraglenoid tubercle, ask the client to extend his or her forearm at the elbow joint against resistance to bring out the infraglenoid attachment of the long head of the triceps brachii. (You can provide the resistance to extension of the forearm at the elbow joint, or the resistance can be provided by the client pressing the forearm against his or her own thigh.)

PLEASE NOTE: The teres major and teres minor muscles attach to the lateral border of the scapula; the long head of the triceps brachii attaches to the infraglenoid tubercle of the scapula. On the anterior side, the subscapularis muscle attaches onto or near the lateral border of the scapula.

Superior Border of the Scapula. The **superior border of the scapula** is more challenging to palpate than the medial and lateral borders. First, trace the medial border of the scapula up to the superior angle once again. Once the superior angle has been located, continue to palpate laterally along the

superior border with your pressure directed inferiorly against the superior border (Figure 8-15). Elevating the scapula (at the scapulocostal joint) may help to bring out the superior border a bit more. Palpating the entire length of the superior border of the scapula is usually not possible.

PLEASE NOTE: The omohyoid muscle attaches to the superior border of the scapula. The levator scapulae muscle also attaches onto the superior border of the scapula at the superior angle.

Subscapular Fossa of the Scapula. The **subscapular fossa** is located on the anterior surface of the scapula and can be slightly challenging to palpate. With the client supine, grasp the medial border of the client's scapula with one hand and passively protract the scapula. With your other hand, palpate slowly but firmly against the anterior surface of the scapula (Figure 8-16).

PLEASE NOTE: The subscapularis muscle attaches to the subscapular fossa on the anterior side of the scapula; the serratus anterior muscle also attaches to the anterior side of the scapula, along the medial border.

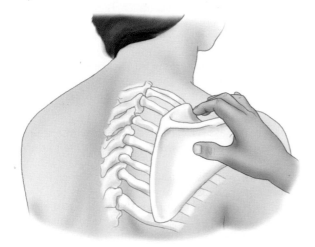

Posterolateral view

Figure 8-15 Superior border of the scapula.

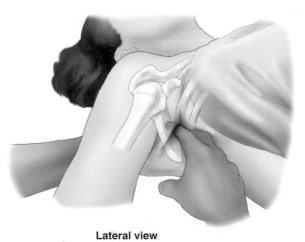

Lateral view

Figure 8-16 Subscapular fossa of the scapula.

SECTION 2: ARM AND FOREARM

Greater Tubercle, Bicipital Groove, and Lesser Tubercle of the Humerus. The **greater tubercle** is located on the lateral side of the **bicipital groove**; the **lesser tubercle** is located on the medial side. First locate the anterolateral margin of the acromion process of the scapula and then drop immediately off it onto the head of the humerus; you should be on the greater tubercle of the humerus. Figure 8-17, *A*, is an anterolateral view of the proximal arm; Figure 8-17, *B*, is a superior view looking down the arm in which we see the contours of the greater and lesser tubercles and the bicipital groove between. Now, with a flat finger pad palpation across the anterior surface of the head of the humerus, passively move the client's arm into lateral rotation at the shoulder joint. You should be able to feel your palpating finger dropping into the bicipital groove as it passes under your finger pads (see Figure 8-17, *C*). As you continue to passively move the client's arm into lateral rotation, you will feel the lesser tubercle under your fingers, just medial to the bicipital groove (see Figure 8-17, *D*). If you do not successfully feel the tubercles and bicipital groove,

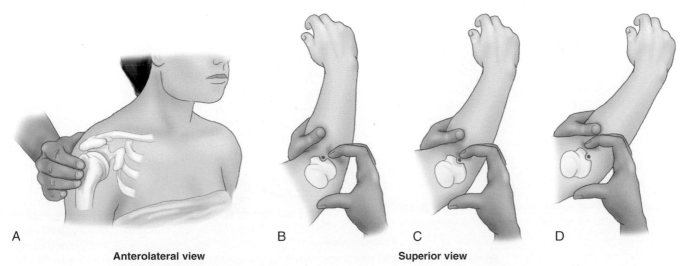

A   B   C   D

Anterolateral view   **Superior view**

Figure 8-17 Greater tubercle, bicipital groove, and lesser tubercle of the humerus.

alternately move the client's arm through medial and lateral rotation, feeling for them.

PLEASE NOTE: The long head of the biceps brachii muscle runs through the bicipital groove; the supraspinatus, infraspinatus, and teres minor muscles attach onto the greater tubercle; the subscapularis muscle attaches onto the lesser tubercle.

Deltoid Tuberosity. From the tubercles on the head of the humerus, move distally down the lateral surface of the shaft of the humerus until you feel a bony prominence approximately ⅓ of the way down the lateral surface of the shaft of the humerus. This is the **deltoid tuberosity** (Figure 8-18). This landmark can often be located by following the deltoid muscle distally to its attachment into the deltoid tuberosity.

PLEASE NOTE: The deltoid attaches to the deltoid tuberosity of the humerus. Also attaching very close to the deltoid tuberosity is the proximal attachment of the brachialis.

Medial and Lateral Epicondyles of the Humerus. To locate the **medial and lateral epicondyles of the humerus**, ask the client to flex the forearm at the elbow joint to approximately 90 degrees; place your palpating fingers (thumb and middle finger) on the medial and lateral sides of the client's arm

(Figure 8-19, *A*). Now move distally down the client's arm with your palpating fingers, and you will clearly run into the medial and lateral epicondyles of the humerus (see Figure 8-19, *B*). They are prominently the widest points along the sides of the humerus near the elbow joint.

PLEASE NOTE: Five muscles attach onto the medial epicondyle of the humerus: pronator teres, flexor carpi radialis, palmaris longus, flexor carpi ulnaris, and flexor digitorum superficialis; the flexor pollicis longus also usually attaches onto the medial epicondyle. Six muscles attach to the lateral epicondyle of the humerus: the extensor carpi radialis brevis, extensor digitorum, extensor digiti minimi, extensor carpi ulnaris, anconeus, and supinator.

Olecranon Process of the Ulna. The **olecranon process of the ulna** is extremely easy to locate. With the thumb and middle finger on the medial and lateral epicondyles of the humerus, place your index finger on the point of the elbow (the olecranon process), located halfway between the two epicondyles (Figure 8-20). Note: If the client's elbow joint is flexed, the olecranon process will be located farther distally than the two epicondyles of the humerus. Be careful with palpatory pressure between the medial epicondyle of the humerus and the olecranon process of the ulna due to the presence of the ulnar nerve, which is known in lay terms as the "funny bone."

PLEASE NOTE: The triceps brachii and anconeus muscles attach onto the olecranon process.

Olecranon Fossa of the Humerus. Once the olecranon process of the ulna has been located, the **olecranon fossa of the humerus** is fairly easy to locate. The client's forearm must be partially flexed at the elbow joint so that the olecranon fossa of the humerus is exposed (in full extension, the olecranon process of the ulna is located in and obstructs palpation of the olecranon fossa of the humerus). Find the most proximal midline point of the olecranon process of the ulna and drop off it just proximally, and you will feel the olecranon fossa of the humerus (Figure 8-21).

PLEASE NOTE: The distal tendon of the triceps brachii muscle overlies the olecranon fossa of the humerus.

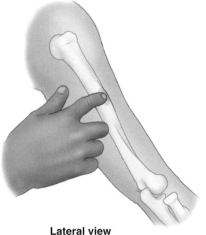

Lateral view
Figure 8-18 Deltoid tuberosity.

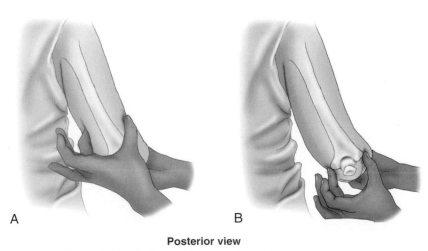

A   B

Posterior view
Figure 8-19 Medial and lateral epicondyles of the humerus.

Lateral Supracondylar Ridge of the Humerus. From the lateral epicondyle of the humerus (Figure 8-22, *A*), palpate just proximally onto the **lateral supracondylar ridge of the humerus** with your pressure directed medially against it (see Figure 8-22, *B*).

PLEASE NOTE: The brachioradialis and extensor carpi radialis longus muscles attach onto the lateral supracondylar ridge of the humerus.

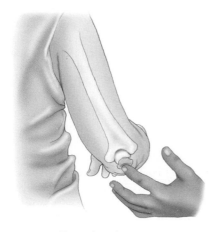

Posterior view

Figure 8-20 Olecranon process of the ulna.

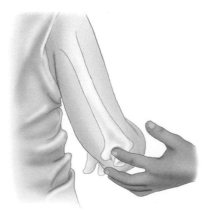

Posterior view

Figure 8-21 Olecranon fossa of the humerus.

Lateral Humeral Shaft. The majority of the **humeral shaft** is deep to musculature and difficult to directly palpate. However, the lateral shaft may be palpated. From the lateral supracondylar ridge, continue palpating the lateral shaft of the humerus proximally with your pressure directed medially against the shaft between the brachialis and triceps brachii muscles (Figure 8-23).

PLEASE NOTE: Attaching onto or near the lateral shaft of the humerus are the deltoid, brachialis, and triceps brachii muscles.

Radial Head. The **radial head** lies at the proximal end of the radius. To palpate it, begin at the lateral epicondyle of the humerus and drop immediately distal to it (Figure 8-24). It is possible to feel the joint space between the head of the radius and the humerus. (The capitulum is the landmark of the humerus at the elbow joint that is directly next to the head of the radius and is also palpable here.) To bring out the radial head, place two fingers on either side (proximal and distal) of it and ask the client to alternately pronate and supinate the forearm at the radioulnar joints; the spinning of the head of the radius can be felt under your fingers.

Medial Supracondylar Ridge of the Humerus. Now move over to the medial side of the elbow. Begin on the medial epicondyle of the humerus (Figure 8-25, *A*). Now palpate just proximally onto the **medial supracondylar ridge of the humerus** with your pressure directed laterally against it (see Figure 8-25, *B*).

PLEASE NOTE: The pronator teres attaches to the most distal end of the medial supracondylar ridge of the humerus (as well as to the medial epicondyle).

Medial Shaft of the Humerus. The majority of the medial shaft of the humerus is also palpable. However, you must be careful with your palpatory pressure here because of the presence of a number of neurovascular structures (median, ulnar, and musculocutaneous nerves and the brachial artery). To palpate the medial shaft of the humerus, continue palpating proximally from the medial supracondylar ridge of the humerus with your pressure directed laterally against the medial shaft (Figure 8-26).

PLEASE NOTE: Attaching onto or near the medial shaft of the humerus are the brachialis, coracobrachialis, and triceps brachii muscles. Farther proximally, the latissimus dorsi and teres major muscles also attach near the medial shaft of the humerus.

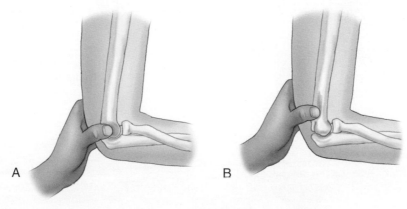

A   B

Lateral view

Figure 8-22 Lateral supracondylar ridge of the humerus.

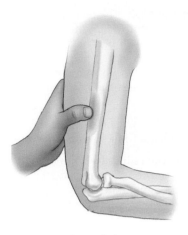

Lateral view

Figure 8-23 Lateral humeral shaft.

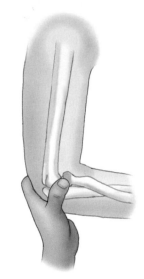

Lateral view

Figure 8-24 Radial head.

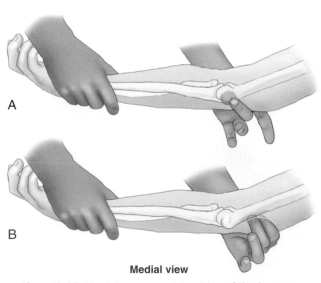

A

B

Medial view

Figure 8-25 Medial supracondylar ridge of the humerus.

Ulnar Shaft. The entire medial border of the **ulnar shaft** is easily palpable. Begin on the medial side of the olecranon process and continue palpating distally with your pressure directed laterally against the medial border of the ulna until you reach the distal end of the ulna (Figure 8-27).

PLEASE NOTE: Three muscles attach onto the medial border of the shaft of the ulna: the ulnar head of the flexor carpi ulnaris, the ulnar head of the extensor carpi ulnaris, and the flexor digitorum profundus.

Lateral Shaft of the Radius. The majority of the lateral **radial shaft** is palpable. Begin approximately midshaft and palpate into the lateral radius with your pressure directed medially against the lateral shaft of the radius (Figure 8-28). Asking the client to alternately pronate and supinate the forearm at the radioulnar joints helps bring out the shaft of the radius. Continue palpating the lateral shaft of the radius proximally until you reach the head of the radius. (Note: A part of the proximal, lateral radial shaft is difficult to palpate because it is deep to the supinator muscle.) Beginning again from the midshaft, continue to palpate the radial shaft to its distal end on the styloid process. (Note: A small part of the distal radial shaft is slightly challenging to palpate, because two deeper muscles of the forearm that move the thumb cross the shaft here.)

PLEASE NOTE: The supinator, pronator teres, and flexor pollicis longus muscles attach onto the lateral shaft of the radius. The abductor pollicis longus (APL) and extensor pollicis brevis

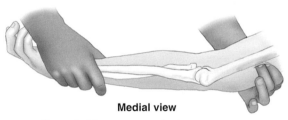

Medial view

Figure 8-26 Medial shaft of the humerus.

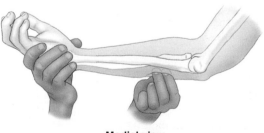

Medial view

Figure 8-27 Ulnar shaft.

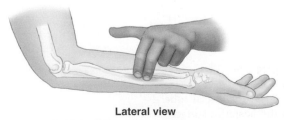

Lateral view

Figure 8-28 Lateral shaft of the radius.

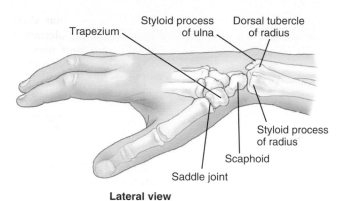

Trapezium — Styloid process of ulna — Dorsal tubercle of radius

Styloid process of radius

Scaphoid

Saddle joint

Lateral view

Figure 8-29 Lateral view of the wrist/hand.

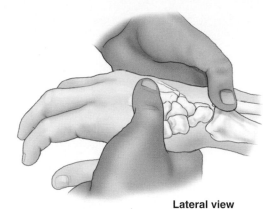

Lateral view

Figure 8-31 Dorsal (Lister's) tubercle.

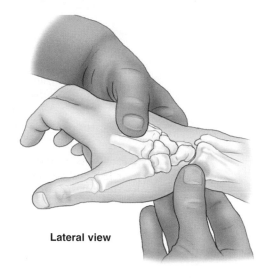

Lateral view

Figure 8-30 Styloid process of the radius.

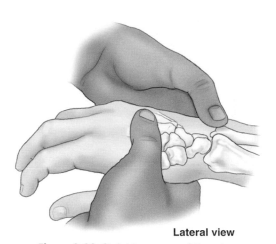

Lateral view

Figure 8-32 Styloid process of the ulna.

SECTION 3: RADIAL SIDE OF THE WRIST (SCAPHOID AND TRAPEZIUM)

(EPB) cross over (superficial to) the distal lateral radial shaft near the radial styloid.

Lateral View of the Wrist/Hand (Figure 8-29)

Styloid Process of the Radius. Now that the lateral shaft of the radius has been located, continue palpating it distally until you reach the **styloid process of the radius** located at the distal end of the lateral radial shaft (Figure 8-30).

PLEASE NOTE: The brachioradialis muscle attaches onto the styloid process of the radius.

Dorsal (Lister's) Tubercle. The **dorsal tubercle** (also known as **Lister's tubercle**) is located on the posterior side of the distal end of the radius. From the radial styloid, palpate posteriorly onto the radius; the dorsal tubercle is a prominence located in the middle of the distal posterior radial shaft (Figure 8-31).

PLEASE NOTE: The dorsal tubercle separates the distal tendons of the extensors carpi radialis longus and brevis muscles (located on the radial/lateral side) from the distal tendon of the extensor pollicis longus (EPL) muscle (located on the ulnar/medial side).

Styloid Process of the Ulna. The **styloid process of the ulna** is located at the distal end of the ulna on the posterior side. From the dorsal tubercle of the radius, move medially onto the posterior surface of the distal ulna, and feel for the prominence of the ulnar styloid (Figure 8-32).

The carpals are small but can be easily palpated if the placement of your palpating finger pads is precise. As a general rule, moving the hand at the wrist joint "away" from your palpation placement contact helps to move the carpal bone into your contact so as to be more easily felt. So, if you are palpating a carpal bone on the ulnar side of the wrist, ask the client to radially deviate; if you are palpating on the radial side, ask the client to ulnar deviate. If palpating on the posterior side, ask the client to flex; and if palpating on the anterior side, ask the client to extend.

Scaphoid. The **scaphoid** is the carpal bone located in the proximal row of carpals on the lateral (radial) side, directly distal to the lateral side of the radius. It can be palpated dorsally, laterally, and anteriorly. Begin palpating the scaphoid laterally by dropping distally onto it from the radial styloid (Figure 8-33, A). To bring out the scaphoid, ask the client to alternately do active radial and ulnar deviation of the hand at the wrist joint; the scaphoid alternately presses into your palpating finger with ulnar deviation and then disappears with radial deviation. To palpate the scaphoid on the dorsal side, ask the client to extend and abduct the thumb; this brings out the **anatomic snuffbox**, a depression bordered by the distal tendons of three thumb muscles (abductor pollicis longus [APL], extensor pollicis brevis [EPB], and extensor pollicis longus [EPL]) (see Figure 8-33, B). The scaphoid forms the floor of the anatomic snuffbox. Palpate

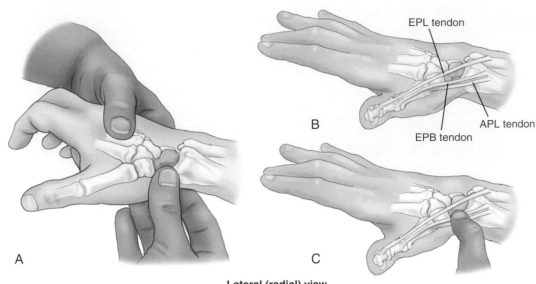

Lateral (radial) view
Figure 8-33 Scaphoid.

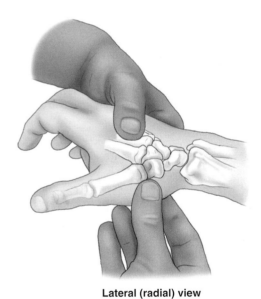

Lateral (radial) view
Figure 8-34 Saddle joint of the thumb.

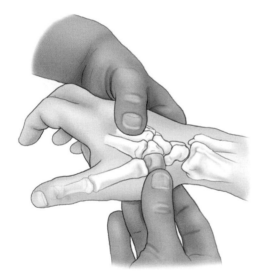

Lateral (radial) view
Figure 8-35 Trapezium.

the scaphoid by palpating between the tendons that border the anatomic snuffbox (see Figure 8-33, *C*). Asking the client to alternately do active ulnar and radial deviation of the hand at the wrist joint also helps to bring out the scaphoid here. However, be careful with palpation pressure into the anatomic snuffbox because of the presence of the radial artery and a branch of the radial nerve. (Note: To palpate the scaphoid anteriorly, see Figure 8-37, *A*.)

PLEASE NOTE: The three muscles whose distal tendons border and define the anatomic snuffbox are the APL and EPB on the lateral side, and the EPL on the medial side.

Saddle Joint of the Thumb. The **saddle joint of the thumb** is the carpometacarpal joint of the thumb and is located between the trapezium and the base of the metacarpal of the thumb. To palpate it, begin proximally from the palpation of the lateral side of the scaphoid (see Figure 8-33, *A*) and palpate distally until you feel the joint line between the trapezium and the metacarpal

of the thumb (Figure 8-34). Perhaps even easier is to begin distally by first locating the lateral shaft of the metacarpal of the thumb and then palpating proximally until you feel the joint line between the metacarpal of the thumb and the trapezium. If you are unsure whether you are on this joint, ask the client to actively move the thumb, and feel for the movement of the metacarpal of the thumb relative to the trapezium at the joint line.

Trapezium. Once the saddle joint of the thumb has been located, palpate just proximally to it, and you will be directly on the lateral surface of the **trapezium** (Figure 8-35). The tubercle of the trapezium can also be palpated anteriorly (see Figure 8-37, *B*).

Anterior (Palmar) View of the Wrist (Figure 8-36)

Tubercles of Scaphoid and Trapezium. The tubercles of the scaphoid and trapezium are prominent and palpable anteriorly. To locate the **tubercle of the scaphoid**, begin on the lateral surface of the scaphoid (see Figure 8-33, *A*) and move approximately ¼ to ½ inch (.5 to 1 cm) anteriorly until you feel the tubercle of the scaphoid (Figure 8-37, *A*). Alternately, palpate immediately distal to the crease of the wrist joint on the anterior side, slightly to the radial side of the midline, and feel for a bony prominence. To locate the **tubercle of the trapezium**, begin on the lateral surface of the trapezium (see Figure 8-35) and move approximately ½ inch (1 cm) anteriorly until you feel the tubercle of the trapezium (see Figure 8-37, *B*). Note: The tubercle of the trapezium is located approximately ¼ inch (½ cm) distal to the tubercle of the scaphoid and slightly toward the radial side.

PLEASE NOTE: The opponens pollicis muscle attaches onto the tubercle of the trapezium. The abductor pollicis brevis muscle attaches onto both the tubercle of the scaphoid and the tubercle of the trapezium. The flexor pollicis brevis muscle attaches onto the anterior surface of the trapezium. The transverse carpal ligament (flexor retinaculum) that forms the roof of the carpal tunnel also attaches to the tubercles of the scaphoid and trapezium.

SECTION 4: CENTRAL CARPAL BONES OF THE WRIST (CAPITATE, LUNATE, AND TRAPEZOID)

Third Metacarpal Base and the Capitate. The dorsal (Lister's) tubercle of the radius, base of the third metacarpal, and **capitate** (of the distal row of carpal bones) are all located in a straight line on the dorsal side of the wrist/hand region (Figure 8-38, *A*). First locate the dorsal tubercle of the radius (see Figure 8-31); from there, palpate distally for the base of the third metacarpal (see Figure 8-38, *B*). A **metacarpal base** is the expanded proximal end of a metacarpal. (The base of the third metacarpal is the largest and most prominent of the metacarpal bases and is located directly medial to the base of the head of the second metacarpal.) Once the base of the third metacarpal has been located, drop just off it proximally onto the capitate (see Figure 8-38, *C*). To bring out the capitate, ask the client to do active flexion and ulnar deviation of the hand at the wrist joint, and the capitate can be felt pressing up into your palpating finger.

PLEASE NOTE: The adductor pollicis muscle attaches onto the anterior side of the capitate.

Lunate. The **lunate** is the carpal bone located in the proximal row of carpals between the scaphoid (on the radial side) and the triquetrum (on the ulnar side). The best place to palpate the lunate is posteriorly. To find the lunate, move proximally from the capitate and slightly in the ulnar direction. This area feels like a depression. Now ask the client to alternately do active flexion and extension of the hand at the wrist joint. Upon wrist joint flexion, the lunate can be felt pressing up into your palpating finger (Figure 8-39). Upon wrist joint extension, the lunate disappears from palpation.

Second Metacarpal Base and the Trapezoid (Figure 8-40). The **trapezoid** is the carpal bone that is located in the distal row of carpals, directly next to the trapezium and just proximal to the base of the second metacarpal. The best place to palpate the trapezoid is posteriorly. First locate the base of the third metacarpal (see Figure 8-38, *B*) and drop off it in the radial direction onto the base of the second metacarpal (see Figure 8-40, *A*). Once the base of the second metacarpal has been found, drop off it proximally and you will be on the trapezoid (see Figure 8-40, *B*). To bring out the trapezoid, ask the client to do active flexion and ulnar deviation of the hand at the wrist joint, and the trapezoid can be felt to press up against your palpating finger.

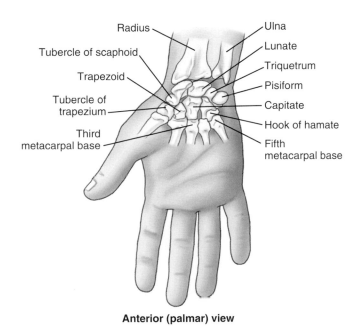

Radius — Ulna
Tubercle of scaphoid — Lunate
Trapezoid — Triquetrum
Tubercle of trapezium — Pisiform
Third metacarpal base — Capitate
— Hook of hamate
— Fifth metacarpal base

Anterior (palmar) view

Figure 8-36 Anterior (palmar) view of the wrist.

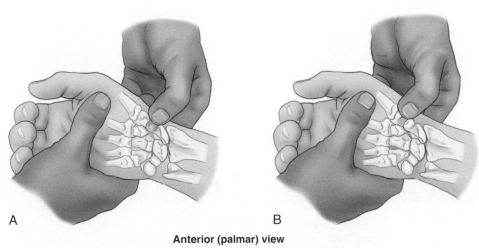

A   B

Anterior (palmar) view

Figure 8-37 Tubercles of scaphoid and trapezium.

8

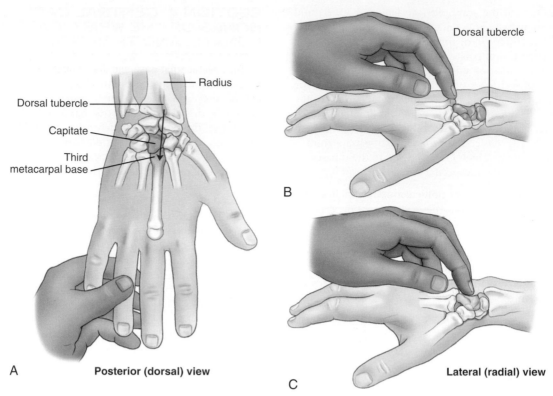

A   **Posterior (dorsal) view**

B

C   **Lateral (radial) view**

Figure 8-38 Third metacarpal base and the capitate.

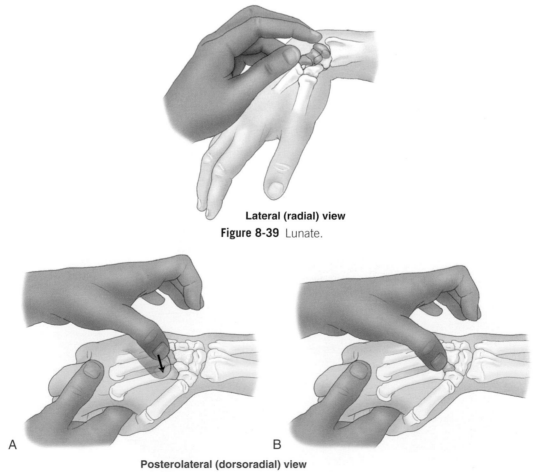

Lateral (radial) view
Figure 8-39 Lunate.

A   B

Posterolateral (dorsoradial) view
Figure 8-40 Second metacarpal base and the trapezoid.

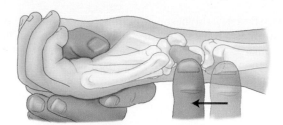

Medial (ulnar) view

Figure 8-41 Triquetrum.

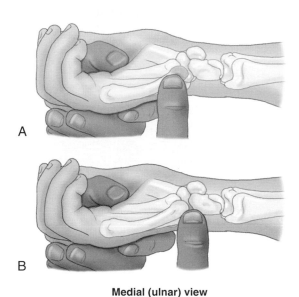

A

B

Medial (ulnar) view

Figure 8-42 Fifth metacarpal base and the hamate.

SECTION 5: ULNAR SIDE OF THE WRIST (TRIQUETRUM AND HAMATE)

Triquetrum. The **triquetrum** is a carpal bone located in the proximal row of carpals on the medial (ulnar) side, directly distal to the styloid process of the ulna on the posterior side of the wrist. The easiest way to palpate the triquetrum is to locate the medial border of the styloid process of the ulna, then drop distally off the ulnar styloid, and you will be directly on the triquetrum (Figure 8-41). To bring out the borders of the triquetrum, ask the client to alternately do active radial and ulnar deviation of the hand at the wrist joint; the triquetrum presses against your palpating finger with radial deviation and disappears from palpation with ulnar deviation.

Fifth Metacarpal Base and the Hamate. It is challenging, but the **hamate** can often be palpated on the ulnar side of the wrist. After locating the triquetrum on the ulnar side, palpate farther distal for the base of the fifth metacarpal (Figure 8-42, A). From the base of the fifth metacarpal, drop immediately proximal into a little depression that is located between the base of the fifth metacarpal and the triquetrum; the ulnar surface of the hamate may be palpated there (see Figure 8-42, B).

Fourth Metacarpal Base and Hamate and Triquetrum Dorsally. First find the dorsal side of the base of the fifth metacarpal (Figure 8-43, A). Now move radially onto the base of the fourth metacarpal (see Figure 8-43, B). From there, drop proximally onto the dorsal surface of the hamate (see Figure 8-43, C). From the dorsal surface of the hamate, drop proximally (and stay toward the ulnar side) onto the dorsal surface of the triquetrum (see Figure 8-43, D).

8

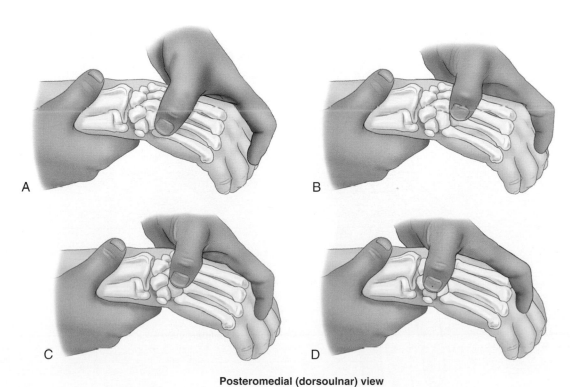

A

B

C

D

Posteromedial (dorsoulnar) view

Figure 8-43 Fourth metacarpal base and hamate and triquetrum dorsally.

SECTION 6: ANTERIOR WRIST

Anterior (Palmar) View of the Wrist (Figure 8-44)

Pisiform and Hook of the Hamate. The **pisiform** is a carpal bone located anteriorly on top of the triquetrum in the proximal row of carpals on the ulnar side. The pisiform is prominent and easily palpated on the anterior side of the wrist, just distal to the ulna (Figure 8-45, *A*). The hamate is also easily palpated anteriorly in the palm. Specifically, the **hook of the hamate** is palpable here. Begin by locating the pisiform; then palpate approximately ½ to ¾ inch (1 to 1.5 cm) distal and lateral (i.e., toward the midline of the hand) from the pisiform (see Figure 8-45, *B*). Note: The hook of the hamate is fairly pointy and can be somewhat tender to palpation.

PLEASE NOTE: The flexor carpi ulnaris and abductor digiti minimi manus muscles attach onto the pisiform. The flexor carpi ulnaris, flexor digiti minimi manus, and opponens digiti minimi muscles attach onto the hook of the hamate. The transverse carpal ligament (flexor retinaculum) that forms the roof of the carpal tunnel also attaches to the pisiform and hook of the hamate.

Most Prominent Landmarks of the Anterior Wrist. There are four carpal landmarks that are prominent and fairly easy to palpate in the anterior wrist. They are the pisiform and hook of the hamate on the ulnar side, and the tubercle of the scaphoid and tubercle of the trapezium on the radial side (Figure 8-46).

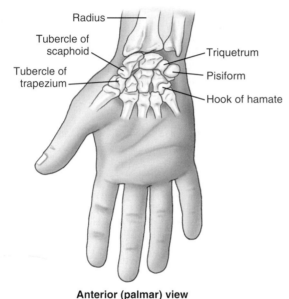

Anterior (palmar) view

Figure 8-44 Anterior (palmar) view of the wrist.

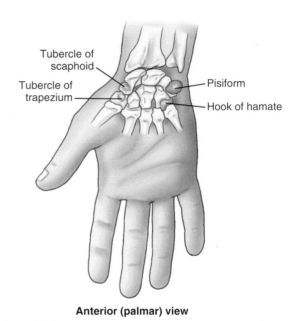

Anterior (palmar) view

Figure 8-46 Most prominent landmarks of the anterior wrist.

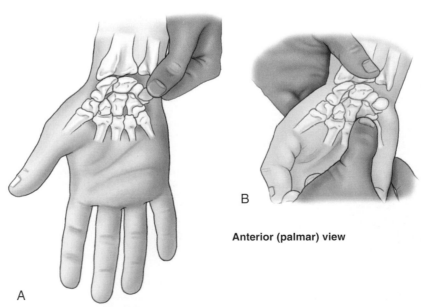

Anterior (palmar) view

Figure 8-45 Pisiform and hook of the hamate.

SECTION 7: HAND

Metacarpals and Metacarpophalangeal Joints. There are five **metacarpals**, located distal to the carpal bones and proximal to the phalanges of the fingers. All five metacarpals are easily palpable on the dorsal, ulnar, and radial sides. For each metacarpal, first locate its dorsal side anywhere along the middle of the **metacarpal shaft**. (Note: The radial side of the second metacarpal and the second **metacarpophalangeal [MCP] joint** are illustrated being palpated in Figure 8-47.) Once the shaft has been located, follow the metacarpal shaft proximally until you feel the expanded base. (The base of the third metacarpal is the largest of the five.) If you palpate just proximal to each base, the carpometacarpal joint for each individual metacarpal bone can be palpated. (The palpation of all five metacarpal bases has already been covered in this chapter.) Now palpate each metacarpal shaft on either its dorsal or radial side moving distally until you feel the expanded **metacarpal head**. Palpating just distal to the head of each metacarpal, the MCP joints can be discerned.

PLEASE NOTE: The flexor carpi radialis, flexor carpi ulnaris, extensor carpi radialis longus, extensor carpi radialis brevis, extensor carpi ulnaris, opponens digiti minimi, adductor pollicis, palmar interossei, and dorsal interossei manus muscles attach onto the second through fifth metacarpals. The APL, opponens pollicis, and dorsal interossei manus muscles attach onto the first metacarpal.

Phalanges and Interphalangeal Joints of Fingers Two through Five. There are three **phalanges** for each of the fingers (except the thumb, which has only two phalanges). Furthermore, each phalanx has a proximal expanded **base**, a **shaft**, and a distal expanded **head**. The bases, shafts, and heads of each of the phalanges are easily palpable on the dorsal, ulnar, and radial sides. (Note: Because of the presence of the fingernail, the distal phalanx is moderately more difficult to palpate.) Between the

proximal and middle phalanges of each finger is the **proximal interphalangeal (PIP) joint**. Between the middle and distal phalanges of each finger is the **distal interphalangeal (DIP) joint**. Between the proximal and distal phalanges of the thumb is the **interphalangeal (IP) joint**. Figure 8-48 illustrates palpation of the radial (lateral) side of the shaft of the proximal phalanx and the PIP joint of the index finger. Figure 8-49 illustrates palpation of the radial (lateral) side of the shaft of the middle phalanx and the DIP joint of the index finger. And Figure 8-50 illustrates palpation of the radial (lateral) side of the shaft of the distal phalanx of the index finger.

PLEASE NOTE: The abductor digiti minimi manus, flexor digiti minimi manus, palmar interossei, and dorsal interossei manus muscles attach onto the proximal phalanges of fingers two through five. The flexor digitorum superficialis, extensor digitorum, extensor digiti minimi, and extensor indicis muscles attach onto the middle phalanges of fingers two through five. And the flexor digitorum profundus, extensor digitorum, extensor digiti minimi, and extensor indicis muscles attach onto the distal phalanges of fingers two through five.

Phalanges and Interphalangeal Joints of the Thumb. Similar to the palpation of fingers two through five, the phalanges and IP joints of the thumb can be palpated. Figure 8-51 illustrates palpation of the radial (lateral) side of the shaft of the metacarpal and the MCP joint of the thumb. Figure 8-52 illustrates palpation of the radial (lateral) side of the shaft of the proximal phalanx and the IP joint of the thumb. And Figure 8-53 illustrates palpation of the radial (lateral) side of the shaft of the distal phalanx of the thumb.

PLEASE NOTE: The abductor pollicis brevis, flexor pollicis brevis, adductor pollicis, and extensor pollicis brevis (EPB) muscles attach onto the proximal phalanx of the thumb. And the flexor pollicis longus and extensor pollicis longus (EPL) muscles attach onto the distal phalanx of the thumb.

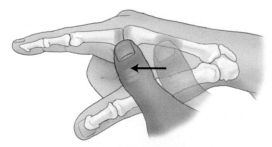

Lateral (radial) view

Figure 8-47 Metacarpals and metacarpophalangeal (MCP) joints.

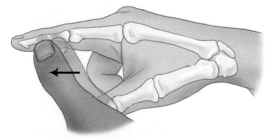

Lateral (radial) view

Figure 8-49 Palpation of the radial (lateral) side of the shaft of the middle phalanx and the distal interphalangeal (DIP) joint of the index finger.

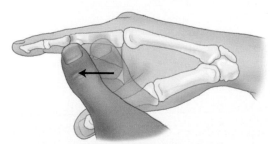

Lateral (radial) view

Figure 8-48 Palpation of the radial (lateral) side of the shaft of the proximal phalanx and the proximal interphalangeal (PIP) joint of the index finger.

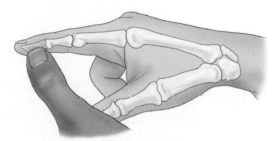

Lateral (radial) view

Figure 8-50 Palpation of the radial (lateral) side of the shaft of the distal phalanx of the index finger.

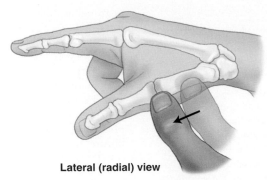

Lateral (radial) view

Figure 8-51 Palpation of the radial (lateral) side of the shaft of the metacarpal and the metacarpophalangeal (MCP) joint of the thumb.

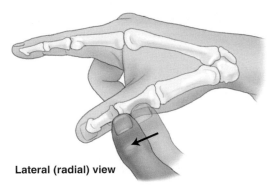

Lateral (radial) view

Figure 8-52 Palpation of the radial (lateral) side of the shaft of the proximal phalanx and the interphalangeal (IP) joint of the thumb.

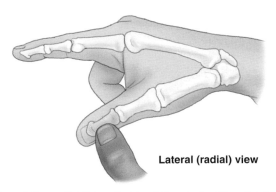

Lateral (radial) view

Figure 8-53 Palpation of the radial (lateral) side of the shaft of the distal phalanx of the thumb.

SECTION 8: LIGAMENTS OF THE UPPER EXTREMITY

Ligaments are fibrous fascial tissue that connects bones at a joint. The function of a ligament is to maintain stability of a joint by limiting motion. Figure 8-54 is an anterior view of the ligaments of the right upper extremity. Figure 8-55 is an anterior view of the ligaments of the right wrist and hand. Figure 8-56 is a posterior view of the ligaments of the right upper extremity. Figure 8-57 is a posterior view of the ligaments of the right wrist and hand.

8

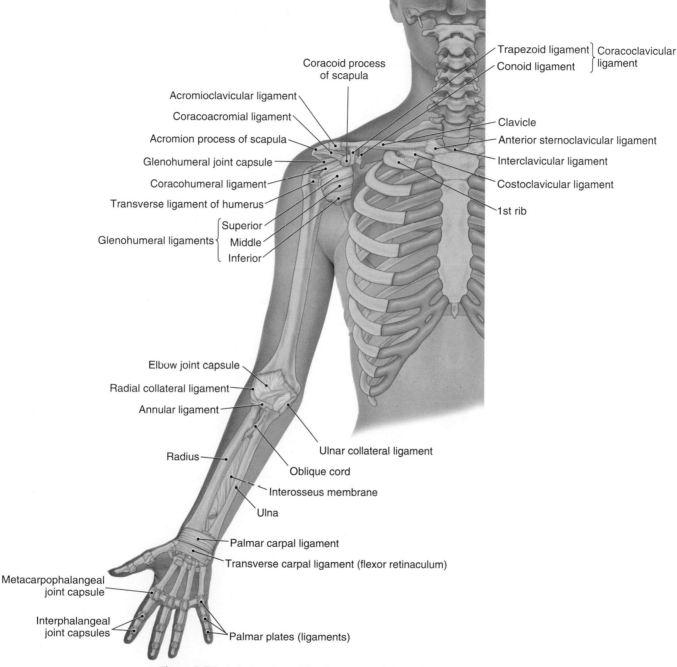

Figure 8-54 Anterior view of the ligaments of the right upper extremity.

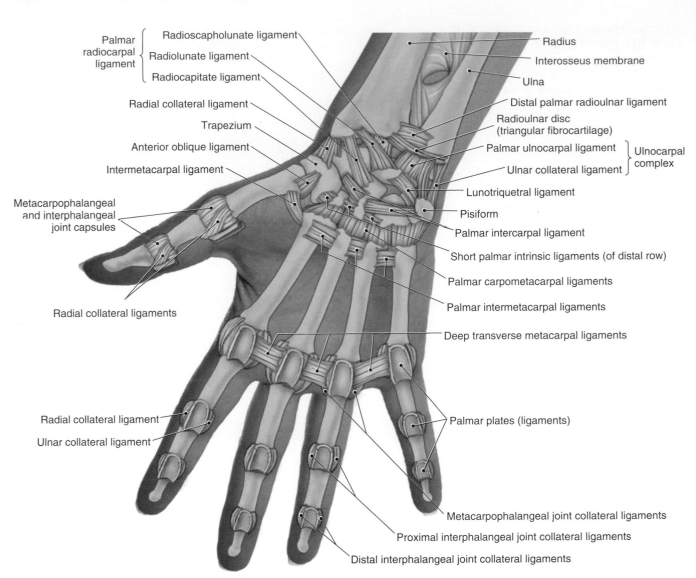

Figure 8-55 Anterior view of the ligaments of the right wrist and hand.

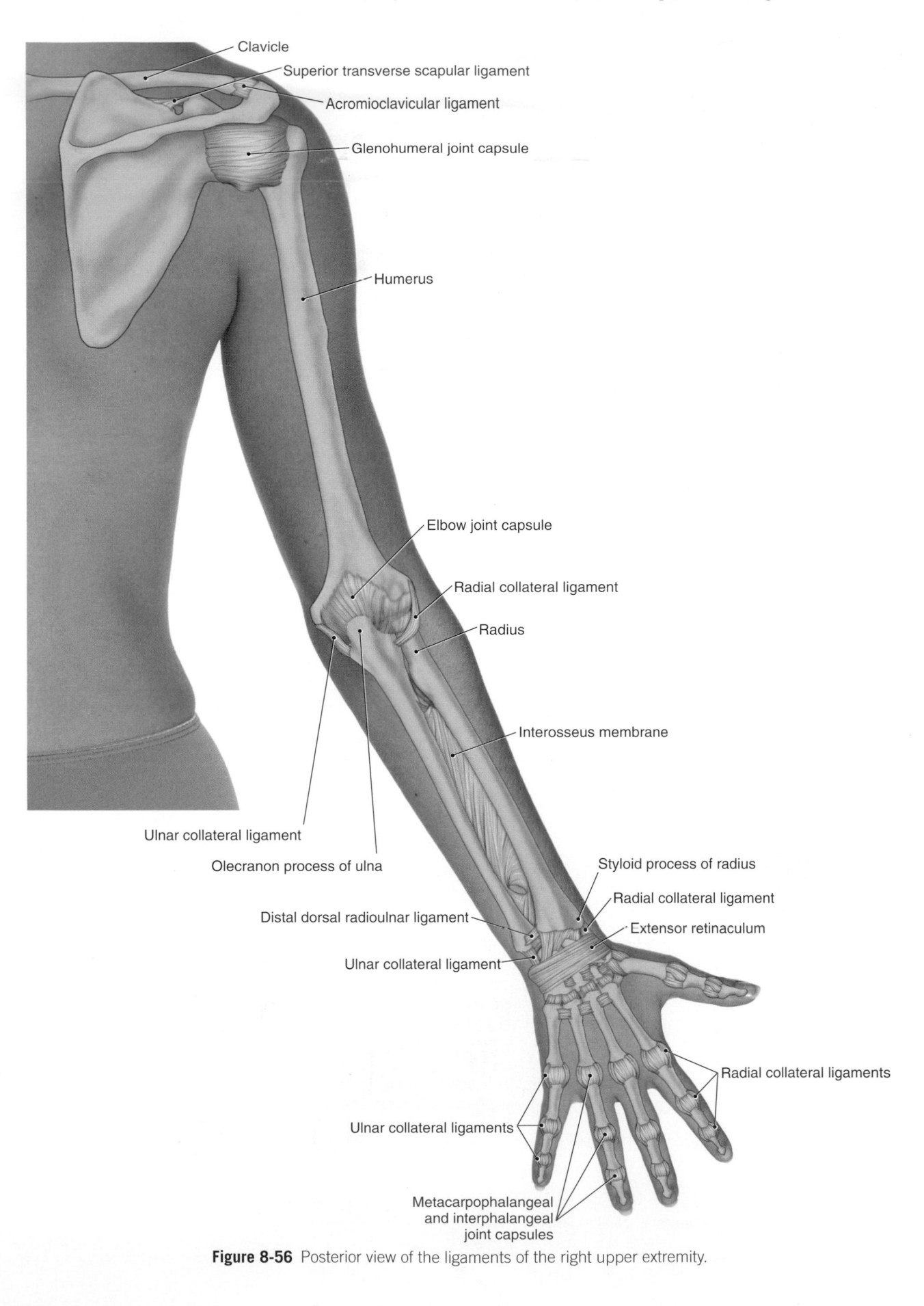

Figure 8-56 Posterior view of the ligaments of the right upper extremity.

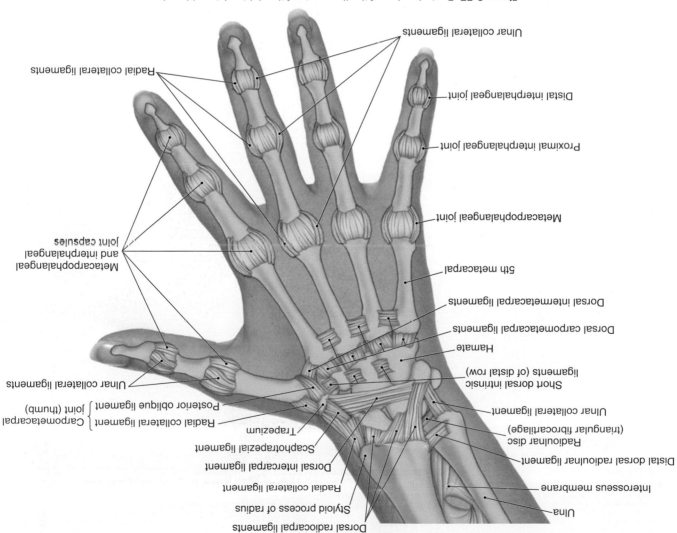

Figure 8-57 Posterior view of the ligaments of the right wrist and hand.

Ulnar collateral ligaments

Radial collateral ligaments

Distal interphalangeal joint

Proximal interphalangeal joint

Metacarpophalangeal joint

5th metacarpal

Dorsal intermetacarpal ligaments

Dorsal carpometacarpal ligaments

Hamate

Short dorsal intrinsic ligaments (of distal row)

Ulnar collateral ligament

Distal dorsal radioulnar ligament

Interosseus membrane

Ulna

Metacarpophalangeal and interphalangeal joint capsules

Ulnar collateral ligaments

Carpometacarpal joint (thumb) { Posterior oblique ligament
Radial collateral ligament }

Trapezium

Scaphotrapezial ligament

Dorsal intercarpal ligament

Radial collateral ligament

Styloid process of radius

Dorsal radiocarpal ligaments

Radioulnar disc (triangular fibrocartilage)

Review Questions

1. What muscle lies superficial to the coracoid process of the scapula? What three muscles attach to the coracoid process of the scapula?
2. The spine of the scapula is a continuation of what bony structure?
3. Confirmation of what bony structure can be obtained by having the client extend the forearm at the elbow joint against resistance?
4. What two muscles does a therapist need to be aware of when palpating the subscapular fossa?
5. What bony structure is located on the medial side of the bicipital groove of the humerus? On the lateral side?
6. What three muscles have attachments at the greater tubercle of the humerus?
7. Name any four of the six muscles that attach onto the lateral epicondyle of the humerus.
8. What sensitive structure runs between the medial epicondyle of the humerus and the olecranon process of the ulna?
9. Why must a client's forearm be partially flexed at the elbow joint during palpation of the olecranon fossa of the humerus?
10. The anatomic snuffbox is bordered by the tendons of what three muscles?
11. List the carpal bones in the order of their proximal and distal rows, from lateral to medial.
12. The hook of the hamate serves as an attachment for what three muscles?

8

CHAPTER 9

Axial Body Bone Palpation and Ligaments

Overview

Chapter 9 is one of three chapters of Part III of this book that addresses palpation of the skeleton. This chapter is a palpation tour of the bones, bony landmarks, and joints of the axial body. The tour begins with the face, then addresses the cranium and anterior and posterior neck, and concludes with the anterior and posterior trunk. Although any one bone or bony landmark can be independently palpated, this chapter is set up sequentially to flow from one landmark to another, so following the order presented here is recommended. Muscle attachments for each of the palpated structures are also given. Even though specific palpations for these muscles are covered in Part IV of this book, now would also be a good time to palpate and explore these muscle attachments. The ligaments of the axial body are presented at the end of this chapter.

Chapter 8 presents the ligaments of the upper extremity and the palpation of the bones, bony landmarks, and joints of the upper extremity. Chapter 10 presents the ligaments of the lower extremity and the palpation of the bones, bony landmarks, and joints of the lower extremity.

Chapter Outline

The bones, bony landmarks, and joints of the following regions are covered:

Section 1: Face
Section 2: Cranium
Section 3: Anterior Neck
Section 4: Posterior Neck
Section 5: Anterior Trunk
Section 6: Posterior Trunk
Section 7: Ligaments of the Axial Body

Chapter Objectives

After completing this chapter, the student/therapist should be able to perform the following:

1. Define the key terms of this chapter.
2. Palpate each of the bones, bony landmarks, and joints of this chapter, which are listed as key terms.
3. State the muscle or muscles that attach to each of the bony landmarks of this chapter.
4. Describe the location of each of the ligaments of the axial body.

Key Terms

Angle of Louis
Angle of the mandible
Anterior tubercles (of cervical transverse processes)
Articular pillar
Articular processes
Body of the mandible
Carotid tubercle (of C6)
Cervical pillar
Condyle (of the ramus) of the mandible
Coronoid process (of the ramus) of the mandible
Costal cartilages
Cricoid cartilages
External occipital protuberance (EOP)
Facet joints (of the spine)
Frontal bone
Hyoid bone
Inferior nuchal line of the occiput
Intercostal spaces
Interscapular region
Interspinous space
Jugular notch
Laminar groove (of the spine)
Mastoid process of the temporal bone
Maxilla
Nasal bone
Occipital bone
Parietal bone
Posterior tubercle of C1
Posterior tubercles (of cervical transverse processes)
Ramus of the mandible
Rib cage
Ribs
Spinous processes (SPs)
Sternomanubrial joint
Superior nuchal line of the occiput

Suprasternal notch of the manubrium of the sternum	Thyroid cartilage	Xiphoid process of the sternum
Temporal bone	Transverse process (TP) of C1	Zygomatic arch of the temporal bone
Temporomandibular joint (TMJ)	Transverse processes (TPs)	Zygomatic bone
	Vertebra prominens (of C7)	

ⓔ Go to http://evolve.elsevier.com/Muscolino/palpation for identification of bony landmark exercises.

SECTION 1: FACE

Oblique (Inferolateral) View of the Face (Figure 9-1)

Body and Angle of the Mandible. The **body of the mandible** is subcutaneous and easily palpable. Begin palpating the inferior border of the body of the mandible anteriorly and continue palpating it laterally and posteriorly until the **angle of the mandible** is reached (Figure 9-2). The angle of the mandible is the transition area where the body of the mandible becomes the ramus of the mandible.

PLEASE NOTE: The following muscles attach onto the external surface of the body of the mandible: depressor anguli oris, depressor labii inferioris, mentalis, and platysma. The digastric, mylohyoid, and geniohyoid muscles attach onto the internal surface of the body of the mandible. The masseter and medial pterygoid muscles attach onto the angle of the mandible.

Ramus (Posterior Border) and Condyle of the Mandible. The **ramus of the mandible** branches off from the body of the mandible at the angle of the mandible. The posterior border of the ramus is fairly easily palpable for its entire course and gives rise to the **condyle (of the ramus) of the mandible**. To palpate the ramus, begin at the angle of the mandible and palpate superiorly along the posterior border until the condyle is reached, anterior to the ear (Figure 9-3). To bring out the condyle, ask the client to alternately open and close the mouth. This allows you to feel the movement of the condyle of the mandible at the **temporomandibular joint (TMJ)**. (Note: The condyle can also be palpated from within the ear. Wearing a finger cot or glove, gently place your palpating finger inside the client's ear, press anteromedially, and ask the client to alternately open and close the mouth. The movement of the condyle of the mandible at the TMJ is clearly palpable.)

PLEASE NOTE: The lateral pterygoid muscle attaches onto the condyle of the mandible.

Coronoid Process of the Mandible. The anterior border of the ramus of the mandible gives rise to the **coronoid process (of the ramus) of the mandible**. From outside the mouth, the coronoid process is difficult to palpate but can be felt if the mandible is depressed (i.e., the mouth is opened). Find the zygomatic bone and palpate directly inferior to it while asking the client to slightly move the mandible up and down, maintaining a position of the mouth that is nearly fully open (Figure 9-4).

PLEASE NOTE: The temporalis and masseter muscles attach onto the coronoid process of the mandible.

Ramus and Coronoid Process From Inside the Mouth. The anterior border of the ramus is easily palpable from the inside.

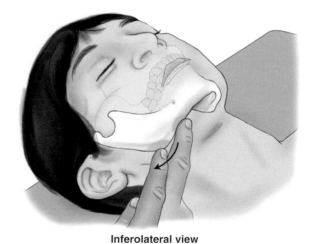

Inferolateral view

Figure 9-2 Body and angle of the mandible.

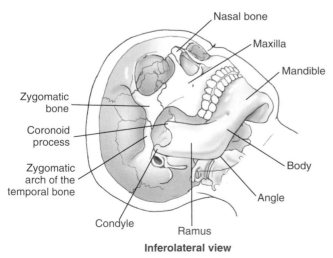

Inferolateral view

Figure 9-1 An oblique (inferolateral) view of the face.

Labels on Figure 9-1: Nasal bone, Maxilla, Mandible, Zygomatic bone, Coronoid process, Zygomatic arch of the temporal bone, Condyle, Ramus, Angle, Body

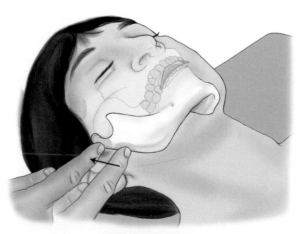

Inferolateral view

Figure 9-3 Ramus (posterior border) and condyle of the mandible.

To palpate the anterior border of the mandible inside the mouth, use a finger cot or glove and gently press posterolaterally (Figure 9-5). To palpate the coronoid process from inside the mouth, simply continue palpating along the anterior border of the ramus superiorly to the coronoid process.

Maxilla. The **maxilla**, also known as the *upper jaw*, is subcutaneous and easily palpated. First locate the maxilla superior to the mouth and then continue exploring all aspects of the maxilla (Figure 9-6).

PLEASE NOTE: The orbicularis oris, nasalis, depressor septi nasi, levator labii superioris alaeque nasi, levator labii superioris, and levator anguli oris muscles attach onto the maxilla.

Zygomatic Bone. The **zygomatic bone**, commonly referred to as the *cheek bone*, is easily palpated inferolateral to the eye. Once located, explore the zygomatic bone to its borders with the maxilla, frontal bone, and temporal bone (Figure 9-7).

PLEASE NOTE: The masseter, zygomaticus minor, and zygomaticus major muscles attach onto the zygomatic bone.

Nasal Bone. The **nasal bone** is easily palpable at the superior end of the nose (Figure 9-8). Note: The inferior end of the nose, which is composed of cartilage, is softer and more pliable.

PLEASE NOTE: The procerus muscle overlies the nasal bone.

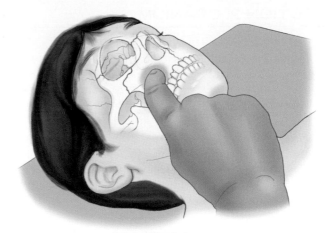

Inferolateral view
Figure 9-6 Maxilla.

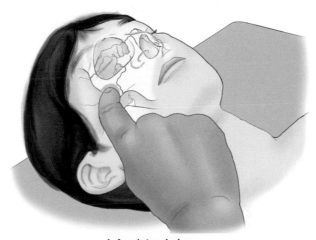

Inferolateral view
Figure 9-7 Zygomatic bone.

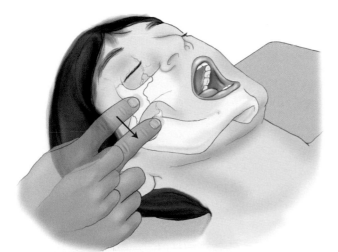

Inferolateral view
Figure 9-4 Coronoid process of the mandible.

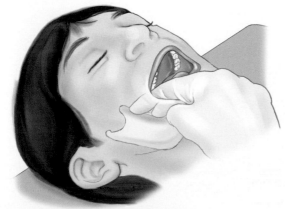

Inferolateral view
Figure 9-5 Ramus and coronoid process from inside the mouth.

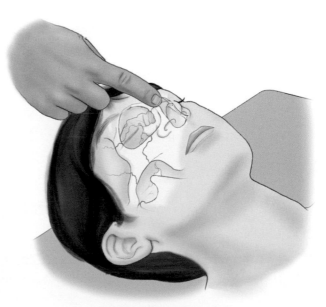

Inferolateral view
Figure 9-8 Nasal bone.

SECTION 2: CRANIUM

Lateral View of the Head (Figure 9-9)

Frontal and Parietal Bones. The frontal and parietal bones are subcutaneous and easily palpable. First locate the **frontal bone** superior to the eye (Figure 9-10). Then continue to palpate posteriorly onto the **parietal bone**, which is located at the top of the head (see Figure 9-10).

PLEASE NOTE: The orbicularis oculi and corrugator supercilii muscles attach onto the frontal bone; the frontalis muscle overlies the frontal bone. The temporalis muscle attaches onto the parietal bone. The temporoparietalis muscle and the galea aponeurotica of the occipitofrontalis muscle overlie the parietal bone.

Temporal Bone. The **temporal bone** is located on the side of the head (inferior to the parietal bone) (Figure 9-11, A).

To palpate the zygomatic arch of the temporal bone, first find the zygomatic bone (see Figure 9-7). Once located, continue palpating the zygomatic bone posteriorly until you reach the **zygomatic arch of the temporal bone** (see Figure 9-11, B). It can be helpful to strum your fingers vertically over the zygomatic arch. The entire length of the zygomatic arch of the temporal bone can be palpated.

To palpate the **mastoid process of the temporal bone**, palpate just posterior to the earlobe, then press medially and strum over the mastoid process by moving your palpating finger anteriorly and posteriorly (see Figure 9-11, C).

PLEASE NOTE: The temporalis muscle attaches to the majority of the temporal bone, making it more difficult to palpate this bone directly. Also, the temporoparietalis muscle overlies the temporal bone. The masseter muscle attaches onto the zygomatic arch of the temporal bone. The sternocleidomastoid, splenius capitis, and longissimus capitis muscles attach onto the mastoid process of the temporal bone.

Occipital Bone. The **occipital bone** is located at the back of the skull; it is subcutaneous and easily palpable (Figure 9-12, A). The **external occipital protuberance (EOP)** is a midline bump on the superior nuchal line of the occiput at the back of the head.

The EOP is usually fairly large and prominent and therefore readily palpable (see Figure 9-12, B).

To palpate the **superior nuchal line of the occiput**, begin by locating the EOP at the center of the superior nuchal line; then palpate laterally for the superior nuchal line. It should feel like a raised ridge of bone running horizontally. It can be helpful to strum your fingers vertically over the superior nuchal line (see Figure 9-12, C). The superior nuchal line is fairly prominent and easily palpable on some people and much more challenging to palpate on others. Note: The **inferior nuchal line of the occiput** runs parallel and is located inferiorly to the superior nuchal line. It is usually difficult to palpate. If its palpation is attempted, first locate the superior nuchal line and then palpate inferior to it for the inferior nuchal line.

PLEASE NOTE: The occipitalis muscle attaches to the occipital bone. The upper trapezius muscle attaches to the EOP and the superior nuchal line. The splenius capitis and sternocleidomastoid muscles also attach to the superior nuchal line of the occiput. The rectus capitis posterior major, rectus capitis posterior minor, and obliquus capitis superior also attach to the occipital bone.

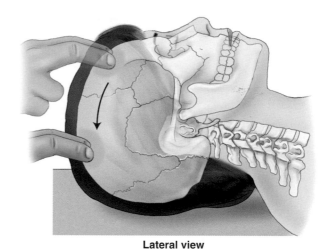

Lateral view

Figure 9-10 Frontal and parietal bones.

Zygomatic arch
of temporal bone

Mastoid process
of temporal bone

Frontal bone

Parietal bone

Temporal bone

Occipital bone

Superior nuchal line

External occipital
protuberance (EOP)

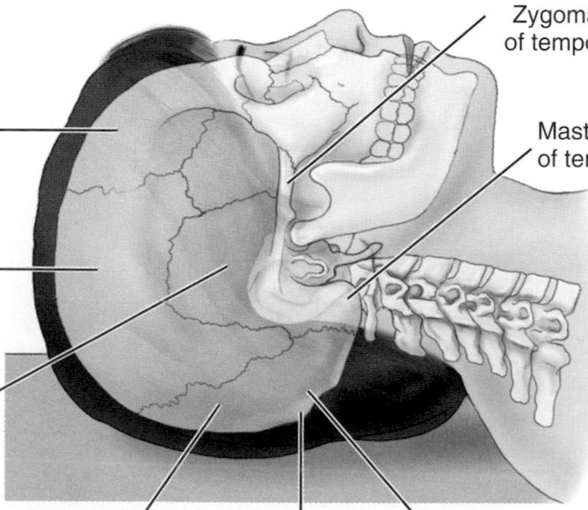

Lateral view

Figure 9-9 A lateral view of the head.

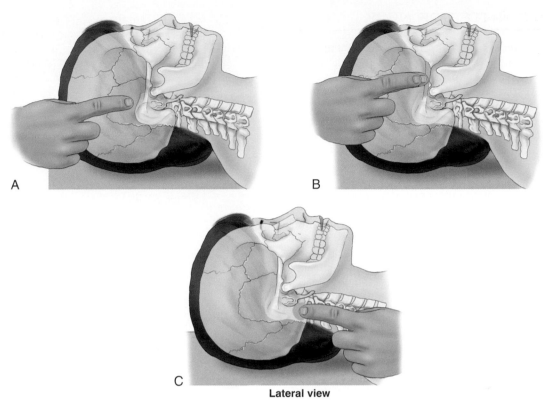

Lateral view

Figure 9-11 Temporal bone.

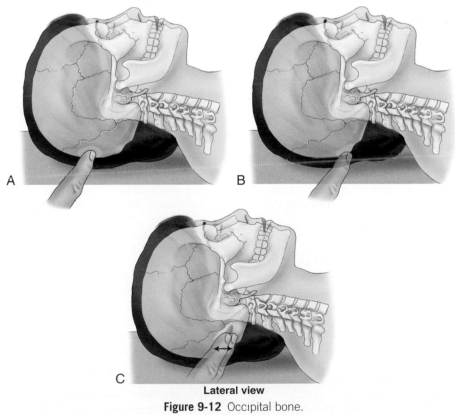

Lateral view

Figure 9-12 Occipital bone.

SECTION 3: ANTERIOR NECK

With all palpations in the anterior neck, a careful and sensitive touch is necessary, and palpatory pressure must be applied gradually. There are many structures in the anterior neck that are very sensitive and can be tender. Furthermore, the carotid arteries are found in the anterior neck and pressure upon them can not only potentially restrict blood flow within them to the anterior brain, but can also trigger a neurologic reflex (the carotid reflex) that can lower blood pressure. For this reason, it is best to palpate the anterior neck unilaterally (i.e., one side at a time). If you feel that your palpating fingers are on the carotid artery (with gentle to moderate pressure on an artery, you will detect a pulse), either move slightly off it, or gently displace it from your palpating fingers. Generally, palpation of the structures of the anterior neck is best accomplished if the client's neck is relaxed and either in a neutral position or a position of slight passive flexion. Note: Some of the following palpations are cartilage structures, not bony landmarks.

Lateral View of the Neck (Figure 9-13)

Hyoid Bone. The **hyoid bone** is found in the anterior neck, inferior to the mandible (located at the level of the third cervical vertebra). To find the hyoid bone, begin at the mandible and move inferiorly in the anterior neck until you feel hard bony tissue (Figure 9-14). Once on the hyoid bone, ask the client to swallow, and movement of the hyoid bone will be felt. The hyoid bone is very mobile, and it is possible to passively move it from left to right. A note of trivia: The hyoid bone is the only bone in the human body that does not articulate (form a joint) with another bone.

PLEASE NOTE: All four suprahyoid muscles and all four infrahyoid muscles (except the sternothyroid) attach onto the hyoid bone.

Thyroid Cartilage. The **thyroid cartilage** is located in the anterior neck, inferior to the hyoid bone. (The thyroid cartilage is located at the level of the fourth and fifth cervical vertebrae.) Once the hyoid bone has been located, drop off it inferiorly; you will feel a joint space and then the thyroid cartilage will be felt. Palpate the small midline superior notch (Figure 9-15, *A*). Then gently palpate both sides of the thyroid cartilage (see Figure 9-15, *B*). Movement of the thyroid cartilage is clearly felt if the client is asked to swallow. Palpation of the thyroid cartilage must be done gently and carefully, because the thyroid gland often overlies part of the thyroid cartilage.

PLEASE NOTE: The sternothyroid and thyrohyoid muscles attach onto the thyroid cartilage.

First Cricoid Cartilage and the Carotid Tubercle of C6. Directly inferior to the thyroid cartilage in the anterior neck is the first cricoid ring of cartilage at the sixth cervical vertebral level. To palpate the first cricoid cartilage, first locate the thyroid cartilage and continue to palpate along it inferiorly until a small joint line is felt. Immediately inferior to this joint line is the first cricoid cartilage (Figure 9-16, *A*). Subsequent **cricoid cartilages** are located inferior to the first cricoid cartilage and may be palpated until their palpation is no longer possible at the level of the suprasternal notch of the manubrium of the sternum. Palpation of the cricoid cartilages must be done gently and carefully because the thyroid gland overlies them.

The **carotid tubercle** is the anterior tubercle of the transverse process of the sixth cervical vertebra. It is the largest

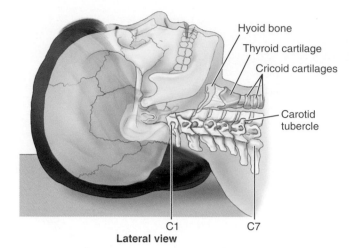

Figure 9-13 A lateral view of the neck.

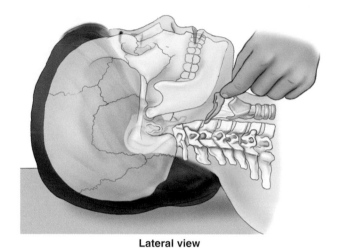

Figure 9-14 Hyoid bone.

anterior tubercle and is palpable in the anterior neck. To palpate the carotid tubercle, find the first cricoid cartilage and then drop off it laterally approximately ½ inch (1 cm); the carotid tubercle is felt by pressing firmly but gently in a posterior direction (see Figure 9-16, *B*).

Transverse Processes of C1 through C7. The **transverse processes (TPs)** of C2 through C7 are bifid and have **anterior tubercles** and **posterior tubercles**. These TPs may be palpated but must be palpated with gentle pressure because their tubercles are pointy, and pressing the overlying musculature into them can be tender for the client. Also, caution should be observed because the spinal nerves that enter/exit the spinal cord pass through the intervertebral foramina, which are located between the anterior and posterior tubercles. Begin by finding the carotid tubercle (anterior tubercle of the TP of C6) (see Figure 9-16, *B*), then palpate inferiorly and superiorly to find the other TPs. The direction of your pressure should be posterior and/or posteromedial (Figure 9-17, *A*).

The **transverse process (TP) of C1** (the atlas) has the widest TP of the cervical spine. The TP of C1 can be palpated at a point that is directly posterior to the posterior border of the ramus of the mandible, directly anterior to the mastoid process of the temporal bone, and directly inferior to the ear. In this depression of surrounding soft tissue, the hard TP of C1 is readily palpable (see Figure 9-17, *B*).

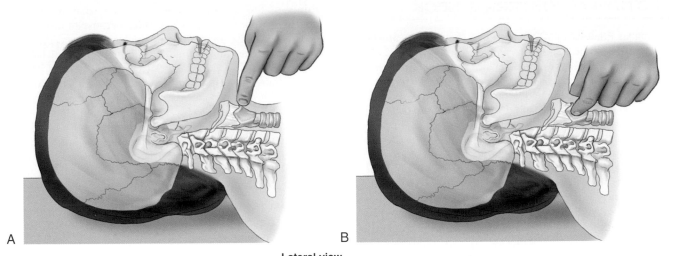

Lateral view

Figure 9-15 Thyroid cartilage.

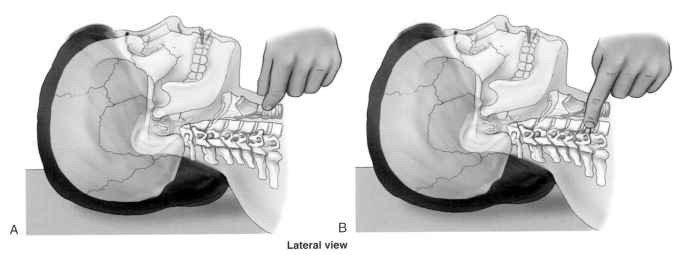

Lateral view

Figure 9-16 First cricoid cartilage and the carotid tubercle of C6.

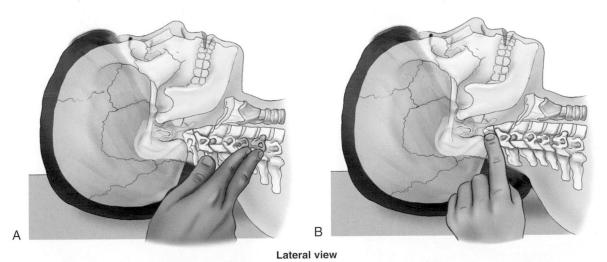

Lateral view

Figure 9-17 Transverse processes (TPs) of C1 through C7.

Pressure should be gentle because this landmark is often sensitive and tender to pressure, and the facial nerve (CN VII) is located nearby.

PLEASE NOTE: The following muscles attach onto the TPs of C2 through C7: the levator scapulae, scalene group, longus colli, longus capitis, erector spinae group, transversospinalis group, intertransversarii, and levatores costarum. The following muscles attach onto the TP of C1: the levator scapulae, splenius cervicis, obliquus capitis inferior, obliquus capitis superior, rectus capitis anterior, rectus capitis lateralis, and intertransversarii.

SECTION 4: POSTERIOR NECK

Spinous Processes of C2 through C7. The **spinous processes (SPs)** of the cervical spine are palpated in the midline of the posterior neck. There are seven cervical vertebrae; however, not all of the cervical SPs are always palpable. Because of the lordotic curve of the spine of the neck (concave posteriorly), the SPs are often deep in the concavity and therefore difficult to palpate. The exact number of cervical SPs that can be palpated is primarily determined by the degree of the cervical curve of the client. The most prominent cervical SPs are those of C2 and C7; these two are always palpable. Begin by finding the EOP in the midline of the occiput. From there, drop inferiorly off the occiput onto the cervical spine; the first cervical SP that is palpable is the SP of C2. As with most cervical SPs, the C2 SP is bifid (i.e., it has two points instead of one). It should be noted that these bifid points are not always symmetrical; one may be larger than the other. From C2, continue palpating inferiorly, feeling for additional cervical SPs (Figure 9-18). In some individuals, the next SP that is readily palpable is the one on C7 at the inferior end of the cervical spine.

The SP of C7 is clearly larger than the other lower cervical SPs, giving C7 the name **vertebra prominens**. In other individuals who have a decreased cervical spinal curve, it may be possible to palpate and count all the SPs from C2 to C7. Note: C1 (the atlas) does not have a SP; it has what is called a *posterior tubercle*. To palpate the **posterior tubercle of C1**, palpate between the SP of C2 and the occiput, pressing anteriorly into the soft tissue.

PLEASE NOTE: The following muscles either attach directly onto the SPs of the cervical spine, or attach into the nuchal ligament that overlies the SPs of the cervical spine: the upper trapezius, splenius capitis, splenius cervicis, interspinales, erector spinae group, and transversospinalis group. Furthermore, the rhomboid minor and serratus posterior superior muscles attach onto the SP of C7, the rectus capitis posterior major and obliquus capitis inferior muscles attach onto the SP of C2, and the rectus capitis posterior minor muscle attaches onto the posterior tubercle of C1.

Articular Processes (Facet Joints) of the Cervical Spine. The inferior and superior **articular processes** that create the **facet joints** of the cervical spine also create what is called the **articular pillar** or the **cervical pillar** because of the way they are stacked. They are easily palpable at the lateral side of the laminar groove (approximately one inch [2.5 cm] lateral to the SPs) and feel like broad flat bone just beyond the bulk of the transversospinalis musculature that attaches into and overlies the laminar groove. The client must be supine and relaxed for palpation to be successful. Begin palpation at the SP of C2, and palpate laterally for the articular process of C2 (Figure 9-19). Continue to palpate inferiorly until you reach the bottom of the neck. Note: The articular processes of the cervical spine are an excellent contact point when performing specific joint mobilizations to the cervical spine.

PLEASE NOTE: Muscles of the erector spinae group and the transversospinalis group attach onto the articular processes of the cervical spine.

Laminar Groove of the Cervical Spine. The **laminar groove** of the cervical spine is the groove that is found between the SPs medially and the articular processes laterally (i.e., the laminar groove overlies the laminae of the vertebrae). A number of muscles lie in the laminar groove, so direct palpation of the laminae at the floor of the laminar groove is difficult. Palpate just lateral to the SPs and you will be in the laminar groove (Figure 9-20).

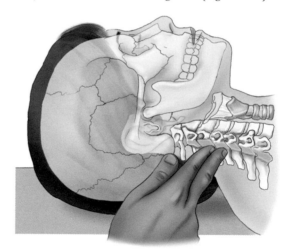

Lateral view

Figure 9-19 Articular processes (facet joints) of the cervical spine.

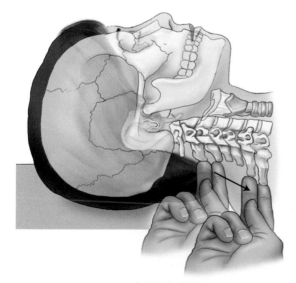

Lateral view

Figure 9-18 Spinous processes (SPs) of C2 through C7.

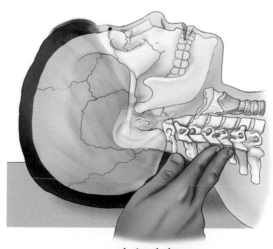

Lateral view

Figure 9-20 Laminar groove of the cervical spine.

PLEASE NOTE: The transversospinalis group attaches into the laminar groove of the neck. Many other muscles overlie the laminar groove.

SECTION 5: ANTERIOR TRUNK

Superolateral View of the Anterior Trunk (Figure 9-21)

Suprasternal Notch of the Sternum. The **suprasternal notch of the manubrium of the sternum** is subcutaneous and easily palpable. Simply palpate at the superior border of the sternum, and the depression of the suprasternal notch is readily felt between the medial ends of the two clavicles (Figure 9-22). Note: The suprasternal notch is also known as the **jugular notch**.

Angle of Louis. The **angle of Louis** is a horizontal prominence of bone on the sternum, formed by the **sternomanubrial joint**, which is the junction between the manubrium and the body of the sternum. (Note: The second sternocostal joint—in other words, where the second rib meets the sternum—is at the level of the angle of Louis.) To locate the angle of Louis, begin at the suprasternal notch of the manubrium and palpate inferiorly along the anterior surface of the manubrium until you feel a slight horizontal prominence of bone (Figure 9-23). It can be helpful to feel the angle of Louis by strumming vertically across it.

Xiphoid Process of the Sternum. The **xiphoid process of the sternum** is at the inferior end of the sternum. The xiphoid process is cartilaginous but may calcify into bone as a person ages. To locate the xiphoid process, continue palpating inferiorly along the anterior surface of the sternum from the angle of Louis until you feel the small, pointy xiphoid process at the inferior end (Figure 9-24). Because the xiphoid process is made of cartilage, it is usually possible to exert mild pressure upon it and feel it move. Note: The xiphoid process is a landmark often used to find the proper hand position to administer CPR.

PLEASE NOTE: The rectus abdominis muscle attaches to the external surface of the xiphoid process; the transversus thoracis and diaphragm muscles attach to its internal surface.

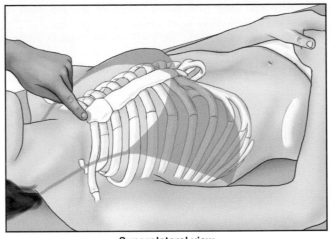

Superolateral view

Figure 9-22 Suprasternal notch of the sternum.

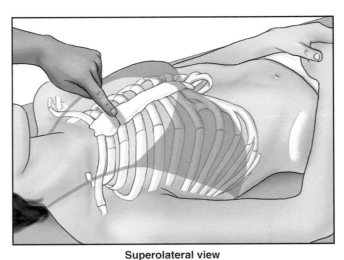

Superolateral view

Figure 9-23 Angle of Louis.

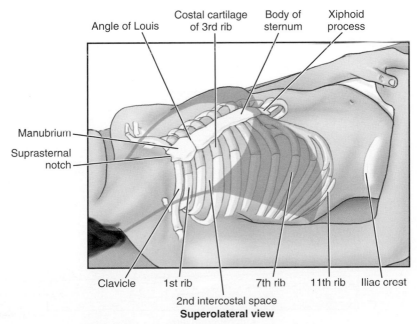

Angle of Louis   Costal cartilage of 3rd rib   Body of sternum   Xiphoid process

Manubrium

Suprasternal notch

Clavicle   1st rib   7th rib   11th rib   Iliac crest

2nd intercostal space

Superolateral view

Figure 9-21 Superolateral view of the anterior trunk.

Anterior Rib Cage. The anterior side of the **rib cage** is composed of twelve **ribs**, seven **costal cartilages** that join the ribs to the sternum, and the eleven **intercostal spaces** located between the adjacent ribs and/or costal cartilages. All ribs, costal cartilages, and intercostal spaces can be palpated anteriorly and anterolaterally (except where the breast tissue of female clients interferes with palpation). The ribs and/or costal cartilages are sensed as hard bony/cartilaginous tissue located subcutaneously, and the intercostal spaces are sensed as depressions of soft tissue located between the ribs and/or the costal cartilages. Once each rib has been successfully palpated, try to follow it medially and laterally for its entire course, as far as possible.

To palpate ribs two through ten: Palpate the anterior rib cage lateral to the sternum. Generally, for ribs two through ten, it is easiest to identify them by strumming across them in a superior to inferior manner. Inferior to the medial end of the clavicle is the first intercostal space. The second rib is located at the level of the angle of Louis (Figure 9-25, *A*). From there, palpate inferiorly and count the intercostal spaces and ribs until you find the seventh costal cartilage. Because of the contour of the rib cage, it is best to continue palpating ribs seven through ten and their costal cartilages more laterally in the anterior trunk (see Figure 9-25, *B*).

To palpate ribs eleven and twelve: Ribs eleven and twelve are called *floating ribs* because they do not articulate with the sternum. They must be palpated at the bottom of the rib cage, superior to the iliac crest, in the lateral and/or posterolateral trunk. It is often easiest to palpate the eleventh and twelfth ribs by pressing directly into and feeling for their pointy ends. (Note: This pressure should be firm but gentle because you are pressing soft tissue into the hard pointy end of a bone.)

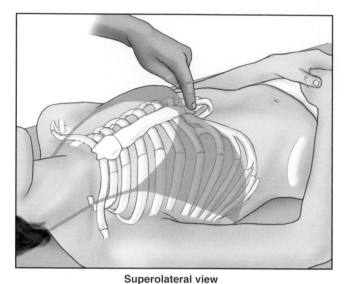

Superolateral view

Figure 9-24 Xiphoid process of the sternum.

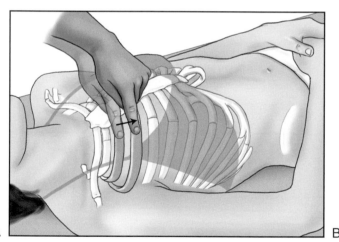

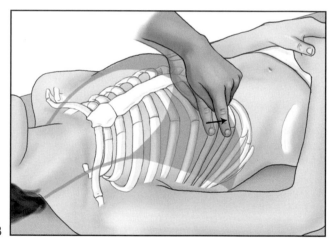

A   B

Superolateral view

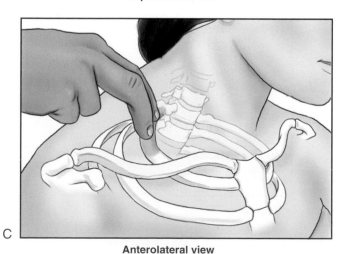

C

Anterolateral view

Figure 9-25 Anterior rib cage.

To palpate the first rib: The first rib is probably the most challenging to palpate, but it can be felt. To palpate the first rib, find the superior border of the upper trapezius muscle and then drop off it anteriorly and direct your palpatory pressure inferiorly against the first rib (see Figure 9-25, C). Asking the client to take in a deep breath elevates the first rib up against your palpating fingers and makes palpation easier.

PLEASE NOTE: Many muscles attach to and/or overlie the anterior rib cage, including the serratus anterior, pectoralis major, pectoralis minor, subclavius, external intercostals, internal intercostals, rectus abdominis, external abdominal oblique, internal abdominal oblique, and transversus abdominis. The transversus thoracis and diaphragm attach to the internal surface of the anterior rib cage.

SECTION 6: POSTERIOR TRUNK

Note: Palpation of the scapula is covered in Chapter 8.

Superolateral View of the Posterior Trunk (Figure 9-26)
Spinous Processes of the Trunk. The SPs of the twelve thoracic and five lumbar vertebrae are all palpable. Begin by locating the SP of C7 (also known as the *vertebra prominens*). It is usually the first very prominent SP inferior to the SP of C2.

When the client is prone, if there is confusion as to which SP is C7, the following is a method to determine it. Palpate the SPs of the lower cervical spine with fingers on two or three of the prominent ones. Then passively flex and extend the client's head and neck. The SP of C6 disappears from palpation with extension; the SP of C7 does not (i.e., the SP of C7 will be the highest SP palpable during flexion and extension).

Once the SP of C7 has been located, palpate each vertebral SP by placing your middle finger on the SP of that vertebra and your index finger in the **interspinous space** between that vertebra and the vertebra below. Continue palpating down the spine in this manner. It is usually possible to count the SPs from C7 to L5 (Figure 9-27). Note: The SPs of the thoracic region are usually easily palpable because of the kyphotic thoracic spinal curve. However, palpating the lumbar SPs is a bit more challenging

because of the lordotic lumbar spinal curve; to accomplish this, deeper pressure may be needed in the lumbar region.

PLEASE NOTE: The following muscles attach onto SPs of the trunk (thoracic and/or lumbar spine): the trapezius, splenius capitis, splenius cervicis, latissimus dorsi, rhomboids major and minor, serratus posterior superior, serratus posterior inferior, erector spinae group, transversospinalis group, and interspinales.

Transverse Processes of the Trunk. The TPs of the trunk can be challenging to discern, but many of them can be palpated. Usually the TPs of the thoracic region can be felt approximately 1 inch (2.5 cm) lateral to the SPs. However, determining the exact vertebral level of a TP can be difficult, because it is not located at the same level as the SP of the same vertebra. To determine the level of the TP that is being palpated, use the following method. Place one palpating finger on an SP, and then press down onto the TPs nearby one at a time until you feel the pressure upon a TP move the SP that is under the palpating finger (Figure 9-28). The vertebral level of that TP will be the same as that of the SP that moved. This method is usually successful for the thoracic spine; palpation of the TPs of the lumbar spine is much more challenging.

PLEASE NOTE: The following muscles attach onto TPs of the trunk (thoracic and/or lumbar spine): the erector spinae group, transversospinalis group, quadratus lumborum, intertransversarii, levatores costarum, and psoas major.

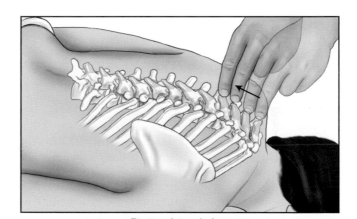

Posterolateral view
Figure 9-27 Spinous processes (SPs) of the trunk.

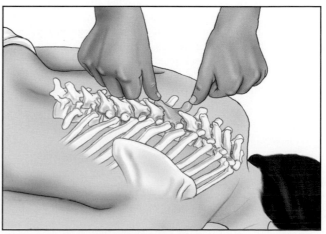

Posterolateral view
Figure 9-28 Transverse processes (TPs) of the trunk.

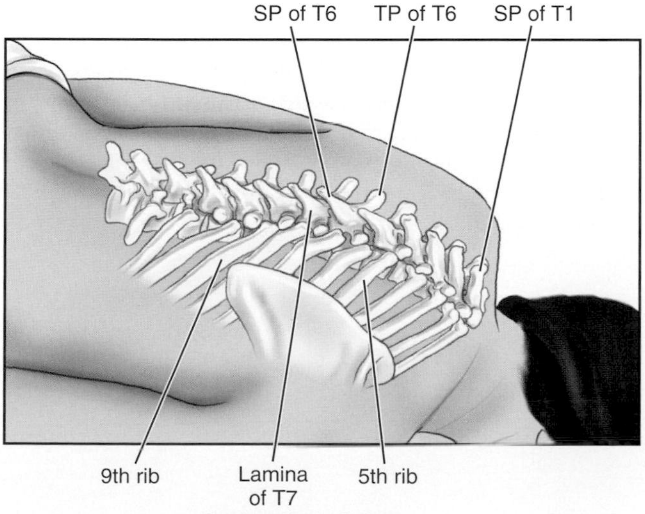

SP of T6   TP of T6   SP of T1

9th rib   Lamina of T7   5th rib
Posterolateral view
Figure 9-26 Superolateral view of the posterior trunk.

9

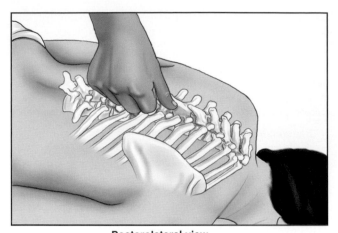

Posterolateral view

Figure 9-29 Laminar groove of the trunk.

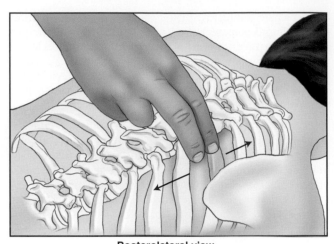

Posterolateral view

Figure 9-30 Posterior rib cage.

Laminar Groove of the Trunk. The laminar groove of the thoracic and lumbar regions is the groove that is found between the SPs medially and the TPs laterally (i.e., the laminar groove overlies the laminae of the vertebrae). Palpate just lateral to the SPs and you will be in the laminar groove (Figure 9-29).

PLEASE NOTE: The transversospinalis group attaches into the laminar groove of the trunk. Many other muscles overlie the laminar groove.

Posterior Rib Cage. The ribs and intercostal spaces of the rib cage can be palpated in the posterior trunk in the **interscapular region** (between the scapulae) of the upper thoracic spine and in the region of the lower thoracic spine as well. Begin palpating in the interscapular region of the posterior trunk by vertically strumming across the ribs (up and down). Once you have gotten the feel of the ribs and intercostal spaces in this region, palpate each rib by simultaneously placing one finger pad on it and another finger pad on the adjacent intercostal space (Figure 9-30). Palpate all twelve ribs (at, above, and below your starting point) in this manner. Depending upon the musculature of the client, it may be easy or somewhat difficult to discern all the ribs. Where the scapulae are not in the way, follow the ribs and intercostal spaces as far lateral as possible.

PLEASE NOTE: The following muscles attach onto the rib cage posteriorly: the latissimus dorsi, serratus posterior superior, serratus posterior inferior, erector spinae group, quadratus lumborum, levatores costarum, external intercostals, and internal intercostals. The subcostales and the diaphragm attach to the internal side of the posterior rib cage. Although primarily anterior, the external abdominal oblique, internal abdominal oblique, and transversus abdominis are located somewhat posteriorly on the rib cage as well.

SECTION 7: LIGAMENTS OF THE AXIAL BODY

Ligaments are fibrous fascial tissue that connects bones at a joint. The function of a ligament is to maintain stability of a joint by limiting motion. Figure 9-31 is an anterior view of the ligaments of the axial skeleton. One vertebral body has been removed. Figure 9-32 is a posterior view of the ligaments of the axial skeleton. Note: The posterior atlanto-occipital membrane is the superior continuation of the ligamentum flavum. Figure 9-33 is a posterior view of the ligaments of the upper cervical region. The atlas and axis have been cut. Notes: 1) The posterior atlanto-occipital membrane is the superior continuation of the ligamentum flavum. 2) The tectorial membrane is the superior continuation of the posterior longitudinal ligament. 3) The occiput has been cut on the right side to expose the tectorial membrane. 4) The tectorial membrane has been cut to expose the cruciate ligament of the dens, alar, and accessory atlantoaxial ligaments. And Figure 9-34 depicts right lateral views of the ligaments of the spine. Figure 9-34, *A*, is a sagittal section that shows the ligaments of the cervical spine. Note: The tectorial membrane is the superior continuation of the posterior longitudinal ligament. Figure 9-34, *B*, shows ligaments of the thoracic spine. The ribs have been cut; one rib has been entirely removed to show the TP attachment of a superior costotransverse ligament; the facets for the rib are also seen. Figure 9-34, *C*, shows the ligaments of the lumbar spine.

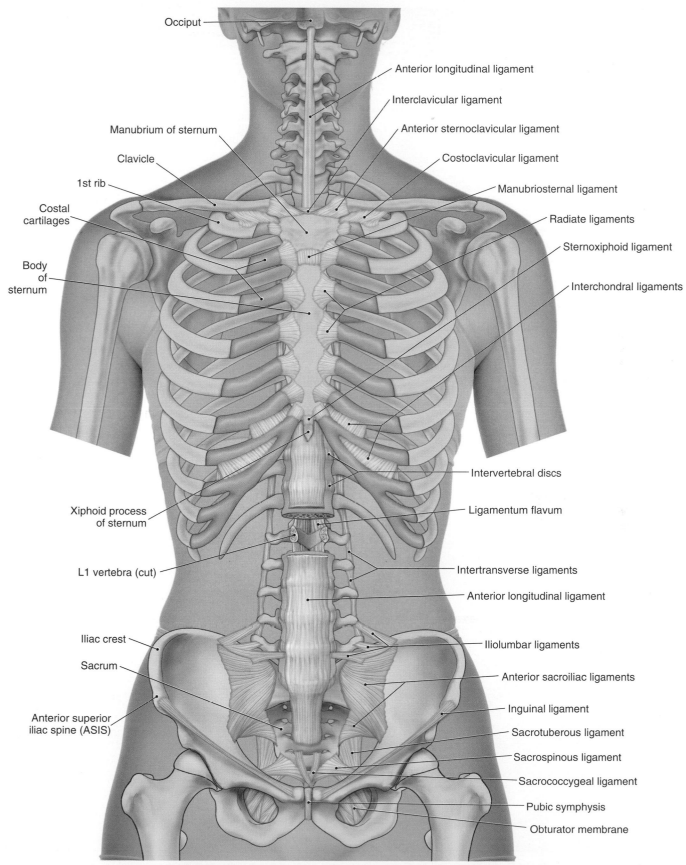

Figure 9-31 Anterior view of the ligaments of the axial skeleton.

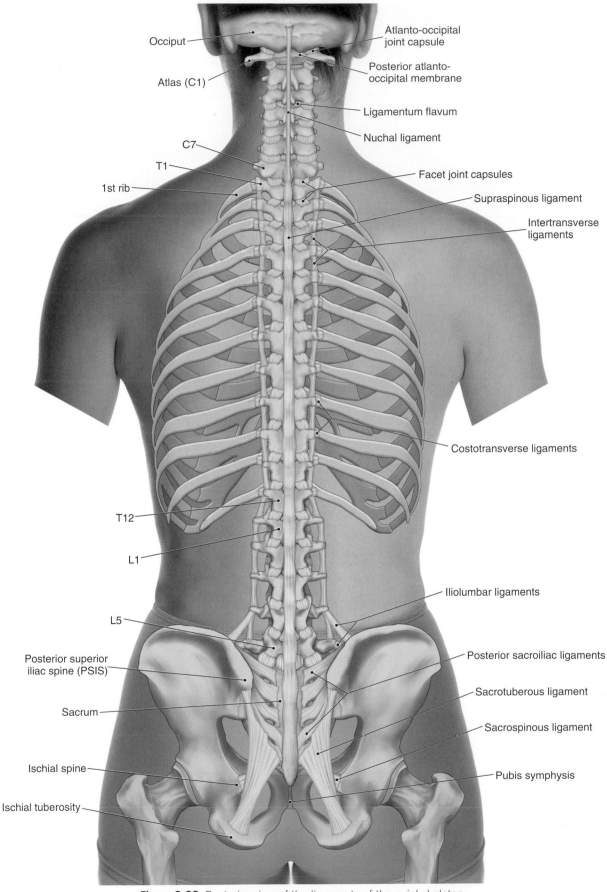

Occiput

Atlas (C1)

C7

T1

1st rib

T12

L1

L5

Posterior superior
iliac spine (PSIS)

Sacrum

Ischial spine

Ischial tuberosity

Atlanto-occipital
joint capsule

Posterior atlanto-
occipital membrane

Ligamentum flavum

Nuchal ligament

Facet joint capsules

Supraspinous ligament

Intertransverse
ligaments

Costotransverse ligaments

Iliolumbar ligaments

Posterior sacroiliac ligaments

Sacrotuberous ligament

Sacrospinous ligament

Pubis symphysis

Figure 9-32 Posterior view of the ligaments of the axial skeleton.

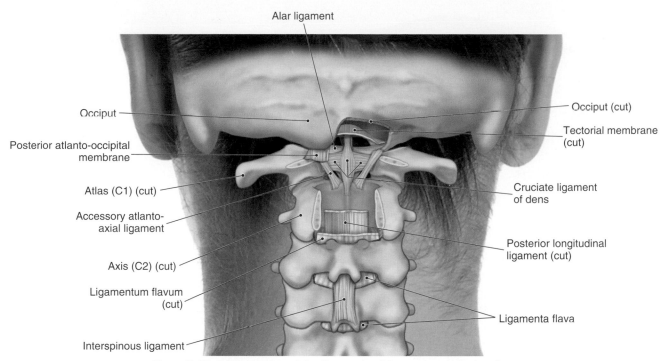

Alar ligament

Occiput

Occiput (cut)

Tectorial membrane
(cut)

Posterior atlanto-occipital
membrane

Atlas (C1) (cut)

Cruciate ligament
of dens

Accessory atlanto-
axial ligament

Posterior longitudinal
ligament (cut)

Axis (C2) (cut)

Ligamentum flavum
(cut)

Ligamenta flava

Interspinous ligament

Figure 9-33 Posterior view of the ligaments of the upper cervical region.

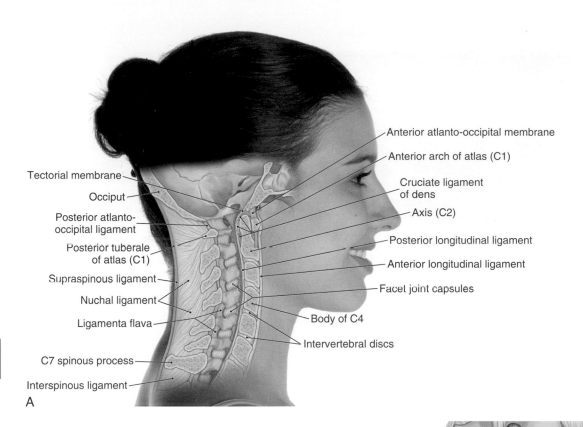

Anterior atlanto-occipital membrane

Anterior arch of atlas (C1)

Cruciate ligament of dens

Axis (C2)

Posterior longitudinal ligament

Anterior longitudinal ligament

Facet joint capsules

Body of C4

Intervertebral discs

Tectorial membrane

Occiput

Posterior atlanto-occipital ligament

Posterior tuberale of atlas (C1)

Supraspinous ligament

Nuchal ligament

Ligamenta flava

C7 spinous process

Interspinous ligament

A

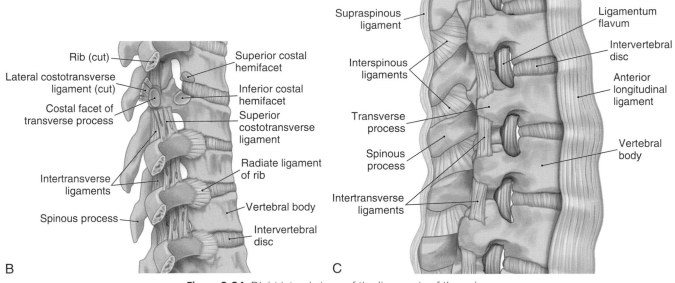

Rib (cut)

Lateral costotransverse ligament (cut)

Costal facet of transverse process

Intertransverse ligaments

Spinous process

Superior costal hemifacet

Inferior costal hemifacet

Superior costotransverse ligament

Radiate ligament of rib

Vertebral body

Intervertebral disc

B

Supraspinous ligament

Interspinous ligaments

Transverse process

Spinous process

Intertransverse ligaments

Ligamentum flavum

Intervertebral disc

Anterior longitudinal ligament

Vertebral body

C

Figure 9-34 Right lateral views of the ligaments of the spine.

Review Questions

1. Palpating along the superior posterior border of the ramus of the mandible anterior to the ear is the way to locate what bony structure? What else can be done to increase the accuracy of the palpation?
2. The coronoid process of the mandible serves as an attachment point for which two muscles?
3. What bone is commonly referred to as the cheek bone? What three bones share a border with this bone?
4. Pressing medially while palpating posterior to the earlobe is the procedure for palpating what bony structure?
5. To more easily palpate the superior nuchal line of the occiput, what bony structure should be located first?
6. What distinction does the hyoid bone hold?
7. What is the location of the carotid tubercle?
8. Care must be observed during palpation of the transverse process (TP) of C1 due to what sensitive nearby structure?
9. What structures make up the facet joints?
10. What is the procedure for locating the angle of Louis?
11. How do the natural curves of the spine impact the ease of palpation of the spinous processes (SPs)?
12. The laminar groove is found between what structures?
13. What primarily anterior abdominal wall muscles are also located somewhat posteriorly?

9

Lower Extremity Bone Palpation and Ligaments

Overview

Chapter 10 is one of three chapters of Part III of this book, which addresses palpation of the skeleton. This chapter is a palpation tour of the bones, bony landmarks, and joints of the lower extremity. The tour begins with the pelvis, then addresses the thigh and leg, and concludes with the foot. Although any one bone or bony landmark can be independently palpated, this chapter is set up sequentially to flow from one landmark to another, so following the order presented here is recommended. Muscle attachments for each of the palpated structures are also given. Even though specific palpations for these muscles are covered in Part IV of this book, now would also be a good time to palpate and explore these muscle attachments. The ligaments of the lower extremity are presented at the end of this chapter.

Chapter 8 presents the ligaments of the upper extremity and the palpation of the bones, bony landmarks, and joints of the upper extremity. Chapter 9 presents the ligaments of the axial body and the palpation of the bones, bony landmarks, and joints of the axial body.

Chapter Outline

The bones, bony landmarks, and joints of the following regions are covered:
Section 1: Pelvis
Section 2: Thigh and Leg
Section 3: Medial Foot
Section 4: Lateral Foot
Section 5: Dorsal Foot
Section 6: Plantar Foot
Section 7: Ligaments of the Lower Extremity

Chapter Objectives

After completing this chapter, the student/therapist should be able to perform the following:
1. Define the key terms of this chapter.
2. Palpate each of the bones, bony landmarks, and joints of this chapter, which are listed as key terms.
3. State the muscle or muscles that attach to each of the bony landmarks of this chapter.
4. Describe the location of each of the ligaments of the lower extremity.

Key Terms

Anterior inferior iliac spine (AIIS)
Anterior superior iliac spine (ASIS)
Calcaneal tuberosity
Calcaneus
Coccyx
Cuboid
Distal interphalangeal (DIP) joint
Distal phalanx
Femoral condyles
Fibular shaft
Fibular tubercle of the calcaneus
First cuneiform
Gluteal fold
Greater trochanter of the femur
Head of the fibula

Head of the talus
Iliac crest
Interphalangeal (IP) joint
Ischial tuberosity
Knee joint
Lateral femoral condyle
Lateral malleolus of the fibula
Lateral tibial condyle
Lesser trochanter of the femur
Medial femoral condyle
Medial malleolus of the tibia
Medial tibial condyle
Medial tubercle of the talus
Metatarsal
Metatarsal base
Metatarsal head

Metatarsophalangeal (MTP) joint
Middle phalanx
Navicular tuberosity
Patella
Phalanges (singular:phalanx)
Posterior superior iliac spine (PSIS)
Proximal interphalangeal (PIP) joint
Proximal phalanx
Pubic bone
Pubic tubercle
Sacral tubercles
Sacrococcygeal joint
Sacroiliac (SI) joint

Sacrum	Sustentaculum tali of the	Tibial condyles
Second cuneiform	calcaneus	Tibial shaft
Sesamoid bones	Talonavicular joint	Tibial tuberosity
Styloid process of the fifth	Tarsal sinus	Trochlea of the talus
metatarsal	Tarsometatarsal joint	Trochlear groove of the femur
Subtalar joint	Third cuneiform	

ⓔ Go to http://evolve.elsevier.com/Muscolino/palpation for identification of bony landmark exercises.

SECTION 1: PELVIS

An Inferolateral Oblique View of the Posterior Pelvis (Figure 10-1)

Iliac Crest. The **iliac crest** is subcutaneous and easily palpable. With the client prone, place your palpating fingers on the iliac crest and follow it as far anterior as possible (Figure 10-2). It ends at the anterior superior iliac spine (ASIS). Then follow the iliac crest posteriorly to the posterior superior iliac spine (PSIS).

PLEASE NOTE: The following muscles attach onto the iliac crest: the latissimus dorsi, erector spinae group, quadratus lumborum, external abdominal oblique, internal abdominal oblique, transversus abdominis, gluteus maximus, and tensor fasciae latae.

The Posterior Superior Iliac Spine. The **posterior superior iliac spine (PSIS)** is the most posterior aspect of the iliac crest and is usually visually prominent as well as easily palpable. Locate it by following the iliac crest posteriorly until the PSIS is felt (Figure 10-3). The PSIS is located approximately 2 inches (5 cm) from the midline of the superior aspect (the base) of the sacrum, and it is easily located because the skin drops in around the medial side of it, forming a dimple in most individuals. First visually locate the dimple; then palpate into it, pressing slightly laterally against the PSIS.

PLEASE NOTE: The latissimus dorsi and gluteus maximus muscles attach onto the PSIS.

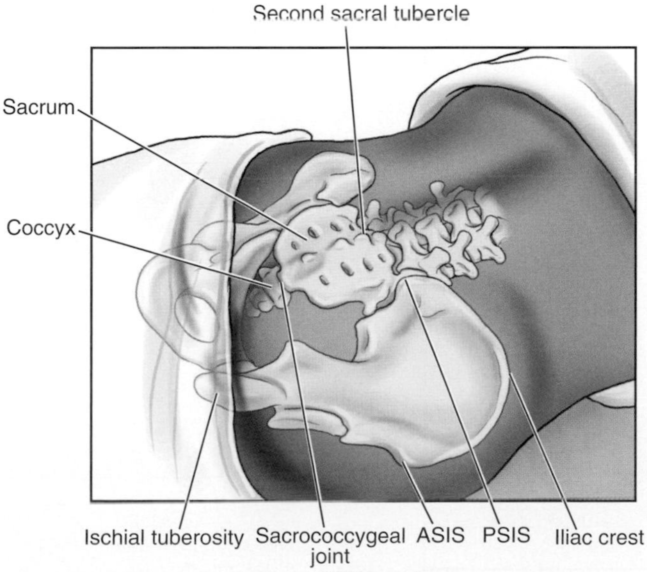

Sacrum and Sacral Tubercles. From the PSIS, palpate the midline of the **sacrum**, feeling for the **sacral tubercles**. Once a sacral tubercle is located, continue palpating superiorly and inferiorly for the other sacral tubercles (Figure 10-4). The second sacral tubercle is usually at the level of the PSISs. Note: The **sacroiliac (SI) joint**, located between the sacrum and ilium on each side, is not directly palpable because of the overhang of the PSIS and the presence of the musculature and joint ligaments.

PLEASE NOTE: The following muscles attach onto the posterior sacrum: the latissimus dorsi, erector spinae group, transversospinalis group, gluteus maximus, and coccygeus. The piriformis

10

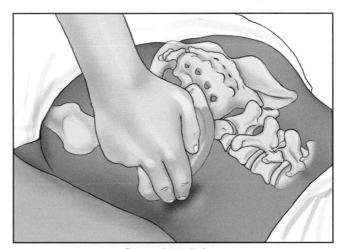

Superolateral view
Figure 10-2 Iliac crest.

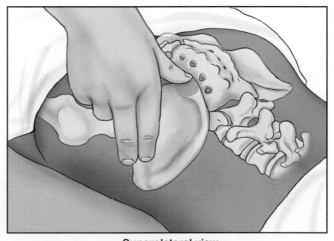

Superolateral view
Figure 10-3 The posterior superior iliac spine (PSIS).

Second sacral tubercle

Sacrum

Coccyx

Ischial tuberosity   Sacrococcygeal   ASIS   PSIS   Iliac crest
joint
Oblique view
Figure 10-1 An inferolateral oblique view of the posterior pelvis.

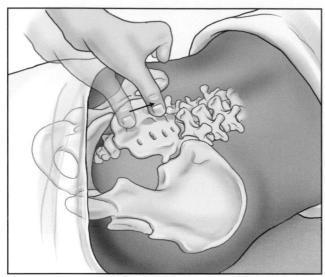

Inferolateral view
Figure 10-4 Sacrum.

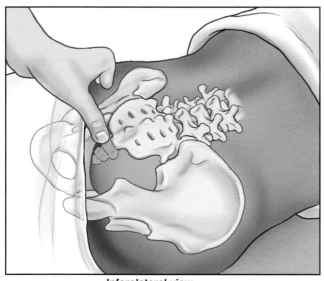

Inferolateral view
Figure 10-5 Coccyx.

and iliacus attach onto the anterior sacrum. The sacrotuberous and sacrospinous ligaments also attach to the sacrum.

Coccyx. The **coccyx** is located directly inferior to the sacrum (Figure 10-5). It is subcutaneous and usually easily palpable. At the most superior aspect of the coccyx, the **sacrococcygeal joint** can usually be palpated.

PLEASE NOTE: The gluteus maximus and coccygeus muscles attach onto the coccyx. The sacrotuberous and sacrospinous ligaments also attach to the coccyx.

Ischial Tuberosity. The **ischial tuberosity** is located deep to the **gluteal fold**, slightly medial to the midpoint of the buttock. Palpating it from the inferior perspective is best so that the palpating fingers do not have to palpate through the gluteus maximus (Figure 10-6). Moderate to deep pressure is necessary to palpate the ischial tuberosity; however, it is not difficult to feel and is usually not tender for the client. Once located, strum across the ischial tuberosity both horizontally and vertically to palpate it in its entirety. Specifically, the ischial tuberosity can be palpated superiorly onto its lateral border and superiorly onto its medial border.

PLEASE NOTE: The adductor magnus, inferior gemellus, quadratus femoris, and hamstring muscles attach onto the ischial tuberosity. The sacrotuberous ligament also attaches to the ischial tuberosity. Note: The levator ani muscle is located at the medial border of the ischial tuberosity.

Greater Trochanter of the Femur. The **greater trochanter of the femur** is valuable to palpate along with the bony landmarks of the posterior pelvis because the majority of the muscles of the posterior pelvis attach distally onto the greater trochanter. It is fairly large (approximately 1.5 × 1.5 inches [4 × 4 cm]) and subcutaneous; hence it is fairly easy to palpate. From the ischial tuberosity, palpate at the same level (or slightly superior) on the lateral proximal thigh and the greater trochanter can be found; strum along it vertically and horizontally to feel the entire greater trochanter (Figure 10-7).

PLEASE NOTE: The following muscles attach onto the greater trochanter: the gluteus medius, gluteus minimus, piriformis, superior gemellus, obturator internus, inferior gemellus, and vastus lateralis.

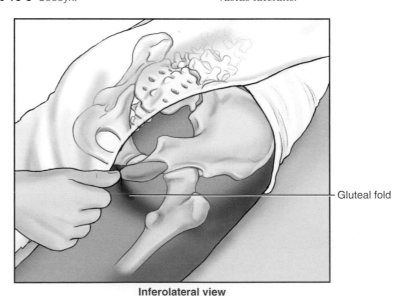

Gluteal fold

Inferolateral view
Figure 10-6 Ischial tuberosity.

Inferolateral Oblique View of the Anterior Pelvis (Figure 10-8)

Anterior Superior Iliac Spine. The **anterior superior iliac spine (ASIS)** is the most anterior aspect of the iliac crest. It is usually visually prominent as well as easily palpable. From the iliac crest (see Figure 10-2), continue palpating anteriorly until you reach the ASIS (Figure 10-9).

PLEASE NOTE: The tensor fasciae latae and sartorius muscles attach onto the ASIS.

Anterior Inferior Iliac Spine. Because of the thickness of musculature that overlies the **anterior inferior iliac spine (AIIS)**, it can be challenging to palpate. One method to locate it is to drop inferiorly from the ASIS and feel for the AIIS deeper into the tissue (Figure 10-10). However, the best method is to first locate the rectus femoris muscle of the quadriceps femoris group and then follow it proximally to its attachment onto the AIIS with the client's hip joint passively flexed. Note: this requires comfort and familiarity with muscle palpation of the rectus femoris.

PLEASE NOTE: The rectus femoris muscle attaches onto the AIIS.

Pubic Bone and Pubic Tubercle. The **pubic bone** is located at the most inferior aspect of the anterior abdomen. The **pubic tubercle** is on the anterior surface of the body of the pubic bone near the pubic symphysis joint and is at approximately the same level as the superior aspect of the greater trochanter of the femur. To locate the pubic bone, begin by palpating more superiorly on the anterior abdominal wall, then carefully and gradually palpate farther inferiorly, pressing gently into the abdominal wall until the pubic bone is felt (Figure 10-11). It helps to use the ulnar side of the hand and direct the pressure posteriorly and inferiorly. It is important that the abdominal wall muscles are relaxed so that when the pubic bone is reached, it will be readily felt.

PLEASE NOTE: The following muscles attach onto the superior ramus of the pubis and/or the body of the pubis: the rectus abdominis, pectineus, adductor longus, gracilis, and adductor brevis.

Greater trochanter of femur

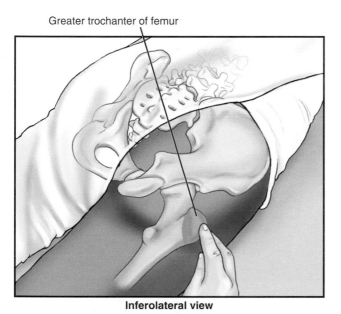

Inferolateral view

Figure 10-7 Greater trochanter of the femur.

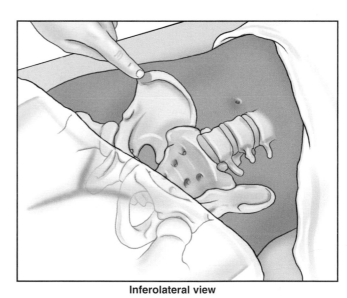

Inferolateral view

Figure 10-9 Anterior superior iliac spine (ASIS).

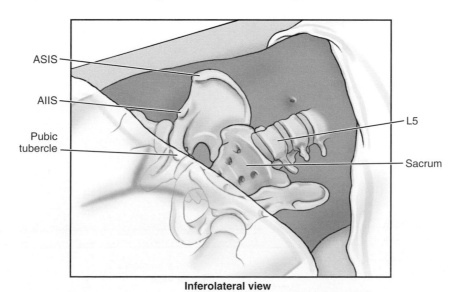

ASIS

AIIS

Pubic tubercle

L5

Sacrum

Inferolateral view

Figure 10-8 An inferolateral oblique view of the anterior pelvis.

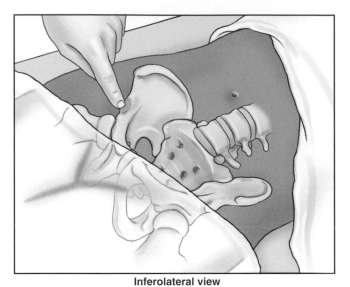

Inferolateral view

Figure 10-10 Anterior inferior iliac spine (AIIS).

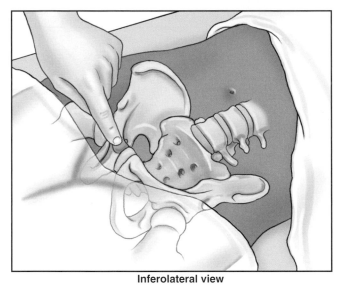

Inferolateral view

Figure 10-11 Pubic bone and pubic tubercle.

SECTION 2: THIGH AND LEG

Distal View of the Proximal Anterior Thigh
(Figure 10-12)

Greater Trochanter. Begin palpation of the thigh by locating again the greater trochanter of the femur. The greater trochanter is located in the proximal lateral thigh, at approximately the same level as the pubic tubercle. It is fairly large (approximately 1.5 × 1.5 inches [4 × 4 cm]) and subcutaneous, hence it is fairly easy to palpate; strum along it vertically and horizontally to feel the entire greater trochanter (Figure 10-13).

PLEASE NOTE: The following muscles attach onto the greater trochanter: the gluteus medius, gluteus minimus, piriformis, superior gemellus, obturator internus, inferior gemellus, and vastus lateralis.

Lesser Trochanter. The **lesser trochanter of the femur** is located in the proximal medial thigh. It is a palpable landmark, but is appreciably more challenging to discern, so palpating it with certainty requires more advanced palpation skills and

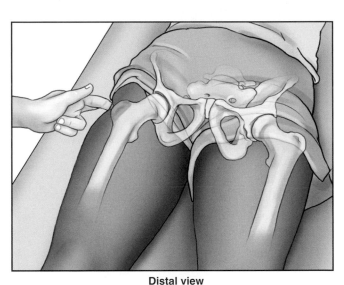

Distal view

Figure 10-13 Greater trochanter.

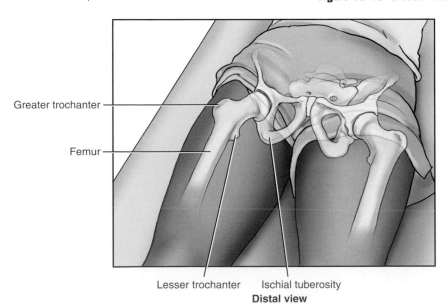

Greater trochanter

Femur

Lesser trochanter   Ischial tuberosity
Distal view

Figure 10-12 Distal view of the proximal anterior thigh.

knowledge of the psoas major muscle. To locate the lesser trochanter of the femur, the distal aspect of the psoas major muscle must be located. Once located, follow the psoas major distally as far as possible. Then have the client relax their thigh in a position of flexion and slight lateral rotation of the thigh at the hip joint to relax and slacken the psoas major; then press in against the femur, feeling for the lesser trochanter (Figure 10-14).

PLEASE NOTE: The psoas major and iliacus muscles (iliopsoas muscle) attach onto the lesser trochanter.

Patella. The **patella** (kneecap) is a prominent sesamoid bone located anterior to the distal femur. To best palpate the patella, have the client supine with the lower extremity relaxed

(Figure 10-15). Palpate the entire patella, gently gliding along the patella horizontally and vertically.

PLEASE NOTE: The quadriceps femoris group attaches onto the patella.

Anterolateral View of the Leg with the Knee Joint Flexed to 90 Degrees (Figure 10-16)

Trochlear Groove of the Femur. To palpate the **trochlear groove of the femur,** the knee joint should be flexed approximately 90 degrees and the quadriceps femoris musculature relaxed. (When the knee joint is fully extended, the patella moves proximally within the trochlear groove and obstructs its palpation.) Now palpate immediately proximal to the patella in the midline of the anterior femur, and the trochlear groove

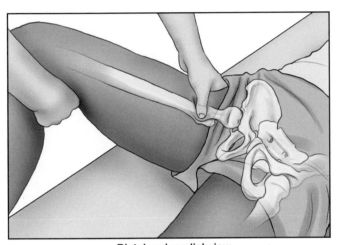

Distal and medial view

Figure 10-14 Lesser trochanter.

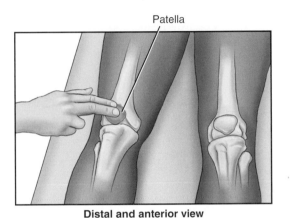

Distal and anterior view

Figure 10-15 Patella.

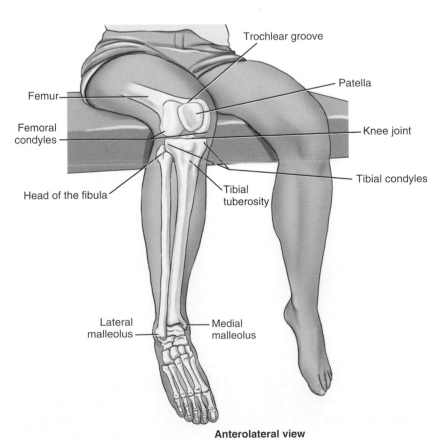

Anterolateral view

Figure 10-16 Anterolateral view of the leg with the knee joint flexed to 90 degrees.

will be evident (Figure 10-17). (Note: The patella is not shown in this figure.)

Knee Joint. With the client's **knee joint** flexed to approximately 90 degrees, drop off the inferior aspect of the patella and the joint line of the knee will be palpable both medially and laterally (Figure 10-18). Palpate within the joint space as well as superiorly against the femur and inferiorly against the tibia as you continue to palpate the knee joint toward the posterior side, medially and laterally.

PLEASE NOTE: The medial and lateral menisci are palpable against the anterior tibia within the joint line of the knee.

Femoral Condyles. The inferior margins of the **medial femoral condyle** and **lateral femoral condyle** are palpable by pressing proximally up against the femur from the joint line of the knee, on both sides of the patella (Figure 10-19). Once located, palpate farther proximally onto the medial and lateral **femoral condyles.**

PLEASE NOTE: The following muscles attach onto the femoral condyles: the adductor magnus, gastrocnemius, plantaris, and popliteus.

Tibial Condyles. The superior margins of the **medial tibial condyle** and **lateral tibial condyle** are palpable by pressing distally down against the tibia from the joint line of the knee on both sides of the patella (Figure 10-20). Once located, palpate farther distally onto the medial and lateral **tibial condyles.**

PLEASE NOTE: The biceps femoris and semimembranosus muscles attach onto the posterior surface of the tibial condyles. The gluteus maximus and tensor fasciae latae attach onto the lateral tibial condyle via the iliotibial band.

Head of the Fibula. As you continue palpating along the superior margin of the lateral condyle of the tibia, you will reach the head of the fibula (Figure 10-21). The **head of the**

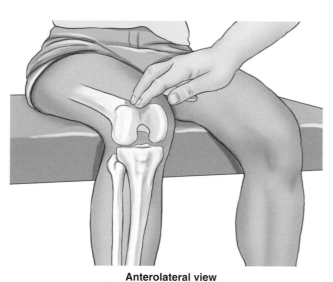

Anterolateral view
Figure 10-17 Trochlear groove of the femur.

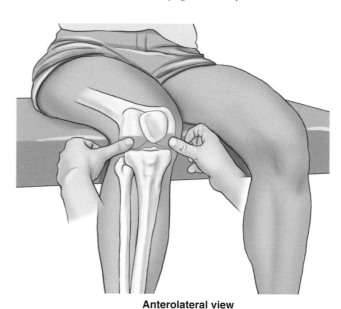

Anterolateral view
Figure 10-19 Femoral condyles.

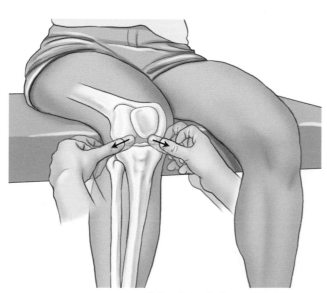

Anterolateral view
Figure 10-18 Knee joint.

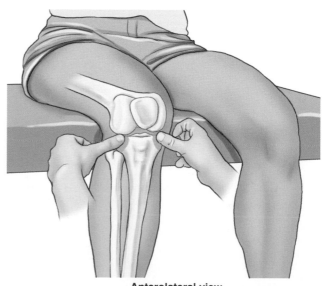

Anterolateral view
Figure 10-20 Tibial condyles.

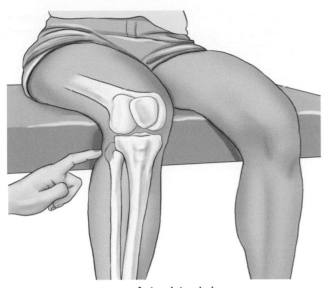

Anterolateral view

Figure 10-21 Head of the fibula.

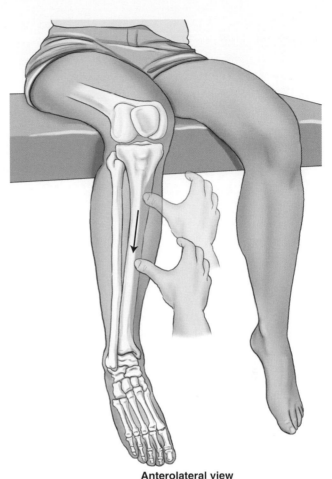

Anterolateral view

Figure 10-23 Tibial shaft.

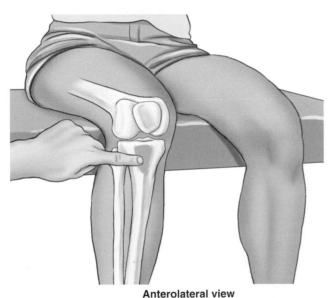

Anterolateral view

Figure 10-22 Tibial tuberosity.

fibula is the most proximal landmark of the fibula, located on the posterolateral side of the knee, and can be palpated anteriorly, laterally, and posteriorly. Note: The common fibular nerve is superficial near the head of the fibula, so care should be taken when palpating here.

PLEASE NOTE: The biceps femoris, fibularis longus, soleus, and extensor digitorum longus muscles attach onto the head of the fibula.

Tibial Tuberosity. The **tibial tuberosity** is a prominent landmark located at the center of the proximal shaft of the anterior tibia, approximately 1 to 2 inches (2.5 to 5 cm) distal to the inferior margin of the patella (Figure 10-22).

PLEASE NOTE: The quadriceps femoris muscle group attaches onto the tibial tuberosity.

Tibial Shaft. From the tibial tuberosity, the entire anteromedial **tibial shaft** is subcutaneous and easily palpable (Figure 10-23).

Begin palpating at the tibial tuberosity and continue palpating distally until you reach the medial malleolus at the end of the anteromedial tibial shaft.

PLEASE NOTE: The tibialis anterior, pes anserine group (sartorius, gracilis, semitendinosus), and quadriceps femoris group of muscles attach onto the anterior tibial shaft. The popliteus, soleus, tibialis posterior, and flexor digitorum longus muscles attach onto the posterior tibial shaft.

Medial Malleolus. The **medial malleolus of the tibia** is the very prominent bony landmark at the ankle region that is located on the medial side. As you palpate down the anteromedial shaft of the tibia, you will reach the medial malleolus (Figure 10-24). Palpate the circumference of this large bony landmark.

PLEASE NOTE: The deltoid ligament attaches onto the medial malleolus.

Lateral Malleolus. The **lateral malleolus of the fibula** is the very prominent bony landmark that is located at the lateral side of the ankle region. The lateral malleolus is the distal expanded end of the fibula (Figure 10-25). Notice that the lateral malleolus of the fibula is located somewhat farther distal than is the medial malleolus of the tibia.

PLEASE NOTE: The anterior talofibular, posterior talofibular, and calcaneofibular ligaments all attach onto the lateral malleolus.

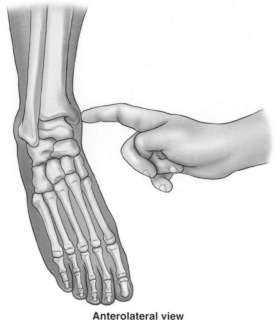

Anterolateral view
Figure 10-24 Medial malleolus.

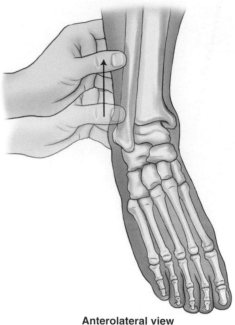

Anterolateral view
Figure 10-26 Fibular shaft.

10

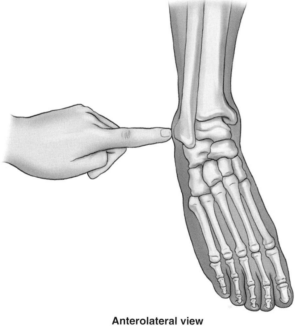

Anterolateral view
Figure 10-25 Lateral malleolus.

Fibular Shaft. The distal **fibular shaft** is palpable in the distal leg. Begin palpating the fibula at the lateral malleolus, and continue palpating the lateral shaft of the fibula proximally until you can no longer feel it deep to the overlying musculature (Figure 10-26).

PLEASE NOTE: The fibularis longus and brevis muscles attach to the lateral fibular shaft. The extensor digitorum longus, extensor hallucis longus, and fibularis tertius muscles attach to the anterior fibular shaft. The soleus, tibialis posterior, and flexor hallucis longus muscles attach to the posterior fibular shaft.

SECTION 3: MEDIAL FOOT

Medial View of the Foot (Figure 10-27)
Phalanges and Interphalangeal Joint of the Big Toe. Begin palpating the medial side of the foot distally at the proximal and distal phalanges of the big toe (Figure 10-28, *A*). The **interphalangeal (IP) joint** between them can be palpated as well (see Figure 10-28, *B*).

PLEASE NOTE: The extensor hallucis longus and extensor hallucis brevis muscles attach onto the dorsal side of the phalanges of the big toe; the flexor hallucis longus, flexor hallucis brevis, adductor hallucis, and abductor hallucis muscles attach onto the plantar side of the phalanges of the big toe.

First Metatarsophalangeal Joint. From the proximal phalanx of the big toe, continue palpating proximally along the medial surface of the foot and you will feel the joint line of the first **metatarsophalangeal (MTP) joint** (Figure 10-29).

First Metatarsal. The dorsal and medial surfaces of the first **metatarsal** are subcutaneous and easily palpable (Figure 10-30). As with the metacarpals of the hand, the expanded distal head and expanded proximal base of the metatarsals are palpable. (Note: The distal head of the first metatarsal is palpable on the dorsal, medial, and planter sides of the foot.)

PLEASE NOTE: The tibialis anterior, fibularis longus, and first dorsal interosseus muscles attach to the first metatarsal.

First Cuneiform. Just proximal to the base of the first metatarsal on the medial and dorsal sides, the joint line between the first metatarsal and first cuneiform is palpable. Move just proximal to the joint line, and the **first cuneiform** is palpable (Figure 10-31).

PLEASE NOTE: The tibialis anterior, fibularis longus, and tibialis posterior muscles attach to the first cuneiform.

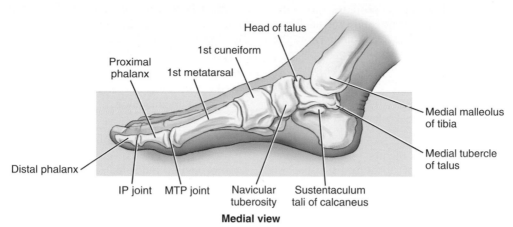

Figure 10-27 Medial view of the foot.

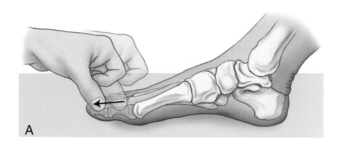

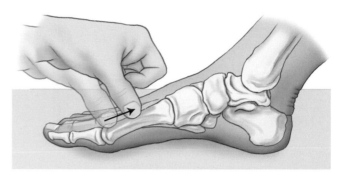

Medial view
Figure 10-30 First metatarsal.

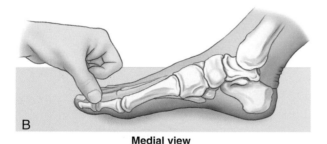

Medial view
Figure 10-28 Phalanges and interphalangeal (IP) joint of the big toe.

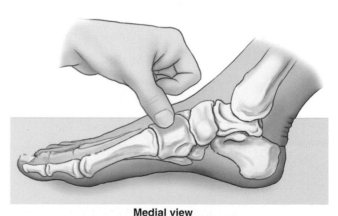

Medial view
Figure 10-31 First cuneiform.

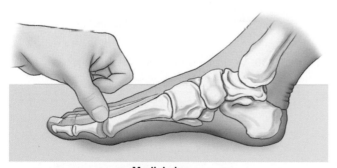

Medial view
Figure 10-29 First metatarsophalangeal (MTP) joint.

Navicular Tuberosity. Continuing proximal from the first cuneiform, the **navicular tuberosity** is quite prominent and palpable (Figure 10-32).

PLEASE NOTE: The tibialis posterior muscle attaches to the navicular tuberosity. The spring ligament also attaches to the navicular tuberosity.

Head of the Talus. The **head of the talus** is immediately posterior to the navicular (Figure 10-33). The **talonavicular joint** between these two bones is most evident if you have the client invert and evert the foot.

PLEASE NOTE: The talus is the only tarsal bone that has no muscle attachments.

Sustentaculum Tali of the Calcaneus. From the navicular tuberosity (see Figure 10-32), move your palpating finger approximately 1 inch (2.5 cm) directly posterior, and the **sustentaculum tali of the calcaneus** should be palpable (or

10

from the head of the talus, drop slightly posterior and in the plantar direction) (Figure 10-34). The sustentaculum tali forms a shelf upon which the talus sits. The joint line between the sustentaculum tali and the talus above is often palpable. As a point of reference, the medial malleolus of the tibia is located approximately 1 inch (2.5 cm) directly above (proximal to) the sustentaculum tali.

PLEASE NOTE: The spring ligament attaches to the sustentaculum tali.

Medial Tubercle of the Talus. Slightly posterior to the sustentaculum tali (posterior and plantar to the medial malleolus) the **medial tubercle of the talus** can be palpated (Figure 10-35).

Most Prominent Landmarks of the Medial Foot. The three most prominent landmarks of the medial foot are the medial malleolus of the tibia, sustentaculum tali of the calcaneus, and the navicular tuberosity (Figure 10-36).

Posterior Surface of the Calcaneus. The posterior surface of the **calcaneus** is palpable as you continue palpating along the medial side to the posterior side of the foot (Figure 10-37).

PLEASE NOTE: The gastrocnemius, soleus, and plantaris muscles attach to the posterior surface of the calcaneus. The gastrocnemius and soleus attach via the calcaneal (Achilles) tendon.

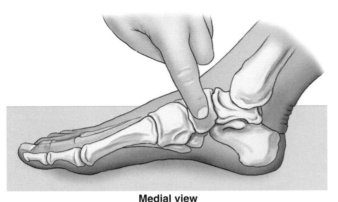

Medial view
Figure 10-32 Navicular tuberosity.

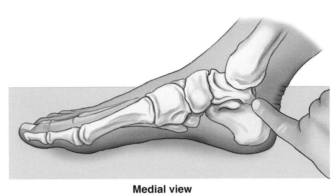

Medial view
Figure 10-35 Medial tubercle of the talus.

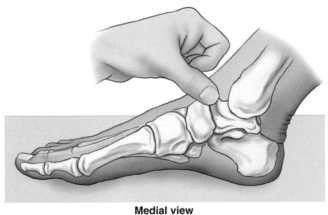

Medial view
Figure 10-33 Head of the talus.

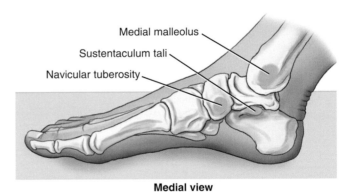

Medial malleolus
Sustentaculum tali
Navicular tuberosity

Medial view
Figure 10-36 Most prominent landmarks of the medial foot.

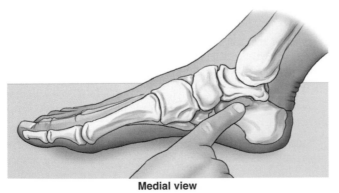

Medial view
Figure 10-34 Sustentaculum tali of the calcaneus.

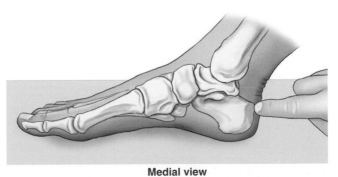

Medial view
Figure 10-37 Posterior surface of the calcaneus.

10

SECTION 4: LATERAL FOOT

Lateral View of the Foot (Figure 10-38)

Phalanges and Interphalangeal Joints of the Little Toe. Begin palpating the lateral side of the foot distally at the proximal, middle, and distal phalanges of the little toe (Figure 10-39, *A*). The **proximal interphalangeal (PIP) joint** and **distal interphalangeal (DIP) joint** between the phalanges can be palpated as well (see Figure 10-39, *B*). Singular of the term *phalanges* is *phalanx*.

PLEASE NOTE: The extensor digitorum brevis and extensor digitorum longus muscles attach to the dorsal surface of the phalanges of the little toe. The flexor digitorum brevis, flexor digitorum longus, flexor digiti minimi pedis, abductor digiti minimi pedis, and third plantar interosseus muscles attach to the plantar surface of the phalanges of the little toe.

Fifth Metatarsophalangeal Joint. From the proximal phalanx of the little toe, continue palpating proximally along the lateral surface of the foot and you will feel the joint line of the fifth MTP joint (Figure 10-40). Note: The proximal phalanx of the little toe extends quite a bit more proximally than do the other proximal phalanges of the foot; therefore the fifth MTP joint is found more proximally than are the other MTP joints of the foot.

Fifth Metatarsal. Proximally from the fifth MTP joint is the fifth metatarsal. The dorsal and lateral surfaces of the fifth metatarsal are readily palpable. Palpate from the expanded distal head to the middle of the shaft of the fifth metatarsal (Figure 10-41, *A*). Continue palpating proximally until you

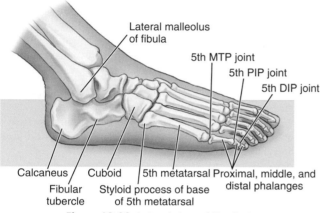

Figure labels: Lateral malleolus of fibula; 5th MTP joint; 5th PIP joint; 5th DIP joint; Calcaneus; Fibular tubercle; Cuboid; Styloid process of base of 5th metatarsal; 5th metatarsal; Proximal, middle, and distal phalanges

Figure 10-38 Lateral view of the foot.

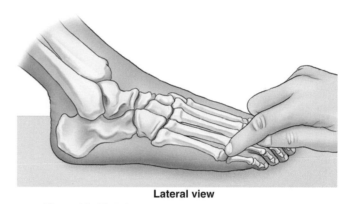

Lateral view

Figure 10-40 Fifth metatarsophalangeal (MTP) joint.

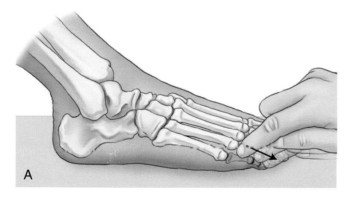

A

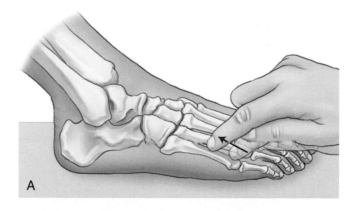

A

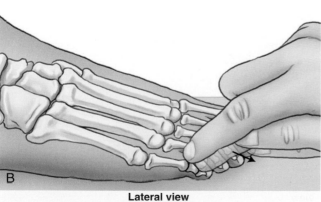

B

Lateral view

Figure 10-39 Phalanges and interphalangeal (IP) joints of the little toe.

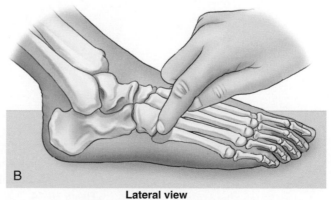

B

Lateral view

Figure 10-41 Fifth metatarsal.

10

reach the large expanded proximal base (see Figure 10-41, B). The base of the fifth metatarsal flares out and is called the **styloid process of the fifth metatarsal.**

PLEASE NOTE: The dorsal surface of the base of the fifth metatarsal is the attachment site of the fibularis brevis and

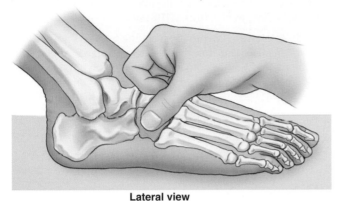

Lateral view
Figure 10-42 Cuboid.

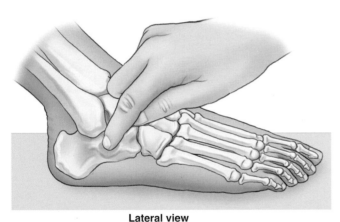

Lateral view
Figure 10-43 Lateral calcaneus.

fibularis tertius muscles. The flexor digiti minimi pedis muscle attaches to the plantar surface of the base of the fifth metatarsal.

Cuboid. Just proximal to the fifth metatarsal along the lateral side of the foot is a depression where the **cuboid** lies. The depression is created by a combination of the flaring of the base of the fifth metatarsal (the styloid process of the fifth metatarsal) and the concave shape of the lateral border of the cuboid. Palpate with firm pressure medially into this depression, and the cuboid can be felt (Figure 10-42).

PLEASE NOTE: The tibialis posterior and flexor hallucis brevis muscles attach to the plantar surface of the cuboid. A groove in the lateral border of the cuboid is created by the passage of the distal tendon of the fibularis longus muscle from the dorsal to the plantar surface of the foot.

Lateral Calcaneus. From the cuboid, continue palpating proximally along the lateral surface of the foot and the lateral surface of the calcaneus will be evident; it is subcutaneous and easily palpable. The **fibular tubercle of the calcaneus** is palpable distal to the lateral malleolus of the fibula (Figure 10-43).

PLEASE NOTE: The extensor digitorum brevis and extensor hallucis brevis muscles attach to the lateral surface of the calcaneus. The fibular tubercle is a valuable landmark because it separates the distal tendons of the fibularis longus and fibularis brevis muscles.

SECTION 5: DORSAL FOOT

Lateral View of the Dorsal Foot (Figure 10-44)
Anterior Talus. The anterior aspect of the talus, especially on the lateral side, can be palpated distal to the tibia. The anterior aspect of the **trochlea of the talus** is fairly easily palpated directly medial to the distal end of the lateral malleolus of the fibula (Figure 10-45). A greater portion of the anterior talus becomes palpable if the client's foot is passively inverted and plantarflexed.

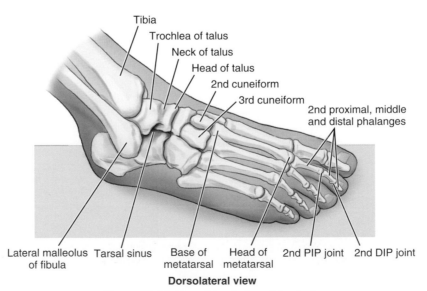

Dorsolateral view
Figure 10-44 Dorsolateral view of the foot.

Tarsal Sinus. If you palpate directly distal and anteromedial to the lateral malleolus of the fibula, you will feel a depression. This depression overlies the **tarsal sinus**, which is the space that leads into the **subtalar joint** cavity between the talus and the calcaneus (Figure 10-46). To best palpate the tarsal sinus, direct your palpatory pressure medially and inferiorly.

PLEASE NOTE: The extensor digitorum brevis and extensor hallucis brevis muscles overlie the tarsal sinus.

Phalanges and Interphalangeal Joints of Toes Two through Four. The **phalanges** and metatarsals of toes two through four

are easily palpable on the dorsum of the foot. Start distally and palpate the **distal phalanx, middle phalanx,** and **proximal phalanx** of each toe (Figure 10-47, *A*). Now palpate the joint lines between these phalanges: the PIP and DIP joints (see Figure 10-47, *B*). Singular of the term *phalanges* is *phalanx*.

PLEASE NOTE: The extensor digitorum brevis, extensor digitorum longus, and dorsal interossei pedis muscles attach to the dorsal surfaces of the phalanges of toes two through four. The flexor digitorum brevis, flexor digitorum longus, and first and second plantar interossei muscles attach to the plantar surfaces of the phalanges of toes two through four.

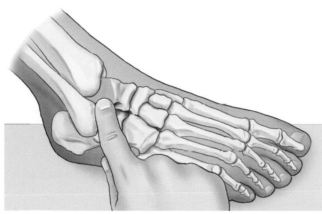

Dorsolateral view

Figure 10-45 Anterior talus.

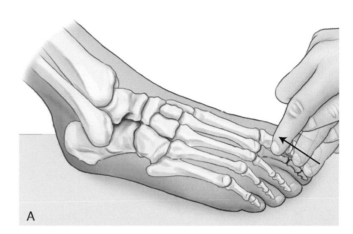

A

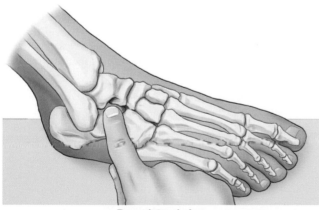

Dorsolateral view

Figure 10-46 Tarsal sinus.

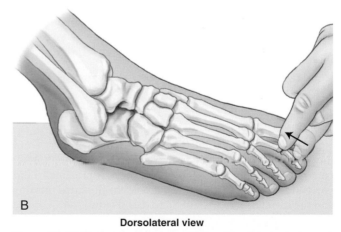

B

Dorsolateral view

Figure 10-47 Phalanges (singular: phalanx) and interphalangeal joints of toes two through four.

10

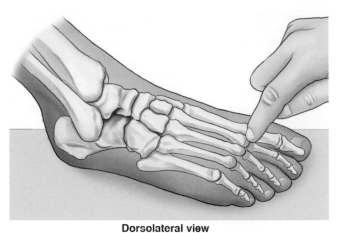

Dorsolateral view

Figure 10-48 Metatarsophalangeal (MTP) joints of toes two through four.

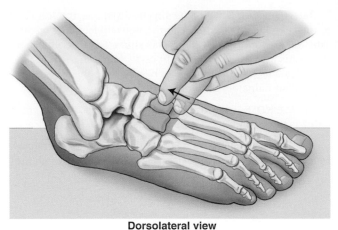

Dorsolateral view

Figure 10-50 Second and third cuneiforms.

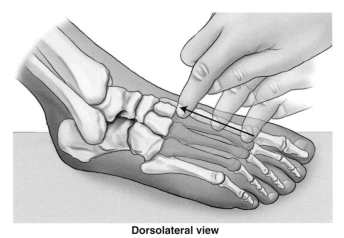

Dorsolateral view

Figure 10-49 Metatarsals of toes two through four.

Metatarsophalangeal Joints of Toes Two through Four. From the proximal phalanx of each of toes two through four, continue palpating the dorsal side of the foot proximally and you will feel the MTP joint line between the proximal phalanx and the metatarsal of each of these toes (Figure 10-48).

Metatarsals of Toes Two through Four. Proximally from the MTP joint line of each toe, the metatarsal can be palpated. The distal expanded **metatarsal head**, shaft, and proximal expanded **metatarsal base** are all subcutaneous and easily palpable (Figure 10-49).

PLEASE NOTE: The dorsal interossei pedis, plantar interossei, adductor hallucis, and tibialis posterior muscles attach to the metatarsals of toes two through four.

Second and Third Cuneiforms. The second and third cuneiforms can be palpated on the dorsal side of the foot. The **second cuneiform** is directly proximal to the second metatarsal; the **third cuneiform** is directly proximal to the third metatarsal. From the base of the second and third metatarsals, palpate directly proximally and you will feel the **tarsometatarsal joint** line between the metatarsal and the cuneiform; proximal to the joint line, the cuneiform itself is palpable (Figure 10-50).

PLEASE NOTE: The tibialis posterior muscle attaches to the plantar surfaces of the second and third cuneiforms.

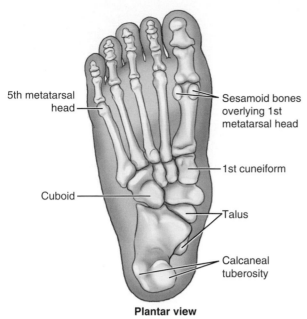

5th metatarsal head

Cuboid

Sesamoid bones overlying 1st metatarsal head

1st cuneiform

Talus

Calcaneal tuberosity

Plantar view

Figure 10-51 Plantar view of the foot.

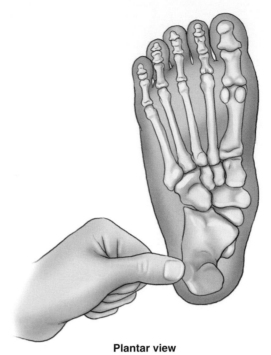

Plantar view

Figure 10-53 Calcaneal tuberosity.

10

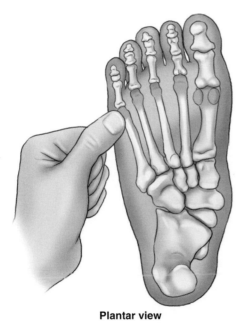

Plantar view

Figure 10-52 Metatarsal heads of toes one through five.

palpating the head of the first metatarsal on the plantar side, it is actually the two sesamoids that are felt.

PLEASE NOTE: The flexor hallucis brevis attaches into the sesamoid bones that overlie the head of the first metatarsal.

Calcaneal Tuberosity. The **calcaneal tuberosity** can often be palpated on the plantar side of the foot. With the client's foot relaxed, palpate with firm pressure on either side of the midline of the plantar side of the calcaneus. The medial aspect of the calcaneal tuberosity is often more prominent than the lateral aspect (Figure 10-53).

PLEASE NOTE: The abductor hallucis, abductor digiti minimi pedis, and flexor digitorum brevis muscles attach to the calcaneal tuberosity on the plantar surface of the calcaneus. The quadratus plantae and tibialis posterior muscles also attach onto the plantar surface of the calcaneus (but not the calcaneal tuberosity). The plantar aponeurosis (fascia) attaches onto the calcaneal tuberosity. The spring, long plantar, and short plantar ligaments attach onto the plantar surface of the calcaneus.

SECTION 6: PLANTAR FOOT

Plantar View of the Foot (Figure 10-51)

Metatarsal Heads of Toes One through Five. The heads of all five metatarsals are palpable on the plantar surface of the foot. Although all five metatarsals are palpable, because of the concavity of the transverse arch of the foot, the heads of the first and fifth metatarsals are most prominent. Begin by palpating the head of the fifth metatarsal and then continue medially, palpating each of the other four metatarsal heads (Figure 10-52). Overlying the plantar surface of the head of the first metatarsal are two small **sesamoid bones**. When

SECTION 7: LIGAMENTS OF THE LOWER EXTREMITY

Ligaments are fibrous fascial tissue that connects bones at a joint. The function of a ligament is to maintain stability of a joint by limiting motion. Figure 10-54 is an anterior view of the ligaments of the right lower extremity. Figure 10-55 is a posterior view of the ligaments of the right lower extremity. Figure 10-56 is a plantar view of the ligaments of the right foot. Figure 10-57 is a medial view of the ligaments of the right foot. And Figure 10-58 is a lateral view of the ligaments of the right foot.

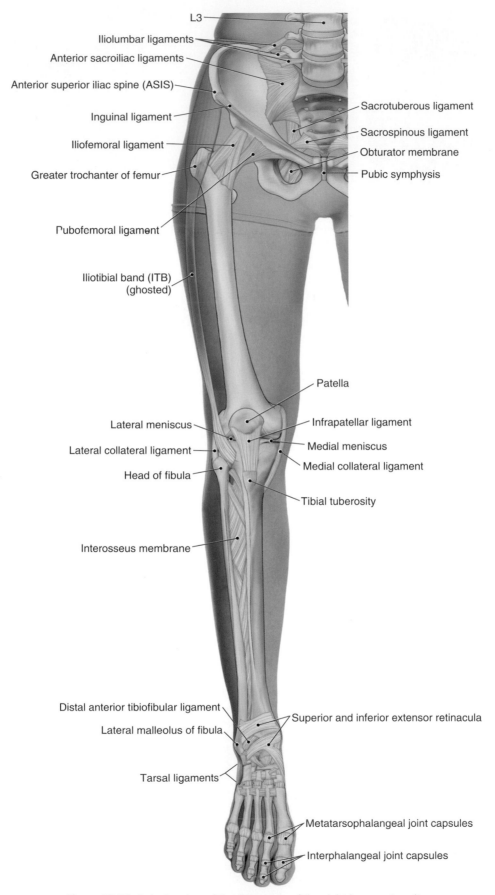

Figure 10-54 Anterior view of the ligaments of the right lower extremity.

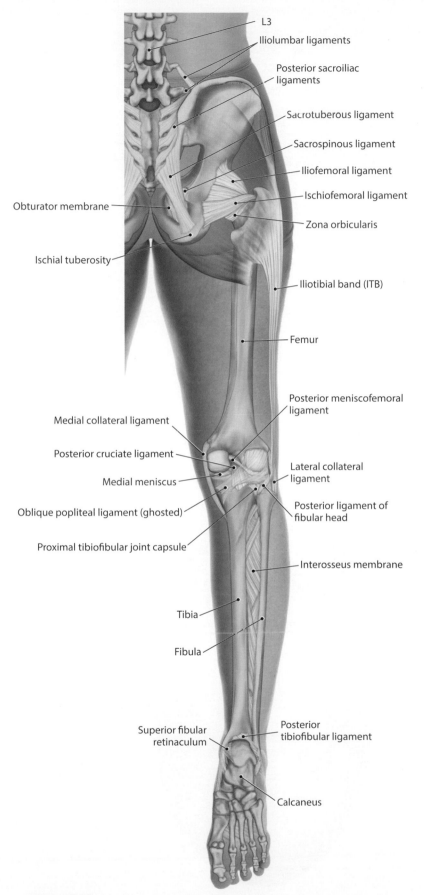

Figure 10-55 Posterior view of the ligaments of the right lower extremity.

10

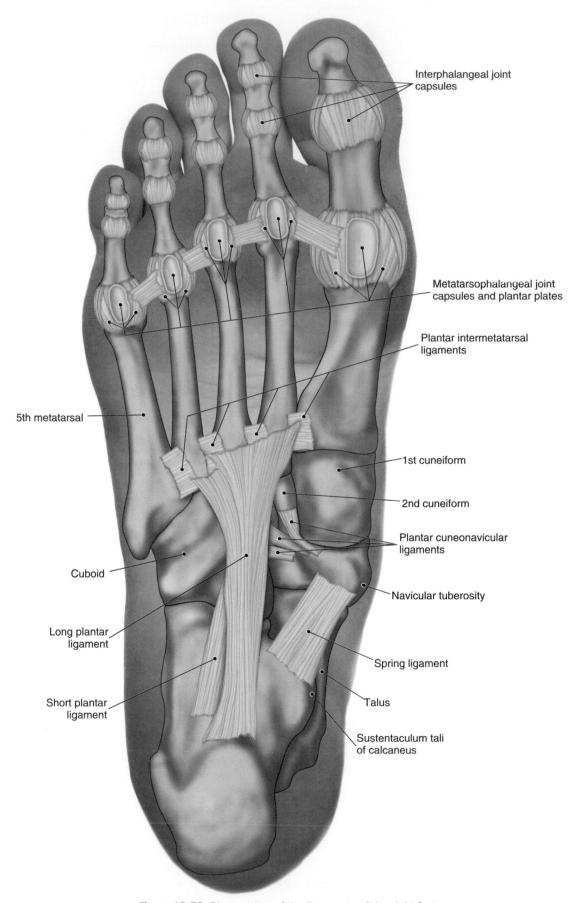

Interphalangeal joint capsules

Metatarsophalangeal joint capsules and plantar plates

Plantar intermetatarsal ligaments

5th metatarsal

1st cuneiform

2nd cuneiform

Plantar cuneonavicular ligaments

Cuboid

Navicular tuberosity

Long plantar ligament

Spring ligament

Short plantar ligament

Talus

Sustentaculum tali of calcaneus

Figure 10-56 Plantar view of the ligaments of the right foot.

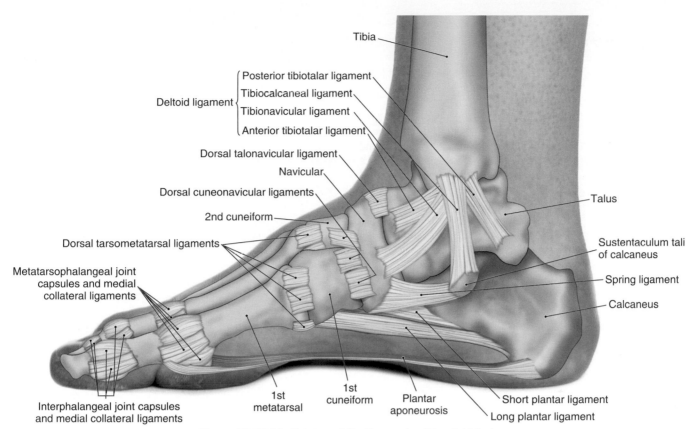

Figure 10-57 Medial view of the ligaments of the right foot.

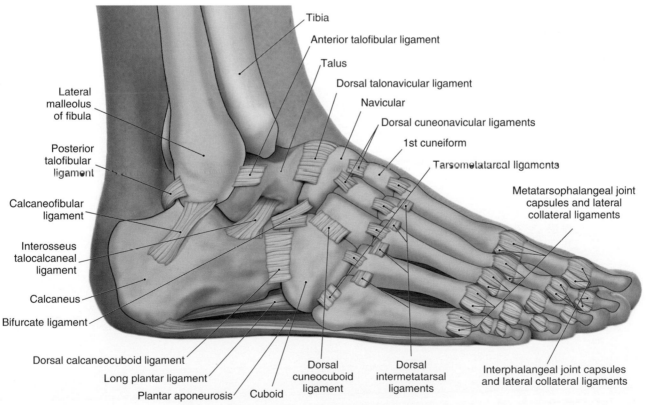

Figure 10-58 Lateral view of the ligaments of the right foot.

10

Review Questions

1. What bony structure serves as an attachment point for both the latissimus dorsi and the gluteus maximus?
2. What two muscles have attachments on the anterior sacrum?
3. What is the location of the ischial tuberosity?
4. What two muscles attach onto the anterior superior iliac spine (ASIS)?
5. Palpating the anterior inferior iliac spine (AIIS) may be made easier by first palpating what muscle?
6. Describe an effective method for locating the pubic bone.
7. In what position should the supine client's thigh be placed in order to palpate the lesser trochanter of the femur?
8. Where are the medial and lateral menisci palpable?
9. What sensitive structure lies superficially near the head of the fibula?
10. What three muscles attach to the posterior surface of the calcaneus?
11. What landmark separates the distal tendons of the fibularis longus and the fibularis brevis?
12. What is the common bony attachment of the abductor hallucis, abductor digiti minimi pedis, and the flexor digitorum brevis?
13. What is the name of the space that leads directly into the subtalar joint cavity between the talus and the calcaneus?
14. Which metatarsal heads are most prominent? Why?

10

CHAPTER 11

Tour #1 Palpation of the Muscles of the Shoulder Girdle

Overview

This chapter is a palpation tour of the muscles of the shoulder girdle. The tour begins with muscles on the posterior side and then addresses the muscles on the anterior side. Palpation of the posterior shoulder girdle muscles is shown in the prone position, and palpation of the anterior shoulder girdle muscles is shown in the supine position. Alternate palpation positions are also described. The major muscles or muscle groups of the region are each given a separate layout, and there are also a few detours to other muscles of the region. Trigger point (TrP) information and stretching, both therapist-assisted and self-care stretching, are given for each of the muscles covered in this chapter. The chapter closes with an advanced *Whirlwind Tour* that explains the sequential palpation of all of the muscles of the chapter.

Chapter Outline

Trapezius
Rhomboids
    Detour to the Serratus Posterior Superior
Levator Scapulae
Posterior Deltoid
Infraspinatus and Teres Minor
Teres Major
    Detour to the Latissimus Dorsi
Supraspinatus
Anterior Deltoid
Subscapularis
Serratus Anterior
Pectoralis Major
Pectoralis Minor
Subclavius
Whirlwind Tour: Muscles of the Shoulder Girdle

Chapter Objectives

After completing this chapter, the student/therapist should be able to perform the following for each of the muscles covered in this chapter:
1. State the attachments.
2. State the actions.
3. Describe the starting position for palpation.
4. Describe and explain the purpose of each of the palpation steps.
5. Palpate each muscle.
6. State the "Palpation Key."
7. Describe alternate palpation positions.
8. State the locations of the most common TrP(s).
9. Describe the TrP referral zones.
10. State the most common factors that create and/or perpetuate TrPs.
11. State the symptoms most commonly caused by TrPs.
12. Describe and perform the therapist-assisted and self-care stretches.

e Go to http://evolve.elsevier.com/Muscolino/palpation for video demonstrations of the muscle palpations presented in this chapter.

11

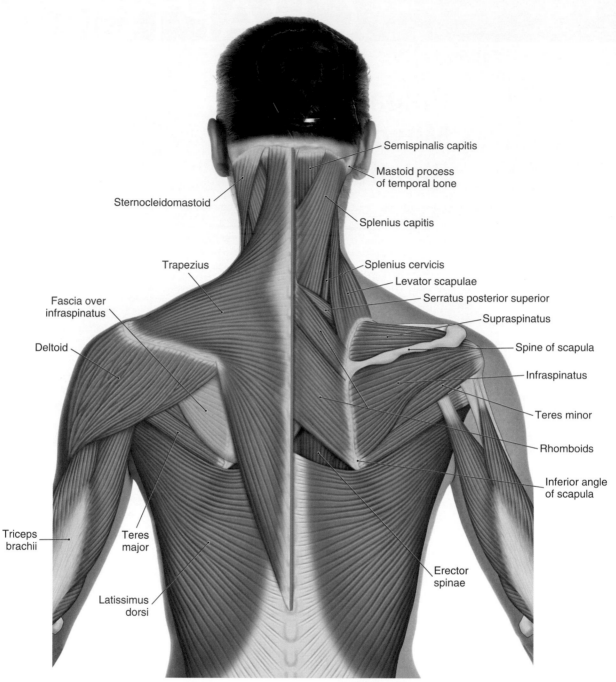

Semispinalis capitis

Mastoid process
of temporal bone

Sternocleidomastoid

Splenius capitis

Splenius cervicis

Trapezius

Levator scapulae

Fascia over
infraspinatus

Serratus posterior superior

Supraspinatus

Deltoid

Spine of scapula

Infraspinatus

Teres minor

Rhomboids

Inferior angle
of scapula

Triceps
brachii

Teres
major

Erector
spinae

Latissimus
dorsi

Figure 11-1 Posterior view of the posterior shoulder girdle region. The left side is superficial. The right side is deep. (The deltoid, trapezius, sternocleidomastoid (SCM), and infraspinatus fascia have been removed.)

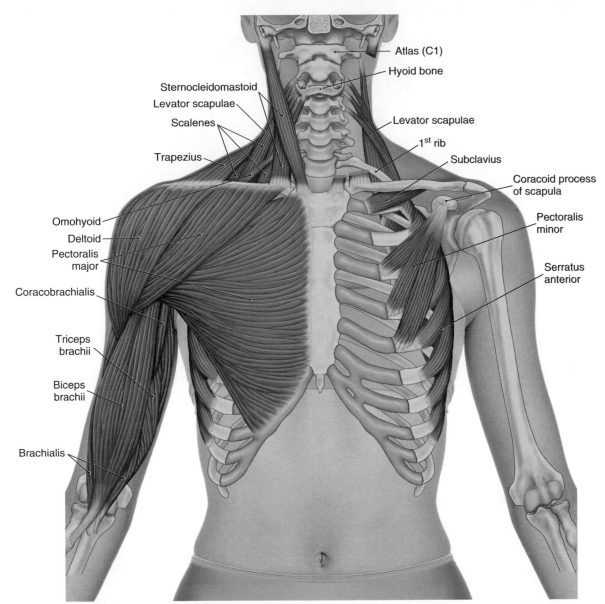

Figure 11-2 Anterior view of the posterior shoulder girdle region. The right side is superficial. The left side is deep. (The deltoid, pectoralis major, trapezius, scalenes, omohyoid, and muscles of the arm have been removed; the sternocleidomastoid [SCM] has been cut.)

11

11

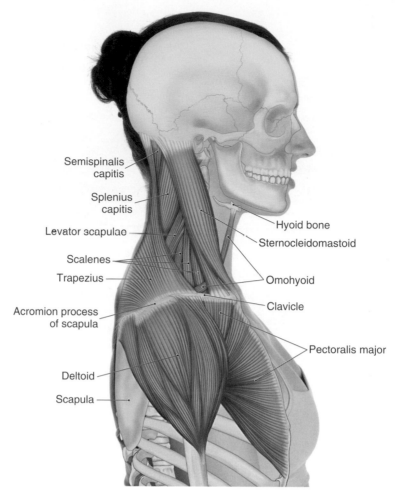

Figure 11-3 Right lateral view of the shoulder girdle and neck region.

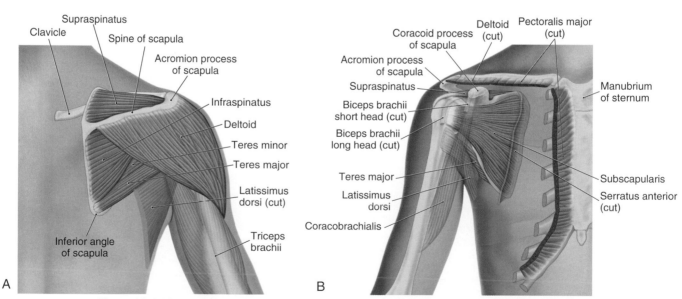

Figure 11-4 Views of the right shoulder girdle region. **A,** Posterior view. **B,** Anterior view; the majority of the deltoid and pectoralis major have been cut and removed.

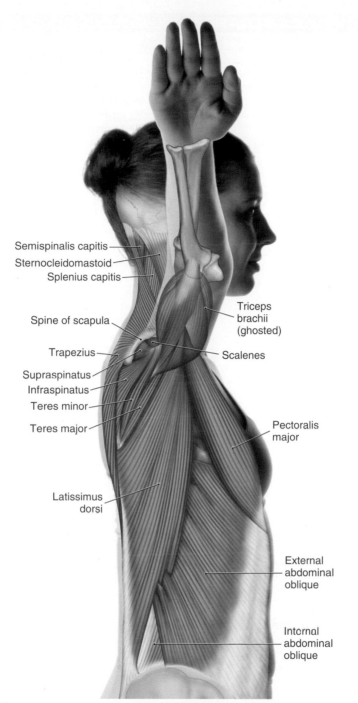

Figure 11-5 Right lateral view of the shoulder girdle and trunk region.

11

TRAPEZIUS—PRONE

✅ ATTACHMENTS

☐ External occipital protuberance, medial ⅓ of the superior nuchal line, nuchal ligament, and the spinous processes of C7 through T12

to the

☐ lateral ⅓ of the clavicle, acromion process, and spine of the scapula

✅ ACTIONS

Upper Trapezius
☐ Elevates the scapula at the scapulocostal (ScC) joint
☐ Retracts the scapula at the ScC joint
☐ Upwardly rotates the scapula at the ScC joint
☐ Extends the head and neck at the spinal joints
☐ Laterally flexes the head and neck at the spinal joints
☐ Contralaterally rotates the head and neck at the spinal joints

Middle Trapezius
☐ Retracts the scapula at the ScC joint

Lower Trapezius
☐ Depresses the scapula at the ScC joint
☐ Retracts the scapula at the ScC joint
☐ Upwardly rotates the scapula at the ScC joint

Starting Position (Figure 11-7)

■ Client prone with arm resting on the table at the side of the body
■ Therapist standing to the side of the client
■ Palpating hand placed just lateral to the lower thoracic spine (on the lower trapezius)

Palpation Steps

1. Ask the client to abduct the arm at the glenohumeral (GH) joint to 90 degrees with the elbow joint extended, and to slightly retract the scapula at the ScC joint by pinching the shoulder blade toward the spine (Figure 11-8). Adding gentle resistance to the client's arm abduction with your support hand might be helpful.
2. Palpate the lower trapezius. To locate the lateral border, palpate perpendicular to it (Figure 11-9, *A*). Once located, palpate the entire lower trapezius.

3. Repeat for the middle trapezius between the scapula and the spine. Strum perpendicular to the direction of the fibers (i.e., strum vertically) (see Figure 11-9, *B*).
4. Repeat for the upper trapezius.
5. To further engage the upper trapezius, ask the client to do slight extension of the head and neck at the spinal joints. Then palpate the entire upper trapezius (see Figure 11-9, *C*).
6. Once the trapezius has been located, have the client relax it and palpate to assess its baseline tone.

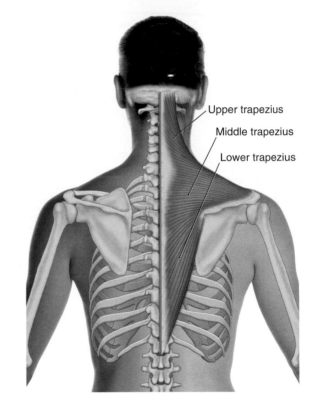

Figure 11-6 Posterior view of the right trapezius. The sternocleidomastoid (SCM), levator scapulae, and splenius capitis are ghosted in.

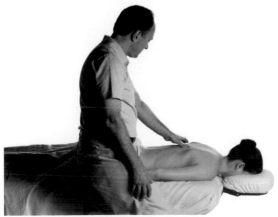

Figure 11-7 Starting position for prone palpation of the right trapezius.

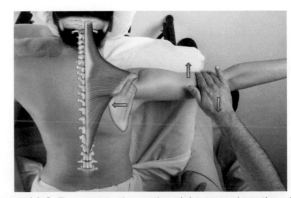

Figure 11-8 To engage the entire right trapezius, the client abducts the arm at the glenohumeral (GH) joint (resistance can be added as shown) and slightly retracts the scapula at the scapulocostal (ScC) joint.

TRAPEZIUS—PRONE—*cont'd*

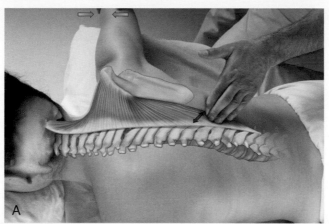

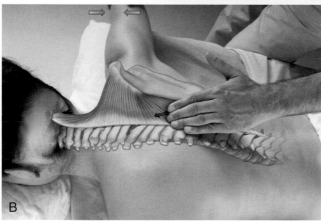

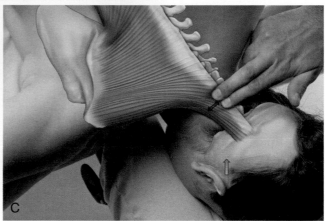

Figure 11-9 Palpation of the right trapezius. **A** shows palpation of the lower trapezius. **B** shows palpation of the middle trapezius. **C** shows palpation of the upper trapezius. Palpation of the upper trapezius is facilitated by asking the client to slightly extend the head and neck at the spinal joints. For all three parts of the trapezius, palpate while strumming perpendicular to the fiber direction as shown.

PALPATION NOTES

1. Abducting the arm at the glenohumeral (GH) joint requires an upward rotation force by the upper and lower trapezius to first stabilize the scapula and then move the scapula into upward rotation. Retracting the scapula engages the entire trapezius, especially the middle trapezius.
2. Clients often lift the arm up into the air when asked to retract the scapula. Emphasize that the client should "pinch the shoulder blade back." However, the client should not retract the scapula excessively, or the scapula moves too close to the spine, and the retractor musculature in the interscapular region bunches up, making it difficult to palpate the middle trapezius.
3. When asking the client to extend the head and neck to further engage the upper trapezius, do not have the client extend very far or it will be difficult to palpate into the neck.
4. The lateral border of the lower trapezius is often visible; look for it before placing your palpating hands on the client.

Palpation Key:
Fly like an airplane:
If both trapezius muscles are palpated at the same time, both arms out to the sides make the client appear to be flying like an airplane.

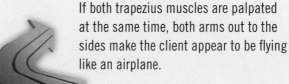

TRAPEZIUS—PRONE—*cont'd*

TRIGGER POINTS

1. Trigger points (TrPs) in the upper trapezius often result from or are perpetuated by acute or chronic overuse of the muscle. Examples include chronic postures of elevation of the shoulder girdle; anteriorly held head; any chronic posture due to poor ergonomics, especially while sitting at the computer or crimping the phone between the shoulder and ear; resisting depression of the shoulder girdle when the upper extremity is hanging, especially when the upper extremity is carrying a weight; trauma (e.g., whiplash); compression forces (e.g., carrying a heavy purse or backpack on the shoulder, having a tight bra strap); or chronic stress/tension (holding the shoulder girdles uptight). Middle trapezius TrPs are activated/perpetuated by a chronic rounded shoulder posture, or when driving and holding the top of the steering wheel. Lower trapezius TrPs are activated/perpetuated by chronically pressing the shoulder girdles down (e.g., supporting the chin in the hand, pressing the hands down on the sitting surface when seated).

2. TrPs in the upper trapezius tend to produce a classic stiff neck with restricted contralateral lateral flexion and ipsilateral rotation of the neck at the spinal joints, a posture of an elevated shoulder girdle, pain at the end of contralateral rotation of the neck, and tension headaches. Middle trapezius TrPs tend to produce inhibition and weakness of the middle trapezius resulting in chronically protracted shoulder girdles (rounder shoulders), and goose bumps on the arm (and sometimes on the thigh). Lower trapezius TrPs tend to produce burning pain, and inhibition and weakness of the lower trapezius resulting in elevated shoulders. TrPs in all parts of the trapezius may produce spinal joint dysfunction of the vertebrae to which they are attached.

3. The referral patterns of upper trapezius TrPs must be distinguished from the referral patterns of TrPs in the sternocleidomastoid (SCM), masseter, temporalis, occipitalis, splenius cervicis, levator scapulae, semispinalis capitis, cervical multifidus, and lower trapezius. Middle trapezius referral patterns must be distinguished from the levator scapulae, erector spinae and transversospinalis of the trunk, and lower trapezius. Lower trapezius referral patterns must be distinguished from the cervical multifidus, levator scapulae, rhomboids, scalenes, infraspinatus, latissimus dorsi, serratus anterior, erector spinae and transversospinalis of the trunk, intercostals, and upper trapezius.

4. TrPs in the trapezius are often incorrectly assessed as cervical disc syndrome, temporomandibular joint (TMJ) syndrome, or occipital neuralgia.

5. Associated TrPs of the upper trapezius often occur in the scalenes, splenius capitis and cervicis, levator scapulae, rhomboids, semispinalis capitis, temporalis, masseter, and the contralateral upper trapezius. Associated TrPs of the middle trapezius often occur in the pectoralis major and minor, and the erector spinae and transversospinalis muscles of the trunk. Associated TrPs of the lower trapezius often occur in the latissimus dorsi and ipsilateral upper trapezius.

6. Note: The trapezius is considered to be the muscle most commonly found to have TrPs. Specifically, the upper trapezius has the most commonly found TrP in the body; further, the referral symptoms of this common TrP have occasionally spread to the other side of the body.

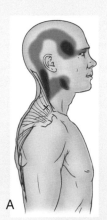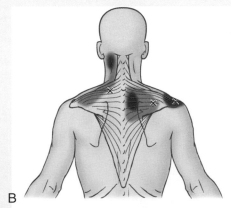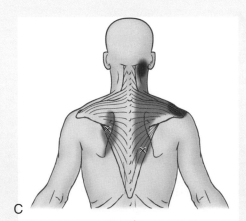

Figure 11-10 Common trapezius trigger points (TrPs) and their corresponding referral zones. **A** is a lateral view showing the location of a TrP in the most vertical fibers of the upper trapezius. **B** shows another upper trapezius TrP on the left side; the *right side* illustrates middle trapezius TrP locations. **C** shows two lower trapezius TrPs and their referral zones.

TRAPEZIUS—PRONE—*cont'd*

STRETCHING THE TRAPEZIUS

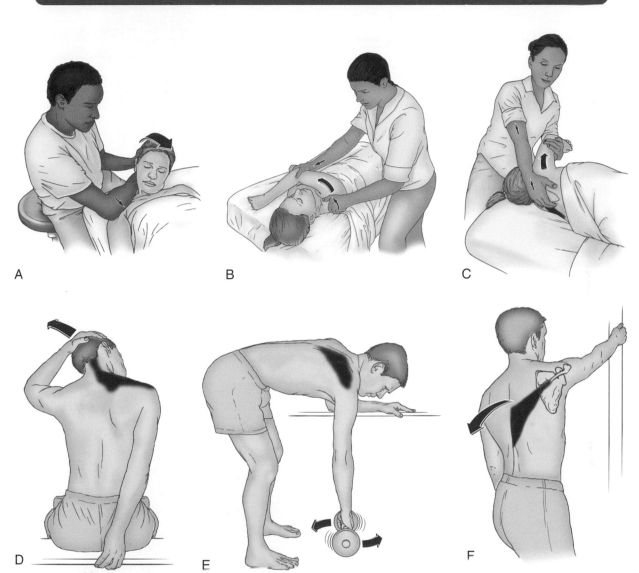

A   B   C

D   E   F

Figure 11-11 Stretching the three functional parts of the right trapezius. **A, B,** and **C,** Therapist-assisted stretching of the upper, middle, and lower trapezius respectively. **A,** The client's neck is flexed, left laterally flexed, and rotated (ipsilaterally) to the right. Note that the therapist stabilizes the client's shoulder girdle and trunk with the right forearm. **B,** The client's right arm is horizontally flexed to protract the scapula. Note that the therapist assists scapular protraction by curling the fingertips around the medial border of the scapula and pulling. **C,** The client's arm and scapula are moved as in **B,** but are pulled in a more upward direction so that the scapula is protracted and elevated. **D, E,** and **F,** Self-care stretching of the right upper, middle, and lower trapezius respectively. **D,** The client uses the left hand to passively flex, left laterally flex, and right (ipsilaterally) rotate the head and neck. To keep the shoulder girdle down, the right hand holds on to the bench/chair. **E,** A weight is held in the right hand; its traction force protracts the scapula. Medially rotating the right arm enhances the stretch. **F,** A pole is grasped at approximately head height and the client leans back, causing protraction and elevation of the scapula.

RHOMBOIDS—PRONE

☑ ATTACHMENTS

☐ Spinous processes of C7 through T5

to the

☐ medial border of the scapula from the root of the spine to the inferior angle

☑ ACTIONS

☐ Retracts the scapula at the scapulocostal (ScC) joint
☐ Elevates the scapula at the ScC joint
☐ Downwardly rotates the scapula at the ScC joint

Starting Position (Figure 11-13)

■ Client prone with the hand resting in the small of the back
■ Therapist standing to the side of the client
■ Palpating hand placed between the spinal column and the scapula at the midscapular level

Palpation Steps

1. Ask the client to lift the hand away from the small of the back (Figure 11-14).
2. Look for the lower border of the rhomboids to become visible (Figure 11-15); make sure you are not covering the lower border with your palpating hand.
3. Palpate the rhomboids from the inferior aspect to the superior aspect. When palpating, strum perpendicular to the direction of the fibers.
4. Once the rhomboids have been located, have the client relax them and palpate to assess their baseline tone.

11

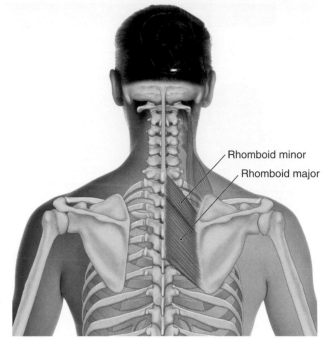

Figure 11-12 Posterior view of the right rhomboids major and minor. The levator scapulae has been ghosted in.

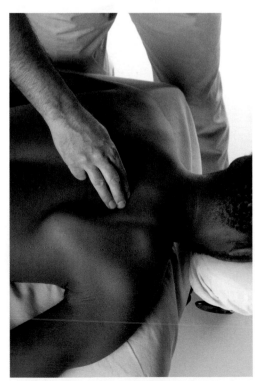

Figure 11-13 Starting position for prone palpation of the right rhomboids. Note: The client's right hand is in the small of the back, as seen in Figure 11-15.

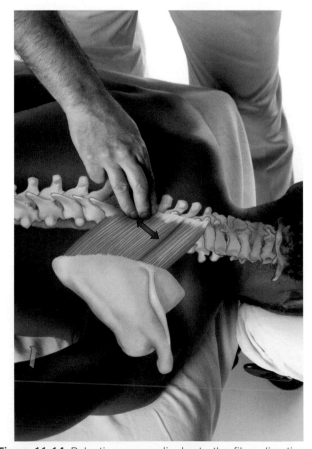

Figure 11-14 Palpating perpendicular to the fiber direction of the right rhomboids.

RHOMBOIDS—PRONE—*cont'd*

Alternate Palpation Position—Seated

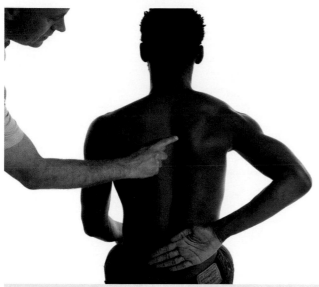

Figure 11-15 The rhomboids can also be easily palpated in the seated position. Note that the inferior border of the rhomboids is often visible.

PALPATION NOTES

1. Having the client place the hand in the small of the back requires extension of the arm at the glenohumeral (GH) joint. This requires the coupled action of downward rotation of the scapula at the scapulocostal (ScC) joint, which causes the trapezius to relax (because of reciprocal inhibition) so that we can palpate through it. It also engages the rhomboids so that their contraction is clearly felt.
2. The superior border of the rhomboids is more challenging to visualize and palpate than the inferior border. However, it can usually be palpated. Feel for a gap between the rhomboids and the levator scapulae.
3. It is usually not possible to clearly distinguish the border between the rhomboid major and rhomboid minor.

Palpation Key:
Client's hand in the small of the back.

11

TRIGGER POINTS

1. Trigger points (TrPs) in the rhomboids often result from or are perpetuated by acute or chronic overuse of the muscle (both as movers of scapular retraction and as stabilizers of the scapula when the arm is moved at the glenohumeral [GH] joint), a chronic stretch caused by a rounded-shoulder posture due to tight pectoralis muscles anteriorly, and TrPs in the trapezius.
2. TrPs in the rhomboids tend to produce pain that is felt superficially at rest and with use of the muscles; they can also cause joint dysfunction of the vertebrae to which they are attached.
3. The referral patterns of rhomboids TrPs must be distinguished from the referral patterns of TrPs in the levator scapulae, scalenes, middle trapezius, infraspinatus, latissimus dorsi, serratus posterior superior (SPS), thoracic transversospinalis, and serratus anterior.
4. TrPs in the rhomboids are often incorrectly assessed as fibromyalgia.
5. Associated TrPs often occur in the trapezius, levator scapulae, pectoralis major and minor, serratus anterior, and infraspinatus.

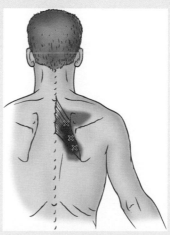

Figure 11-16 Posterior view illustrating common rhomboids trigger points (TrPs) and their corresponding referral zone.

RHOMBOIDS—PRONE—*cont'd*

STRETCHING THE RHOMBOIDS

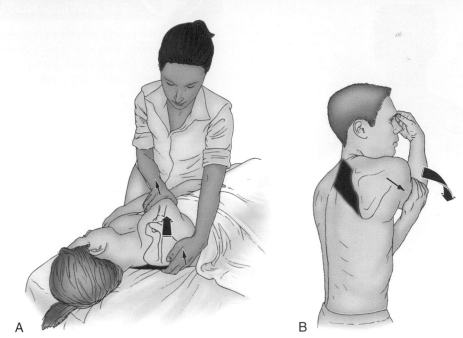

A   B

Figure 11-17 Stretching the right rhomboids. The client's arm is used to protract and depress the right scapula while the trunk remains facing forward. **A,** Therapist-assisted stretch. Note that the therapist assists scapular protraction by curling the fingertips around the medial border of the scapula and pulling. **B,** Self-care stretch.

11

RHOMBOIDS—PRONE—*cont'd*

DETOUR

Serratus posterior superior trigger point notes:

1. Trigger points (TrPs) in the serratus posterior superior (SPS) often result from or are perpetuated by acute or chronic overuse of the muscle (e.g., in clients who have labored breathing due to chronic obstructive respiratory diseases, such as asthma, bronchitis, and emphysema) and TrPs in the scalenes.

2. TrPs in the SPS tend to produce a deep ache that is felt deep to the scapula (pain is often felt at rest, but increased with motions of the arm that cause the scapula to compress the SPS against the rib cage), difficulty sleeping on the affected side due to pressure on the TrP, a feeling of numbness in the little finger of the hand, or C7 to T3 spinal joint dysfunction.

3. The referral patterns of SPS TrPs must be distinguished from the referral patterns of TrPs in the erector spinae and transversospinalis muscles of the trunk, scalenes, rhomboids, levator scapulae, posterior deltoid, supraspinatus, infraspinatus, teres minor, latissimus dorsi, teres major, subscapularis, triceps brachii, all three wrist extensors, and extensor digitorum.

4. TrPs in the SPS are often incorrectly assessed as cervical disc syndrome, thoracic outlet syndrome, or elbow joint dysfunction.

5. Associated TrPs often occur in the scalenes, rhomboids, and erector spinae and transversospinalis muscles of the trunk.

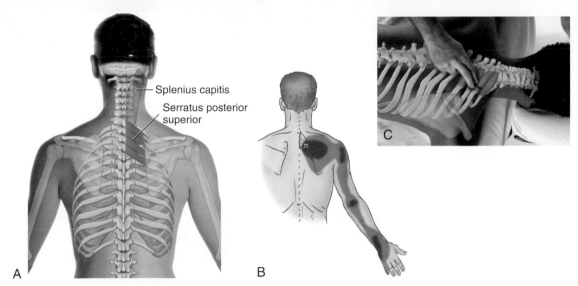

A

Splenius capitis
Serratus posterior superior

B

C

Figure 11-18 Serratus posterior superior (SPS). **A,** Posterior view of the right SPS; the splenius capitis has been ghosted in. The SPS attaches from the spinous processes of C7-T3 to ribs two through five. **B,** Posterior view illustrating a common SPS trigger point (TrP) and its corresponding referral zone. **C,** Palpation of the SPS. The arm is hanging off the table to protract the scapula at the scapulocostal (ScC) joint, exposing the entire SPS.

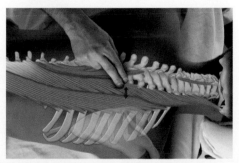

Figure 11-19 Palpation of the right erector spinae group in the thoracic region. The client is asked to extend the head, neck, and trunk to engage the erector spinae musculature. For more information on palpation of the erector spinae, please see Tour #7 in Chapter 17.

LEVATOR SCAPULAE—PRONE

☑ATTACHMENTS

☐ Transverse processes of C1 through C4

to the

☐ medial border of the scapula from the root of the spine to the superior angle

☑ACTIONS

☐ Elevates the scapula at the scapulocostal (ScC) joint
☐ Downwardly rotates the scapula at the ScC joint
☐ Extends the neck at the spinal joints
☐ Laterally flexes the neck at the spinal joints
☐ Ipsilaterally rotates the neck at the spinal joints

Starting Position (Figure 11-21)

◼ Client prone with hand resting in the small of the back
◼ Therapist standing or seated to the side of the client
◼ Palpating hand placed just superior and medial to the superior angle of the scapula

Palpation Steps

1. With the client's hand in the small of the back, the client is asked to perform a gentle, very short range of motion of elevation of the scapula at the ScC joint. Feel for the levator scapulae's contraction deep to the trapezius (Figure 11-22, *A*).
2. Continue palpating the levator scapulae toward its superior attachment while strumming perpendicular to its fibers.
3. Once you are palpating the levator scapulae in the posterior triangle (superior to the trapezius), the client's hand no longer needs to be in the small of the back. It is also possible to ask the client to elevate the scapula more forcefully now; resistance can also be added (see Figure 11-22, *B*).
4. Palpate the levator scapulae as far superiorly as possible. (Near its superior attachment, it lies deep to the sternocleidomastoid [SCM].)
5. Once the levator scapulae has been located, have the client relax it and palpate to assess its baseline tone.

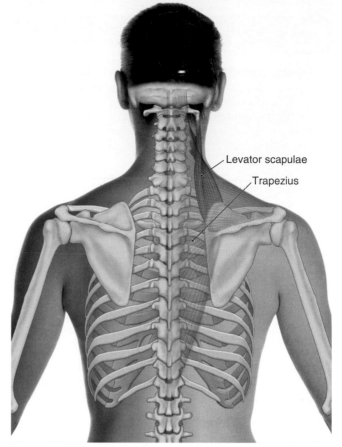

Figure 11-20 Posterior view of the right levator scapulae. The trapezius has been ghosted in.

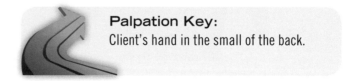

Palpation Key:
Client's hand in the small of the back.

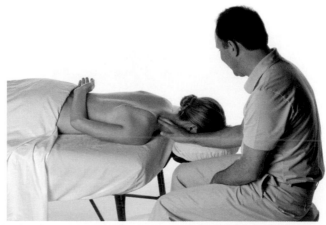

Figure 11-21 Starting position for prone palpation of the right levator scapulae.

LEVATOR SCAPULAE—PRONE—cont'd

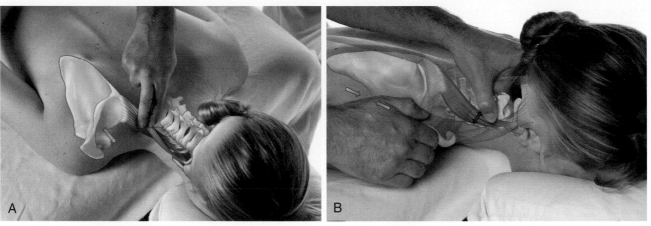

Figure 11-22 Palpation of the right levator scapulae. **A** shows palpation near the superior angle of the scapula (where the levator scapulae is deep to the trapezius). **B** shows palpation where the levator scapulae is superficial in the posterior triangle of the neck.

 PALPATION NOTES

1. Having the client place the hand in the small of the back requires extension and adduction of the arm at the glenohumeral (GH) joint. This requires the coupled action of downward rotation of the scapula at the scapulocostal (ScC) joint, which causes the upper trapezius to relax (because of reciprocal inhibition) so that the inferior attachment of the levator scapulae can be clearly felt when it contracts. It also engages the levator scapulae, so its contraction is more clearly felt.
2. Do not have the client perform a forceful elevation of the scapula or the reflex of reciprocal inhibition will be overcome and the upper trapezius will contract, blocking palpation of the levator scapulae at its inferior attachment.
3. Once the levator scapulae is being palpated in the posterior triangle of the neck, the client can remove the hand from the small of the back, because it is no longer necessary to inhibit (relax) the upper trapezius. Furthermore, once we are palpating the levator scapulae in the posterior triangle, a forceful contraction of the levator scapulae can be engaged to better palpate and locate it.
4. In middle-aged or older adults, the levator scapulae is often visible in the posterior triangle of the neck (Figure 11-23).
5. It can be difficult to palpate the most superior aspect of the levator scapulae deep to the sternocleidomastoid (SCM). To do so, slacken the SCM by slightly flexing and ipsilaterally laterally flexing the neck and try to palpate deep to the SCM, reaching for the transverse processes of C1 through C4 (see Figure 12-39).
6. Note that the transverse process of C1 is directly inferior to the ear (between the mastoid process and the ramus of the mandible)!

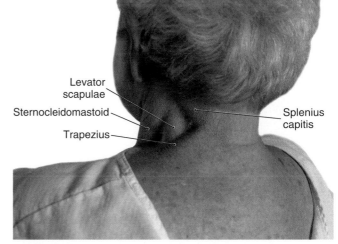

Figure 11-23 Posterolateral view showing the levator scapulae and splenius capitis in the posterior triangle of the neck. (Courtesy of Joseph E. Muscolino.)

LEVATOR SCAPULAE—PRONE—*cont'd*

Alternate Palpation Position—Seated

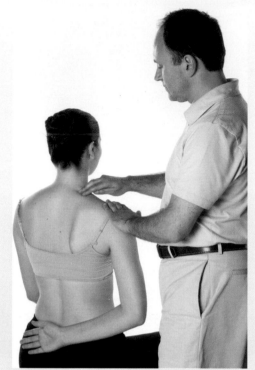

Figure 11-24 The levator scapulae can also be easily palpated with the client seated.

TRIGGER POINTS

1. Trigger points (TrPs) in the levator scapulae often result from or are perpetuated by acute or chronic overuse of the muscle (e.g., carrying a bag or purse on the shoulder, crimping a phone between the shoulder and ear, excessive exercise such as playing tennis, holding the shoulders uptight), chronic shortening or stretching of the muscle due to poor work or leisure postures (e.g., having a poorly placed computer monitor, reading with the head inclined forward), motor vehicle accidents, having a cold draft on the neck, or being overly stressed psychologically.
2. TrPs in the levator scapulae tend to produce a classic stiff neck (often called *torticollis* or *wry neck*) with restricted contralateral rotation of the neck.
3. The referral patterns of levator scapulae TrPs must be distinguished from the referral patterns of TrPs in the scalenes, rhomboids, supraspinatus, and infraspinatus.
4. TrPs in the levator scapulae are often incorrectly assessed as joint dysfunction of the cervical spine.
5. Associated TrPs often occur in the upper trapezius, splenius cervicis, scalenes, and erector spinae of the cervical spine.

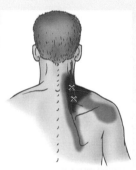

Figure 11-25 Posterior view illustrating common levator scapulae trigger points (TrPs) and their corresponding referral zone.

LEVATOR SCAPULAE—PRONE—cont'd

STRETCHING THE LEVATOR SCAPULAE

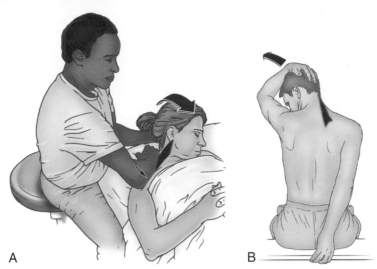

A   B

Figure 11-26 Stretching the right levator scapulae. The client's neck is flexed, left laterally flexed, and rotated (contralaterally) to the left. The right shoulder girdle must be stabilized to prevent it from elevating, and the trunk must be stabilized to prevent it from rotating to the left. **A,** Therapist-assisted stretch. Note that the therapist stabilizes the client's shoulder girdle and trunk with the right forearm. **B,** Self-care stretch. The client holds on to the bench/chair behind him to stabilize the shoulder girdle and trunk.

11

POSTERIOR DELTOID—PRONE

☑ ATTACHMENTS

☐ Spine of the scapula

to the

☐ deltoid tuberosity of the humerus

☑ ACTIONS

☐ Extends the arm at the glenohumeral (GH) joint
☐ Abducts the arm at the GH joint
☐ Adducts the arm at the GH joint (lowest fibers)
☐ Laterally rotates the arm at the GH joint
☐ Horizontally extends the arm at the GH joint

Starting Position (Figure 11-28)

■ Client prone with arm abducted 90 degrees to the side and resting on the table, and the forearm hanging off the table
■ Therapist standing or seated to the side of the client
■ Palpating hand placed just inferior to the lateral end of the spine of the scapula
■ Support hand placed on the distal end of the client's arm

Palpation Steps

1. Ask the client to horizontally extend the arm at the GH joint (by lifting it straight up toward the ceiling) and feel for the contraction of the posterior fibers of the deltoid. Resistance can be added (Figure 11-29).
2. Palpate from the spine of the scapula to the deltoid tuberosity.
3. Once the posterior deltoid has been located, have the client relax it and palpate to assess its baseline tone.

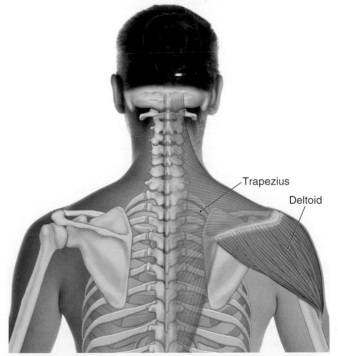

Trapezius

Deltoid

Figure 11-27 Posterior view of the right deltoid. The trapezius has been ghosted in.

POSTERIOR DELTOID—PRONE—*cont'd*

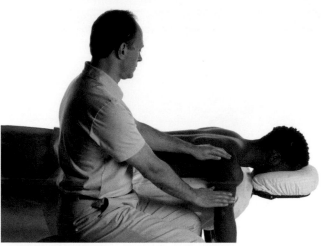

Figure 11-28 Starting position for prone palpation of the right posterior deltoid.

Figure 11-29 Palpation of the right posterior deltoid as the client horizontally extends the arm against resistance.

Alternate Palpation Position—Seated

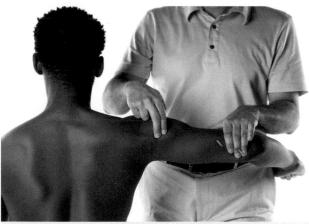

Figure 11-30 The posterior deltoid can also be easily palpated with the client seated or standing. To engage the posterior fibers of the deltoid, have the client horizontally extend the arm at the glenohumeral (GH) joint against resistance.

Palpation Key:
Resist horizontal extension of the arm.

TRIGGER POINTS

1. Trigger points (TrPs) in the posterior deltoid often result from or are perpetuated by acute or chronic overuse (e.g., holding the arm up in abduction or extension for prolonged periods, such as when working at a computer keyboard), direct trauma (e.g., impact during sports), and TrPs in the infraspinatus.
2. TrPs in the posterior deltoid tend to produce weakness when performing abduction or extension of the arm at the glenohumeral (GH) joint.
3. The referral patterns of posterior deltoid TrPs must be distinguished from the referral patterns of TrPs in the levator scapulae, scalenes, supraspinatus, infraspinatus, teres minor, subscapularis, teres major, triceps brachii, and serratus posterior superior (SPS).
4. TrPs in the posterior deltoid are often incorrectly assessed as a rotator cuff tear, subdeltoid/subacromial bursitis, or GH or acromioclavicular joint arthritis.
5. Associated TrPs often occur in the supraspinatus, teres major, infraspinatus, teres minor, triceps brachii, and latissimus dorsi.

PALPATION NOTES

1. Even though the posterior fibers of the deltoid laterally rotate the arm at the glenohumeral (GH) joint, when palpating the posterior deltoid, do not ask the client to do this action because the infraspinatus and teres minor muscles will also be engaged, making it more difficult to discern the posterior deltoid from these muscles.
2. The posterior deltoid attaches on the spine of the scapula nearly to the root of the spine of the scapula at the medial border.

POSTERIOR DELTOID—PRONE—*cont'd*

TRIGGER POINTS—*cont'd*

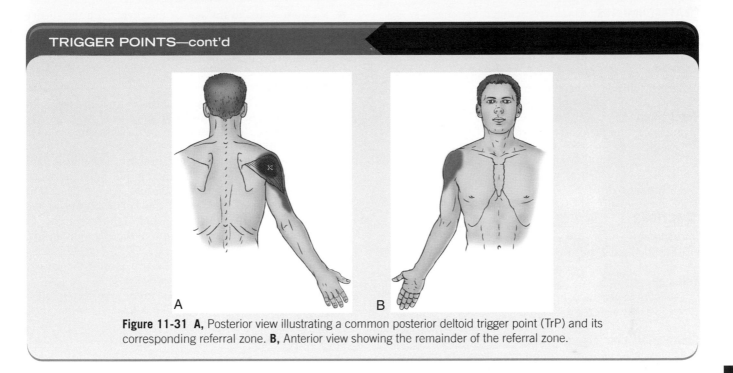

Figure 11-31 A, Posterior view illustrating a common posterior deltoid trigger point (TrP) and its corresponding referral zone. **B,** Anterior view showing the remainder of the referral zone.

STRETCHING THE POSTERIOR DELTOID

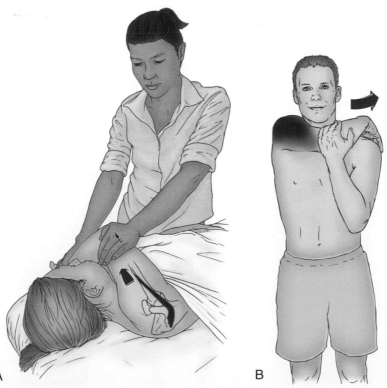

Figure 11-32 Stretching the right posterior deltoid. The client's right arm is horizontally flexed, keeping the trunk facing forward. **A,** Therapist-assisted stretch. **B,** Self-care stretch.

11

INFRASPINATUS AND TERES MINOR—PRONE

☑ ATTACHMENTS

Infraspinatus
- ☐ Infraspinous fossa of the scapula

  to the

- ☐ greater tubercle of the humerus

Teres Minor
- ☐ Superior ⅔ of the dorsal surface of the lateral border of the scapula

  to the

- ☐ greater tubercle of the humerus

☑ ACTIONS

Infraspinatus
- ☐ Laterally rotates the arm at the glenohumeral (GH) joint

Teres Minor
- ☐ Laterally rotates the arm at the GH joint
- ☐ Adducts the arm at the GH joint

Starting Position (Figure 11-34)
- ■ Client prone with arm abducted 90 degrees to the side and resting on the table, and the forearm hanging off the table

- ■ Therapist seated to the side of the client, with the client's forearm between the knees
- ■ Palpating hand placed just inferior to the spine of the scapula in the infraspinous fossa

Palpation Steps
1. Ask the client to laterally rotate the arm at the GH joint against the resistance of your knee, and feel for the contraction of the infraspinatus in the infraspinous fossa (Figure 11-35, *A*).
2. Continue palpating the infraspinatus distally toward the greater tubercle attachment on the humerus while strumming perpendicular to its fibers.
3. Locate the superior aspect of the lateral border of the scapula, and feel for the contraction of the teres minor as the client laterally rotates the arm at the GH joint against your knee (see Figure 11-35, *B*).
4. Continue palpating its distal tendon toward the greater tubercle while strumming perpendicular to it.
5. Once the infraspinatus and teres minor have been located, have the client relax them and palpate to assess their baseline tone.

11

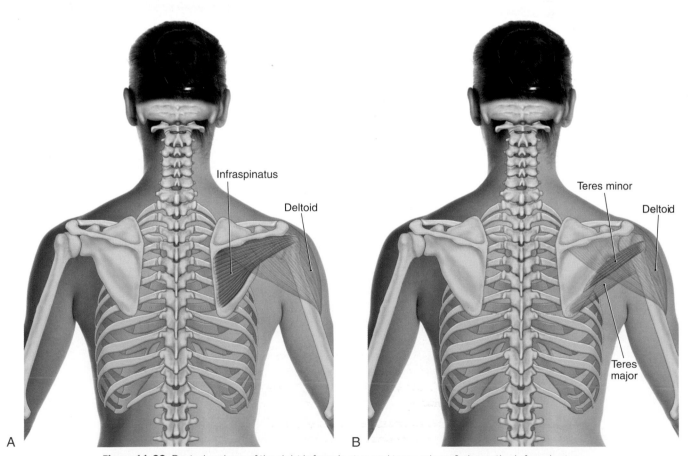

A   B

Figure 11-33 Posterior views of the right infraspinatus and teres minor. **A** shows the infraspinatus; the deltoid has been ghosted in. **B** shows the teres minor; the deltoid and teres major have been ghosted in.

INFRASPINATUS AND TERES MINOR—PRONE—*cont'd*

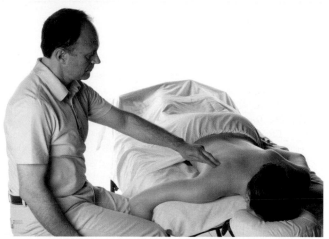

Figure 11-34 Starting position for prone palpation of the right infraspinatus.

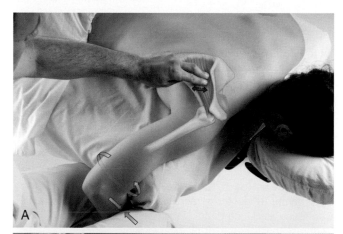

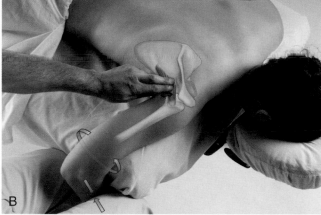

Figure 11-35 Palpation of the right infraspinatus and teres minor as the client laterally rotates the arm against resistance. **A** shows palpation of the infraspinatus. **B** shows teres minor palpation.

PALPATION NOTES

1. It can be difficult to palpate the distal tendons of the infraspinatus and teres minor all the way to the greater tubercle of the humerus, because they run deep to the posterior deltoid, which also contracts with lateral rotation of the arm at the glenohumeral (GH) joint. To better palpate the distal tendons, either ask the client to do a very gentle lateral rotation contraction of the arm so that the posterior deltoid is not engaged, or place the client's arm in flexion (This requires the client to be seated instead of lying prone.) to reciprocally inhibit the posterior deltoid as the gentle lateral rotation of the arm contraction is performed.

2. It can be difficult to discern the border between the bellies of the infraspinatus and teres minor because they usually blend together. Their distal tendons are easier to discern. Feel for the gap between them; the teres minor is more inferior, and the infraspinatus is more superior.

3. It is easy to discern the inferior border of the teres minor from the superior border of the teres major. To do so, simply have the client alternate between lateral rotation of the arm and medial rotation of the arm at the GH joint (in each case against the resistance of your knee). The teres minor is felt to contract with lateral rotation, and the teres major is felt to contract with medial rotation.

Palpation Key:
Place client's forearm between your knees; use your knee to provide resistance.

11

INFRASPINATUS AND TERES MINOR—PRONE—*cont'd*
Alternate Palpation Position—Seated

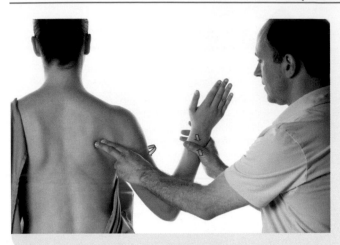

Figure 11-36 The infraspinatus and teres minor can also be easily palpated with the client seated. To engage these muscles, have the client perform lateral rotation of the arm at the glenohumeral (GH) joint against resistance. Note: Given that it is usually uncomfortable to resist rotation of the arm by resisting motion of the arm itself, the client can be asked to flex the elbow joint to 90 degrees and then the resistance can be given to the forearm. It is important that the client's resistance against the therapist's hand is not coming from horizontal extension of the arm at the GH joint, but rather lateral rotation of the arm.

TRIGGER POINTS

1. Trigger points (TrPs) in the infraspinatus and teres minor often result from or are perpetuated by acute or chronic overuse of the muscle (e.g., reaching behind the body with lateral rotation of the arm at the glenohumeral [GH] joint) and trauma (e.g., GH joint dislocation).

2. TrPs in the infraspinatus and teres minor both tend to restrict medial rotation of the arm at the GH joint (e.g., reaching behind to the lower back) and cause discomfort when sleeping on the affected side. TrPs in the infraspinatus tend to also produce strong deep pain in the anterior shoulder or discomfort sleeping on the back due to pressure on the TrPs. (When sleeping on the unaffected side, it may be necessary to support the affected arm on a pillow.) TrPs in the teres minor tend to also produce deep pain that is well localized, altered sensation in the ring and little fingers, or cause quadrilateral space syndrome (entrapment of the axillary nerve between the teres minor and teres major).

3. Infraspinatus: The referral patterns of infraspinatus TrPs must be distinguished from the referral patterns of TrPs in the teres minor, supraspinatus, latissimus dorsi, teres major, subscapularis, rhomboids, deltoid, coracobrachialis, biceps brachii, triceps brachii, scalenes, pectoralis major and minor, subclavius, serratus posterior superior (SPS), and thoracic transversospinalis.

Teres minor: The referral patterns of teres minor TrPs must be distinguished from the referral patterns of TrPs in the infraspinatus, supraspinatus, teres major, subscapularis, deltoid, triceps brachii, SPS, levator scapulae, and scalenes.

4. TrPs in the infraspinatus and teres minor are often incorrectly assessed as rotator cuff lesions or cervical disc syndrome. TrPs in the infraspinatus are also often incorrectly assessed as osteoarthritis of the GH joint, entrapment of the suprascapular nerve, or bicipital tendinitis. TrPs in the teres minor are also often incorrectly assessed as shoulder bursitis or cervical disc syndrome.

5. Associated TrPs of the infraspinatus and teres minor often occur in each other, as well as the teres major, supraspinatus, anterior deltoid, subscapularis, and pectoralis major.

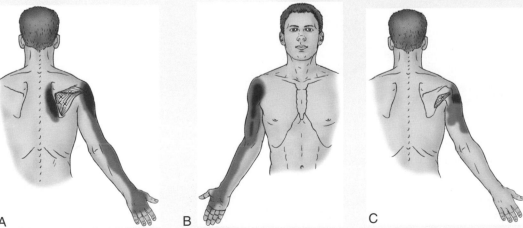

Figure 11-37 A, Posterior view illustrating common infraspinatus trigger points (TrPs) and their corresponding referral zone. **B,** Anterior view showing the remainder of the referral zone. **C,** Posterior view illustrating a common teres minor TrP and its corresponding referral zone.

INFRASPINATUS AND TERES MINOR—PRONE—*cont'd*

STRETCHING THE INFRASPINATUS AND TERES MINOR

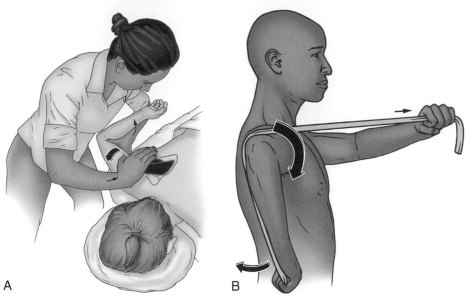

A   B

Figure 11-38 Stretching the right infraspinatus and teres minor. The arm is medially rotated at the glenohumeral (GH) joint. **A,** Therapist-assisted stretch. Note that the client's scapula is stabilized by the therapist's right hand. **B,** Self-care stretch. The client's right arm is medially rotated using a rope.

11

TERES MAJOR—PRONE

☑ ATTACHMENTS

☐ Inferior angle and inferior ⅓ of the dorsal surface of the lateral border of the scapula

to the

☐ medial lip of the bicipital groove of the humerus

☑ ACTIONS

☐ Medially rotates the arm at the glenohumeral (GH) joint
☐ Adducts the arm at the GH joint
☐ Extends the arm at the GH joint
☐ Upwardly rotates the scapula at the scapulocostal (ScC) and GH joints

Starting Position (Figure 11-40)

■ Client prone with arm abducted 90 degrees to the side and resting on the table, and the forearm hanging off the table
■ Therapist seated to the side of the client with the client's forearm between the knees
■ Palpating hand placed just lateral to the lower aspect of the lateral border of the scapula

Palpation Steps

1. Ask the client to medially rotate the arm at the GH joint against the resistance of your knee, and feel for the contraction of the teres major at the inferior aspect of the lateral border of the scapula (Figure 11-41).

2. Continue palpating the teres major distally toward the humerus while strumming perpendicular to its fibers.
3. Once the teres major muscle has been located, have the client relax it and palpate to assess its baseline tone.

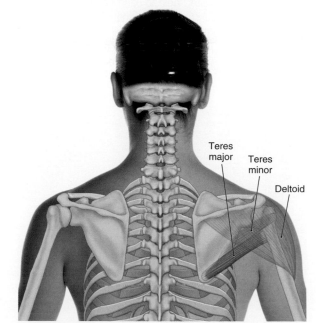

Teres major
Teres minor
Deltoid

Figure 11-39 Posterior view of the right teres major. The deltoid and teres minor have been ghosted in.

TERES MAJOR—PRONE—*cont'd*

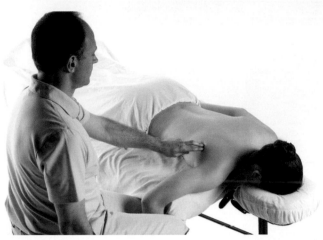

Figure 11-40 Starting position for prone palpation of the right teres major.

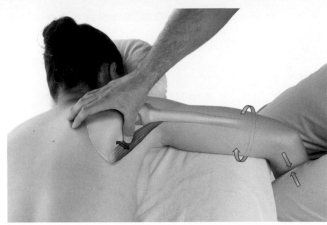

Figure 11-41 Palpation of the right teres major as the client medially rotates the arm against resistance.

PALPATION NOTES

1. It is easy to discern the superior border of the teres major from the inferior border of the teres minor. To do so, simply have the client alternate between medial rotation of the arm and lateral rotation of the arm at the glenohumeral (GH) joint (in each case against the resistance of your knee). The teres major contracts with medial rotation, and the teres minor contracts with lateral rotation.
2. It is sometimes challenging to discern the border between the bellies of the teres major and latissimus dorsi. They are located next to each other and they engage with the same actions of the arm at the GH joint. On the humerus, the latissimus dorsi attaches more anteriorly on the humerus than the teres major, but the teres major does attach slightly further distal.

Alternate Palpation Position—Seated

The teres major can also be easily palpated with the client seated. This palpation should be carried out in a similar manner to the seated palpation of the teres minor and infraspinatus (see Figure 11-36), except that medial rotation of the arm at the GH joint is resisted. If the resistance is given to the forearm (with the elbow joint flexed to 90 degrees), be sure that the client is providing the resistance with medial rotation of the arm at the GH joint and not horizontal flexion of the arm at the GH joint.

Palpation Key:
Place client's forearm between your knees; use your knee to provide resistance.

11

TERES MAJOR—PRONE—*cont'd*

TRIGGER POINTS

1. Trigger points (TrPs) in the teres major often result from or are perpetuated by acute or chronic overuse of the muscle (e.g., forceful extension of the arm, such as when rowing).
2. TrPs in the teres major tend to produce deep pain in the posterior shoulder when contracting or stretching the muscle, restricted arm abduction at the glenohumeral (GH) joint, or winging (lateral tilt) of the scapula.
3. The referral patterns of teres major TrPs must be distinguished from the referral patterns of TrPs in the deltoid, triceps brachii, serratus posterior superior (SPS), supraspinatus, infraspinatus, teres minor, and subscapularis.
4. TrPs in the teres major are often incorrectly assessed as joint dysfunction of the GH or acromioclavicular joints, deltoid strain, or rotator cuff disease.
5. Associated TrPs often occur in the latissimus dorsi, triceps brachii, posterior deltoid, teres minor, subscapularis, rhomboids, middle trapezius, or serratus anterior.

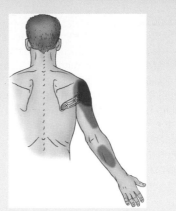

Figure 11-42 Posterior view illustrating common teres major trigger points (TrPs) and their corresponding referral zone.

STRETCHING THE TERES MAJOR

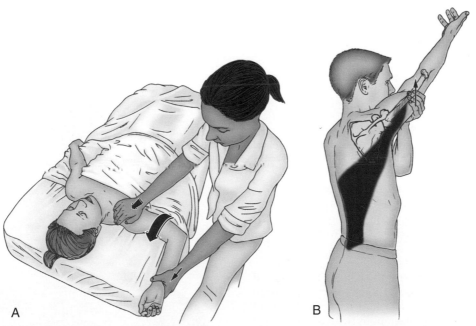

Figure 11-43 Stretching the right teres major. The arm is laterally rotated at the glenohumeral (GH) joint. **A,** Therapist-assisted stretch. Note that the client's scapula is stabilized by the therapist's right hand. **B,** Self-care stretch. The client passively moves his arm into lateral rotation, flexion, and adduction in front of the body. (Note: The latissimus dorsi is also stretched.)

11

TERES MAJOR—PRONE—*cont'd*

↻ DETOUR

Latissimus dorsi:

With the client prone, it is easy to palpate the latissimus dorsi along with the teres major. To do so, have the client perform either resisted extension or medial rotation of the arm at the GH joint (medial rotation shown in Figure 11-44). Even though the teres major and latissimus dorsi both attach together onto the medial lip of the bicipital groove of the humerus, the distal tendon of the latissimus dorsi is more easily palpated at the humerus because it is the more anterior (superficial) of the two tendons. For more information on palpation of the latissimus dorsi, please see Tour #7 in Chapter 17.

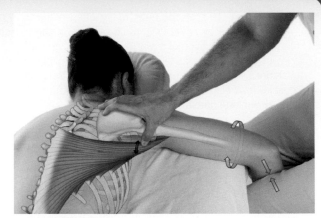

Figure 11-44 Palpation of the right latissimus dorsi as the client medially rotates the arm against resistance. The teres major is ghosted in.

SUPRASPINATUS—PRONE

☑ ATTACHMENTS

☐ Supraspinous fossa of the scapula

to the

☐ greater tubercle of the humerus

☑ ACTIONS

☐ Abducts the arm at the glenohumeral (GH) joint
☐ Flexes the arm at the GH joint

Starting Position (Figure 11-46)

■ Client prone with the arm resting on the table at the side of the client
■ Therapist seated to the side of the client
■ Palpating hand placed just superior to the spine of the scapula in the supraspinous fossa
■ Support hand placed on distal arm (just proximal to the elbow joint); only needed if resistance is given

Palpation Steps

1. Ask the client to perform a very short range of motion of abduction of the arm at the GH joint (approximately 10 to 20 degrees) and feel for the contraction of the belly of the supraspinatus in the supraspinous fossa of the scapula (Figure 11-47, *A*).
2. To further bring out the contraction of the supraspinatus, the therapist can provide gentle resistance with the support hand to the client's arm abduction.
3. The distal tendon can be palpated deep to the deltoid. This can be done by locating the acromion process of the scapula and dropping just distally and laterally off it onto the distal

tendon of the supraspinatus (see Palpation Note #2). Strum perpendicular to the distal tendon with the supraspinatus either relaxed or contracting gently (see Figure 11-47, *B*).
4. Once the supraspinatus muscle has been located, have the client relax it and palpate to assess its baseline tone.

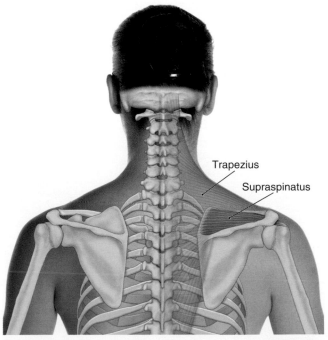

Trapezius

Supraspinatus

Figure 11-45 Posterior view of the right supraspinatus. The trapezius has been ghosted in.

SUPRASPINATUS—PRONE—*cont'd*

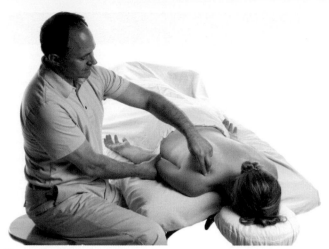

Figure 11-46 Starting position for prone palpation of the right supraspinatus.

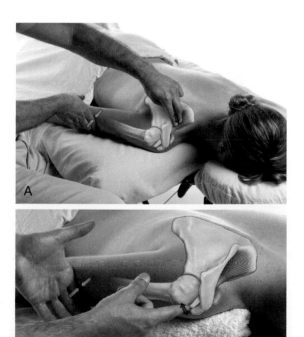

Figure 11-47 Palpation of the right supraspinatus. **A** shows palpation of the belly superior to the spine of the scapula. **B** shows palpation of the distal tendon just distal to the acromion process of the scapula.

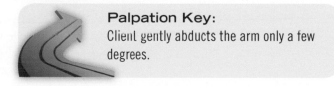

Palpation Key:
Client gently abducts the arm only a few degrees.

PALPATION NOTES

1. One difficulty with palpating the belly of the supraspinatus is that the upper trapezius, which lies superficial to it, contracts to stabilize the scapula whenever the arm is abducted. To minimize contraction of the upper trapezius, the client can be asked to actively move the arm halfway between abduction and flexion. This is difficult with the client prone, but it can be easily done if the supraspinatus is palpated with the client seated (Figure 11-48).
2. There are two ways to find the distal tendon of the supraspinatus. One method is to follow the line of the spine of the scapula to the head of the humerus (just distal to the acromion process) and then palpate just anterior to that line. The other method is to find the bicipital groove and then palpate just posterior to that point on the greater tubercle.
3. Medially rotating the arm at the glenohumeral (GH) joint may help increase access to the greater tubercle attachment of the supraspinatus.

Alternate Palpation Position—Seated

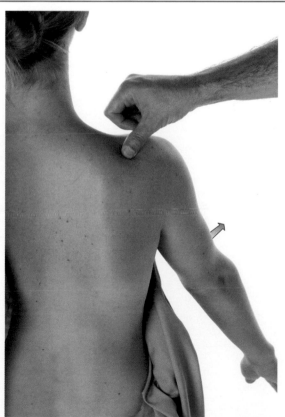

Figure 11-48 The supraspinatus can also be easily palpated with the client seated. To engage the supraspinatus, have the client either perform a very short range of motion (approximately 10 to 20 degrees) of abduction of the arm at the glenohumeral (GH) joint with the hand in the small of the back (to reciprocally inhibit the upper trapezius), or perform a short range of motion (approximately 10 to 20 degrees) of the arm halfway between abduction and flexion at the GH joint as seen here.

11

SUPRASPINATUS—PRONE—*cont'd*

TRIGGER POINTS

1. Trigger points (TrPs) in the supraspinatus often result from or are perpetuated by acute or chronic overuse of the muscle (e.g., postures requiring the arm to be held in abduction for extended periods, especially at or above shoulder height), holding heavy objects in the hand when the arm is hanging down by the side of the body or walking a dog that constantly pulls at the leash (both of which require the supraspinatus to contract to hold the head of the humerus in the glenoid fossa), and trauma (e.g., shoulder dislocation).

2. TrPs in the supraspinatus tend to produce joint crepitus, difficulty performing and strong pain during shoulder abduction, dull pain at rest, stiff shoulder, difficulty sleeping because of pain, and extreme tenderness at the humeral attachment.

3. The referral patterns of supraspinatus TrPs must be distinguished from the referral patterns of TrPs in the infraspinatus, teres minor, teres major, deltoid, coracobrachialis, biceps brachii, triceps brachii, brachioradialis, extensor carpi radialis longus, extensor digitorum, supinator, pectoralis major, pectoralis minor, subclavius, scalenes, and serratus posterior superior (SPS).

4. TrPs in the supraspinatus are often incorrectly assessed as rotator cuff tendinitis or tears, shoulder bursitis, cervical disc syndrome, frozen shoulder, or lateral epicondylitis/epicondylosis.

5. Associated TrPs often occur in the infraspinatus, teres minor, subscapularis, upper trapezius, deltoid, and latissimus dorsi.

6. Note: The supraspinatus and infraspinatus share the referral zone at the outside of the glenohumeral (GH) joint. However, referral pain from the infraspinatus is usually experienced as a deeper ache than is the referral pain of the supraspinatus.

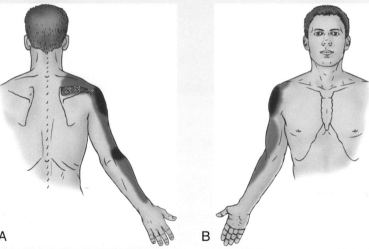

A   B

Figure 11-49 A, Posterior view illustrating common supraspinatus trigger points (TrPs) and their corresponding referral zone. **B,** Anterior view showing the remainder of the referral zone.

11

SUPRASPINATUS—PRONE—*cont'd*

STRETCHING THE SUPRASPINATUS

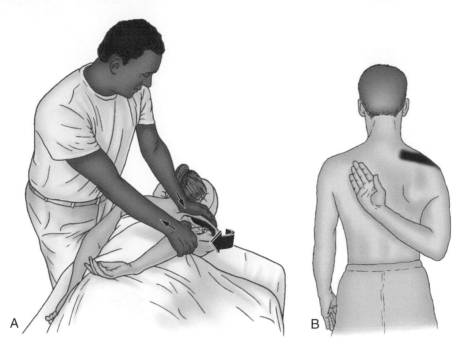

Figure 11-50 Stretching the right supraspinatus. The arm is extended and adducted behind the body. **A,** Therapist-assisted stretch. Note that the client's scapula is stabilized by the therapist's left hand. **B,** Self-care stretch. (See also Figure 14-10, *F,* for another self-care stretch of the supraspinatus.)

11

ANTERIOR DELTOID—SUPINE

☑ ATTACHMENTS

☐ Lateral ⅓ of the clavicle
  to the
☐ deltoid tuberosity of the humerus

☑ ACTIONS

☐ Flexes the arm at the glenohumeral (GH) joint
☐ Abducts the arm at the GH joint
☐ Adducts the arm at the GH joint (lowest fibers)
☐ Medially rotates the arm at the GH joint
☐ Horizontally flexes the arm at the GH joint

Starting Position (Figure 11-52)

- Client supine with arm resting on table against the body
- Therapist seated at the head of the table
- Palpating hand placed just inferior to the lateral end of the clavicle
- Support hand placed on the distal end of the arm (just proximal to the elbow joint)

Palpation Steps

1. Ask the client to lift the arm at the GH joint halfway between flexion and abduction, and feel for the contraction of the anterior deltoid (Figure 11-53).
2. To further bring out the contraction of the anterior deltoid, the therapist can provide gentle resistance with the support hand.
3. Strum the fibers of the anterior deltoid perpendicularly from the lateral clavicle to the deltoid tuberosity.
4. Once the anterior deltoid has been located, have the client relax it and palpate to assess its baseline tone.

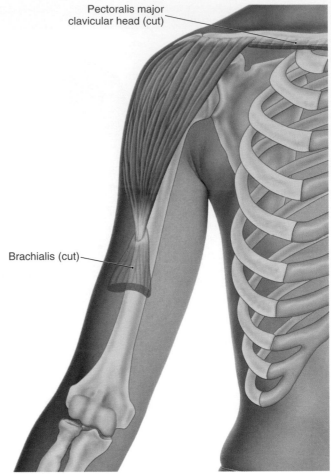

Figure 11-51 Anterior view of the right deltoid. The brachialis and pectoralis major have been cut and ghosted in.

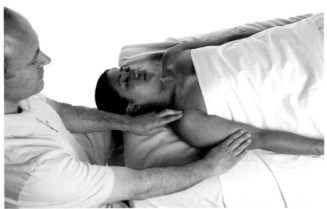

Figure 11-52 Starting position for supine palpation of the right anterior deltoid.

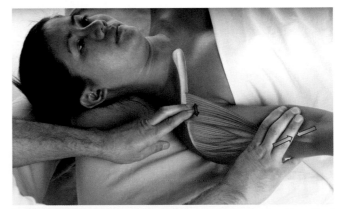

Figure 11-53 Palpation of the right anterior deltoid as the client moves the arm obliquely into flexion and abduction.

ANTERIOR DELTOID—SUPINE—*cont'd*

PALPATION NOTES

1. In the supine position, the anterior deltoid can also be engaged and palpated by asking the client to horizontally flex the arm at the glenohumeral (GH) joint. In this position, gravity often provides adequate resistance, but further resistance may be added with the therapist's hand.
2. The clavicular head of the pectoralis major also usually contracts with horizontal flexion of the arm at the GH joint.
3. When the anterior deltoid and the clavicular head of the pectoralis major are contracted, there is usually a small gap located between them that is visible.

Palpation Key:
Arm moves halfway between flexion and abduction.

Alternate Palpation Position—Seated or Standing

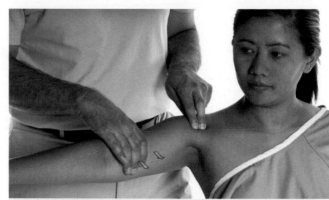

Figure 11-54 The anterior deltoid can also be easily palpated with the client seated or standing. To engage the anterior fibers of the deltoid, have the client perform horizontal flexion of the arm at the glenohumeral (GH) joint against resistance.

11

TRIGGER POINTS

1. Trigger points (TrPs) in the anterior deltoid often result from or are perpetuated by acute overuse, chronic overuse (e.g., holding the arm up in abduction or flexion for prolonged periods, such as when working at a computer keyboard), direct trauma (e.g., impact during sports), and TrPs in the supraspinatus.
2. TrPs in the anterior deltoid may produce weakness when performing abduction or flexion of the arm at the glenohumeral (GH) joint.
3. The referral patterns of anterior deltoid TrPs must be distinguished from the referral patterns of TrPs in the scalenes, pectoralis major, pectoralis minor, coracobrachialis, supraspinatus, infraspinatus, and biceps brachii.
4. TrPs in the anterior deltoid are often incorrectly assessed as a rotator cuff tear, bicipital tendinitis, subdeltoid/subacromial bursitis, GH or acromioclavicular joint arthritis, or C5 nerve compression.
5. Associated TrPs often occur in the clavicular head of the pectoralis major, supraspinatus, biceps brachii, latissimus dorsi, and teres major.

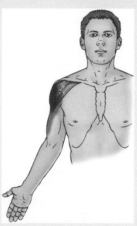

Figure 11-55 Anterior view illustrating a common anterior deltoid trigger point (TrP) and its corresponding referral zone.

ANTERIOR DELTOID—SUPINE—*cont'd*

STRETCHING THE ANTERIOR DELTOID

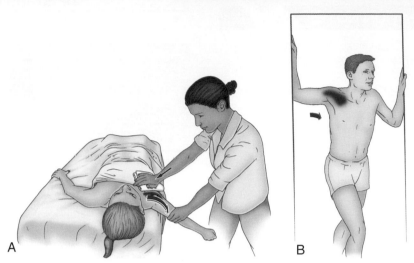

Figure 11-56 Stretching the right anterior deltoid. The arm is abducted to 90 degrees and horizontally extended. **A,** Therapist-assisted stretch. Note that the client's trunk/shoulder girdle is stabilized by the therapist's right hand; a cushion is used for comfort. **B,** Self-care stretch. The client stabilizes the forearm against the doorframe and leans in. (Note: The pectoralis major is also stretched.)

11

SUBSCAPULARIS—SUPINE

☑ ATTACHMENTS

☐ Subscapular fossa of the scapula

   to the

☐ lesser tubercle of the humerus

☑ ACTIONS

☐ Medially rotates the arm at the glenohumeral (GH) joint

Starting Position (Figure 11-58)
■ Client supine with the arm resting on the trunk and the other side hand gently holding the elbow of the side being palpated
■ Therapist seated to the side of the client
■ Palpating finger pads placed against the anterior surface of the scapula
■ Support hand reaching under the client's body to grip the medial border of the scapula

Palpation Steps
1. Passively protract the client's scapula with your support hand.
2. Ask the client to take in a deep breath and as the client exhales, slowly but firmly press your finger pads in against the anterior surface of the client's scapula (Figure 11-59, *A*) (see Palpation Note #1).
3. To verify that you are on the subscapularis, ask the client to medially rotate the arm at the GH joint (This will cause the arm to lift slightly off the trunk.) (see Figure 11-59, *B*).
4. Palpate as much of the subscapularis as possible by pressing in deeper toward the medial border of the scapula.
5. Once the subscapularis has been located, have the client relax it and palpate to assess its baseline tone.

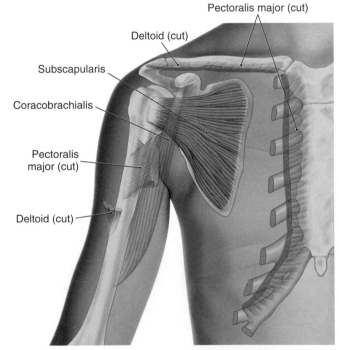

Figure 11-57 Anterior view of the right subscapularis. The coracobrachialis and cut deltoid and pectoralis major have been ghosted in.

SUBSCAPULARIS—SUPINE—*cont'd*

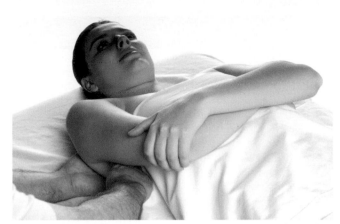

Figure 11-58 Starting position for supine palpation of the right subscapularis.

Palpation Key:
Client rests in peace; pull scapula out with support hand.

PALPATION NOTES

1. Working deep to access the subscapularis need not be painful for the client if you have the client breathe and you sink into the tissue *slowly* with a firm confident touch.
2. To locate the subscapularis tendon's distal attachment on the lesser tubercle of the humerus, have the client rest the arm on your shoulder against the crook of your neck and follow the muscle from the subscapular fossa toward the humerus in baby steps, confirming that you are still on it by asking the client to medially rotate the arm at the glenohumeral (GH) joint. When you have reached the site of distal attachment, have the client fully relax the subscapularis and the rest of the musculature of the arm so that it is easier to feel the lesser tubercle attachment and discern it from the distal tendon of the subscapularis (Figure 11-60).
3. The subscapularis and serratus anterior are both located between the scapula and the rib cage. To palpate the subscapularis, orient your finger pads against the anterior surface of the scapula; to palpate the serratus anterior, orient your finger pads against the rib cage wall.
4. The humeral attachment of the subscapularis can also be palpated through the anterior deltoid. This can be done by locating the lesser tubercle of the humerus and then strumming vertically along it, feeling for the tendon of the subscapularis. Alternately, locate the two heads of the biceps brachii and then palpate between them for the subscapularis tendon.

11

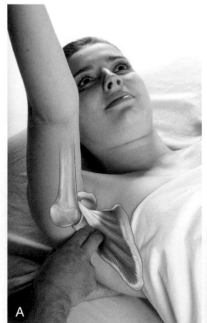
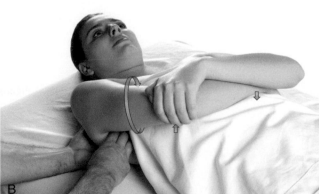

Figure 11-59 Palpation of the right subscapularis. **A,** shows palpation of the belly. Note: The client's arm is up so that the reader can visualize the belly of the muscle; the arm may be down and resting on the chest as seen in **B,** which shows the client medially rotating the arm to engage the subscapularis.

SUBSCAPULARIS—SUPINE—*cont'd*

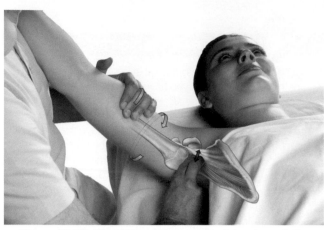

Figure 11-60 Palpation of the humeral tendon of the right subscapularis as the client medially rotates the arm against resistance (see Palpation Note #2).

Alternate Palpation Position—Side Lying

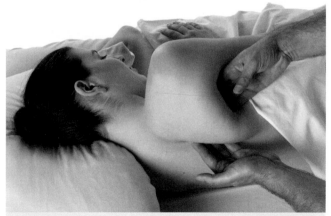

Figure 11-61 The subscapularis can also be palpated with the client side lying.

TRIGGER POINTS

1. Trigger points (TrPs) in the subscapularis often result from or are perpetuated by acute or chronic overuse of the muscle (e.g., swimming), trauma (e.g., glenohumeral [GH] joint dislocation), prolonged immobilization (e.g., when the arm is held medially rotated in a sling or cast), and chronic shortening of the muscle (e.g., when the client has chronic rounded shoulders posture with the arms medially rotated).
2. TrPs in the subscapularis tend to produce restricted and painful lateral rotation of the arm at the GH joint (Because lateral rotation of the arm is required for full abduction of the arm, arm abduction is also often restricted.), pain when the client is at rest, or extreme tenderness at the humeral attachment.
3. The referral patterns of subscapularis TrPs must be distinguished from the referral patterns of TrPs in the scalenes, teres minor, teres major, posterior deltoid, triceps brachii, extensor carpi radialis brevis, extensor carpi ulnaris, extensor carpi radialis longus, extensor indicis, and serratus posterior superior (SPS).
4. TrPs in the subscapularis are often incorrectly assessed as frozen shoulder, rotator cuff lesions, cervical disc syndrome, or thoracic outlet syndrome.
5. Associated TrPs often occur in the pectoralis major, latissimus dorsi, teres major, and anterior deltoid.

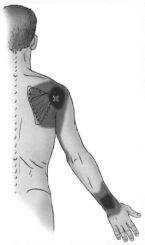

Figure 11-62 Posterior view illustrating a common subscapularis trigger point (TrP) and its corresponding referral zone.

SUBSCAPULARIS—SUPINE—*cont'd*

STRETCHING THE SUBSCAPULARIS

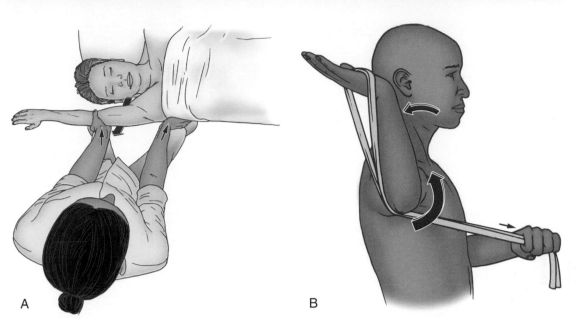

A   B

Figure 11-63 Stretching the right subscapularis. The arm is laterally rotated. **A,** Therapist-assisted stretch. Note that the client's shoulder girdle is stabilized by the therapist's right hand. **B,** Self-care stretch. The client's right arm is laterally rotated using a rope.

11

SERRATUS ANTERIOR—SUPINE

☑ATTACHMENTS

☐ Anterolateral surfaces of ribs one through nine

to the

☐ anterior surface of the entire medial border of the scapula

☑ACTIONS

☐ Protracts the scapula at the scapulocostal (ScC) joint
☐ Upwardly rotates the scapula at the ScC joint
☐ Upper fibers can also elevate the scapula at the ScC joint
☐ Lower fibers can also depress the scapula at the ScC joint

Starting Position (Figure 11-65)

■ Client supine with the arm straight up in the air pointed toward the ceiling
■ Therapist seated to the side of the client
■ Palpating hand placed with finger pads oriented against the lateral rib cage wall, directly inferior to the axilla (armpit)
■ Support hand placed on top of the client's fist; only needed if resistance is given

Palpation Steps

1. Ask the client to reach the hand toward the ceiling (This requires protraction of the scapula at the ScC joint.) and feel for the contraction of the serratus anterior (Figure 11-66).
2. If desired, resistance to the client's action can be given with your support hand.
3. Continue palpating as much of the serratus anterior as possible (Figure 11-67).
4. Once the serratus anterior has been located, have the client relax it and palpate to assess its baseline tone.

11

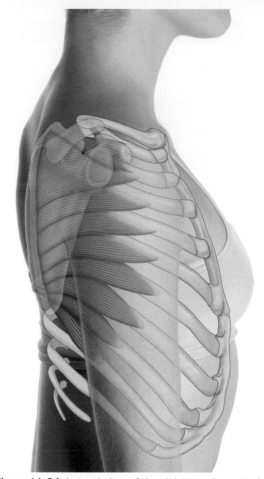

Figure 11-64 Lateral view of the right serratus anterior.

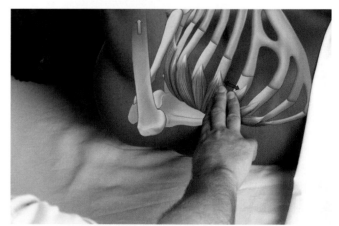

Figure 11-66 Palpation of the right serratus anterior against the lateral rib cage wall.

Alternate Palpation Position—Side Lying

The serratus anterior can also be easily palpated with the client side lying. As with the supine palpation, the client's upper extremity should be moved to allow access to the serratus anterior.

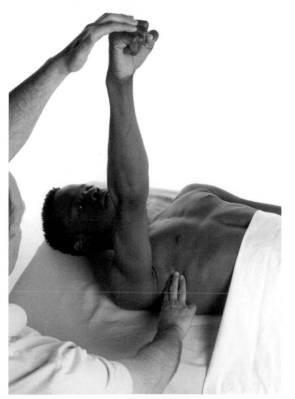

Figure 11-65 Starting position for supine palpation of the right serratus anterior.

SERRATUS ANTERIOR—SUPINE—*cont'd*

PALPATION NOTES

1. To palpate the upper fibers at their rib cage attachment, slowly but firmly sink in against the rib cage deep to the pectoralis major (see Figure 11-67); it can be extremely challenging to access the fibers on the upper two ribs. To palpate the upper fibers closer to the scapular attachment, slowly but firmly sink in against the rib cage between the scapula and rib cage.
2. To better engage the upper fibers of the serratus anterior, have the client angle the arm upward (approximately 135 degrees of flexion) so that the scapula protracts and elevates at the scapulocostal (ScC) joint (Figure 11-68, *A*). Similarly, to better engage the lower fibers, have the client angle the arm downward (approximately 45 degrees of flexion) so that the scapula protracts and depresses at the ScC joint (see Figure 11-68, *B*).
3. The serratus anterior and subscapularis are both located between the scapula and rib cage. To palpate the serratus anterior, orient your finger pads against the rib cage wall; to palpate the subscapularis, orient your finger pads against the anterior surface of the scapula.

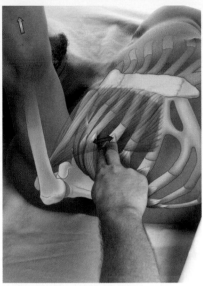

Figure 11-67 Palpation of the right serratus anterior deep to the pectoralis major.

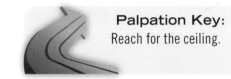

Palpation Key:
Reach for the ceiling.

11

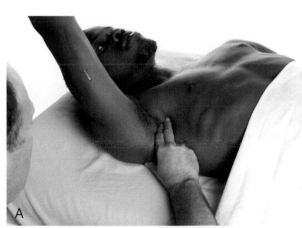

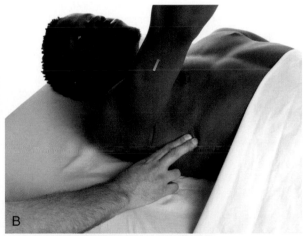

Figure 11-68 To better engage the upper fibers of the serratus anterior, orient the client's arm more superiorly as it is protracted, as seen in **A.** To better engage the lower fibers of the serratus anterior, orient the client's arm more inferiorly during protraction, as seen in **B.**

SERRATUS ANTERIOR—SUPINE—*cont'd*

TRIGGER POINTS

1. Trigger points (TrPs) in the serratus anterior often result from or are perpetuated by acute or chronic overuse of the muscle (e.g., push ups or any motion that requires the scapula to protract, such as throwing a punch in martial arts, swinging a tennis racquet, throwing a ball, or forceful pushing motions) or labored breathing (because of its accessory role in breathing).

2. TrPs in the serratus anterior tend to restrict scapular retraction at the scapulocostal (ScC) joint; make it difficult to sleep if lying on the affected side due to compression on the TrP(s), or on the other side if the scapula falls (protracts) forward, resulting in shortening of the muscle; make it difficult to take a deep breath; or cause a "stitch in the side" when "pumping the arms" while running fast.

3. The referral patterns of serratus anterior TrPs must be distinguished from the referral patterns of TrPs in the intercostal muscles, middle trapezius, rhomboids, erector spinae/transversospinalis muscles of the thoracic spine, latissimus dorsi, infraspinatus, and diaphragm.

4. TrPs in the serratus anterior are often incorrectly assessed as angina pectoris or heart attack referral pain (if the muscle on the left side is affected), rib joint dysfunction or fracture, entrapment of the intercostal nerves, costochondritis, cervical disc syndrome, thoracic outlet syndrome, herpes zoster, and TrPs of the intercostal muscles.

5. Associated TrPs often occur in the erector spinae/transversospinalis muscles of the thoracic spine, rhomboids, middle trapezius, serratus posterior superior (SPS), latissimus dorsi, scalenes, and sternocleidomastoid (SCM).

6. Notes: Central and attachment TrPs can occur in any of the nine digitations of the serratus anterior. TrPs of the serratus anterior may also refer down the ulnar side of the entire upper extremity.

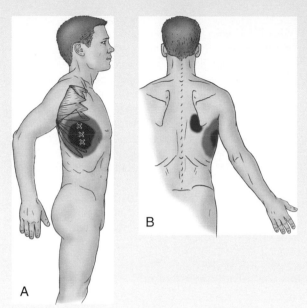

Figure 11-69 A, Lateral view illustrating common serratus anterior trigger points (TrPs) and their corresponding referral zone. **B,** Posterior view showing the remainder of the referral zone.

STRETCHING THE SERRATUS ANTERIOR

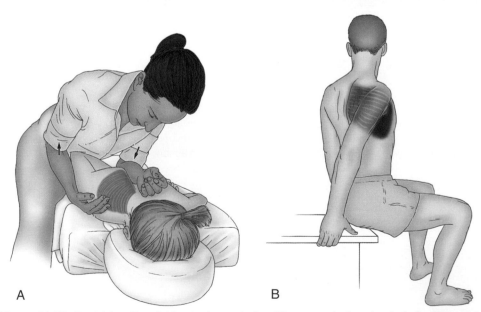

Figure 11-70 Stretching the right serratus anterior. The scapula is retracted. **A,** Therapist-assisted stretch. Note that the client's trunk is stabilized by the therapist's left forearm. **B,** Self-care stretch. The client extends the arm to hold onto the back of the bench and rotates the body to the opposite side (causing retraction of the scapula).

PECTORALIS MAJOR—SUPINE

☑ ATTACHMENTS

☐ Medial half of the clavicle, sternum, and the costal cartilages of ribs one through seven

to the

☐ lateral lip of the bicipital groove of the humerus

☑ ACTIONS

Entire Muscle
☐ Adducts the arm at the glenohumeral (GH) joint
☐ Medially rotates the arm at the GH joint
☐ Horizontally flexes the arm at the GH joint
☐ Protracts the scapula at the scapulocostal (ScC) joint

Clavicular Head (also)
☐ Flexes the arm at the GH joint

Sternocostal Head (also)
☐ Extends the arm at the GH joint (from a position of flexion to anatomic position)
☐ Depresses the scapula at the ScC joint

Starting Position (Figure 11-72)
■ Client supine with the arm resting at the side
■ Therapist seated to the side of the client
■ Palpating hand placed over the lower aspect of the anterior axillary fold of tissue
■ Support hand placed on the distal arm, just proximal to the elbow joint

Palpation Steps
1. Begin by palpating the sternocostal head. Ask the client to adduct the arm at the GH joint against resistance. Resistance can be added either with your support hand or simply by having the client adduct against his body wall (Figure 11-73, *A*).
2. Feel for the contraction of the sternocostal head, and palpate toward its proximal (medial) attachment.
3. To palpate the clavicular head, place the palpating hand just inferior to the medial clavicle, and ask the client to obliquely move the arm at the GH joint between flexion

and adduction against resistance. Resistance can be added with your support hand (see Figure 11-73, *B*).
4. Feel for the contraction of the clavicular head, and palpate toward the distal attachment while strumming perpendicular to the fibers.
5. Once the pectoralis major has been located, have the client relax it and palpate to assess its baseline tone.

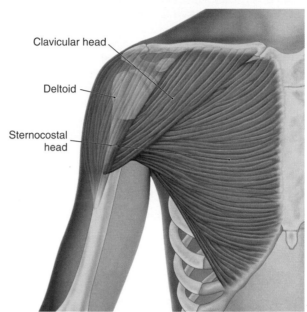

Figure 11-71 Anterior view of the right pectoralis major. The deltoid has been ghosted in.

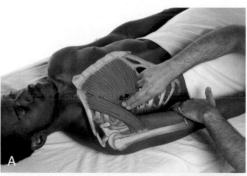

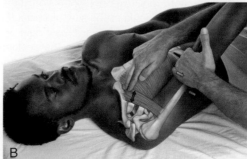

Figure 11-73 Palpation of the right pectoralis major. **A** shows palpation of the sternocostal head as the client performs adduction against resistance. **B** shows palpation of the clavicular head as the client performs an oblique plane motion of flexion and adduction against resistance.

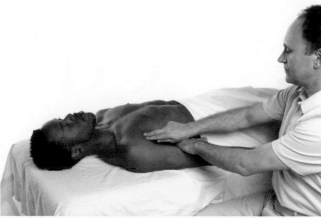

Figure 11-72 Starting position for supine palpation of the right pectoralis major (sternocostal head).

PECTORALIS MAJOR—SUPINE—*cont'd*

PALPATION NOTES

1. Ask the client to abduct the arm at the glenohumeral (GH) joint, and grab the anterior axillary fold of tissue; then have the client relax the arm back against the body. You have the client's pectoralis major in your hand (Figure 11-74, *A*).
2. There is usually a discernable and visible groove between the clavicular head of the pectoralis major and the anterior deltoid.
3. To engage the entire pectoralis major, ask the client to horizontally flex the arm at the GH joint against resistance. (Note: This also engages the anterior deltoid.) This is most easily done with the client seated (see Figure 11-74, *B*).
4. When the client horizontally flexes the arm against resistance, there is usually a discernable and visible groove between the clavicular and sternocostal heads of the pectoralis major.

Palpation Key:
Palpate the anterior axillary fold of tissue.

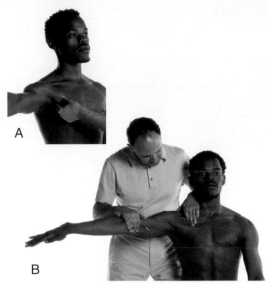

Figure 11-74 If the arm is abducted away from the body, the anterior axillary fold of tissue containing the pectoralis major can be easily grasped between palpating fingers, as seen in **A.** The entire pectoralis major can be easily palpated with the client seated by resisting the client's horizontal flexion of the arm at the glenohumeral (GH) joint, as seen in **B.**

TRIGGER POINTS

1. Trigger points (TrPs) in the pectoralis major often result from or are perpetuated by acute or chronic overuse of the muscle (e.g., repetitive lifting in front of the body, any repetitive adduction of the arm at the glenohumeral [GH] joint), prolonged postures that shorten the muscle (e.g., a chronic rounded shoulder posture, use of a sling or cast, sleeping on the back with the arms folded across the chest, sleeping on the affected side with the shoulder girdle protracted), use of a cane or crutches, excessively tight bra strap that compresses the muscle, or myocardial infarction.
2. TrPs in the pectoralis major tend to produce a rounded shoulder posture (which may cause pain in the interscapular region and may cause costoclavicular syndrome), restricted abduction and horizontal extension of the arm at the GH joint or retraction of the scapula at the scapulocostal (ScC) joint, difficulty sleeping (due to pain), or breast pain or swelling. Additionally, a TrP in the right side of the pectoralis major between the fifth and sixth ribs has been attributed to causing cardiac arrhythmia.
3. The referral patterns of pectoralis major TrPs must be distinguished from the referral patterns of TrPs in the pectoralis minor, subclavius, intercostals, scalenes, anterior deltoid, supraspinatus, infraspinatus, coracobrachialis, and biceps brachii.
4. TrPs in the pectoralis major are often incorrectly assessed as angina pectoris or myocardial infarction (for left-sided TrPs), rib joint dysfunction, costochondritis, hiatal hernia, bicipital tendinitis, GH joint bursitis, cervical disc syndrome, or medial epicondylitis/epicondylosis.

5. Associated TrPs often occur in the anterior deltoid, coracobrachialis, latissimus dorsi, subscapularis, serratus anterior, rhomboids, middle trapezius, sternocleidomastoid (SCM), infraspinatus, teres minor, and posterior deltoid.

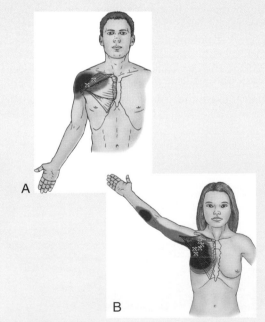

Figure 11-75 Anterior views illustrating common pectoralis major trigger points (TrPs) and their corresponding referral zones. **A** shows the clavicular head; **B** shows the sternocostal head.

PECTORALIS MAJOR—SUPINE—cont'd

STRETCHING THE PECTORALIS MAJOR

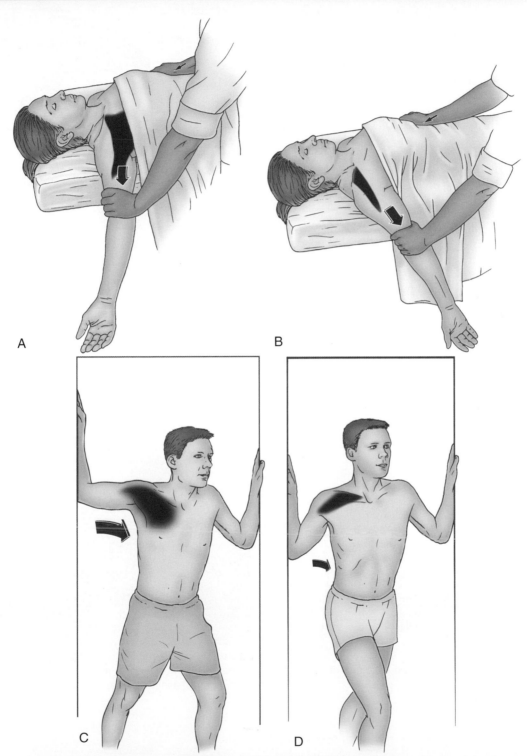

Figure 11-76 Stretching the right pectoralis major. To stretch the sternocostal head, the arm is abducted approximately 90 degrees and horizontally extended. To stretch the clavicular head, the arm is abducted approximately 45 degrees and horizontally extended. **A** and **B,** Therapist-assisted stretching of the sternocostal and clavicular heads respectively. Note that the client's trunk is stabilized by the therapist's right hand. **C** and **D,** Self-care stretches of the sternocostal and clavicular heads respectively. The client stabilizes the forearm against the doorframe and steps/leans in.

PECTORALIS MINOR—SUPINE

☑ ATTACHMENTS

☐ Ribs three through five

to the

☐ medial surface of the coracoid process of the scapula

☑ ACTIONS

☐ Protracts the scapula at the scapulocostal (ScC) joint
☐ Depresses the scapula at the ScC joint
☐ Downwardly rotates the scapula at the ScC joint
☐ Elevates ribs three through five at the sternocostal and costospinal joints

Starting Position (Figure 11-78)

■ Client supine with the hand under the body in the small of the back
■ Therapist seated at the head of the table
■ Palpating hand placed just inferior to the coracoid process of the scapula

Palpation Steps

1. Ask the client to press the hand and forearm down against the table, and feel for the contraction of the pectoralis minor through the pectoralis major (Figure 11-79).
2. Continue palpating toward the rib attachments while strumming perpendicular to the fibers.
3. Once the pectoralis minor has been located, have the client relax it and palpate to assess its baseline tone.

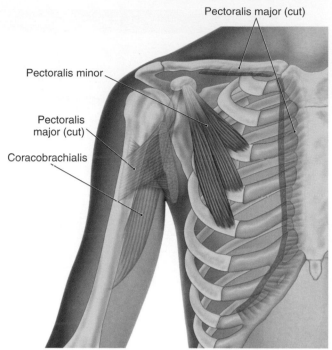

Figure 11-77 Anterior view of the right pectoralis minor. The coracobrachialis and cut pectoralis major have been ghosted in.

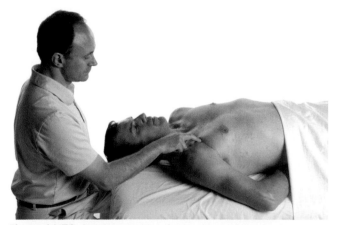

Figure 11-78 Starting position for supine palpation of the right pectoralis minor.

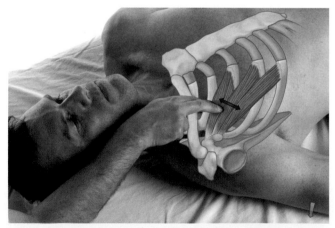

Figure 11-79 Palpation of the right pectoralis minor perpendicular to the fibers as the client presses the hand and forearm down against the table.

11

PECTORALIS MINOR—SUPINE—*cont'd*

Alternate Palpation Position—Seated

PALPATION NOTES

1. The client is asked to press the hand and forearm against the table, because this requires extension of the arm at the glenohumeral (GH) joint, which requires the coupled action of downward rotation of the scapula at the scapulocostal (ScC) joint, an action of the pectoralis minor. This is easiest to perform with the client seated (Figure 11-80).
2. It is usually possible to individually palpate and discern each of the three slips of the pectoralis minor.
3. An alternate method to palpate the lateral-most fibers of the pectoralis minor is to access it from the side by pressing in deep to the pectoralis major. This method does work, but it can be uncomfortable for the client and is not necessary because the pectoralis minor can usually be easily palpated and worked through the pectoralis major.

Palpation Key:
Client's hand in the small of the back.

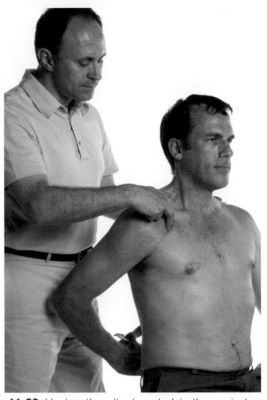

Figure 11-80 Having the client seated is the easiest position for palpating the pectoralis minor, because the client can comfortably place the hand in the small of the back and easily move it posteriorly when asked to do so by the therapist.

TRIGGER POINTS

1. Trigger points (TrPs) in the pectoralis minor often result from or are perpetuated by acute or chronic overuse of the muscle, prolonged postures that shorten the muscle (e.g., a chronic rounded shoulder posture, use of a sling or cast, sleeping on the back with the arms folded across the chest, sleeping on the affected side with the shoulder girdle protracted), use of a cane or crutches, myocardial infarction, labored breathing, compression of the muscle (e.g., due to the straps of a heavy backpack), or from TrPs in the pectoralis major or scalenes.
2. TrPs in the pectoralis minor tend to produce pectoralis minor syndrome (causing neurologic or vascular symptoms in the upper extremity), a rounded shoulder posture (which may cause pain in the interscapular region and may cause costoclavicular syndrome), restricted retraction of the scapula at the scapulocostal (ScC) joint, or winging of the scapula.
3. The referral patterns of pectoralis minor TrPs must be distinguished from the referral patterns of TrPs in the pectoralis major, deltoid, coracobrachialis, scalenes, supraspinatus, infraspinatus, biceps brachii, and triceps brachii.
4. TrPs in the pectoralis minor are often incorrectly assessed as cervical disc syndrome, anterior scalene syndrome, costoclavicular syndrome, carpal tunnel syndrome, bicipital tendinitis, medial epicondylitis/epicondylosis, or angina pectoris or myocardial infarction (for left-sided TrPs).
5. Associated TrPs often occur in the pectoralis major, anterior deltoid, scalenes, and sternocleidomastoid (SCM).

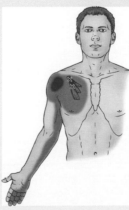

Figure 11-81 Anterior view illustrating common pectoralis minor trigger points (TrPs) and their corresponding referral zone.

PECTORALIS MINOR—SUPINE—*cont'd*

STRETCHING THE PECTORALIS MINOR

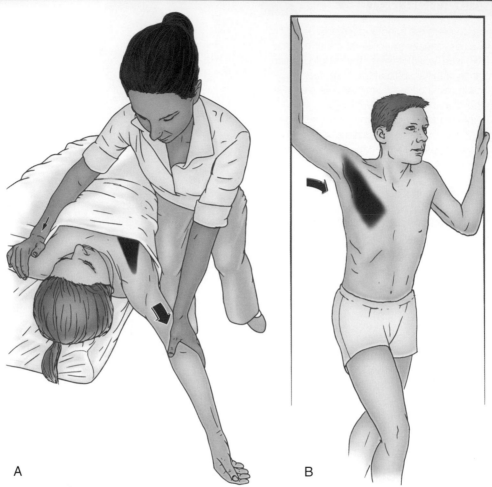

A   B

Figure 11-82 Stretching the right pectoralis minor. The arm is abducted to approximately 135 degrees and horizontally extended. **A,** Therapist-assisted stretch. Note that the client's trunk is stabilized by the therapist's right hand. **B,** Self-care stretch. The client stabilizes the forearm against the doorframe and leans in.

SUBCLAVIUS—SUPINE

✔ ATTACHMENTS

☐ First rib at the junction with its costal cartilage

to the

☐ middle ⅓ of the inferior surface of the clavicle

✔ ACTIONS

☐ Depresses the clavicle at the sternoclavicular (SC) joint
☐ Protracts the clavicle at the SC joint
☐ Downwardly rotates the clavicle at the SC joint
☐ Elevates the first rib at the sternocostal and costospinal joints

Starting Position (Figure 11-84)

■ Client supine with the arm medially rotated at the GH joint and resting on the table at the side of the body
■ Therapist seated at the head of the table
■ Palpating fingers curled around the clavicle so that the finger pads are on the inferior surface of the clavicle

Palpation Steps

1. The subclavius can be challenging to palpate.
2. With the musculature of the region relaxed, feel for the subclavius on the underside of the clavicle.
3. To palpate while engaged, ask the client to depress the clavicle at the SC joint (i.e., to depress the shoulder girdle [scapula and clavicle]) and feel for the contraction of the subclavius (Figure 11-85).
4. Palpate from attachment to attachment.
5. Once the subclavius has been located, have the client relax it and palpate to assess its baseline tone.

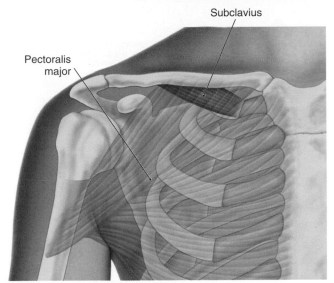

Figure 11-83 Anterior view of the right subclavius. The pectoralis major has been ghosted in.

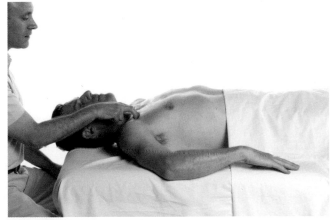

Figure 11-84 Starting position for supine palpation of the right subclavius.

Alternate Palpation Position

The subclavius can also be palpated with the client side-lying or seated.

11

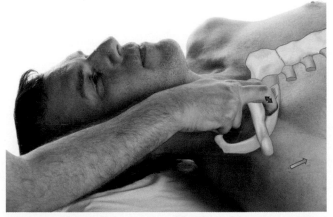

Figure 11-85 Palpation of the right subclavius as the client depresses the shoulder girdle.

SUBCLAVIUS—SUPINE—*cont'd*

PALPATION NOTES

1. Asking the client to have the arm passively medially rotated at the glenohumeral (GH) joint helps to slacken the pectoralis major, which lies superficial to the subclavius. Also, having the arm in adduction further slackens the pectoralis major.
2. When palpating the subclavius, it can also be helpful to hold the client's arm in passive abduction. Abducting the arm at the GH joint requires the clavicle to upwardly rotate at the sternoclavicular (SC) joint, exposing more of the inferior surface of the clavicle to palpation. It is important that the client's arm is passively abducted so that the musculature of the region is relaxed.

Palpation Key
Curl your fingertips around the clavicle.

TRIGGER POINTS

1. Trigger points (TrPs) in the subclavius often result from or are perpetuated by acute or chronic overuse of the muscle, prolonged postures that shorten the muscle (e.g., a chronic rounded shoulder posture, use of a sling or cast, sleeping on the affected side with the shoulder girdle protracted), or use of a cane or crutches.
2. TrPs in the subclavius tend to produce costoclavicular syndrome (causing neurologic or vascular symptoms in the upper extremity).
3. The referral patterns of subclavius TrPs must be distinguished from the referral patterns of TrPs in the biceps brachii, brachialis, scalenes, supraspinatus, infraspinatus, brachioradialis, extensor carpi radialis longus, extensor digitorum, supinator, opponens pollicis, and adductor pollicis.
4. TrPs in the subclavius are often incorrectly assessed as cervical disc syndrome, anterior scalene syndrome, pectoralis minor syndrome, or lateral epicondylitis/epicondylosis.
5. Associated TrPs are likely to occur in the pectoralis major and pectoralis minor.

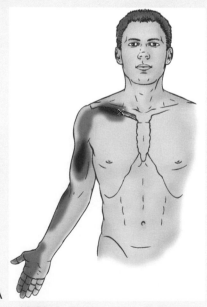
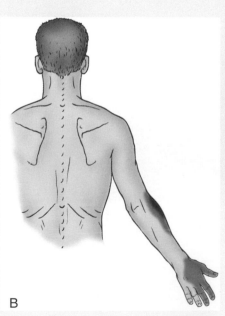

Figure 11-86 A, Anterior view illustrating a common subclavius trigger point (TrP) and its corresponding referral zone. **B,** Posterior view showing the remainder of the referral zone.

SUBCLAVIUS—SUPINE—*cont'd*

STRETCHING THE SUBCLAVIUS

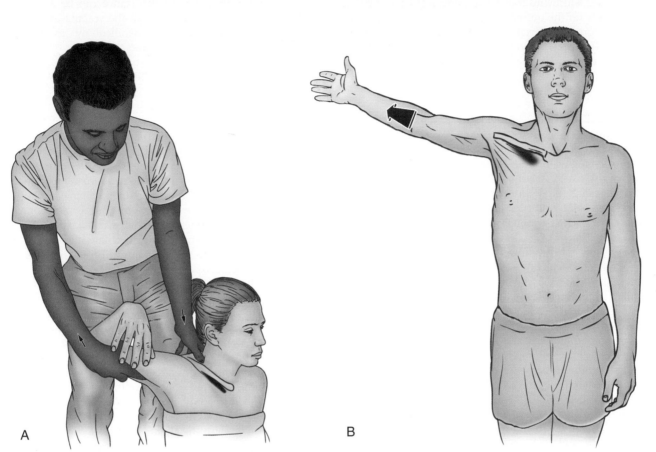

Figure 11-87 Stretching the right subclavius. **A,** Therapist-assisted stretch. The client's arm is abducted and extended back while the therapist stabilizes the client's first rib with the left thumb. **B,** Self-care stretch. The arm is abducted, laterally rotated, and extended back while the trunk remains facing forward.

11

Muscles of the Shoulder Girdle

The following whirlwind tour is an abbreviated set of palpation protocols for the muscles of this chapter. Once you have read and become comfortable with each of the protocols presented thus far, this whirlwind tour allows you to quickly and efficiently run through the palpations protocols for all the muscles of the chapter.

Client Prone

1. **Trapezius:** Begin with the client prone with the arm abducted to 90 degrees and resting on the table and the forearm hanging off the table; you are standing to the side of the client. Ask the client to abduct the arm at the glenohumeral (GH) joint with the forearm extended at the elbow joint, and to slightly retract the scapula at the scapulocostal (ScC) joint. First look for and then feel for the lateral border of the lower trapezius. Once felt, palpate the entirety of the lower trapezius while strumming perpendicular to its fibers as the client alternately contracts and relaxes the muscle. Next, palpate the middle trapezius while strumming perpendicular to its fibers as the client alternately contracts and relaxes the muscle. Then ask the client to slightly extend the head and upper neck at the spinal joints, and feel for the contraction of the upper trapezius. Once felt, palpate the entire upper trapezius while strumming perpendicular to its fibers as the client alternately contracts and relaxes the muscle.

2. **Rhomboids:** The client is prone and places the hand in the small of the back; you are standing to the side of the client. Ask the client to lift the hand up, away from the small of the back, and look for the rhomboids to contract and become visible (especially the lower border). Then palpate all of the rhomboids while strumming perpendicular to its fibers as the client alternately contracts and relaxes the muscle. Remember that the most superior aspect of the medial attachment is C7 at the base of the neck.

3. **Levator scapulae:** The client is prone with the hand in the small of the back; you are standing or seated to the side of the client. Ask the client to perform a gentle, very short range of motion of elevation of the scapula and feel for the contraction of the levator scapulae deep to the trapezius at the superior angle of the scapula. Once felt, strum perpendicular to the fibers, palpating the muscle superiorly as the client gently contracts and relaxes the muscle. Once you are palpating the levator scapulae in the posterior triangle, the hand does not need to be in the small of the back and the client can elevate the scapula more forcefully. Continue strumming perpendicularly with the client contracting and relaxing the muscle until you reach the transverse processes attachment. Remember that the transverse process of C1 is directly below the client's ear.

4. **Posterior deltoid:** The client is prone with the arm abducted to 90 degrees and resting on the table and the forearm hanging off the table; you are standing or seated to the side of the client. Ask the client to horizontally extend the arm at the GH joint, and feel for the contraction of the posterior deltoid. Resistance can be added. Once felt, palpate from the spine of the scapula to the deltoid tuberosity, strumming perpendicularly as the client alternately contracts and relaxes the muscle.

5. **Infraspinatus and teres minor:** To palpate the infraspinatus, have the client prone with the arm abducted to 90 degrees and resting on the table, and the forearm hanging off the table; you are seated to the side of the client with the client's forearm between your knees. Ask the client to laterally rotate the arm at the GH joint, and feel for the contraction of the infraspinatus immediately inferior to the spine of the scapula. Once felt, palpate the entire infraspinatus in the infraspinous fossa as the client alternately contracts and relaxes the muscle. Continue palpating it toward the greater tubercle attachment while strumming perpendicularly as the client contracts and relaxes it. To palpate the teres minor, ask the client to laterally rotate the arm at the GH joint, and palpate for the contraction of the teres minor at the superior aspect of the lateral border of the scapula. Once felt, palpate it toward the greater tubercle attachment while strumming perpendicularly as the client alternately contracts and relaxes it. Note: It can be challenging to locate the border between the infraspinatus and teres minor; however, it is easy to locate the border between the teres minor and the teres major by simply asking the client to alternately perform lateral rotation and medial rotation of the arm. (The teres minor contracts with lateral rotation; the teres major contracts with medial rotation.)

6. **Teres major:** The client is prone; you are seated to the side of the client with the client's forearm between your knees. Palpate as for the teres minor, except that the palpating fingers are placed at the inferior aspect of the lateral border of the scapula and the client is asked to medially rotate the arm at the GH joint. Once the contraction of the teres major is felt, continue palpating it toward the humeral attachment while strumming perpendicularly as the client alternately contracts and relaxes the muscle. To reach the attachment on the medial lip of the bicipital groove, it is necessary to palpate within the axillary region. Note: It can be challenging to discern the teres major from the latissimus dorsi.

7. **Supraspinatus:** The client is prone with the arm resting at the side of the body; you are seated to the side of the client. Ask the client to perform a very short range of motion of abduction of the arm (approximately 10 to 15 degrees) at the GH joint and feel for the contraction of the supraspinatus immediately superior to the spine of the scapula (gentle resistance can be given). Once felt, palpate the entire belly in the supraspinous fossa. To palpate the distal tendon, drop just off the acromion process of the scapula onto the distal tendon. (Draw an imaginary line along the spine of the scapula onto the humerus, and place your palpating fingers just anterior to that point on the humerus.) Strum perpendicular to the distal tendon, and feel for it deep to the deltoid; this may be done with the supraspinatus either relaxed or gently contracted.

11

Muscles of the Shoulder Girdle—*cont'd*

Client Supine

8. **Anterior deltoid:** The client is supine; you are seated at the head of the table. Ask the client to lift the arm at the GH joint halfway between flexion and abduction, and feel for the contraction of the anterior deltoid; resistance can be added if needed. Once felt, palpate the anterior deltoid from the lateral clavicle to the deltoid tuberosity while strumming perpendicular to the fibers as the client alternately contracts and relaxes the muscle.

9. **Subscapularis:** Have the client supine with the arm resting on the trunk and the other side hand gently holding the elbow of the upper extremity on the side being palpated; you are seated to the side of the client. Using your support hand under the client's body, passively protract the client's scapula; ask the client to take in a deep breath and slowly but firmly palpate into the subscapularis as the client slowly exhales. Be sure to press your finger pads against the anterior surface of the client's scapula. To verify that you are palpating the client's subscapularis, ask the client to medially rotate the arm at the GH joint and feel for the muscle's contraction. Palpate as much of the subscapularis as possible by pressing deeper toward the medial border of the scapula. Note: To follow the subscapularis all the way to the lesser tubercle of the humerus, rest the client's arm up in the air (in a position of flexion) against your body and follow the subscapularis toward the humerus as the client alternately contracts and relaxes the muscle. To feel the lesser tubercle attachment, be sure that the muscle is relaxed.

10. **Serratus anterior:** Have the client supine with the arm straight up in the air, pointed toward the ceiling; you are seated to the side of the client. Ask the client to reach toward the ceiling as you palpate against the lateral rib cage wall. If desired, resistance can be given with your support hand. Continue palpating as much of the serratus anterior as possible (including palpating deep to the pectoralis major).

11. **Pectoralis major:** Have the client supine with the arm resting at their side; you are seated to the side of the client. For the sternocostal head, palpate the lower aspect of the axillary fold of tissue as you resist adduction of the client's arm at the GH joint. Palpate the entire sternocostal head while strumming perpendicular to the fibers. For the clavicular head, palpate just inferior to the medial aspect of the clavicle as the client moves the arm at the GH joint obliquely between flexion and adduction. Resistance can be added if desired. Palpate the entire clavicular head while strumming perpendicular to the fibers.

12. **Pectoralis minor:** Have the client supine with the hand under the body in the small of the back; you are seated at the head of the table. Palpate for the contraction of the pectoralis minor just inferior to the coracoid process of the scapula as the client presses the hand and forearm down against the table. Once felt, palpate all three slips of the pectoralis minor to the rib attachments while strumming perpendicular to the fibers as the client alternately contracts and relaxes the muscle.

13. **Subclavius:** Have the client supine with the arm medially rotated and resting at the side of the body; you are seated at the head of the table. Curl your palpating fingers around the clavicle so that your finger pads are on its inferior surface. With the muscle relaxed, feel for the subclavius on the inferior surface of the clavicle. To feel the subclavius while contracting, palpate the muscle while asking the client to depress the shoulder girdle.

11

Review Questions

1. List the actions of the three parts of the trapezius.
2. List the actions of the pectoralis major.
3. What are the attachments of the subscapularis?
4. What are the attachments of the levator scapulae?
5. When palpating the belly of the supraspinatus, what muscle might make palpation difficult? How can this difficulty be negated?
6. When palpating the trapezius, what position should the client be in to engage the entire muscle?
7. When palpating the rhomboids, what is the proper seated positioning and motion to engage the muscle?
8. What is the rationale for placing the hand in the small of the back to palpate the levator scapulae?
9. When palpating the teres minor's inferior border, what other muscle needs to be distinguished? How is this accomplished?
10. What difficulty might a therapist encounter when discerning between the bellies of the teres major and latissimus dorsi?
11. What two ways can the anterior deltoid be engaged while supine?
12. Referral patterns for TrPs in the subclavius must be distinguished from TrP referral patterns in what other muscles? List three.
13. Angina pectoris, rib fracture, and costochondritis are common incorrect assessments for TrPs in what muscle?
14. In what position should the client be placed to fully stretch the right upper trapezius?
15. Describe the method of self-stretching for the infraspinatus and teres minor.
16. What difference, if any, is there between stretching the levator scapulae versus stretching the upper trapezius?
17. Why is it not advantageous to use lateral rotation of the arm at the glenohumeral joint to engage the posterior deltoid during palpation?

11

CASE STUDY

A 21-year-old male arrives for a massage therapy session complaining of pain and stiffness in the right shoulder joint and posterior right neck. The client is a right-handed pitcher on a local university baseball team who was referred for massage therapy by the team's athletic trainer after a decrease in performance over the last 3 weeks was noticed. The client is otherwise healthy with no prior history of injury to his shoulder or neck.

He states that the shoulder pain is located anterior to the shoulder joint with radiation down into the anterior arm and wrapping around to the posterior shoulder with a pain level of three out of ten at rest and rising to seven out of ten during activity. The neck pain is only present during active left rotation of the neck (especially during the preparation stage of pitching) with a pain level of five out of ten. He describes both issues as having a gradual onset with simple stiffness at first but becoming painful beginning approximately 3 weeks ago. For self-care, he has been applying ice as needed and taking 400 mg of ibuprofen every 6-8 hours for the last 2 weeks. The pain has been disruptive enough for him to miss practice and games for the past week.

The physical exam reveals limited left cervical passive and active rotations producing pain at end ranges of motion. Right shoulder joint extension is limited to 20 degrees before onset of pain. Manual resistance to medial and lateral rotation of the right shoulder joint reveal reduced muscle strength. Palpatory assessment shows tightness and spasms in the right pectoralis major, pectoralis minor, anterior deltoid, posterior deltoid, biceps brachii, upper trapezius, and levator scapulae.

1. What further assessments, if any, should be performed? Are there any other questions that could be asked?
2. What treatment plan would you recommend?
3. What self-care activities would you suggest?

CHAPTER 12

Tour #2   **Palpation of the Neck Muscles**

Overview

This chapter is a palpation tour of the muscles of the neck. The tour begins with anterior neck muscles and then moves to the posterior muscles of the neck. Palpation of anterior neck muscles is shown in the supine position. Palpation of most of the posterior neck muscles is shown with the client seated; a few are shown with the client supine. Alternate palpation positions are also described. The major muscles or muscle groups of the region are each given a separate layout; there are also a number of detours to other muscles of the region. Trigger point (TrP) information and stretching, both therapist-assisted and self-care stretching, are given for each of the major muscles covered in this chapter. The chapter closes with an advanced *Whirlwind Tour* that explains the sequential palpation of all of the muscles of the chapter.

Chapter Outline

Sternocleidomastoid (SCM)—Supine
    Detour to the Platysma
Scalene Group—Supine
    Detour to the Omohyoid Inferior Belly
Longus Colli and Longus Capitis—Supine
    Detour to the Rectus Capitis Anterior and Lateralis
Hyoid Group—Supine
Upper Trapezius—Seated
Levator Scapulae—Seated
Splenius Capitis—Seated
    Detour to the Splenius Cervicis
Semispinalis Capitis—Supine
    Detour to the Longissimus Capitis, Semispinalis Cervicis, and Cervical Multifidus
Suboccipital Group—Supine

Chapter Objectives

After completing this chapter, the student/therapist should be able to perform the following for each of the muscles covered in this chapter:
1. State the attachments.
2. State the actions.
3. Describe the starting position for palpation.
4. Describe and explain the purpose of each of the palpation steps.
5. Palpate each muscle.
6. State the "Palpation Key."
7. Describe alternate palpation positions.
8. State the locations of the most common TrP(s).
9. Describe the TrP referral zones.
10. State the most common factors that create and/or perpetuate TrPs.
11. State the symptoms most commonly caused by TrPs.
12. Describe and perform the therapist-assisted and self-care stretches.

e Go to http://evolve.elsevier.com/Muscolino/palpation for video demonstrations of the muscle palpations presented in this chapter.

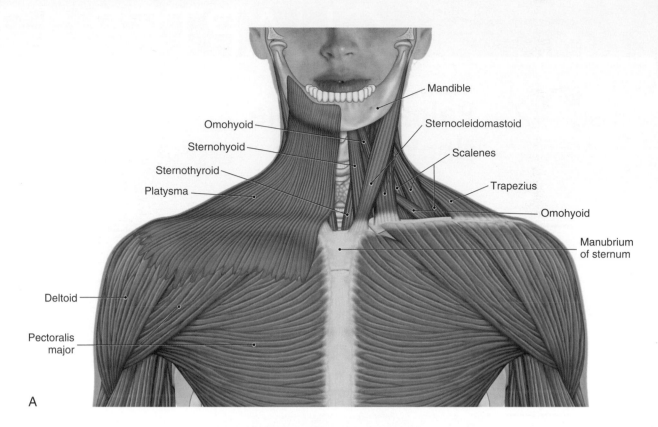

A

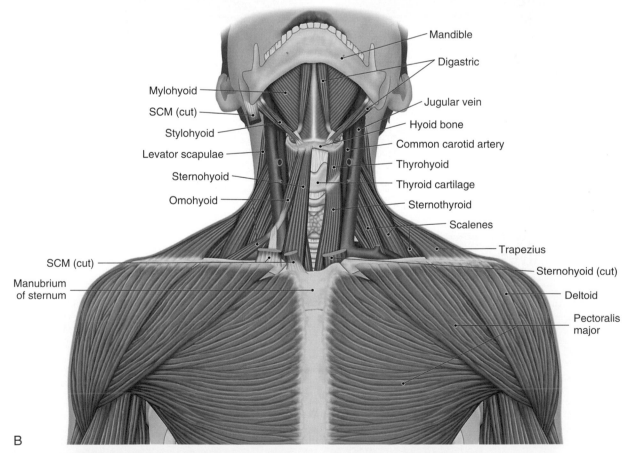

B

Figure 12-1 Anterior views of the neck and upper chest region. **A,** Superficial views; the platysma has been removed on the left side. Note: The *posterior triangle of the neck* is located between the upper trapezius, sternocleidomastoid, and the clavicle. **B,** Intermediate views; the SCM has been cut on the right side; the SCM and omohyoid have been removed, and the sternohyoid has been cut on the left side.

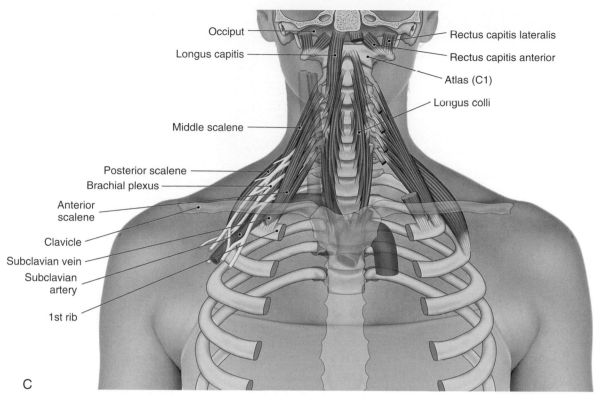

Occiput

Longus capitis

Middle scalene

Posterior scalene

Brachial plexus

Anterior scalene

Clavicle

Subclavian vein

Subclavian artery

1st rib

Rectus capitis lateralis

Rectus capitis anterior

Atlas (C1)

Longus colli

C

Figure 12-1, cont'd C, Deep views; the anterior scalene and longus capitis, as well as the brachial plexus of nerves and subclavian artery and vein, have been cut and/or removed on the left side.

12

12

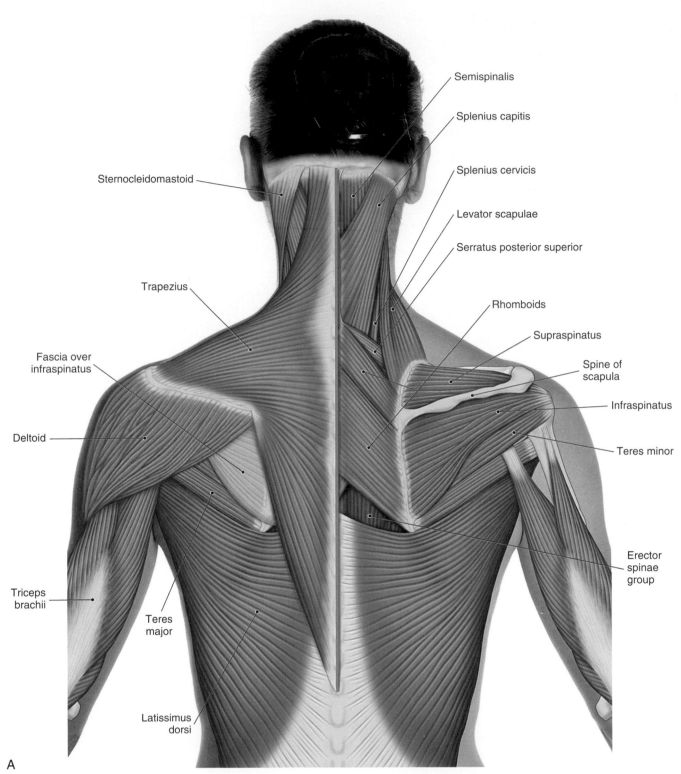

Semispinalis

Splenius capitis

Splenius cervicis

Sternocleidomastoid

Levator scapulae

Serratus posterior superior

Trapezius

Rhomboids

Supraspinatus

Fascia over infraspinatus

Spine of scapula

Infraspinatus

Deltoid

Teres minor

Erector spinae group

Triceps brachii

Teres major

Latissimus dorsi

A

Figure 12-2 Posterior views of the neck and upper back region. **A,** Superficial views; the trapezius, sternocleidomastoid (SCM), and deltoid have been removed on the right side.

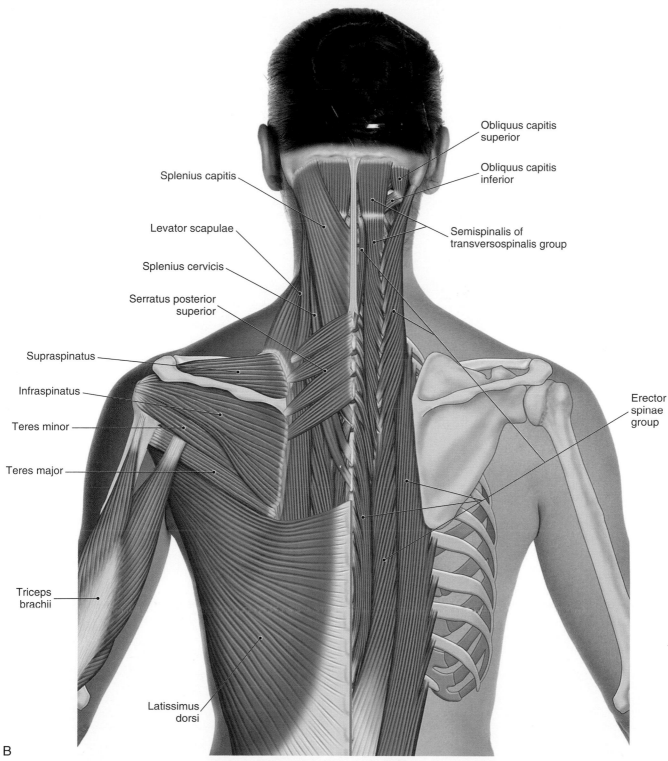

Figure 12-2, cont'd B, Intermediate views; the serratus posterior superior, splenius capitis and cervicis, levator scapulae, supraspinatus, infraspinatus, teres minor and major, and triceps brachii have been removed on the right side.

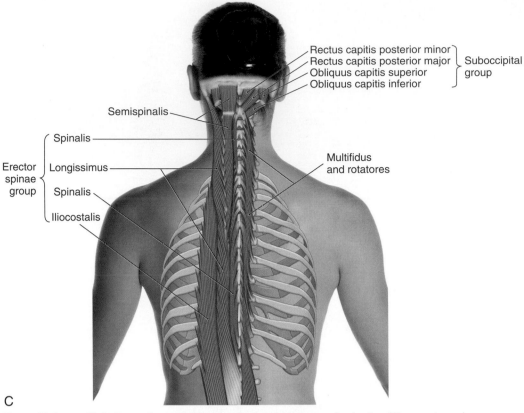

C

Figure 12-2, cont'd C, Deep views; the iliocostalis, longissimus, and spinalis of the erector spinae group and the semispinalis of the transversospinalis group have been removed on the right side.

12

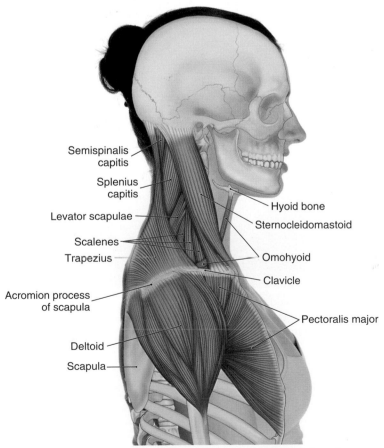

Figure 12-3 Right lateral view of the muscles of the neck region.

STERNOCLEIDOMASTOID (SCM)—SUPINE

☑ ATTACHMENTS

☐ Manubrium of the sternum and the medial ⅓ of the clavicle

to the

☐ mastoid process of the temporal bone and the lateral ½ of the superior nuchal line of the occiput

☑ ACTIONS

☐ Flexes the lower neck at the spinal joints
☐ Extends the head and upper neck at the spinal joints
☐ Laterally flexes the head and neck at the spinal joints
☐ Contralaterally rotates the head and neck at the spinal joints
☐ Elevates the sternum and clavicle

Starting Position (Figure 12-5)

■ Client supine with the head and neck contralaterally rotated
■ Therapist seated at the head of the table
■ Palpating hand placed just superior to the sternoclavicular joint

Palpation Steps

1. Ask the client to lift the head and neck from the table, and look for the sternocleidomastoid (SCM) to become visible (Figure 12-6).
2. Although resistance could be added by the support hand, it is often unnecessary because lifting the head and neck against gravity usually provides sufficient resistance.
3. Palpate toward the superior attachment while strumming perpendicular to the fibers.
4. Once the SCM has been located, have the client relax it and palpate to assess its baseline tone.

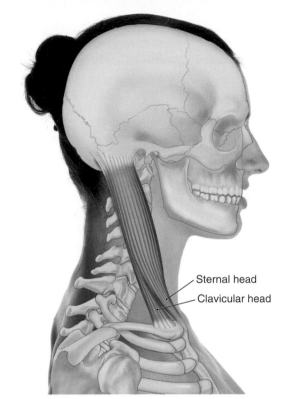

Figure 12-4 Lateral view of the right sternocleidomastoid (SCM).

Sternal head
Clavicular head

12

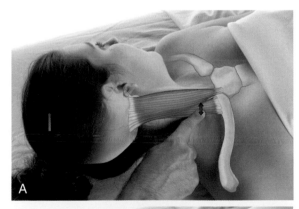

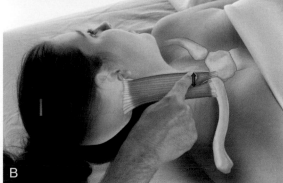

Figure 12-6 Supine palpation of the right sternocleidomastoid (SCM) as the client raises the head and neck from the table. **A,** Palpation of the clavicular head. **B,** Palpation of the sternal head.

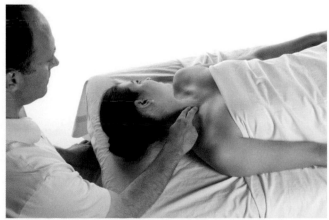

Figure 12-5 Starting position for supine palpation of the right sternocleidomastoid (SCM).

STERNOCLEIDOMASTOID (SCM)—SUPINE—*cont'd*

PALPATION NOTES

1. The sternal head of the SCM is usually much more visible than the clavicular head. If the clavicular head is not visible, palpate for it just lateral to the inferior aspect of the sternal head. Note: Although it is common to have a small gap between the sternal and clavicular heads, some people have a large gap and other people have no gap at all.
2. Palpation of the SCM must be done somewhat carefully, because the carotid sinus of the common carotid artery lies deep to the SCM (see Figure 12-1, *B*), and pressure against the carotid sinus can create a reflex that lowers blood pressure. For this reason, pincer palpation is often recommended for palpating the SCM, rather than flat palpation.
3. The SCM forms the anterior border of the posterior triangle of the neck, and is an excellent landmark for locating the scalenes. It also forms the posterior border of the anterior triangle of the neck, and is an excellent landmark for locating the longus colli and longus capitis muscles.

Palpation Key:
Turn to the opposite side and lift the head.

Alternate Palpation Position—Seated

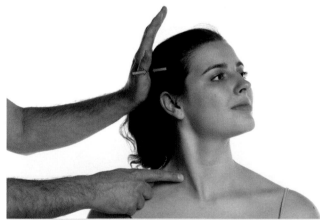

Figure 12-7 The sternocleidomastoid (SCM) can be easily palpated with the client seated. Ask the client to rotate the head and neck to the opposite side (contralaterally rotate) and slightly laterally flex to the same side; then resist any further lateral flexion to the same side. The sternal head often becomes visible with contralateral rotation. Resistance to same side lateral flexion usually brings out the clavicular head (indicated). If the clavicular head is not visible, try increasing the resistance to lateral flexion.

TRIGGER POINTS

1. Trigger points (TrPs) in the sternocleidomastoid (SCM) often result from or are perpetuated by acute or chronic overuse of the muscle (e.g., chronic postures of sitting with the head turned to one side or looking upward to paint a ceiling, a chronic cough using the muscle for its respiratory function), chronic postures that result in shortening of the muscle (e.g., having a protracted head posture, looking downward to read a book in the lap by flexing the lower cervical spine, sleeping with a pillow that is too thick), irritation from wearing a tie or a shirt with a tight collar, or trauma (e.g., whiplash, fall).
2. TrPs in the SCM tend to produce headaches, altered posture of ipsilateral lateral flexion of the head and neck, restricted range of motion of the neck and head, a sore throat, autonomic nervous system symptoms (sternal head: eye symptoms, such as ptosis of the upper eyelid, loss of visual acuity, and excessive tear formation; clavicular head: localized vasoconstriction and increased sweating), proprioceptive symptoms (sternal head: dizziness, vertigo, nausea, and ataxia; clavicular head: hearing loss), and even entrapment of cranial nerve XI (spinal accessory nerve).
3. The referral patterns of SCM TrPs must be distinguished from the referral patterns of TrPs in the trapezius, semispinalis capitis, suboccipitals, temporalis, masseter, digastric (due to pain referral and possible throat symptoms), lateral and medial pterygoids, occipitofrontalis, platysma, longus colli and capitis (due to possible throat symptoms), and some muscles of facial expression.
4. TrPs in the SCM are often incorrectly assessed as swollen lymph nodes, sinus or migraine headaches, osteoarthritis of the sternoclavicular joint, trigeminal neuralgia, tic douloureux, or neurogenic spasmodic torticollis.
5. Associated TrPs often occur in the scalenes, platysma, levator scapulae, trapezius, splenius capitis and cervicis, semispinalis capitis, temporalis, masseter, digastric, and contralateral SCM.
6. The referral pain of SCM TrPs can cross over to the other side of the body.

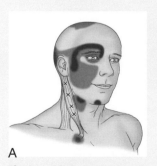
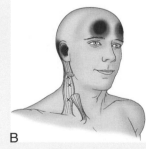

A   B

Figure 12-8 Anterolateral views illustrating common sternocleidomastoid (SCM) trigger points (TrPs) and their corresponding referral zones. **A,** Sternal head. **B,** Clavicular head.

STERNOCLEIDOMASTOID (SCM)—SUPINE—*cont'd*

STRETCHING THE STERNOCLEIDOMASTOID

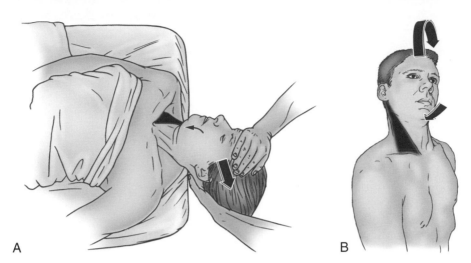

A   B

Figure 12-9 Stretching the right sternocleidomastoid (SCM). The client's head and neck are left laterally flexed and rotated to the right, and the lower neck is extended but the chin is tucked (to flex the head). **A,** Therapist-assisted stretch. Note: Caution is advised whenever bringing the client's head down into extension. **B,** Self-care stretch.

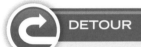 **DETOUR**

Platysma:

The platysma is a very thin superficial sheet of muscle that attaches from the subcutaneous fascia of the superior chest to the mandible and subcutaneous fascia of the lower face (Figure 12-10, *A*). When it contracts, it creates wrinkles in the skin of the neck. It can be engaged by asking the client to forcefully depress and draw the lower lip laterally while keeping the mandible in a position of slight depression (see Figure 12-10, *B*).

Trigger Points

1. Trigger points (TrPs) in the platysma (Figure 12-10, *C*) often result from or are perpetuated by acute or chronic overuse of the muscle (e.g., habitual expression of disgust or horror) and TrPs in the SCM and scalene muscles.
2. TrPs in the platysma tend to produce prickly pain over the mandible.
3. The referral patterns of platysma TrPs must be distinguished from the referral patterns of TrPs in the SCM, masseter, temporalis, and medial pterygoid.
4. TrPs in the platysma are often incorrectly assessed as temporomandibular joint (TMJ) dysfunction.
5. Associated TrPs often occur in other muscles of facial expression.
6. Note: TrPs in the platysma are usually located over the SCM.

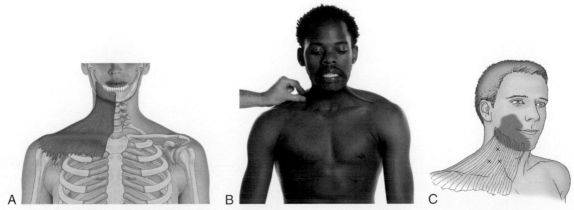

A   B   C

Figure 12-10 Views of the platysma. **A,** Anterior view of the right platysma. **B,** Anterior view of the platysma contracted and being palpated. **C,** Anterolateral view illustrating common platysma trigger points (TrPs) and their corresponding referral zone.

SCALENE GROUP—SUPINE

✅ ATTACHMENTS

Anterior Scalene
- ☐ First rib

  to the

- ☐ transverse processes of C3-C6

Middle Scalene
- ☐ First rib

  to the

- ☐ transverse processes of C2-C7

Posterior Scalene
- ☐ Second rib

  to the

- ☐ transverse processes of C5-C7

✅ ACTIONS

Anterior Scalene
- ☐ Flexes the neck at the spinal joints
- ☐ Laterally flexes the neck at the spinal joints
- ☐ Contralaterally rotates the neck at the spinal joints
- ☐ Elevates the first rib at the sternocostal and costovertebral joints

Middle Scalene
- ☐ Flexes the neck at the spinal joints
- ☐ Laterally flexes the neck at the spinal joints
- ☐ Elevates the first rib at the sternocostal and costovertebral joints

Posterior Scalene
- ☐ Laterally flexes the neck at the spinal joints
- ☐ Elevates the second rib at the sternocostal and costovertebral joints

Starting Position (Figure 12-12)
- ■ Client supine
- ■ Therapist seated at the head of the table
- ■ Palpating hand placed in the posterior triangle of the neck, just superior to the clavicle and just lateral to the inferior aspect of the lateral border of the clavicular head of the sternocleidomastoid (SCM)

Palpation Steps
1. Begin by locating the lateral border of the clavicular head of the SCM muscle (see Figure 12-6, *A*); then drop immediately off it laterally onto the scalenes in the posterior triangle of the neck.
2. With your finger pads pressing into the scalene muscle group, ask the client to take in short, quick breaths through the nose and feel for the contraction of the scalene musculature (Figure 12-13).
3. Palpate as much of the scalenes in the posterior triangle of the neck between the SCM, upper trapezius, levator scapulae, and clavicle as possible. To best palpate the scalenes, remember to strum perpendicular to the fiber direction of the muscles.
4. Once the scalenes have been located, have the client relax them and palpate to assess their baseline tone.

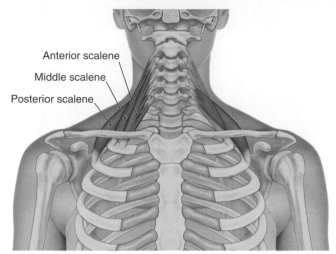

Figure 12-12 Anterior view of the scalenes. All three scalenes are seen on the right; the posterior scalene and ghosted-in middle scalene are seen on the left.

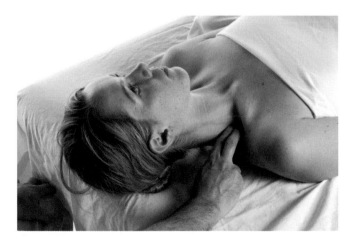

Figure 12-12 Starting position for supine palpation of the right scalenes, lateral to the lateral border of the clavicular head of the sternocleidomastoid (SCM).

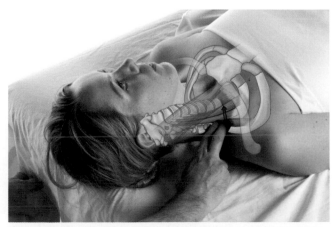

Figure 12-13 Palpation of the right scalenes as the client takes in short, quick breaths through the nose.

12

SCALENE GROUP—SUPINE—*cont'd*

PALPATION NOTES

1. Taking in short, quick breaths requires the scalenes to contract to elevate the first and second ribs to expand the ribcage for inhalation.

2. It can be challenging to discern the anterior, middle, and posterior scalenes from each other. Knowing their location and the direction of their fibers helps. Much of the anterior scalene is deep to the SCM and its fibers are directed toward C3-C6. The middle scalene is located just lateral to the anterior scalene and has the greatest presence in the posterior triangle of the neck; its fibers are directed toward C2-C7. There is usually a small palpable depression between the anterior and middle scalenes. The posterior scalene is the most difficult to palpate of the three, because it is mostly deep to other musculature. Feel for it just anterior to the upper trapezius and levator scapulae; its fibers are directed nearly horizontally toward C5-C7.

3. The scalene attachments on the transverse processes of the cervical spine can be palpated deep to the SCM if the SCM is first relaxed and slackened. To achieve this, passively move the client's head and neck into flexion and lateral flexion to the same side, and perhaps some contralateral rotation. Then slowly sink in deep to the SCM, pressing with your finger pads toward the transverse processes of the spine, and feel for the scalene attachments.

4. To better access the inferior attachments of the scalenes on the first and second ribs posterior to the clavicle, it can be helpful to slacken the soft tissue of the area by passively bringing the client's neck into flexion and lateral flexion to the side that is being palpated. This usually affords more space for the palpating fingers to reach down behind the clavicle toward the first and second ribs.

5. Palpation of the scalenes must be done carefully because the brachial plexus of nerves and the subclavian artery are located between the anterior and middle scalenes (see Figure 12-1, *C*).

Alternate Palpation Position—Seated

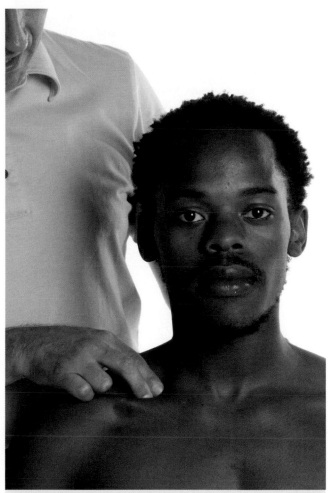

Figure 12-14 The scalenes can be easily palpated with the client seated. Locate the lateral border of the clavicular head of the sternocleidomastoid (SCM); then drop off it onto the scalenes and follow the supine scalene palpation directions.

12

Palpation Key:
Drop laterally off the SCM and have the client take in short, quick breaths through the nose.

SCALENE GROUP—SUPINE—*cont'd*

TRIGGER POINTS

1. Trigger points (TrPs) in the scalenes often result from or are perpetuated by acute or chronic overuse of the muscles (e.g., coughing, labored breathing, especially due to chronic obstructive respiratory disease) or motor vehicle accidents.

2. TrPs in the scalenes tend to produce thoracic outlet syndrome (especially anterior scalene syndrome but also may contribute to costoclavicular syndrome, causing neurologic or vascular symptoms in the upper extremity), restricted lateral flexion and/or ipsilateral rotation of the neck, entrapment of nerve roots that contribute to the long thoracic nerve (that innervates the serratus anterior muscle), joint dysfunction of the first or second ribs, or painful sleeping.

3. The referral patterns of scalene TrPs must be distinguished from the referral patterns of TrPs in the levator scapulae, rhomboids, serratus posterior superior, subclavius, supraspinatus, infraspinatus, teres minor, subscapularis, latissimus dorsi, teres major, deltoid, coracobrachialis, biceps brachii, brachialis, triceps brachii, extensor carpi radialis brevis, extensor indicis, and supinator.

4. TrPs in the scalenes are often incorrectly assessed as cervical disc syndrome, cervical spine joint dysfunction, angina (from left-sided TrPs), costoclavicular syndrome, pectoralis minor syndrome, or carpal tunnel syndrome.

5. Associated TrPs often occur in the SCM, upper trapezius, splenius capitis, pectoralis major, pectoralis minor, deltoid, triceps brachii, posterior forearm extensor muscles, and brachialis.

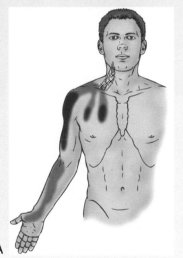 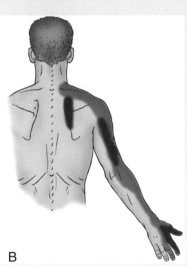

A   B

Figure 12-15 A, Anterior view illustrating common scalene trigger points (TrPs) and their corresponding referral zone. **B,** Posterior view showing the remainder of the referral zone.

SCALENE GROUP—SUPINE—*cont'd*

STRETCHING THE SCALENE GROUP

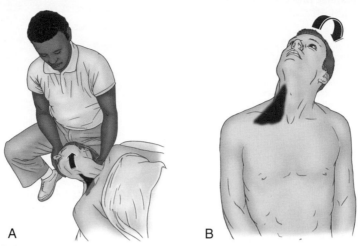

A   B

Figure 12-16 Stretching the right scalene group. The client's neck is extended, left laterally flexed, and rotated (ipsilaterally) to the right. **A,** Therapist-assisted stretch. Note: Caution is advised when bringing the client's head down into extension. **B,** Self-care stretch.

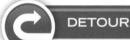

DETOUR

Omohyoid inferior belly:
The inferior belly of the omohyoid is fairly easily palpable in the posterior triangle of the neck. Palpate just lateral to the SCM and superior to the clavicle, feeling for the horizontal fibers of the omohyoid as the client depresses the mandible at the temporomandibular joints (TMJs) against resistance.

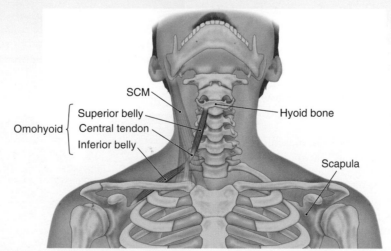

Figure 12-17 Anterior view of the right omohyoid. The sternocleidomastoid (SCM) has been ghosted in.

LONGUS COLLI AND LONGUS CAPITIS—SUPINE

☑ ATTACHMENTS

Longus Colli
☐ Between T3 and C1, from transverse processes and anterior surfaces of vertebral bodies inferiorly

to the

☐ transverse processes and anterior surfaces of vertebral bodies superiorly

Longus Capitis
☐ Transverse processes of C3-C5

to the

☐ occiput

☑ ACTIONS

Longus Colli
☐ Flexes the neck at the spinal joints
☐ Laterally flexes the neck at the spinal joints
☐ Contralaterally rotates the neck at the spinal joints

Longus Capitis
☐ Flexes the head and neck at the spinal joints
☐ Laterally flexes the head and neck at the spinal joints

Starting Position (Figure 12-19)
■ Client supine
■ Therapist seated at the head of the table
■ Place palpating hand just medial to the sternocleidomastoid (SCM) muscle
■ Place support hand on the client's forehead (if resistance will be added)

Palpation Steps
1. Begin by locating the medial border of the sternal head of the SCM muscle; then drop immediately off it medially onto the longus muscles in the anterior neck.
2. Gently and slowly but firmly sink in toward the anterior surface of the vertebral bodies of the cervical spine. Note: If you feel a pulse under your fingers, you are on the common carotid artery; either gently move it out of the way, or move your fingers slightly to one side of it or the other, continuing to aim for the longus muscles.
3. To confirm that you are on the longus musculature, ask the client to flex the head and neck at the spinal joints by lifting the head up from the table, and feel for their contraction (Figure 12-20). Note: Lifting the head and neck up into flexion against gravity usually creates a fairly strong contraction of the longus muscles. However, if necessary, resistance can be given with your support hand (as seen in Figure 12-21).
4. Once located, strum perpendicular to the fibers and palpate as far superiorly as possible and as far inferiorly as possible.
5. Once the longus muscles have been located, have the client relax them and palpate to assess their baseline tone.

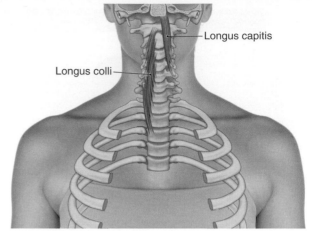

Figure 12-18 Anterior view of the longus colli and capitis. The longus colli is seen on the right; the longus capitis is seen on the left.

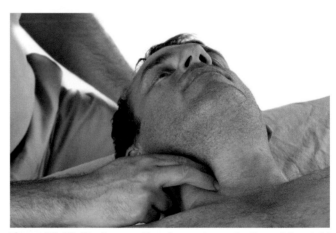

Figure 12-19 Starting position for supine palpation of the right longus colli and capitis.

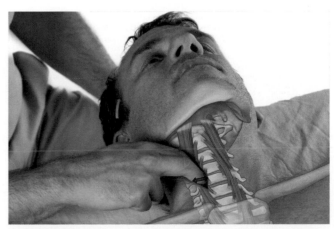

Figure 12-20 Palpation of the right longus colli and capitis as the client engages the muscles by lifting his head and neck into flexion.

LONGUS COLLI AND LONGUS CAPITIS—SUPINE—*cont'd*

PALPATION NOTES

1. The anterior neck has a number of fragile structures; therefore palpation into this region must be done carefully. When palpating, sink into the tissue slowly and gently, but with pressure that is firm enough to reach the longus musculature.
2. One precaution when palpating the longus musculature is the carotid sinus of the common carotid artery, located just lateral to the spine. Pressure against the carotid sinus can create a neurologic reflex that lowers blood pressure.
3. If the common carotid artery is blocking access to the longus musculature, one method to access the musculature is to gently displace the trachea toward the opposite side of the body, and then drop posteriorly down toward the longus muscles. Be careful to not exert excessive pressure against the trachea or you may cause the client to involuntarily cough.
4. Even though there are many fragile and sensitive structures in the anterior neck, palpation/treatment of the longus muscles should not be avoided, because it can be very beneficial for the client.
5. If you find it difficult to discern the longus musculature from the SCM, ask the person to rotate the head and neck to the same side as where you are palpating; this will inhibit and relax the SCM.
6. The longus musculature of the spine is often injured in whiplash accidents.

Alternate Palpation Position—Seated

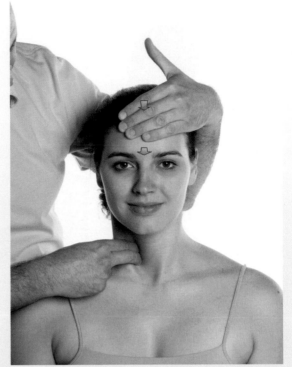

Figure 12-21 The longus muscles can be easily palpated with the client seated. Follow the supine directions; the only difference in this position is that it is necessary to resist flexion of the client's head and neck with your support hand to make the longus musculature contract (because flexion of the head and neck is not against gravity when seated).

TRIGGER POINTS

1. Trigger points (TrPs) in the longus muscles often result from or are perpetuated by acute or chronic overuse of the muscle, and trauma such as whiplash.
2. TrPs in the longus muscles tend to produce a sore throat, difficulty swallowing, and tight posterior neck muscles (working harder to oppose the tension of tight longus muscles).
3. The referral patterns of longus muscle TrPs must be distinguished from the referral patterns of TrPs in the anterior belly of the digastric and the SCM (due to the possible throat symptoms).
4. TrPs in the longus muscles are often incorrectly assessed as a sore throat.
5. Associated TrPs often occur in the posterior cervical muscles (e.g., upper trapezius, semispinalis capitis).
6. Note: Referral pain patterns for the longus colli and capitis have not been well mapped out.

LONGUS COLLI AND LONGUS CAPITIS—SUPINE—*cont'd*

STRETCHING THE LONGUS COLLI AND CAPITIS

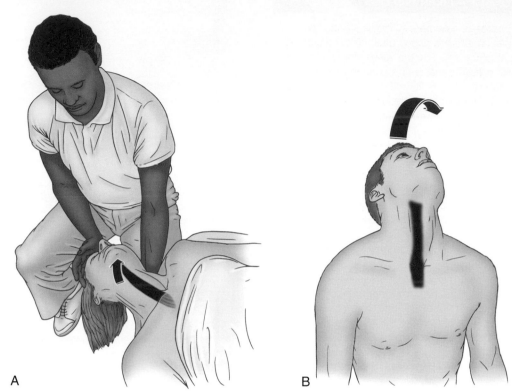

A   B

Figure 12-22 Stretching the right longus colli and capitis muscles. The client's head and neck are extended and laterally flexed to the opposite (left) side. **A,** Therapist-assisted stretch. Note: Caution is advised whenever bringing the client's head down into extension. **B,** Self-care stretch.

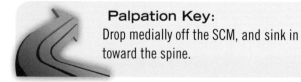

Palpation Key:
Drop medially off the SCM, and sink in toward the spine.

LONGUS COLLI AND LONGUS CAPITIS—SUPINE—*cont'd*

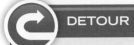
DETOUR

Rectus capitis anterior and lateralis:
The rectus capitis anterior attaches from the occiput to the transverse process of the atlas (C1) and is extremely deep and usually not palpable; its action is flexion of the head at the atlanto-occipital joint. The rectus capitis lateralis also attaches from the occiput to the transverse process of the atlas and is also located quite deep, but can sometimes be palpated; its action is lateral flexion of the head at the atlanto-occipital joint. To palpate the rectus capitis lateralis in the anterolateral neck, have the client supine or seated and palpate immediately superior to the transverse process

of the atlas (Note: The location of the transverse process of the atlas is often mistaken; it is located immediately posterior to the ramus of the mandible and inferior to the ear, between the atlas and the occiput.) Press gently into the small depression that can often be felt here and feel for the rectus capitis lateralis (Figure 12-24); it can be very difficult to discern this muscle from adjacent soft tissue. Notes: 1) Due to the presence of the facial nerve and styloid process located nearby, be careful to not press too forcefully. 2) Trigger point (TrP) pain referral zones for the rectus capitis anterior and lateralis have not been mapped out.

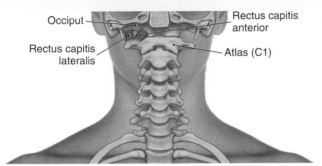

Figure 12-23 Anterior view of the right rectus capitis anterior and rectus capitis lateralis.

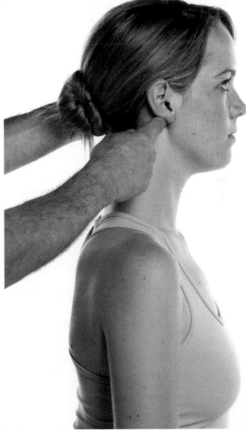

Figure 12-24 Palpation of the right rectus capitis lateralis superior to the transverse process of the atlas.

12

HYOID GROUP—SUPINE

☑ ATTACHMENTS

Infrahyoids
☐ Sternohyoid: Sternum

  to the

☐ hyoid
☐ Sternothyroid: Sternum

  to the

☐ thyroid cartilage
☐ Thyrohyoid: Thyroid cartilage

  to the

☐ hyoid
☐ Omohyoid: Superior border of the scapula

  to the

☐ hyoid (with a central tendon attached to the clavicle)

Suprahyoids
☐ Digastric: Mastoid notch of the temporal bone

  to the

☐ mandible (with a central tendon attached to the hyoid)
☐ Stylohyoid: Styloid process of the temporal bone

  to the

☐ hyoid
☐ Mylohyoid: Hyoid

  to the

☐ inner surface of the mandible
☐ Geniohyoid: Hyoid *to the* inner surface of the mandible

  to the

☐ inner surface of the mandible

☑ ACTIONS

Hyoid Muscle Group
☐ Depresses the mandible at the temporomandibular joints (TMJs)
☐ Flexes the head and neck at the spinal joints
☐ Infrahyoids also depress the hyoid bone
☐ Suprahyoids also elevate the hyoid bone

Starting Position (Figure 12-26)
■ Client supine
■ Therapist seated at the head of the table
■ Palpating hand placed immediately inferior to the hyoid, just off center
■ Support hand placed under the client's chin

Palpation Steps
1. Begin palpating the infrahyoid muscle group by asking the client to depress the mandible at the TMJs while providing resistance with your support hand, and feel for the contraction of the infrahyoid muscles while strumming perpendicular to their fibers (Figure 12-27, *A*).
2. Continue palpating them inferiorly toward the sternum (strumming perpendicular to their fibers).
3. To palpate the suprahyoid muscle group, place your palpating hand just inferior to the mandible; add resistance to prevent the client from depressing the mandible at the TMJs, and feel for the contraction of the suprahyoid muscles (see Figure 12-27, *B*).
4. Continue palpating them toward the hyoid bone while resisting mandibular depression while strumming perpendicular to their fibers.
5. To palpate the stylohyoid and the posterior belly of the digastric of the suprahyoid group, continue palpating laterally from the hyoid toward the mastoid process of the temporal bone while resisting mandibular depression and strumming perpendicular to the fibers (see Figure 12-27, *C*).
6. Once the hyoid muscles have been located, have the client relax them and palpate to assess their baseline tone.

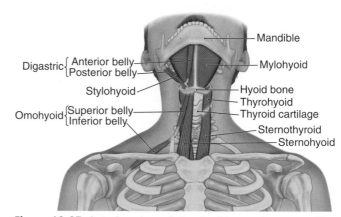

Figure 12-25 Anterior view of the hyoid muscle group. The sternohyoid, omohyoid, stylohyoid, and digastric have been removed on the left. The geniohyoid is not seen.

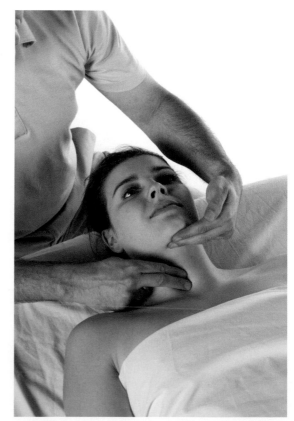

Figure 12-26 Starting position for supine palpation of the right hyoid muscles.

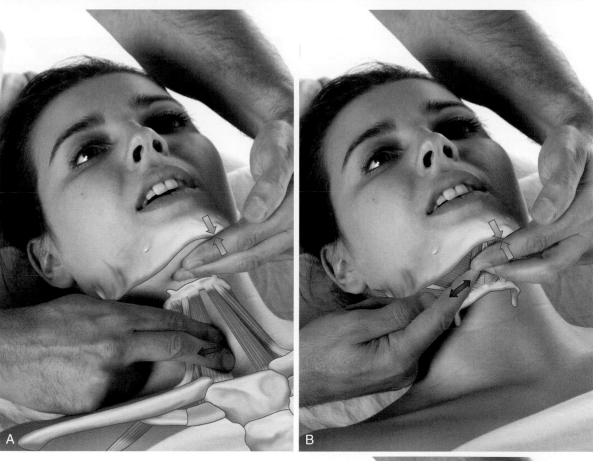

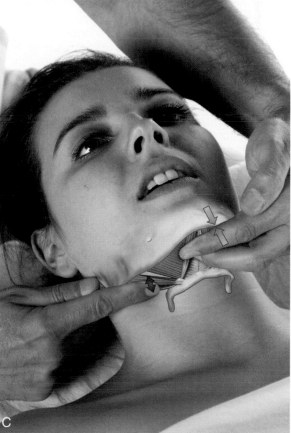

Figure 12-27 Palpation of the right hyoid muscles as the client depresses the mandible against resistance. **A,** Palpation of the right infrahyoids. **B,** Palpation of the right suprahyoids. **C,** Palpation of the right stylohyoid and posterior belly of digastric (of the suprahyoid group).

12

HYOID GROUP—SUPINE—*cont'd*

Alternate Palpation Position

The hyoid muscles can be easily palpated with the client seated.

Palpation Key:
Resist depression of the mandible.

PALPATION NOTES

1. When depression of the mandible is resisted, all hyoid muscles, except the stylohyoid, contract. The digastric, mylohyoid, and geniohyoid contract as movers to depress the mandible at the TMJs. The other hyoid muscles contract to stabilize the hyoid, providing a firm base from which the digastric, mylohyoid, and geniohyoid can pull upon the mandible.
2. If the hyoids contract as a group and the mandible is fixed to the temporal bone (by contraction of elevators of the mandible, such as the temporalis and/or masseter), the hyoids will exert their pull upon the head and cause flexion of the head and neck at the spinal joints.
3. Most of the hyoid muscles are small thin muscles and can be challenging to discern from each other.

TRIGGER POINTS

Of all the hyoid muscles, the referral patterns for the digastric have been best mapped out. Each belly of the digastric has its own typical referral pattern.

1. Trigger points (TrPs) in the digastric often result from or are perpetuated by acute or chronic overuse of the muscle (e.g., having an open-mouthed posture, which is especially common for individuals who habitually breath through their mouth, perhaps because of nasal congestion; excessive tone to oppose tight elevators of the mandible, such as the temporalis, masseter, and medial pterygoid), protracted head posture (which causes a chronic pulling on all the hyoid muscles), or trauma, such as whiplash.
2. TrPs in the anterior belly of the digastric tend to produce pain in the four lower incisor teeth (two on the same side as the TrP and two on the other side), tongue pain, throat discomfort, or difficulty swallowing. TrPs in the posterior belly of the digastric tend to produce TrPs in the occipitofrontalis.
3. The referral patterns of digastric TrPs must be distinguished from the referral patterns of TrPs in the other hyoid muscles, SCM, upper trapezius, medial pterygoid, longus colli and

capitis (because of possible throat symptoms), and the suboccipitals.
4. TrPs in the digastric are often incorrectly assessed as dental conditions of the affected teeth (e.g., cavities) or tight SCM musculature.
5. Associated TrPs often occur in the ipsilateral occipitofrontalis or SCM. They also often occur ipsilaterally or contralaterally in other hyoid muscles and the masseter, temporalis, or medial pterygoid.
6. Notes: 1) The stylohyoid lies next to the posterior belly of the digastric, is difficult to discern from the digastric, and is assumed to have a similar referral pattern to the posterior digastric. Furthermore, the stylohyoid has been known to cause entrapment of the external carotid artery. 2) TrPs in the omohyoid are thought to create tension in the muscle that can press on the brachial plexus of nerves (causing thoracic outlet syndrome) and can contribute via its fascial attachments to dysfunction of the costospinal joints of the first rib. 3) Similar to the anterior belly of the digastric, the mylohyoid has also been reported to refer pain to the tongue.

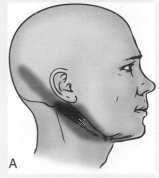
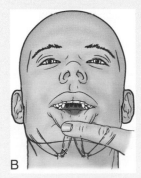

Figure 12-28 Common digastric trigger points (TrPs) and their corresponding referral zones. **A,** Lateral view. **B,** Anterior view.

HYOID GROUP—SUPINE—*cont'd*

STRETCHING THE HYOID GROUP

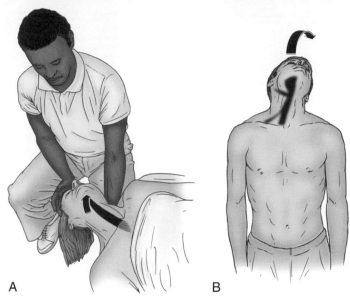

A   B

Figure 12-29 Stretching the right hyoids. The client's neck is extended and left laterally flexed. **A,** Therapist-assisted stretch. Note: Caution is advised whenever bringing the client's head down into extension. **B,** Self-care stretch.

UPPER TRAPEZIUS—SEATED

☑ ATTACHMENTS

☐ External occipital protuberance and medial ⅓ of the superior nuchal line of the occiput, entire nuchal ligament, and the spinous process of C7

   to the

☐ lateral clavicle and the acromion process of the scapula

☑ ACTIONS

☐ Elevates the scapula at the scapulocostal (ScC) joint
☐ Retracts the scapula at the ScC joint
☐ Upwardly rotates the scapula at the ScC joint
☐ Extends the head and neck at the spinal joints
☐ Laterally flexes the head and neck at the spinal joints
☐ Contralaterally rotates the head and neck at the spinal joints

Starting Position (Figure 12-31)
■ Client seated with the head and neck rotated (contralaterally) to the opposite side of the body
■ Therapist standing to the side of the client
■ Place palpating hand on the upper trapezius at the top of the shoulder region
■ Place support hand on the back of the client's head

Palpation Steps
1. Resist extension of the client's head and neck at the spinal joints, and look and feel for the contraction of the upper trapezius (Figure 12-32).

2. Continue palpating the upper trapezius superiorly to the occiput and inferiorly to the scapula and clavicle (strumming perpendicular to its fibers).
3. Once the upper trapezius has been located, have the client relax it and palpate to assess its baseline tone.

12

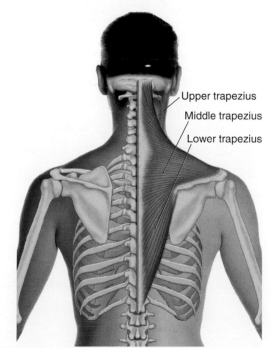

Upper trapezius
Middle trapezius
Lower trapezius

Figure 12-30 Posterior view of the right trapezius. The sternocleidomastoid (SCM), splenius capitis, and levator scapulae have been ghosted in.

UPPER TRAPEZIUS—SEATED—*cont'd*

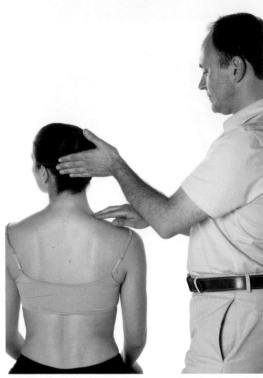

Figure 12-31 Starting position for seated palpation of the right upper trapezius.

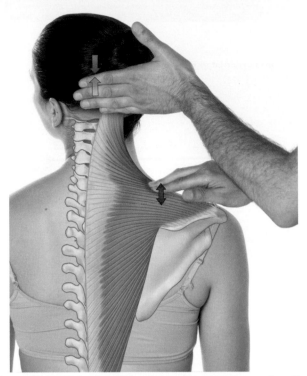

Figure 12-32 Palpation of the right upper trapezius as the client extends the head and neck against resistance.

12

PALPATION NOTE

1. All muscles in the posterior neck contract with resisted extension of the head and neck at the spinal joints. By having the client contralaterally rotate the head and neck (to the opposite side), the splenius capitis and cervicis, and levator scapulae are reciprocally inhibited (relaxed) and the upper trapezius is more forcefully engaged and therefore easier to palpate.

Alternate Palpation Position—Prone

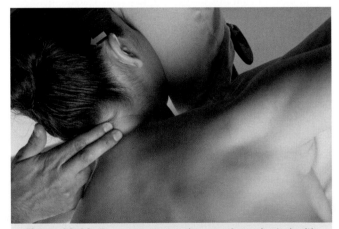

Figure 12-33 The upper trapezius can be palpated with the client prone. Asking the client to lift her head up from the face cradle engages the upper trapezius.

UPPER TRAPEZIUS—SEATED—*cont'd*

TRIGGER POINTS

1. Trigger points (TrPs) in the upper trapezius often result from or are perpetuated by acute or chronic overuse of the muscle (e.g., chronic postures of elevation of the shoulder girdle, anteriorly held head, or any chronic posture due to poor ergonomics, especially at the computer or with crimping the phone between the ear and shoulder; also when working to resist depression of the shoulder girdle when the upper extremity is hanging, and especially when the upper extremity is carrying a weight), trauma (e.g., whiplash), compression forces (e.g., carrying a heavy purse or backpack on the shoulder, having a tight bra strap), irritation from wearing a tie or a shirt with a tight collar, having a cold draft on the neck, or chronic stress/tension (holding the shoulder girdles uptight).
2. TrPs in the upper trapezius tend to produce a classic stiff neck with restricted contralateral lateral flexion and ipsilateral rotation of the neck at the spinal joints, a posture of elevated shoulder girdles, pain at the end of ipsilateral rotation of the neck, and tension headaches.
3. The referral patterns of upper trapezius TrPs must be distinguished from the referral patterns of TrPs in the SCM, masseter, temporalis, occipitalis, splenius cervicis, levator scapulae, semispinalis capitis, cervical multifidus, and lower trapezius.
4. TrPs in the trapezius are often incorrectly assessed as cervical disc syndrome, TMJ syndrome, or greater occipital neuralgia.
5. Associated TrPs of the upper trapezius often occur in the scalenes, splenius capitis and cervicis, levator scapulae, rhomboids, semispinalis capitis, temporalis, masseter, and contralateral upper trapezius.
6. Note: The upper trapezius has the most commonly found TrP in the body. Furthermore, the referral symptoms of this common TrP occasionally spread to the other side of the body.

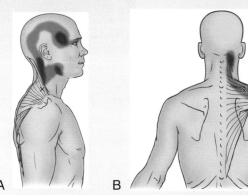

Figure 12-34 Common upper trapezius trigger points (TrPs) and their corresponding referral zones. **A,** Lateral view. **B,** Posterior view.

STRETCHING THE UPPER TRAPEZIUS

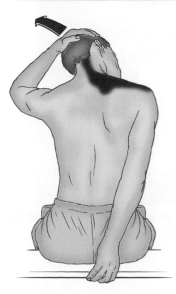

Figure 12-35 A stretch of the right upper trapezius. The client's head and neck are flexed, left laterally flexed (to the opposite side), and (ipsilaterally) rotated to the right. To keep the shoulder girdle down, the right hand holds onto the bench.

Palpation Key:
Contralaterally rotate and push back into extension.

LEVATOR SCAPULAE—SEATED

☑ ATTACHMENTS

☐ Transverse processes of C1-C4

to the

☐ medial border of the scapula from the root of the spine to the superior angle

☑ ACTIONS

☐ Elevates the scapula at the scapulocostal (ScC) joint
☐ Downwardly rotates the scapula at the ScC joint
☐ Extends the neck at the spinal joints
☐ Laterally flexes the neck at the spinal joints
☐ Ipsilaterally rotates the neck at the spinal joints

Starting Position (Figure 12-37)

■ Client seated with the hand in the small of the back
■ Therapist standing behind or to the side of the client
■ Place palpating hand immediately superior and medial to the superior angle of the scapula
■ Place support hand on top of the client's shoulder

Palpation Steps

1. With the client's hand in the small of the back, the client is asked to perform a gentle, very short range of motion of elevation of the scapula at the ScC joint. Feel for the levator scapulae's contraction deep to the trapezius (Figure 12-38, *A*).
2. Continue palpating the levator scapulae toward its superior attachment while strumming perpendicular to its fibers.
3. Once you are palpating the levator scapulae in the posterior triangle of the neck (superior to the trapezius), the client's hand no longer needs to be in the small of the back. It is also possible to ask the client to elevate the scapula more forcefully now; resistance can also be added with your support hand (see Figure 12-38, *B*).
4. Palpate the levator scapulae as far superiorly as possible. (Near its superior attachment, it will go deep to the SCM.)
5. Once the levator scapulae has been located, have the client relax it and palpate to assess its baseline tone.

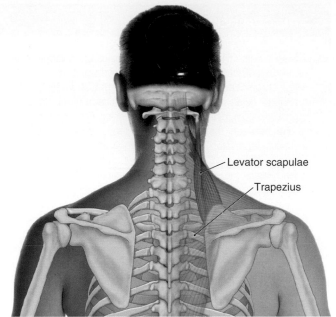

Figure 12-36 Posterior view of the right levator scapulae. The trapezius has been ghosted in.

Levator scapulae

Trapezius

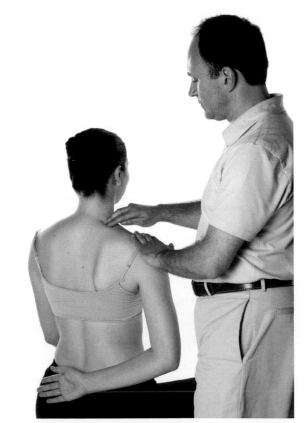

Figure 12-37 Starting position for seated palpation of the right levator scapulae.

12

LEVATOR SCAPULAE—SEATED—*cont'd*

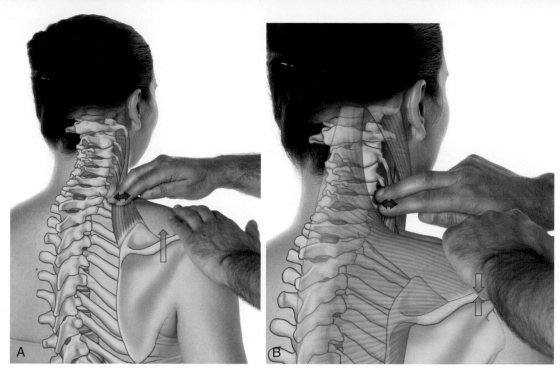

Figure 12-38 Palpation of the right levator scapulae. **A,** Palpation of the levator scapulae deep to the trapezius as the client performs gentle, short ranges of motion of elevation of the scapula with the hand in the small of the back; no resistance is given. **B,** Palpation in the posterior triangle of the neck; resistance can now be added to elevation of the scapula to better engage the levator scapulae.

PALPATION NOTES

1. Having the client place the hand in the small of the back requires extension and adduction of the arm at the shoulder joint. This requires the coupled action of downward rotation of the scapula at the ScC joint, which causes the trapezius to relax (because of reciprocal inhibition) so that the inferior attachment of the levator scapulae can be clearly felt when the levator scapulae contracts. It also engages the levator scapulae, so its contraction is more clearly felt.

2. Do not have the client perform a forceful action of elevation of the scapula, or the reflex of reciprocal inhibition will be overridden and the upper trapezius will contract, blocking palpation of the levator scapulae at its inferior attachment.

3. Once the levator scapulae is being palpated in the posterior triangle of the neck, it is no longer necessary to have the client place the hand in the small of the back, because it is no longer necessary to relax the trapezius. Furthermore, once we are palpating the levator scapulae in the posterior triangle, a forceful contraction of the levator scapulae can be engaged to better palpate and locate it.

4. In middle-aged and older people, the levator scapulae is often visible in the posterior triangle of the neck, even when they are not consciously contracting it (see Figure 12-23).

5. It can be challenging to palpate the most superior aspect of the levator scapulae deep to the sternocleidomastoid (SCM). To do so, slacken the SCM by slightly flexing, ipsilaterally (same-side) laterally flexing, and perhaps contralaterally rotating the neck and try to palpate deep to the SCM (Figure 12-39).

6. Note that the transverse process of C1 is directly inferior to the ear (between the mastoid process and the ramus of the mandible)! (See Figure 12-39.)

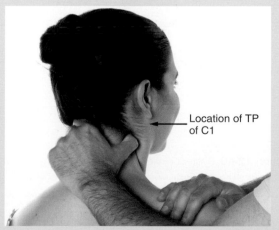

Location of TP of C1

Figure 12-39 The superior attachment of the levator scapulae is accessed by reaching deep to the sternocleidomastoid (SCM) and pressing anteriorly and superiorly toward the transverse process of the atlas (C1). This is best accomplished by first passively slackening the SCM by moving the client's head and neck into flexion and ipsilateral (same side) lateral flexion (not shown). Note the location of the transverse process of C1.

12

LEVATOR SCAPULAE—SEATED—*cont'd*

AlternatePalpation Position

The levator scapulae can be palpated with the client prone (see Figures 11-21 and 11-22).

TRIGGER POINTS

1. Trigger points (TrPs) in the levator scapulae often result from or are perpetuated by acute or chronic overuse of the muscle (e.g., carrying a bag or purse on the shoulder, crimping a phone between the ear and shoulder, excessive exercise such as playing tennis, holding the shoulders uptight), chronic shortening or stretching of the muscle due to poor work or leisure postures (e.g., having a poorly placed computer monitor, reading with the head inclined forward), motor vehicle accidents, having a cold draft on the neck, or being overly stressed psychologically.
2. TrPs in the levator scapulae tend to produce a classic stiff neck (often called *torticollis* or *wry neck*) with restricted contralateral rotation of the neck.
3. The referral patterns of levator scapulae TrPs must be distinguished from the referral patterns of TrPs in the scalenes, rhomboids, supraspinatus, and infraspinatus.
4. TrPs in the levator scapulae are often incorrectly assessed as joint dysfunction of the cervical spine.
5. Associated TrPs often occur in the upper trapezius, splenius cervicis, scalenes, and erector spinae of the cervical spine.

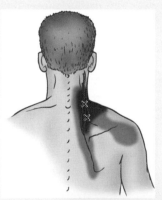

Figure 12-40 Posterior view illustrating common levator scapulae TrPs and their corresponding referral zone.

STRETCHING THE LEVATOR SCAPULAE

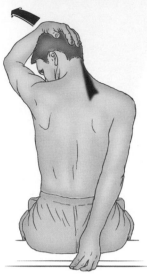

Figure 12-41 A stretch of the right levator scapulae. The client's neck is left laterally flexed, and (contralaterally) rotated to the left. To keep the shoulder girdle down, the right hand holds onto the bench.

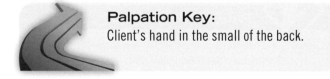

Palpation Key:
Client's hand in the small of the back.

SPLENIUS CAPITIS—SEATED

☑ ATTACHMENTS

☐ Nuchal ligament from the level of C3-C6 and the spinous processes of C7-T4

to the

☐ mastoid process of the temporal bone and the lateral ⅓ of the superior nuchal line of the occiput

☑ ACTIONS

☐ Extends the head and neck at the spinal joints
☐ Laterally flexes the head and neck at the spinal joints
☐ Ipsilaterally rotates the head and neck at the spinal joints

Starting Position (Figure 12-43)

■ Client seated with the head and neck ipsilaterally rotated
■ Therapist standing behind the client
■ Palpating hand placed at the upper aspect of the posterior triangle of the neck just inferior to the occiput and just posterior to the SCM; the splenius capitis is superficial here
■ Support hand placed on the back of the client's head

Palpation Steps

1. With palpating hand in position and the client's head and neck ipsilaterally rotated, resist the client from extending the head and neck at the spinal joints, and feel for the contraction of the splenius capitis (Figure 12-44).
2. Strum perpendicular to the fibers of the splenius capitis in the posterior triangle until you reach the border of the upper trapezius.
3. While asking the client to alternately extend the head and neck against gentle resistance and then relax, feel for the contraction and relaxation of the splenius capitis deep to the upper trapezius. Continue palpating the splenius capitis deep to the trapezius as far inferiorly as possible.
4. Once the splenius capitis has been located, have the client relax it and palpate to assess its baseline tone.

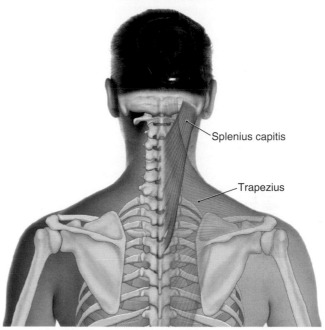

Figure 12-42 Posterior view of the right splenius capitis. The trapezius has been ghosted in.

12

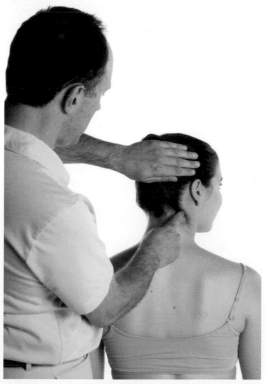

Figure 12-43 Starting position for seated palpation of the right splenius capitis.

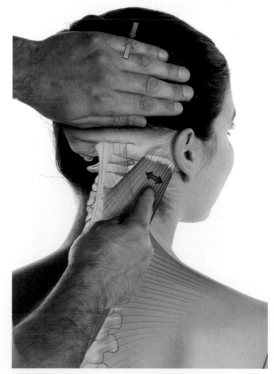

Figure 12-44 Palpation of the right splenius capitis in the posterior triangle of the neck as the client extends the head and neck against resistance.

SPLENIUS CAPITIS—SEATED—*cont'd*

PALPATION NOTES

1. By having the client's head and neck ipsilaterally rotated, the splenius capitis is better engaged to contract. Ipsilateral rotation also reciprocally inhibits and therefore relaxes the SCM and upper trapezius. Relaxing the upper trapezius makes it easier to feel the contraction of the splenius capitis deep to it. However, only gentle resistance should be given to the client's head and neck extension, or the reciprocal inhibition of the upper trapezius will be overridden and it will contract, blocking the ability to palpate the splenius capitis deep to it.
2. The inferior attachment of the splenius capitis on the spinous processes of the upper thoracic spine can be directly accessed by palpating anterior to the border of the upper trapezius and pressing downward toward the spinous processes. Sink slowly into the tissue with your finger pads oriented anteriorly, using firm pressure to palpate deep toward the spinous processes (Figure 12-45).
3. The client's hand can be placed in the small of the back to inhibit and relax the upper trapezius. Placing the hand in this manner requires extension and adduction of the arm at the shoulder joint, which requires downward rotation of the scapula at the scapulocostal (ScC) joint. Because the upper trapezius is an upward rotator of the scapula, it is inhibited and relaxed.

Alternate Palpation Position—Prone or Supine

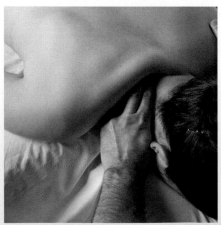

Figure 12-45 The splenius capitis can also be palpated with the client prone or supine. The prone position especially allows easy access to the inferior attachment on the spinous processes, deep to the trapezius (as explained in Palpation Note #2).

Palpation Key:
Begin at the top of the posterior triangle.

TRIGGER POINTS

1. Trigger points (TrPs) in the splenius capitis often result from or are perpetuated by acute or chronic overuse of the muscle (e.g., prolonged forward head posture, or prolonged posture with the head and neck rotated to one side, for example when working on a computer in which the monitor is not located directly in front of the person; or when playing violin), a sudden excessive stretch (e.g., whiplash injury), or a cold draft on the neck.
2. TrPs in the splenius capitis tend to produce restricted flexion and contralateral rotation of the head and neck at the spinal joints, restricted active rotation to the same side (due to pain upon contraction), cervical joint dysfunction, or headaches.
3. The referral patterns of splenius capitis TrPs must be distinguished from the referral patterns of TrPs in the occipitofrontalis and SCM.
4. TrPs in the splenius capitis are often incorrectly assessed as cervical joint dysfunction, migraine headaches, or spasmodic torticollis.
5. Associated TrPs often occur in the splenius cervicis, upper trapezius, levator scapulae, and semispinalis capitis.

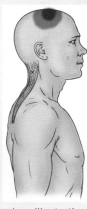

Figure 12-46 Lateral view illustrating a common splenius capitis trigger point (TrP) and its corresponding referral zone.

12

SPLENIUS CAPITIS—SEATED—*cont'd*

STRETCHING THE SPLENIUS CAPITIS

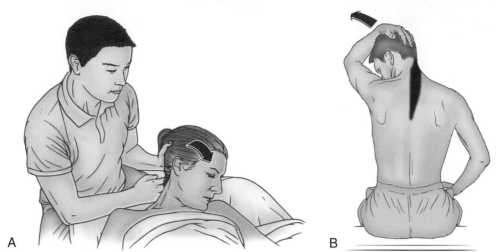

A   B

Figure 12-47 Stretching the right splenius capitis and cervicis. The client's head and neck are flexed, left laterally flexed, and left (contralaterally) rotated. Note: This stretch is identical to the levator scapulae stretch (Figure 11-26) except that there is no need to hold the scapula down with this stretch. **A,** Therapist-assisted stretch. **B,** Self-care stretch.

 DETOUR

Splenius cervicis:

The splenius cervicis attaches from the spinous processes of T3-T6 to the transverse processes of C1-C3 (Figure 12-48, *A*) and is deep to other musculature for its entire course; therefore it can be difficult to palpate and discern. The best place to first locate and palpate the splenius cervicis is between the levator scapulae and splenius capitis muscles (see Figure 12-2, *A*, right side). The actions of the splenius cervicis are the same as the splenius capitis, except that the splenius cervicis only moves the neck, not the head. Ask the client to ipsilaterally rotate the neck (against resistance if necessary) and feel for its contraction. Once located, try to follow toward both attachments.

Palpation Key:

Palpate between the splenius capitis and levator scapulae.

Trigger Points

1. Trigger points (TrPs) in the splenius cervicis often result from or are perpetuated by the same factors that create/perpetuate TrPs in the splenius capitis.
2. TrPs in the splenius cervicis tend to produce headaches, eye pain, or even blurriness of vision in the ipsilateral eye.
3. The referral patterns of splenius cervicis TrPs must be distinguished from the referral patterns of TrPs in the trapezius, SCM, suboccipitals, occipitofrontalis, temporalis, masseter, levator scapulae, and erector spinae and transversospinalis of the upper trunk.
4. TrPs in the splenius cervicis are often incorrectly assessed as cervical joint dysfunction, migraine headaches, or spasmodic torticollis.
5. Associated TrPs often occur in the splenius capitis, upper trapezius, levator scapulae, and semispinalis capitis.

12

SPLENIUS CAPITIS—SEATED—*cont'd*

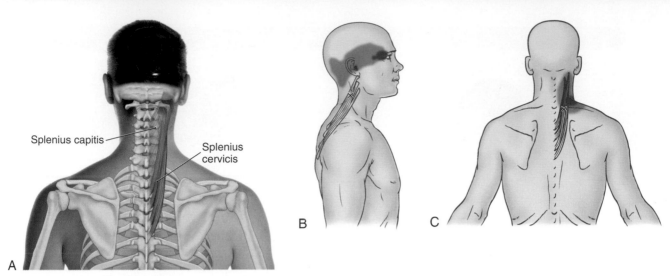

Figure 12-48 The splenius cervicis. **A,** Posterior view of the right splenius cervicis; the splenius capitis has been ghosted in. Common splenius cervicis trigger points (TrPs) and their corresponding referral zones are shown in lateral view **(B)** and posterior view **(C).**

SEMISPINALIS CAPITIS—SUPINE

☑ ATTACHMENTS

☐ Transverse processes of C7-T6 and articular processes of C4-6

to the

☐ medial ½ of the occipital bone between the superior and inferior nuchal lines

☑ ACTIONS

☐ Extends the head and neck at the spinal joints
☐ Laterally flexes the head and neck at the spinal joints

Starting Position (Figure 12-50)

■ Client supine with the hand in the small of the back and/ or the head and neck rotated to the same side (ipsilaterally rotated)
■ Therapist seated at the head of the table
■ Palpating hand placed just inferior to the occiput and just lateral to the midline of the spine (i.e., over the laminar groove)

Palpation Steps

1. Ask the client to extend the head and neck at the spinal joints by gently pressing the head into the table, and feel for the contraction of the semispinalis capitis deep to the upper trapezius (Figure 12-51).
2. Once felt, continue palpating superiorly to the occiput and then inferiorly as far as possible while strumming perpendicular to its fibers.
3. Once the semispinalis capitis has been located, have the client relax it and palpate to assess its baseline tone.

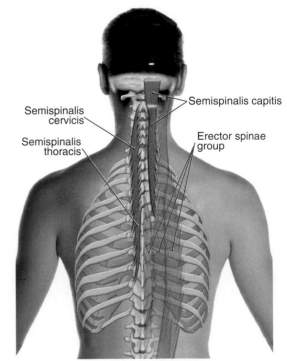

Figure 12-49 Posterior view of the right semispinalis capitis. The semispinalis thoracis and cervicis are seen on the left. The semispinalis capitis is seen on the right; the erector spinae group has been ghosted in on the right.

12

SEMISPINALIS CAPITIS—SUPINE—*cont'd*

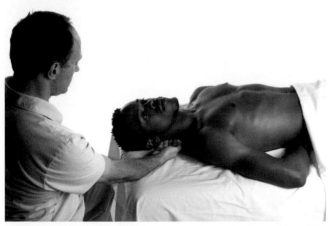

Figure 12-50 Starting position for supine palpation of the right semispinalis capitis.

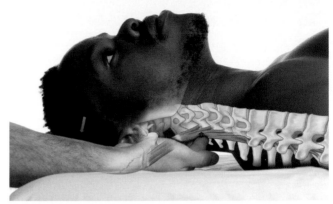

Figure 12-51 Palpation of the right semispinalis capitis as the client extends the head and neck down against the table.

PALPATION NOTES

1. The hand is placed in the small of the back to extend and adduct the arm at the shoulder joint, which requires downward rotation of the scapula at the scapulocostal (ScC) joint; this reciprocally inhibits and relaxes the upper trapezius, making it easier to palpate the semispinalis deep to it. Ipsilaterally rotating the head and neck also reciprocally inhibits the upper trapezius.
2. Be sure that the client does not contract the head and neck into extension too forcefully, or the neurologic reflex of reciprocal inhibition will be overridden and the upper trapezius will contract, blocking the ability to palpate the semispinalis capitis deep to it.
3. Even though the upper trapezius is the best known muscle of the posterior neck, the semispinalis capitis muscle in the neck is appreciably larger and thicker; in fact, it is the largest muscle of the posterior neck.

Alternate Palpation Position—Prone

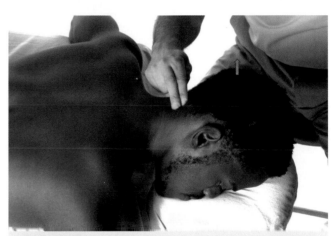

Figure 12-52 The semispinalis capitis can also be palpated with the client prone. In this position, it is also important to reciprocally inhibit the upper trapezius to relax it; this is accomplished by having the client ipsilaterally rotate the head and neck at the spinal joints. Then the head can be lifted up slightly into extension against gravity to engage the semispinalis capitis. Note: The upper trapezius can also be inhibited by having the client place the hand in the small of the back, as seen in Figure 12-50.

12

SEMISPINALIS CAPITIS—SUPINE—*cont'd*

TRIGGER POINTS

1. Trigger points (TrPs) in the semispinalis capitis often result from or are perpetuated by acute or chronic overuse of the muscle (e.g., prolonged protracted head posture, or prolonged posture where the head and neck are flexed with their center of weight imbalanced anterior to the trunk), prolonged postures that result in shortening of the muscle (e.g., propping up on elbows to support the head when watching television or when lying prone and doing homework on a bed), trauma such as a whiplash or a fall, radiculopathy of the cervical spinal nerves, osteoarthritic changes of the cervical spine, irritation from wearing a tie or a shirt with a tight collar, a cold draft on the neck, or secondary to TrPs in the upper trapezius or splenius capitis.

2. TrPs in the semispinalis capitis tend to produce headaches, restricted head and neck flexion or contralateral lateral flexion, entrapment of the greater occipital nerve (which may result in altered sensation in the posterior scalp, such as tingling or pain), or joint dysfunction or osteoarthritis of the cervical spine.

3. The referral patterns of semispinalis capitis TrPs must be distinguished from the referral patterns of TrPs in the trapezius, SCM, temporalis, occipitofrontalis, and the suboccipitals.

4. TrPs in the semispinalis capitis are often incorrectly assessed as osteoarthritis of the cervical spine or sinus or migraine headaches.

5. Associated TrPs often occur in the upper trapezius, semispinalis cervicis, splenius capitis or cervicis, and erector spinae and transversospinalis muscles of the trunk.

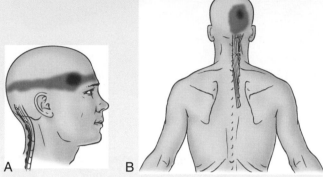

Figure 12-53 Common semispinalis capitis trigger points (TrPs) and their corresponding referral zones. **A,** Lateral view. **B,** Posterior view.

STRETCHING THE SEMISPINALIS CAPITIS

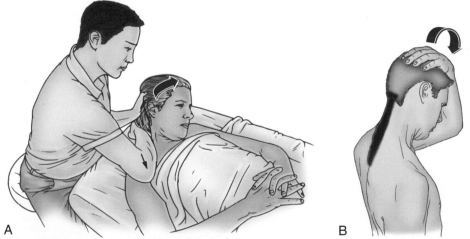

Figure 12-54 Stretching the right semispinalis capitis. The client's head and neck are flexed and left laterally flexed. The trunk must be stabilized to prevent it from flexing and rotating to the left. Note: Flexion is the most important component of this stretch. **A,** Therapist-assisted stretch. **B,** Self-care stretch.

Palpation Key:
Reciprocally inhibit the upper trapezius and palpate deep to it.

SEMISPINALIS CAPITIS—SUPINE—*cont'd*

DETOUR

Longissimus capitis, semispinalis cervicis, and cervical multifidus and rotatores:

The longissimus capitis of the erector spinae group attaches from the transverse or articular processes of C5-T5 to the mastoid process of the temporal bone; it is deep for its entire course and therefore challenging to palpate and discern. Its actions are extension and ipsilateral rotation of the neck and head at the spinal joints. To locate it, with the client supine, palpate lateral to the splenius capitis and deep to the levator scapulae and upper trapezius. Gentle extension of the head against the table with the head and neck ipsilaterally rotated causes it to contract (and reciprocally inhibits the upper trapezius).

The semispinalis cervicis attaches from the transverse processes of T1-T5 to the spinous processes of C2-C5; it is also deep (primarily to the semispinalis capitis) and challenging to palpate and discern.

The cervical multifidus and rotatores are located very deep within the laminar groove of the cervical spine and are also very challenging to palpate and discern.

The semispinalis, multifidus, and rotatores are members of the transversospinalis group and extend and contralaterally rotate the neck at the spinal joints.

Trigger Points

1. Trigger points (TrPs) in the longissimus capitis usually refer pain posterior to the ear. Pain referral may also occur in the neck or around the eye. These TrPs are also often involved in joint dysfunction of the costospinal joints of the first rib (Figure 12-55, *B*).
2. TrPs in the semispinalis cervicis likely refer pain to the occipital region in a pattern similar to the semispinalis capitis (see Figure 12-53, *B*).
3. TrPs in the multifidus of the cervical spine usually refer pain superiorly to the suboccipital region and inferiorly to the medial border of the scapula (see Figure 12-55, *C*).
4. TrPs in the rotatores of the cervical spine usually refer pain to the midline of the spine at the segmental level of the TrP (similar to rotatores TrPs in the thoracic and lumbar regions) (see Figure 12-55, *D*).

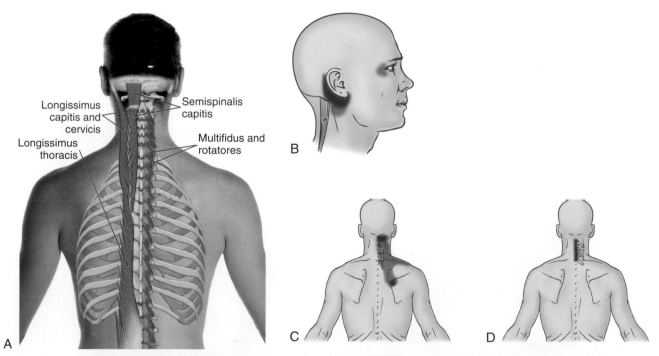

A — Longissimus capitis and cervicis / Semispinalis capitis / Longissimus thoracis / Multifidus and rotatores

B

C

D

Figure 12-55 A, Posterior view of the longissimus, semispinalis, multifidus, and rotatores. The longissimus and semispinalis are seen on the left; the multifidus (ghosted in) and rotatores are seen on the right. **B, C,** and **D,** Common trigger points (TrPs) and their corresponding referral zones. **B,** Lateral view of a common TrP in the longissimus capitis and its referral zone. **C,** Posterior view of a common TrP in the cervical multifidus and its referral zone. **D,** Posterior view of common TrPs in the cervical rotatores and their referral zone.

SUBOCCIPITAL GROUP—SUPINE

The suboccipital group is composed of the following:
- Rectus capitis posterior major (RCPMaj)
- Rectus capitis posterior minor (RCPMin)
- Obliquus capitis inferior (OCI)
- Obliquus capitis superior (OCS)

☑ ATTACHMENTS

☐ RCPMaj: Spinous process of C2

to the

☐ lateral ½ of the inferior nuchal line of the occiput
☐ RCPMin: Posterior tubercle of C1

to the

☐ medial ½ of the inferior nuchal line of the occiput
☐ OCI: Spinous process of C2

to the

☐ transverse process of C1
☐ OCS: Transverse process of C1

to the

☐ lateral occiput between the superior and inferior nuchal lines

☑ ACTIONS

☐ As a group, the suboccipital muscles extend and anteriorly translate the head at the atlanto-occipital joint.
☐ The OCI ipsilaterally rotates the atlas at the atlantoaxial joint.

Starting Position (Figure 12-57)
- Client supine
- Therapist seated at the head of the table
- Palpating hand placed just superior and slightly lateral to the spinous process of C2 (the axis)

Palpation Steps
1. The easiest suboccipital muscle to palpate is the RCPMaj. Begin by finding the spinous process of C2, which is an easy landmark to locate in the upper neck. Then palpate just superolateral to it, and feel for the RCPMaj while strumming perpendicular to its fibers.
2. If located, continue strumming perpendicularly, following it superolaterally toward its occipital attachment (Figure 12-58, *A*).
3. Repeat the same steps for the RCPMin by starting just superolateral to the posterior tubercle of C1. Strum perpendicular to locate the muscle; then follow toward the occipital attachment (see Figure 12-58, *B*). It may be helpful to have the RCPMin contract by asking the client to anteriorly translate the head at the atlanto-occipital joint (see Palpation Note #3).
4. To palpate the OCI, palpate between the spinous process of C2 and the transverse process of C1, strumming perpendicular to the fibers. It may be helpful to have the OCI contract by gently resisting the client's ipsilateral rotation of the head.
5. The OCS is extremely challenging to palpate and discern from adjacent musculature. To attempt its palpation, feel for it just lateral to the superior attachment of the RCPMaj; if felt, try to continue palpating it inferiorly while strumming perpendicular to it.
6. Once the suboccipital muscles have been located, have the client relax them and palpate to assess their baseline tone.

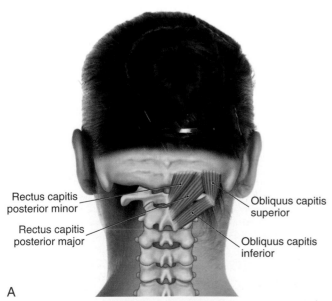

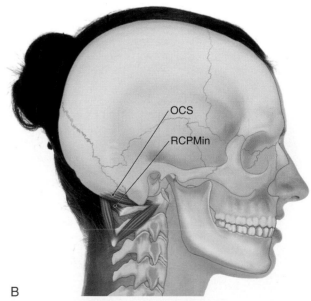

Rectus capitis posterior minor

Rectus capitis posterior major

Obliquus capitis superior

Obliquus capitis inferior

OCS

RCPMin

A

B

Figure 12-56 Views of the right suboccipital group. **A,** Posterior view. **B,** Lateral view. Note the anterior to posterior horizontal direction of the rectus capitis posterior minor (RCPMin) and the obliquus capitis superior (OCS). This fiber direction is ideal for anterior translation of the head at the atlanto-occipital joint.

12

SUBOCCIPITAL GROUP—SUPINE—*cont'd*

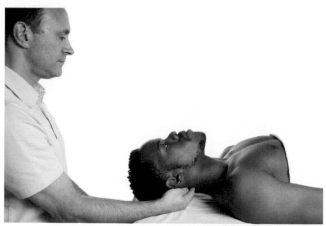

Figure 12-57 Starting position for supine palpation of the right suboccipital muscles.

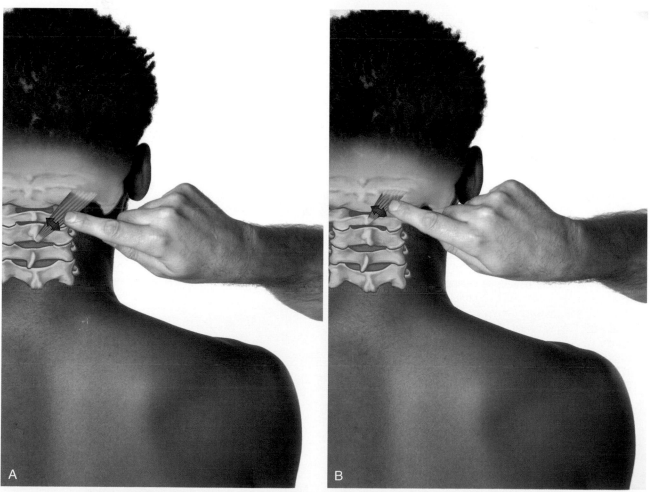

Figure 12-58 Palpation of the suboccipital muscles. **A,** Palpation of the right rectus capitis posterior major (RCPMaj) between the spinous process of the axis (C2) and the occiput. **B,** Palpation of the right rectus capitis posterior minor (RCPMin) between the posterior tubercle of the atlas (C1) and the occiput.

SUBOCCIPITAL GROUP—SUPINE—*cont'd*

PALPATION NOTES

1. Generally it is best to palpate the suboccipital muscles when they are relaxed. They are deep and can be challenging to palpate and discern. However, if the superficial muscles are loose and the suboccipitals are tight, they can be fairly easily palpated.
2. The easiest suboccipital muscle to palpate is the rectus capitis posterior major (RCPMaj). The obliquus capitis superior (OCS) is usually the most difficult to palpate.
3. A certain amount of caution must be exercised when palpating and pressing into the region known as the *suboccipital triangle* (bounded by the RCPMaj and the two obliquus capitis muscles) because of the presence of the vertebral artery and suboccipital nerve. The greater occipital nerve is also located nearby. However, some sources state that when the head and neck are flexed, the tension in the posterior tissues does not allow deep enough access to reach these neurovascular structures; and when the head and neck are extended, these neurovascular structures are not accessible because the occiput drops back to the atlas and blocks pressure into the area located between these two bones.
4. Anterior translation of the head involves the head gliding directly anterior at the atlanto-occipital joint. Asking the client to create this action will cause the rectus capitis posterior minor (RCPMin) and obliquus capitis superior (OCS) to contract and become more easily palpable.

Palpation Key:
Begin at the spinous process of C2 for the RCPMaj.

12

TRIGGER POINTS

1. Trigger points (TrPs) in the suboccipitals often result from or are perpetuated by acute or chronic overuse of the muscle (e.g., sustained extension of the head at the atlanto-occipital joint, perhaps while painting a ceiling or bird-watching, or sustained posture with the head rotated to one side [for the OCI]), chronic forward (anterior translation) head posture, trauma such as whiplash, having a cold draft on the neck, or joint dysfunction of the atlanto-occipital or atlantoaxial joints.
2. TrPs in the suboccipitals tend to produce headache pain that is diffuse and difficult to localize, restrict flexion or contralateral lateral flexion of the head at the atlanto-occipital joint, restrict contralateral rotation of the axis at the atlantoaxial joint (OCI), or cause joint dysfunction of the atlanto-occipital or atlantoaxial joints.
3. The referral patterns of suboccipital TrPs must be distinguished from the referral patterns of TrPs in the SCM, temporalis, splenius cervicis, and semispinalis capitis.

4. TrPs in the suboccipitals are often incorrectly assessed as migraines or greater occipital neuralgia.
5. Associated TrPs often occur in the other posterior cervical muscles or the occipitalis.

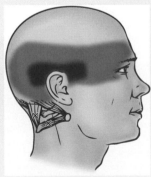

Figure 12-59 Lateral view illustrating common suboccipital trigger points (TrPs) and their corresponding referral zone.

SUBOCCIPITAL GROUP—SUPINE—*cont'd*

STRETCHING THE SUBOCCIPITALS

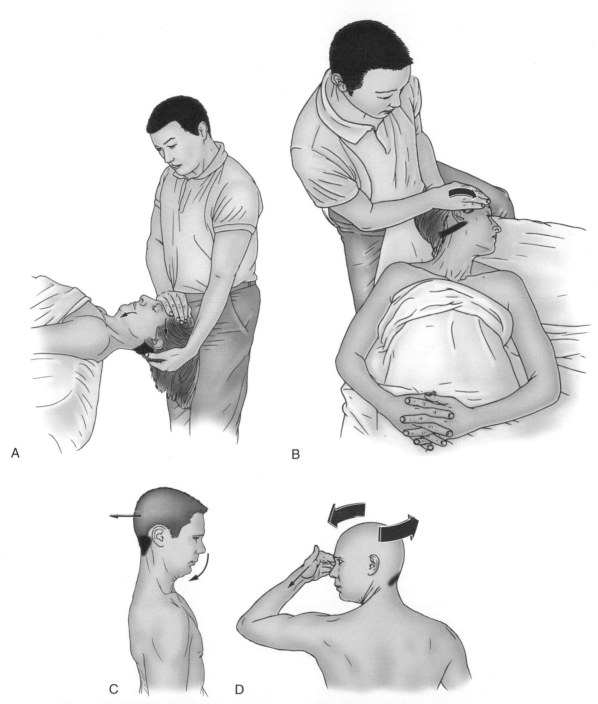

Figure 12-60 Stretching the suboccipital muscles. Stretching the bilateral rectus capitis posterior major and minor (RCPMaj and RCPMin) muscles as well as the bilateral obliquus capitis superior (OCS) muscles is accomplished by both flexing the client's head at the atlanto-occipital joint (by tucking the chin toward the chest) and posteriorly translating the head. To focus this stretch to the right side group, left lateral flexion can be added (not shown). Stretching the right obliquus capitis inferior (OCI) is accomplished by rotating the client's neck as far as possible to the (contralateral) left side. A, Therapist-assisted stretch of the bilateral RCPMaj, RCPMin, and OCS muscles. B, Therapist-assisted stretch of the right OCI muscle. C, Self-care stretch of the bilateral RCPMaj, RCPMin, and OCS muscles. D, Self-care stretch of the right OCI muscle.

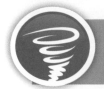

WHIRLWIND TOUR

Muscles of the Neck

The following *Whirlwind Tour* is an abbreviated set of palpation protocols for the muscles of this chapter. Once you have read and become comfortable with each of the protocols presented thus far, this *Whirlwind Tour* allows you to quickly and efficiently run through the palpations protocols for all the muscles of the chapter.

Client Supine

1. **Sternocleidomastoid (SCM):** The client is supine with the head and neck contralaterally rotated; you are seated at the head of the table. Before palpating, first visualize the contraction of the SCM as the client lifts the head from the table. Then palpate the contraction of the SCM just superior to the sternoclavicular joint as the client again lifts the head from the table. Once felt, continue palpating the SCM to the mastoid process of the temporal bone and the superior nuchal line of the occipital bone while strumming perpendicular to the fibers as the client alternately contracts and relaxes the muscle. Note: Look and palpate carefully for the clavicular head; it is usually less obvious than the sternal head.

2. **Scalene group:** The client is supine; you are seated at the head of the table. Locate the lateral border of the clavicular head of the SCM (be sure that it is the lateral border of the clavicular head, not the sternal head that you have located). Place palpating fingers just lateral to the lateral border of the clavicular head of the SCM and just superior to the clavicle, and feel for the contraction of the scalenes as the client takes in short, quick breaths through the nose. Once felt, palpate as much of the scalenes as possible in the posterior triangle of the neck while strumming perpendicular to the fibers. The transverse processes attachment of the scalenes can usually be palpated by pressing in deep to the SCM if it is first slackened by passively flexing and ipsilaterally laterally flexing the client's head and neck. Note: It can be challenging to discern the anterior, middle, and posterior scalenes from each other. A gap can usually be felt between the anterior and middle scalenes. Also, try to feel for the different direction of fibers that each one has. Remember: the anterior scalene goes to C3-C6; the middle scalene goes to C2-C7; and the posterior scalene goes to C5-C7. Also, keep in mind that the posterior scalene is located in the posterior triangle of the neck immediately anterior to the upper trapezius and levator scapulae.

3. **Longus colli/longus capitis:** The client is supine; you are seated at the head of the table. Locate the medial border of the sternal head of the SCM, and then drop off it and place palpating fingers immediately medial to that. Sink in toward the anterior surface of the vertebral bodies slowly and gently, but firmly. If you feel a pulse under your fingers, move your fingers to one side or the other and continue palpating for the vertebral bodies. It is often helpful to gently displace the client's trachea toward the opposite side of the body and then sink down toward the longus

musculature. Once you have reached the vertebral bodies, confirm that you are on the longus colli by asking the client to flex the head and neck by lifting the head up off the table. Palpate as much of the longus colli and capitis as possible superiorly and inferiorly while strumming perpendicular to the fibers. Note: The carotid tubercle on the transverse process of C6 is a good landmark for determining the segmental level of the palpating fingers.

4. **Hyoid group:** For the purpose of palpation, the hyoid group can be divided into the infrahyoid group and the suprahyoid group. The client is supine; you are seated at the head of the table. To palpate the infrahyoids, place your palpating fingers immediately inferior to the hyoid bone and just off center and feel for their contraction as the client is resisted from depressing the mandible at the temporomandibular joints (TMJs). Once felt, palpate these muscles toward their inferior attachments on the sternum while strumming perpendicular to the fibers as the client alternately contracts and relaxes them. The inferior belly of the omohyoid can be palpated in the posterior triangle of the neck while strumming perpendicular to it as the client is resisted from depressing the mandible at the TMJs. To palpate the suprahyoids, place your palpating fingers immediately inferior to the mandible and again feel for their contraction as the client is resisted from depressing the mandible at the TMJs. Once felt, palpate these muscles toward the hyoid bone while strumming perpendicular to the fibers as the client alternately contracts and relaxes them. Palpate the stylohyoid and posterior belly of the digastric while strumming perpendicular to their fibers from the hyoid bone toward the mastoid process of the temporal bone as the client alternately contracts and relaxes them.

Client Seated

5. **Upper trapezius:** The client is seated with the head and neck contralaterally rotated; you are standing to the side of the client. Feel for the contraction of the upper trapezius at the top of the shoulder as the client is resisted from extending the head and neck against the resistance of your support hand on the back of their head (Note: The contraction of the upper trapezius is often visible and palpable; be sure to look for it as well). Continue palpating the upper trapezius toward its medial attachment on the head and neck and its lateral attachment on the lateral clavicle and acromion process while strumming perpendicular to its fibers as the client alternately contracts and relaxes it. Note: The superior aspect of the upper trapezius is actually quite narrow and only attaches to the medial ⅓ of the superior nuchal line of the occipital bone.

6. **Levator scapulae:** Note: The palpation of the levator scapulae can be divided into three parts: where it is deep to the upper trapezius near its scapular attachment, where it is superficial in the posterior triangle of the neck, and where it is deep to the SCM near its spinal attachment. The client is seated

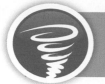

Muscles of the Neck—*cont'd*

with the hand in the small of the back; you are standing behind or to the side of the client. Locate the superior angle of the scapula and place your palpating fingers immediately superior and medial to it. Feel for the contraction of the levator scapulae deep to the upper trapezius as the client performs a gentle, short range of motion of elevation of the scapula at the scapulocostal (ScC) joint. Once felt, continue palpating it until it enters the posterior triangle of the neck (i.e., until it is no longer deep to the upper trapezius) while strumming perpendicular to its fibers as the client alternately gently contracts and relaxes the muscle. Once the levator scapulae is located in the posterior triangle, it is superficial and easily palpable and sometimes visible as well. It is no longer necessary for the client to have the hand in the small of the back, and the client can be asked to perform a more forceful contraction (against resistance if desired) of elevation of the scapula. Continue palpating it superiorly while strumming perpendicular to its fibers as the client alternately contracts and relaxes the muscle. As it approaches its spinal attachment (transverse processes of C1-C4), the levator scapulae lies deep to the SCM. To palpate it all the way to its spinal attachments deep to the SCM, the SCM must be slackened by passively moving the client's head and neck into flexion and ipsilateral lateral flexion. Note: When following the levator scapulae superiorly, be sure that you follow it toward the transverse process of C1, which is located more anteriorly than most people realize; the transverse process of C1 is located immediately inferior to the ear.

7. **Splenius capitis:** The client is seated with the head and neck ipsilaterally rotated; you are standing behind the client. Palpate in the uppermost aspect of the posterior triangle of the neck, just inferior to the occiput and posterior to the SCM. Now feel for the contraction of the splenius capitis as the client is resisted from extending the head and neck at the spinal joints. Once felt, strum perpendicular to its fibers and try to follow it inferiorly as the client alternately contracts and relaxes the muscle. Once you are no longer in the posterior triangle of the neck, the splenius capitis can be palpated two ways: (1) feel for it through the upper trapezius by asking the client to extend the head and neck against *gentle* resistance; once felt, try to follow it as far inferiorly as possible; or (2) feel for it directly: this requires

you to palpate deep (anterior) to the border of the upper trapezius and press anteriorly toward the upper thoracic spinous processes by reaching with your palpating fingers between the upper trapezius and the splenius capitis. To accomplish this, it is best to stand more to the front of the client so that your finger pads are oriented anteriorly toward the splenius capitis. Furthermore, it is important that the upper trapezius is relaxed and slackened; it can be slackened by passively moving the client's head and neck into extension, contralateral rotation, and/or ipsilateral lateral flexion.

Client Supine

8. **Semispinalis capitis:** The client is supine with the hand in the small of the back, and/or the head and neck rotated to the same side (ipsilaterally rotated); you are seated at the head of the table. Ask the client to extend the head and neck at the spinal joints by gently pressing the head into the table and feel for the contraction of the semispinalis capitis deep to the upper trapezius, just below the occiput and just lateral to the spine. Once felt, continue palpating the semispinalis capitis inferiorly as far as possible while the client alternately contracts and relaxes the muscle.

9. **Suboccipital group (RCPMaj, RCPMin, OCI, OCS):** The client is supine; you are seated at the head of the table. Begin by palpating the RCPMaj; palpate just superior and slightly lateral to the spinous process of C2 and strum perpendicular to it fibers. Once felt, continue palpating the RCPMaj to the occiput while strumming perpendicular to its fibers. Palpate the RCPMin in the same manner while strumming perpendicular to it, beginning just superolateral to the posterior tubercle of C1. Once felt, continue palpating the RCPMin to the occiput while strumming perpendicular to it. To palpate the OCI, palpate between the spinous process of C2 and the transverse process of C1, strumming perpendicular to the fibers. It may be helpful to have the OCI contract by gently resisting the client from ipsilaterally rotating the head. The OCS is extremely challenging to palpate and discern from adjacent musculature. To attempt its palpation, feel for it just lateral to the superior attachment of the RCPMaj; if felt, try to continue palpating it inferiorly while strumming perpendicular to it.

12

Review Questions

1. What are the actions of the sternocleidomastoid (SCM)?
2. What are the actions of the hyoid muscles?
3. List the attachments of the longus colli.
4. List the attachments of the anterior, middle, and posterior scalenes.
5. In a seated palpation of the upper trapezius, what client position and actions should be used to engage the muscle?
6. Caution during palpation of the suboccipitals is indicated for what reasons?
7. Briefly describe the procedure for locating the scalenes for palpation. What action can be used to help locate the scalenes?
8. Describe the starting position for palpation of the hyoids.
9. Why is it advantageous for a client's hand to be placed in the small of the back during palpation of the levator scapulae?
10. Where is the easiest place to begin palpation of the splenius capitis?
11. What distinction does the semispinalis capitis hold that is relevant to palpation and function?
12. TrPs in what muscle can produce the following effects: headaches, restricted range of motion of the neck and head, sore throat, ptosis of the upper eyelids, dizziness, vertigo, and entrapment of cranial nerve eleven (CNXI)?
13. Describe the pain pattern produced by TrPs in the anterior belly of the digastric.
14. What is the proper position for stretching the left sternocleidomastoid (SCM)?
15. Describe the proper position for stretching the left upper trapezius.
16. When palpating the longus colli and longus capitis, what structures should a therapist be aware of and why?
17. When using resisted extension of the head and neck as your engaging action, how can a therapist be certain to get a clean palpation of the upper trapezius?

12

CASE STUDY

A new client arrives for a massage therapy session 3 weeks after being involved in a motor vehicle collision complaining of pain and stiffness in the neck, a continuing dull headache, and a general feeling of malaise. The client was a restrained front seat passenger in the middle vehicle of a three-car collision. Clearance by her primary care physician has been given for massage therapy with no restrictions and no specific recommendations for treatment. The client's post-collision exam by the emergency room physician (which included x-rays of the spine) revealed no fractures or dislocations, and she was released with recommendations to rest for a few days and was given a prescription for a low-grade narcotic pain medication. A magnetic resonance imaging (MRI) scan 1 week later also was negative for injury.

History reveals an otherwise physically active woman whose only prior medical issues were an appendectomy over 20 years ago and a cesarean section 5 years ago. Physical exam shows general tenderness to even light palpatory pressure throughout the head and neck area. Active range of motion in all planes is roughly half that of normal; passive range of motion is nearly impossible to discern due to the client not sufficiently relaxing to allow the therapist to passively move their neck.

1. What further information, if any, might you ask of this client before engaging in treatment?
2. What type(s) of treatment may be beneficial for this client?
3. What muscles do you suspect, based upon the type of accident, may be injured/having spasms?

CHAPTER 13

Tour #3   Palpation of the Muscles of the Head

Overview

This chapter is a palpation tour of the muscles of the head. The tour begins with the scalp muscles, then addresses the muscles of mastication, and then concludes with palpation of the muscles of facial expression. Palpation for each of the muscles is shown in the supine position. Alternate palpation positions are also described. The major muscles or muscle groups of the region are each given a separate layout; there is also a detour to other muscles of the scalp. Trigger point (TrP) information and stretching, both therapist-assisted and self-care stretching, are given for each of the muscles covered in this chapter. The chapter closes with an advanced *Whirlwind Tour* that explains the sequential palpation of all of the muscles of the chapter.

Chapter Outline

Occipitofrontalis
  Detour to the Temporoparietalis and Auricularis Muscles
Temporalis
Masseter
Lateral Pterygoid
Medial Pterygoid
Muscles of Facial Expression
Whirlwind Tour: Muscles of the Head

Chapter Objectives

After completing this chapter, the student/therapist should be able to perform the following for each of the muscles covered in this chapter:

1. State the attachments.
2. State the actions.
3. Describe the starting position for palpation.
4. Describe and explain the purpose of each of the palpation steps.
5. Palpate each muscle.
6. State the "Palpation Key."
7. Describe alternate palpation positions.
8. State the locations of the most common TrP(s).
9. Describe the TrP referral zones.
10. State the most common factors that create and/or perpetuate TrPs.
11. State the symptoms most commonly caused by TrPs.
12. Describe and perform the therapist-assisted and self-care stretches.

ⓔ Go to http://evolve.elsevier.com/Muscolino/palpation for video demonstrations of the muscle palpations presented in this chapter.

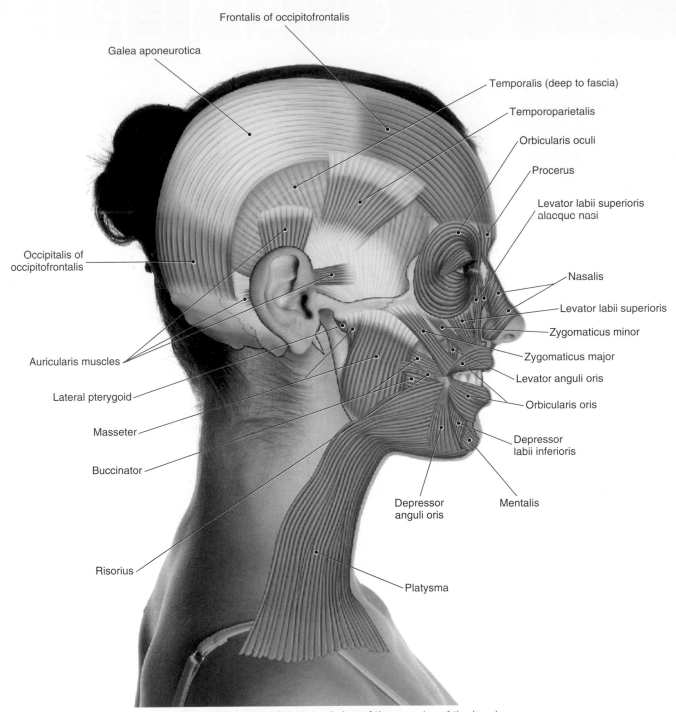

Figure 13-1 Superficial lateral view of the muscles of the head.

13

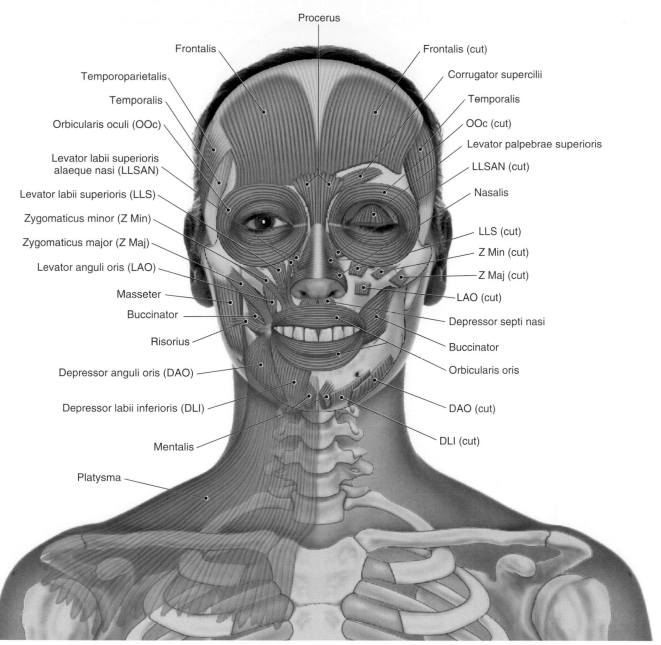

Figure 13-2 Superficial and intermediate anterior views of the muscles of the head. Note: abbreviations are defined on the client's right side.

13

13

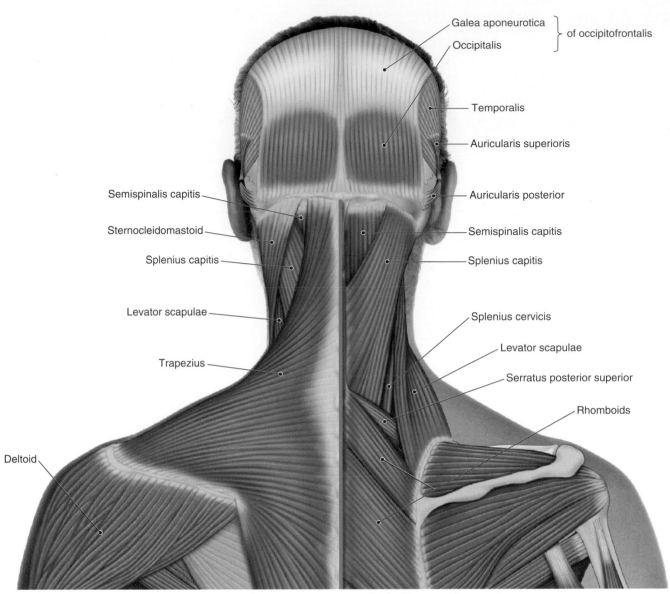

Galea aponeurotica ⎫
                    ⎬ of occipitofrontalis
Occipitalis   ⎭

Temporalis

Auricularis superioris

Auricularis posterior

Semispinalis capitis

Splenius capitis

Splenius cervicis

Levator scapulae

Serratus posterior superior

Rhomboids

Semispinalis capitis

Sternocleidomastoid

Splenius capitis

Levator scapulae

Trapezius

Deltoid

Figure 13-3 Superficial posterior view of the muscles of the head.

OCCIPITOFRONTALIS—SUPINE

☑ ATTACHMENTS

☐ Highest nuchal line of the occiput and the mastoid region of the temporal bone

to the

☐ galea aponeurotica

to the

☐ fascia overlying the frontal bone

☑ ACTIONS

☐ Draws the anterior scalp posteriorly (elevates the eyebrows)
☐ Draws the posterior scalp anteriorly

Starting Position (Figure 13-5)

■ Client supine
■ Therapist seated at head of table
■ Place palpating fingers on the forehead of the client

Palpation Steps

1. With your palpating fingers on the client's forehead, ask the client to elevate the eyebrows and feel for the contraction of the frontalis (see Figure 13-5). Once felt, palpate the entire frontalis belly.
2. Now palpate over the client's occipital bone, ask the client to elevate the eyebrows, and feel for the contraction of the occipitalis (Figure 13-6). Once felt, palpate the entire occipitalis.
3. Once the occipitofrontalis has been located, have the client relax it and palpate to assess its baseline tone.

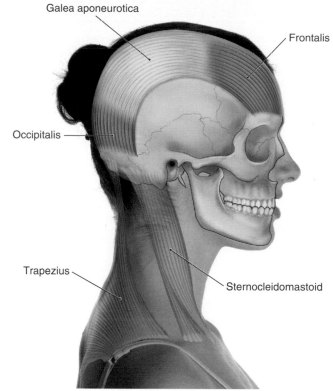

Figure 13-4 Lateral view of the right occipitofrontalis. The trapezius and sternocleidomastoid (SCM) have been ghosted in.

13

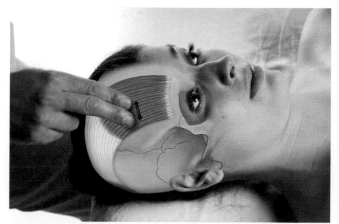

Figure 13-5 Palpation of the right frontalis belly of the occipitofrontalis.

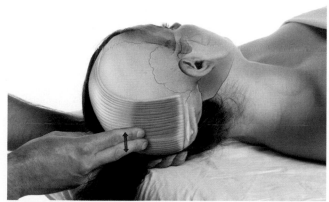

Figure 13-6 Palpation of the right and left occipitalis bellies of the occipitofrontalis muscles.

OCCIPITOFRONTALIS—SUPINE—*cont'd*

Alternate Palpation Position

Both bellies of the occipitofrontalis (the frontalis and the occipitalis) are easily accessible with the client seated. The occipitalis belly can also be easily palpated with the client prone.

Palpation Key:

Palpate over the frontal and occipital bones.

PALPATION NOTES

1. The occipitofrontalis consists of two bellies: the frontalis overlies the frontal bone; the occipitalis overlies the occipital bone. These two bellies are connected to each other by a large aponeurosis called the *galea aponeurotica*.
2. The entire occipitofrontalis is superficial and easily palpable.
3. Because the occipitofrontalis is a thin fascial muscle, feeling its contraction is not always as obvious as feeling the contraction of a thicker larger muscle. For this reason, locating the entire occipitofrontalis by feeling its contraction is not as useful as it is with most other muscles.
4. The occipitofrontalis is often tight in clients who suffer from tension headaches.

TRIGGER POINTS

1. Trigger points (TrPs) in the occipitofrontalis often result from or are perpetuated by acute or chronic overuse of the muscle (from the chronic habit of wrinkling the forehead) or direct trauma. Furthermore, TrPs in the occipitalis belly often result from or are perpetuated by TrPs in the posterior cervical musculature; and TrPs in the frontalis belly often result from or are perpetuated by TrPs in the clavicular head of the sternocleidomastoid (SCM).
2. TrPs in the occipitalis belly tend to produce headache pain in the back of the head and behind the eye, discomfort having pressure against the back of the head (e.g., with pressure against a pillow at night or the back of a chair), and perhaps even an earache. TrPs in the frontalis belly tend to produce headache pain in the forehead and can also entrap the supraorbital nerve (resulting in headache pain in the forehead with symptoms more characteristic of nerve entrapment, such as more of a tingling and prickling pain).
3. The referral patterns of occipitalis TrPs must be distinguished from the referral patterns of TrPs in the splenius cervicis and temporalis; the referral patterns of frontalis TrPs must be distinguished from the referral patterns of TrPs in the SCM, temporalis, masseter, orbicularis oculi, and zygomaticus major.

4. TrPs in the occipitofrontalis are often incorrectly assessed as migraine headaches; furthermore, TrPs in the occipitalis belly are often incorrectly assessed as greater occipital neuralgia.
5. Associated TrPs of the occipitalis often occur in the upper trapezius, semispinalis capitis, and posterior belly of the digastric; associated TrPs of the frontalis often occur in the clavicular head of the SCM.

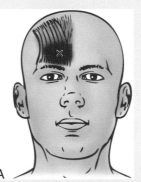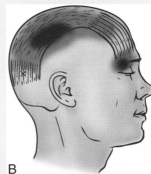

A   B

Figure 13-7 Common occipitofrontalis trigger points (TrPs) and their corresponding referral zones. **A,** Anterior view. **B,** Lateral view.

13

OCCIPITOFRONTALIS—SUPINE—*cont'd*

 DETOUR

Temporoparietalis and auricularis muscles:

The temporoparietalis and the three auricularis muscles (auricularis anterior, superior, and posterior) are other muscles of the scalp. The temporoparietalis attaches from the fascia superior to the ear to the galea aponeurotica; its action is to elevate the ear. The anterior and superior auricularis muscles attach from the galea aponeurotica to the ear; they move the ear anteriorly and superiorly, respectively. The auricularis posterior attaches from the mastoid bone to the ear; it moves the ear posteriorly. The temporoparietalis and all three auricularis muscles can also act to tighten the scalp. Because these scalp muscles are superficial, they are easy to palpate. However, if the client cannot voluntarily control the contraction of these muscles (engaging these muscles requires the ability to move the ear, which most people are unable to do), then they must be palpated based upon location only. However, it can be difficult to be sure of their exact location and discern them from adjacent soft tissue.

To palpate the temporoparietalis, palpate 1 to 2 inches (2.5 to 5 cm) superior and slightly anterior to the ear; ask the client to elevate the ear and feel for the muscle's contraction (Figure 13-8, B).

To palpate the auricularis muscles, palpate either immediately anterior, superior, or posterior to the ear, and ask the client to move the ear in that direction, feeling for the contraction of that particular auricularis muscle. Again, very few people can consciously contract these muscles, so it is usually necessary to palpate them by location while they are relaxed.

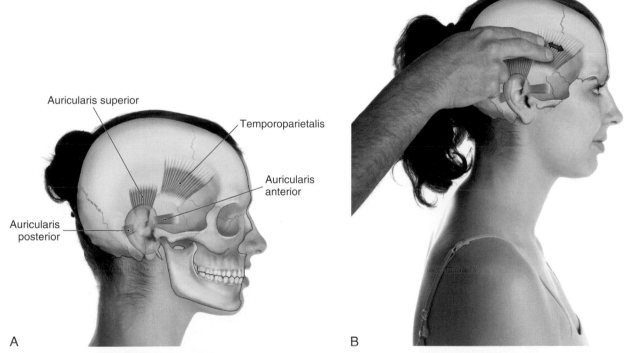

A

B

Figure 13-8 Other muscles of the scalp. **A,** Lateral view of the right temporoparietalis and auricularis muscles. **B,** Palpation of the right temporoparietalis.

13

TEMPORALIS—SUPINE

☑ ATTACHMENTS

☐ Temporal fossa

to the

☐ coronoid process and the anterosuperior aspect of the ramus of the mandible

☑ ACTIONS

☐ Elevates the mandible at the temporomandibular joints (TMJs)
☐ Retracts the mandible at the TMJs

Starting Position (Figure 13-10)

■ Client supine
■ Therapist seated at head of table
■ Palpating fingers placed over the temporal fossa

Palpation Steps

1. With palpating fingers over the temporal fossa, ask the client to alternately contract and relax the temporalis; this is accomplished by alternately clenching the teeth and then relaxing the jaw. Feel for the contraction of the temporalis as the client clenches the teeth (Figure 13-11).
2. Once the contraction of the temporalis has been felt, palpate the entire muscle as the client continues to contract and relax it as indicated in Step 1.
3. Once the temporalis has been located, have the client relax it and palpate to assess its baseline tone.

13

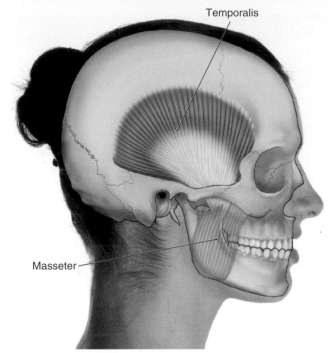

Figure 13-9 Lateral view of the right temporalis. The masseter has been ghosted in.

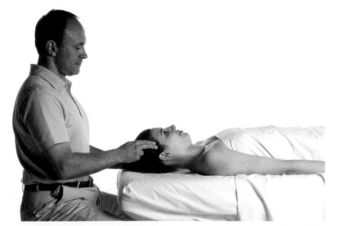

Figure 13-10 Starting position for supine palpation of the right temporalis.

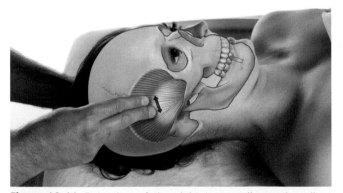

Figure 13-11 Palpation of the right temporalis as the client clenches the teeth.

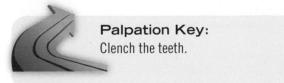

Palpation Key:
Clench the teeth.

TEMPORALIS—SUPINE—*cont'd*

PALPATION NOTES

1. Clenching the teeth requires elevation of the mandible at the TMJs, thereby engaging the temporalis.
2. The vast majority of the temporalis is superficial and easily palpable. Only a small portion at its inferior end (the portion of it that is deep to the zygomatic arch and the inferior attachment on the mandible) is not easily palpable.
3. The inferior attachment of the temporalis on the mandible can be accessed and palpated, especially if the client opens the mouth widely, causing the coronoid process of the mandible to drop down from behind the zygomatic arch. However, if the client is asked to contract the temporalis by elevating the mandible at the TMJs, the more superficial masseter also contracts, making palpation of the mandibular attachment of the temporalis difficult. For this reason, palpation of the mandibular attachment of the temporalis is best attempted with the musculature relaxed.
4. The mandibular attachment of the temporalis is also palpable from inside the mouth. With a gloved hand or a finger cot on your index finger, reach posteriorly into the vestibule of the client's mouth (between the cheeks and the teeth) and feel for the coronoid process of the mandible with the musculature relaxed. Once found, palpate on the anterior and medial surfaces of the coronoid process for the temporalis attachment (Figure 13-12). While palpating the mandibular attachment inside the mouth, it is awkward but possible to have the client contract the temporalis by asking the client to elevate the mandible.

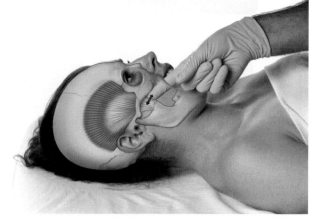

Figure 13-12 Palpation of the mandibular attachment of the right temporalis from inside the mouth.

Alternate Palpation Position—Seated

The temporalis is also easily palpated with the client seated.

13

TRIGGER POINTS

1. Trigger points (TrPs) in the temporalis often result from or are perpetuated by acute or chronic overuse of the muscle (e.g., chronic clenching or grinding of the teeth, excessive gum chewing or fingernail biting), prolonged stretching (e.g., keeping the mouth open during long dental procedures), occlusal asymmetry (poor bite), protracted head posture (creating pull on the hyoid muscles, which then pull on the mandible, requiring the temporalis to contract), TMJ dysfunction, direct trauma, having a cold draft on the head, emotional stress, or TrPs in the upper trapezius or sternocleidomastoid (SCM).
2. TrPs in the temporalis tend to produce headaches, pain and hypersensitivity of the upper teeth and the adjacent gums, occlusal asymmetry, or pain in the TMJ.
3. The referral patterns of temporalis TrPs must be distinguished from the referral patterns of TrPs in the upper trapezius, SCM, masseter, lateral and medial pterygoids, semispinalis capitis, orbicularis oculi, and buccinator.
4. TrPs in the temporalis are often incorrectly assessed as headaches, dental disease, or a TMJ disorder (e.g., osteoarthritis or other internal joint derangement).

5. Associated TrPs often occur in the contralateral temporalis, ipsilateral and contralateral masseters, lateral and medial pterygoids, upper trapezius, and SCM.

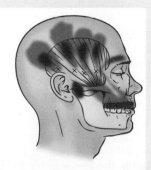

Figure 13-13 Lateral view illustrating common temporalis trigger points (TrPs) and their corresponding referral zones.

MASSETER—SUPINE—*cont'd*

TRIGGER POINTS

1. Trigger points (TrPs) in the masseter often result from or are perpetuated by acute or chronic overuse of the muscle (e.g., chronic clenching or grinding of the teeth, excessive gum chewing or fingernail biting), prolonged stretching (e.g., keeping the mouth open during long dental procedures), occlusal asymmetry (poor bite), protracted head posture (creating pull on the hyoid muscles, which then pull on the mandible, requiring the masseter to contract), TMJ dysfunction, direct trauma, emotional stress, or TrPs in the upper trapezius or sternocleidomastoid (SCM).

2. TrPs in the masseter tend to produce restricted depression of the mandible at the TMJs, pain and hypersensitivity of the upper and lower molar teeth and the adjacent gums, pain in the TMJ, occlusal asymmetry, puffiness of the ipsilateral eye (due to possible entrapment of the maxillary vein), or tinnitus or deeply felt pain in the ipsilateral ear.

3. The referral patterns of masseter TrPs must be distinguished from the referral patterns of TrPs in the upper trapezius, SCM, semispinalis capitis, temporalis, lateral and medial pterygoids, platysma, buccinator, and orbicularis oculi.

4. TrPs in the masseter are often incorrectly assessed as a TMJ disorder (e.g., osteoarthritis or other internal joint derangement), dental disease, headaches, or sinusitis.

5. Associated TrPs often occur in the contralateral masseter, ipsilateral and contralateral temporalis, lateral and medial pterygoids, upper trapezius, and SCM.

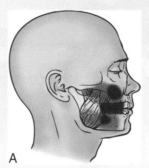 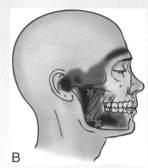

A   B

Figure 13-19 Lateral views illustrating common masseter trigger points (TrPs) and their corresponding referral zones.

STRETCHING THE MASSETER

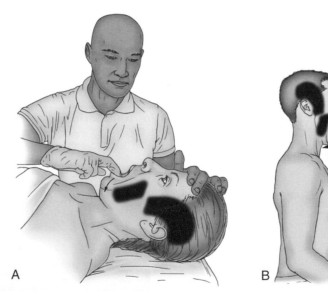

A   B

Figure 13-20 Stretching the right masseter and temporalis. The client's mandible is depressed with the hand as much as possible. **A,** Therapist-assisted stretch. **B,** Self-care stretch.

LATERAL PTERYGOID—SUPINE

☑ ATTACHMENTS

☐ Sphenoid bone

to the

☐ neck of the mandible and the capsule and articular disc of the temporomandibular joint (TMJ)

☑ ACTIONS

☐ Protracts the mandible at the TMJs
☐ Contralaterally deviates the mandible at the TMJs

Starting Position (Figure 13-22, *A*):

■ Client supine
■ Therapist seated at the head or the side of the table
■ Wearing either a glove or a finger cot, place your palpating finger inside the vestibule of the client's mouth (between the cheeks and the teeth), run along the external surfaces of the upper teeth until you reach the back molars; then press posteriorly and superiorly into a little pocket in the tissue between the gum above the upper teeth and the condyle of the mandible (see Palpation Note #2). You will be on the internal surface of the lateral pterygoid (see Figure 13-22, *B*).

Palpation Steps

1. With the palpating finger positioned inside the vestibule of the mouth, ask the client to either protract the mandible at the TMJs or to slowly and carefully contralaterally deviate the mandible (deviate it to the opposite side of the body), and feel for the contraction of the lateral pterygoid (Figure 13-23).
2. Once felt, palpate as much of the lateral pterygoid as possible, from the condyle of the mandible to the inside wall of the mouth (above the gum of the upper teeth).
3. Once the lateral pterygoid has been located, have the client relax it and palpate to assess its baseline tone.

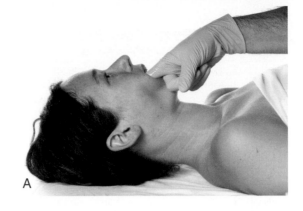

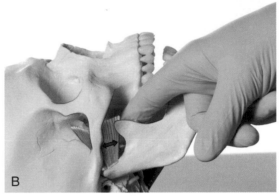

Figure 13-22 Starting position for supine palpation of the right lateral pterygoid. **A,** Palpation with a client. **B,** Palpation with a skull.

13

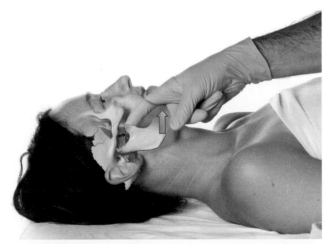

Figure 13-23 Supine palpation of the right lateral pterygoid as the client protracts the mandible.

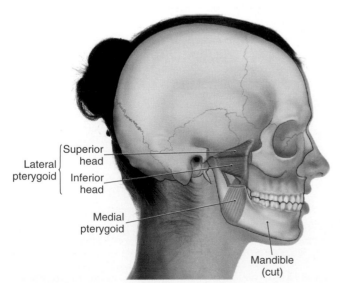

Lateral pterygoid { Superior head / Inferior head }
Medial pterygoid
Mandible (cut)

Figure 13-21 Lateral view of the right lateral pterygoid. The medial pterygoid has been ghosted in. Note: The mandible has been cut to better show the lateral pterygoid.

LATERAL PTERYGOID—SUPINE—cont'd

PALPATION NOTES

1. In addition to the neck of the mandible, the lateral ptery-goid also attaches into the capsule and disc of the TMJ.
2. When placing your palpating finger inside the vestibule of the client's mouth to locate the lateral pterygoid, press posteriorly and superiorly from the back molars, and search for what feels like a little pocket between the upper teeth and the condyle of the mandible. (Food such as peanut butter often gets stuck here!)
3. If you ask the client to contralaterally deviate the man-dible at the TMJs, the client must do so slowly and care-fully; otherwise your palpating finger may be pinched between the client's mandible and upper teeth.
4. The lateral and medial pterygoids are often quite sensi-tive to palpation. One reason for this is that they are covered only by a thin layer of mucosa.
5. Some sources state that the lateral pterygoid can be palpated from outside the mouth between the condyle and coronoid process of the mandible. However, it is difficult to palpate and discern the lateral pterygoid here because it is deep to the masseter. If you do attempt this palpation, ask the client to contralaterally deviate the mandible, and feel for the contraction of the lateral pterygoid.

13

Alternate Palpation Position—Seated

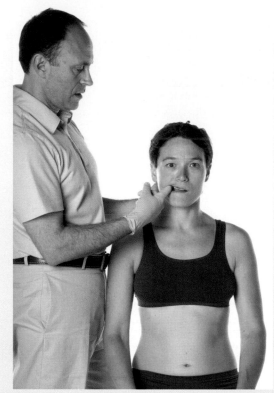

Figure 13-24 The lateral pterygoid is also easily accessed and palpated with the client seated.

TRIGGER POINTS

1. Trigger points (TrPs) in the lateral pterygoid often result from or are perpetuated by acute or chronic overuse of the muscle (e.g., chronic grinding of the teeth, excessive gum chewing or fingernail biting, using the jaw to help hold a violin when playing), occlusal asymmetry (poor bite), or protracted head posture (creating pull on the hyoid muscles, which then pull on the mandible, requiring the lateral pterygoid to contract).
2. TrPs in the lateral pterygoid tend to produce pain felt deeply in the TMJ, joint crepitus in the TMJ, restricted ipsilateral deviation of the mandible at the TMJs, occlusal asymmetry, tingling in the cheek or weakness of the buccinator muscle (if the buccal nerve is entrapped by the lateral pterygoid), or tinnitus.
3. The referral patterns of lateral pterygoid TrPs must be distinguished from the referral patterns of TrPs in the temporalis, masseter, medial pterygoid, sternocleidomastoid (SCM), and zygomaticus major.
4. TrPs in the lateral pterygoid are often incorrectly assessed as TMJ disorder (e.g., osteoarthritis or other internal joint derangement), sinusitis, tic douloureux, or ear infections.

5. Associated TrPs often occur in the contralateral lateral and medial pterygoids, the ipsilateral temporalis and masseter, and the SCM.
6. Notes: 1) The lateral pterygoid is the muscle of mastication most likely to have TrPs. 2) Unlike the temporalis and masseter, the lateral and medial pterygoids do not usually refer pain to the teeth.

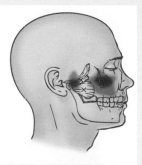

Figure 13-25 Lateral view illustrating common lateral pterygoid trigger points (TrPs) and their corresponding referral zones.

LATERAL PTERYGOID—SUPINE—*cont'd*

Palpation Key:
Find the pocket in the upper vestibule of the mouth where peanut butter gets stuck.

STRETCHING THE LATERAL PTERYGOID

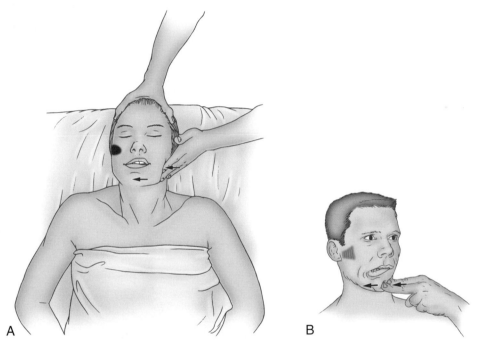

A   B

Figure 13-26 Stretching the right lateral pterygoid. The hand is used to laterally deviate the jaw to the right (same) side. **A,** Therapist-assisted stretch. Note that the therapist's other hand stabilizes the client's head. **B,** Self-care stretch.

13

MEDIAL PTERYGOID—SUPINE

☑ ATTACHMENTS

☐ Sphenoid and maxillary bones

to the

☐ internal surface of the mandible at the angle and inferior aspect of the ramus

☑ ACTIONS

☐ Elevates the mandible at the temporomandibular joints (TMJs)
☐ Protracts the mandible at the TMJs
☐ Contralaterally deviates the mandible at the TMJs

Starting Position (Figure 13-28)

■ Client supine
■ Therapist seated at the head or the side of the table
■ Palpating fingers curled around to the inside surface of the angle of the mandible

Palpation Steps

1. With palpating fingers hooked around to the internal surface of the angle of the mandible, ask the client to elevate the mandible at the TMJs by clenching the teeth, and feel for the contraction of the medial pterygoid (Figure 13-29).
2. Once felt, palpate the medial pterygoid as far superiorly as possible.
3. Once the medial pterygoid has been located, have the client relax it and palpate to assess its baseline tone.

13

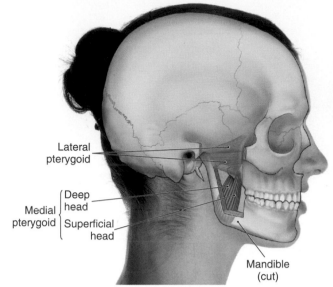

Figure 13-27 Lateral view of the right medial pterygoid. The lateral pterygoid has been ghosted in. Note: The mandible has been cut to better show the medial pterygoid.

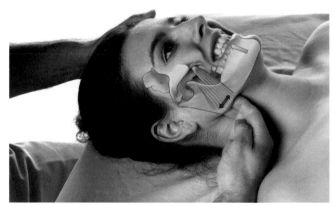

Figure 13-29 Palpation of the right medial pterygoid as the client clenches the teeth.

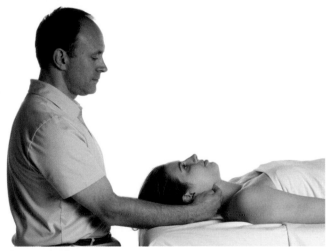

Figure 13-28 Starting position for supine palpation of the right medial pterygoid.

MEDIAL PTERYGOID—SUPINE—*cont'd*

PALPATION NOTES

1. The inferior attachment of the medial pterygoid can be easily palpated from outside the mouth. However, the vast majority of the muscle is palpable only from inside the mouth.
2. To palpate the medial pterygoid from inside the mouth, wearing a glove or finger cot, place your palpating finger along the internal surfaces of the lower teeth until you reach the back molars, then press posterolaterally until you reach the inside wall of the mouth. Now ask the client to protract the mandible and feel for the contraction of the medial pterygoid. Palpate as much of the medial pterygoid as possible by following it toward its attachments as the client alternately contracts and relaxes the muscle (Figure 13-30).
3. When palpating the medial pterygoid toward its attachments from within the mouth, it helps to visualize it as running identically to the masseter (except that the masseter is located on the external surface of the mandible and the medial pterygoid is located on the internal surface of the mandible).
4. The medial and lateral pterygoids are often quite sensitive to palpation. One reason for this is that they are covered only by a thin layer of mucosa.

Alternate Palpation Position—Seated

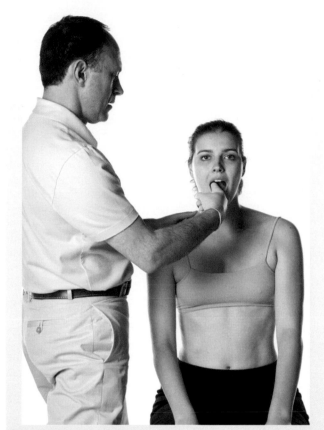

Figure 13-31 The medial pterygoid is also easily accessed and palpated with the client seated.

13

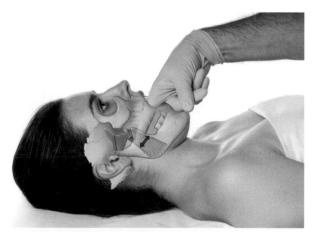

Figure 13-30 Palpation of the right medial pterygoid from inside the mouth (see Palpation Note #2).

MEDIAL PTERYGOID—SUPINE—*cont'd*

TRIGGER POINTS

1. Trigger points (TrPs) in the medial pterygoid often result from or are perpetuated by acute or chronic overuse of the muscle (e.g., chronic clenching or grinding of the teeth, excessive gum chewing or fingernail biting, using the jaw to help hold a violin when playing), prolonged stretching (e.g., keeping the mouth open during long dental procedures), occlusal asymmetry (poor bite), protracted head posture (creating pull on the hyoid muscles, which then pull on the mandible, requiring the medial pterygoid to contract), TMJ dysfunction, direct trauma, emotional stress, or TrPs in the other muscles of mastication.

2. TrPs in the medial pterygoid tend to produce a diffuse aching pain in the mouth (including the tongue) and the throat, TMJ pain, occlusal asymmetry (poor bite), pressure (often described as stuffiness) or pain felt deeply in the ear (when present, the pressure is caused by a eustacian tube blocked by a tight medial pterygoid that prevents the tensor veli palatini from opening the eustacian tube), pain or difficulty when swallowing, or restricted depression of the mandible at the TMJs.

3. The referral patterns of medial pterygoid TrPs must be distinguished from the referral patterns of TrPs in the lateral pterygoid, temporalis, masseter, sternocleidomastoid (SCM), longus colli and capitis, and inferior belly of the digastric.

4. TrPs in the medial pterygoid are often incorrectly assessed as a TMJ disorder (e.g., osteoarthritis or other internal joint derangement), headaches, an ear infection, a head cold, or a sore throat.

5. Associated TrPs often occur in the contralateral medial pterygoid, the ipsilateral and contralateral temporalis, masseter, lateral pterygoids, SCM, longus colli and capitis, and digastric.

6. Note: Unlike the temporalis and masseter, the medial and lateral pterygoids do not usually refer pain to the teeth.

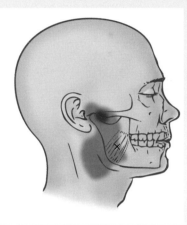

Figure 13-32 Lateral view illustrating a common medial pterygoid trigger point (TrP) and its corresponding referral zone.

STRETCHING THE MEDIAL PTERYGOID

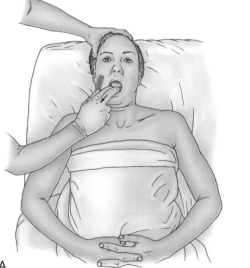

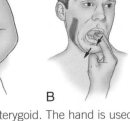

A   B

Figure 13-33 Stretching the right medial pterygoid. The hand is used to depress and slightly deviate the jaw laterally to the right (same) side. **A,** Therapist-assisted stretch. Note that the therapist's other hand stabilizes the client's head. **B,** Self-care stretch.

Palpation Key:
Curl your palpating fingers around to the internal surface of the angle of the mandible.

13

MUSCLES OF FACIAL EXPRESSION—SEATED

Muscles of facial expression are thin superficial muscles located within the skin and fascia of the face. These muscles can be divided into three groups: those that move the eye (three muscles), the nose (three muscles), and the mouth (eleven muscles).

All facial muscle palpations are shown in this chapter with the client seated. These muscles can also be palpated with the client supine and the therapist seated at the head of the table. Furthermore, only the index finger is shown palpating the target muscle so that less of the target muscle is obstructed for the reader. It is often preferable to palpate the muscles of facial expression using the finger pads of two fingers, the index and middle fingers. Palpating facial expression muscles requires gentle pressure and a sensitive touch.

Because muscles of facial expression are small, it may seem unimportant to stretch them. However, like any muscle, a facial expression muscle can become tight, especially

if the same facial expression is habitually created, requiring its repeated contraction. When a muscle of facial expression becomes tight, it pulls the overlying fascia and skin in toward its center, thereby creating wrinkles that are oriented perpendicularly to the direction of the muscle fibers. Examination of the typical pattern of facial wrinkles reveals that the wrinkles are perpendicular to the underlying muscles of facial expression. To stretch the muscles of facial expression, it is necessary to move the face by making a wide variety of strong expressions. Each expression stretches the muscles that create the opposite expression. For this reason, it is especially important to make facial expressions that you do not normally make.

Note: TrPs and their referral patterns have not been mapped out for all the muscles of facial expression. Facial expression muscles that have been investigated and mapped are the orbicularis oculi, zygomaticus major, levator labii superioris, and buccinator.

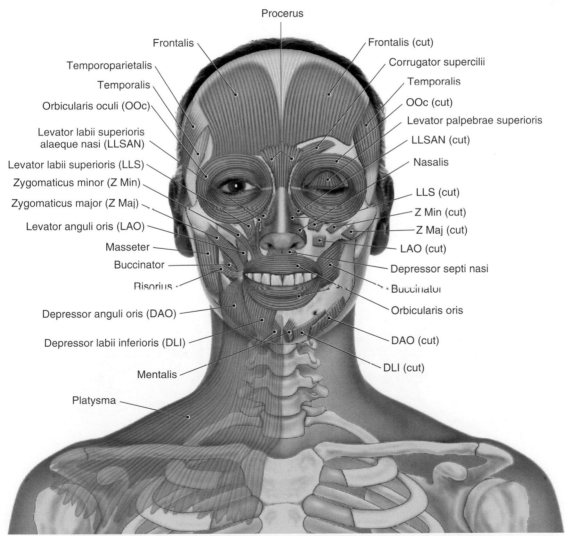

Figure 13-34 Superficial and intermediate anterior views of the muscles of the head.

MUSCLES OF FACIAL EXPRESSION—SEATED—*cont'd*

Facial Expression Muscles of the Eye

Orbicularis Oculi

✔ ATTACHMENTS

☐ The orbicularis oculi encircles the eye (Figure 13-35, *A*).

✔ ACTIONS

☐ Closes and squints the eye
☐ Depresses the upper eyelid
☐ Elevates the lower eyelid

Palpation Steps

1. Gently place palpating finger(s) on the tissue around the client's eye.
2. Ask the client to somewhat forcefully close the eye and feel for the contraction of the orbicularis oculi (see Figure 13-35, *B*).
3. Once felt, palpate the entire muscle as the client alternately contracts and relaxes it. Note: Be sure to distinguish the orbicularis oculi from the nearby corrugator supercilii by having the client try to isolate the actions of closing and squinting the eye, and not also drawing the eyebrows down into a frown.

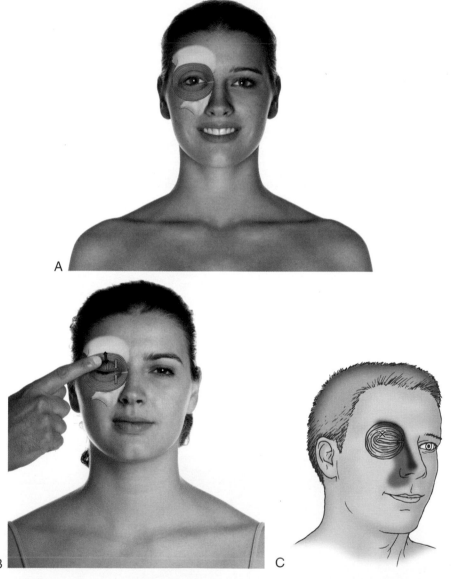

Figure 13-35 A, Anterior view of the right orbicularis oculi. **B,** Palpation of the right orbicularis oculi as the client somewhat forcefully closes the eye as if to squint. **C,** Anterolateral view illustrating a common orbicularis oculi trigger point (TrP) and its corresponding referral zone.

13

MUSCLES OF FACIAL EXPRESSION—SEATED—*cont'd*

TRIGGER POINTS

1. Trigger points (TrPs) in the orbicularis oculi (see Figure 13-35, *C*) often result from or are perpetuated by acute or chronic overuse of the muscle (e.g., habitual squinting or frowning) or TrPs in the sternal head of the sternocleidomastoid (SCM).
2. TrPs in the orbicularis oculi tend to produce pain in the nose.
3. The referral patterns of orbicularis oculi TrPs must be distinguished from the referral patterns of TrPs in the other muscles of facial expression, SCM, temporalis, masseter, and frontalis.
4. TrPs in the orbicularis oculi are often incorrectly assessed as sinusitis or headache.
5. Associated TrPs often occur in the other muscles of facial expression, muscles of mastication (temporalis, masseter, and the lateral and medial pterygoids), SCM, and upper trapezius.

Corrugator Supercilii

☑ ATTACHMENTS

☐ Inferior aspect of the frontal bone

to the

☐ fascia and skin superior to the eyebrow (Figure 13-36, *A*)

☑ ACTIONS

Draws the eyebrow inferomedially

Palpation Steps

- Gently place palpating finger(s) on the medial portion of the client's eyebrow.
- Ask the client to frown, bringing the eyebrows down, and feel for the contraction of the corrugator supercilii (see Figure 13-36, *B*).
- Once felt, palpate the entire muscle as the client alternately contracts and relaxes it. Note: Be sure to distinguish the corrugator supercilii from the nearby orbicularis oculi, which can also draw the eyebrow downward when it contracts.

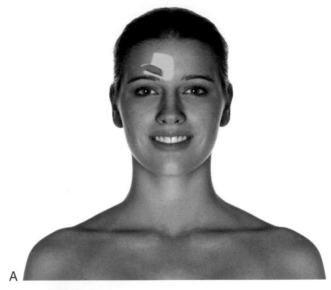

A

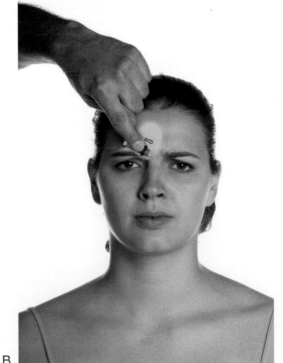

B

13

Figure 13-36 A, Anterior view of the right corrugator supercilii. **B,** Palpation of the right corrugator supercilii as the client frowns.

MUSCLES OF FACIAL EXPRESSION—SEATED—*cont'd*

Levator Palpebrae Superioris

☑ATTACHMENTS

☐ Sphenoid bone

to the

☐ fascia and skin of the upper eyelid (Figure 13-37, *A*)

☑ACTIONS

☐ Elevates the upper eyelid

Palpation Steps

- Gently place palpating finger(s) on the client's upper eyelid; ask the client to elevate the upper eyelid and feel for the contraction of the levator palpebrae superioris (see Figure 13-37, *B*).
- Once felt, palpate as much of the muscle as possible as the client alternately contracts and relaxes it.

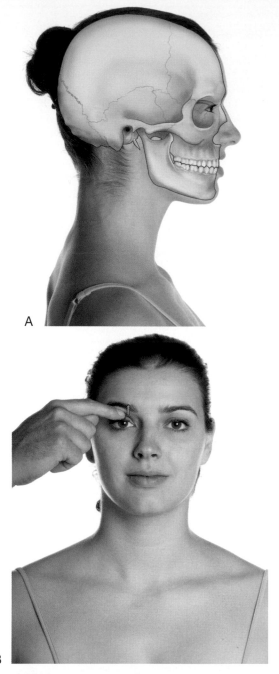

A

B

Figure 13-37 A, Lateral view of the right levator palpebrae superioris. **B,** Palpation of the right levator palpebrae superioris in the upper eyelid as the client elevates the upper eyelid.

MUSCLES OF FACIAL EXPRESSION—SEATED—*cont'd*

Facial Expression Muscles of the Nose

Procerus

☑ ATTACHMENTS

☐ Fascia over the nasal bone

to the

☐ fascia and skin between the eyes (Figure 13-38, *A*)

☑ ACTIONS

☐ Draws down the medial eyebrow
☐ Wrinkles the skin of the nose upward

Palpation Steps

- Gently place palpating finger(s) on the bridge of the client's nose.
- Ask the client to make a look of disdain, bringing the eyebrows down and/or wrinkling the skin of the nose upward, and feel for the contraction of the procerus (see Figure 13-38, *B*).
- Once felt, palpate the entire muscle as the client alternately contracts and relaxes it. Note: Be sure to distinguish the procerus from the nearby corrugator supercilii, which can also result in drawing the medial eyebrow downward when it contracts.

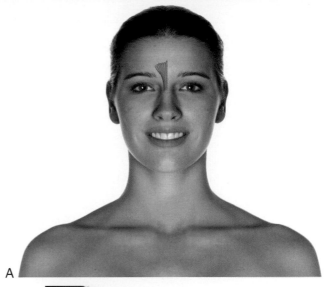

A

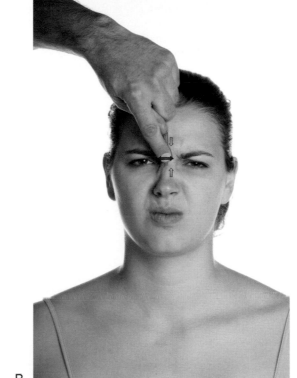

B

Figure 13-38 A, Anterior view of the right procerus. **B,** Palpation of the right procerus as the client makes a look of disdain.

13

MUSCLES OF FACIAL EXPRESSION—SEATED—*cont'd*

Nasalis

☑ ATTACHMENTS

☐ Maxilla

to the

☐ cartilage of the nose (and the opposite-side nasalis muscle) (Figure 13-39, *A*)

☑ ACTIONS

☐ Flares the nostril (alar part)
☐ Constricts the nostril (transverse part)

Palpation Steps

1. Gently place palpating finger(s) on the inferolateral aspect of the client's nose.
2. Ask the client to flare the nostril (as when taking in a deep breath), and feel for the contraction of the alar part of the nasalis (see Figure 13-39, *B*).
3. Once felt, palpate the entire alar part of the muscle as the client alternately contracts and relaxes it. Note: Be sure to distinguish the nasalis from the nearby procerus by making sure that the client does not also elevate the skin of the nose when flaring the nostril. Also, distinguish from the nearby levator labii superioris alaeque nasi, which can also flare the nostril.
4. To palpate the transverse part, place palpating finger(s) on the superolateral aspect of the client's nose and ask the client to constrict the nostril (as if pulling the middle of the nose down toward the mouth). Once felt, palpate the entire transverse part of the muscle as the client alternately contracts and relaxes it.

13

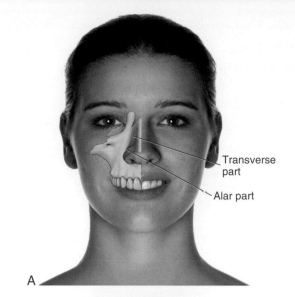

Transverse part

Alar part

A

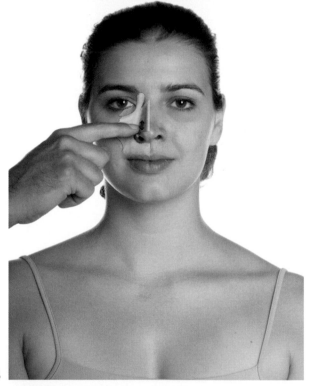

B

Figure 13-39 A, Anterior view of the right nasalis. **B,** Palpation of the alar part of the right nasalis as the client flares her nostril.

MUSCLES OF FACIAL EXPRESSION—SEATED—*cont'd*

Depressor Septi Nasi

☑ ATTACHMENTS

☐ Maxilla

to the

☐ cartilage of the nose (Figure 13-40, *A*)

☑ ACTIONS

☐ Constricts the nostril

Palpation Steps

1. Gently place palpating finger(s) directly inferior to the client's nose.
2. Ask the client to constrict the nostril (as if pulling the middle of the nose down toward the mouth), and feel for the contraction of the depressor septi nasi (see Figure 13-40, *B*).
3. Once felt, palpate the entire muscle as the client alternately contracts and relaxes it. Note: Be sure to distinguish the depressor septi nasi from the nearby orbicularis oris by making sure that the client does not also close and/or protract (protrude) the lips when constricting the nostril.

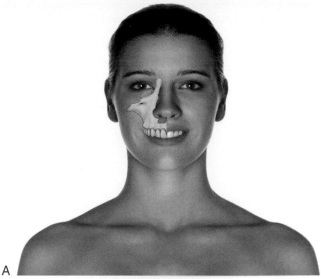

A

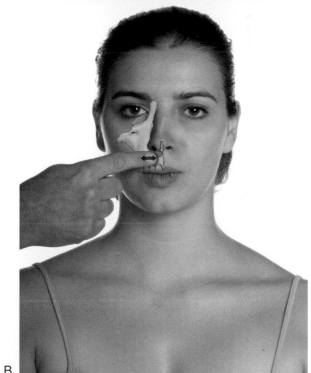

B

Figure 13-40 A, Anterior view of the right depressor septi nasi. **B,** Palpation of the right depressor septi nasi as the client constricts her nostril.

13

MUSCLES OF FACIAL EXPRESSION—SEATED—*cont'd*

Facial Expression Muscles of the Mouth

Levator Labii Superioris Alaeque Nasi

☑ ATTACHMENTS

- ☐ Maxilla

   to the

- ☐ fascia and muscle tissue of the upper lip and the fascia and cartilage of the nose (Figure 13-41, *A*)

☑ ACTIONS

- ☐ Elevates and everts the upper lip
- ☐ Flares the nostril

Palpation Steps

1. Gently place palpating finger(s) just lateral to the client's nose.
2. Ask the client to either elevate the upper lip to show you the upper gum or flare the nostril, and feel for the contraction of the levator labii superioris alaeque nasi (see Figure 13-41, *B*).
3. Once felt, palpate the entire muscle as the client alternately contracts and relaxes it. Note: It can be difficult to distinguish the levator labii superioris alaeque nasi from the nearby nasalis medially (which also flares the nostril), and the nearby levator labii superioris laterally (which also elevates the upper lip).
4. Additional note: The levator labii superioris alaeque nasi is considered to be a muscle of facial expression of the nose as well as of the mouth.

13

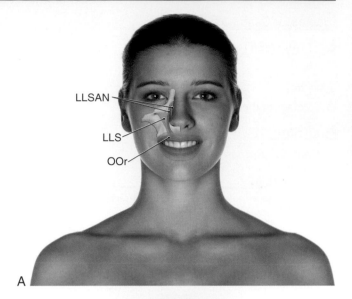

A

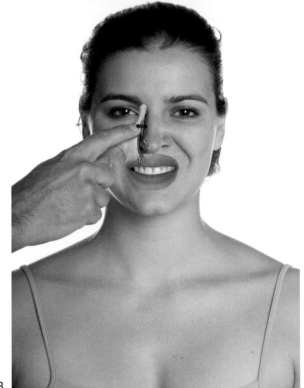

B

Figure 13-41 A, Anterior view of the right levator labii superioris alaeque nasi *(LLSAN)*. The orbicularis oris *(OOr)* and levator labii superioris *(LLS)* have been ghosted in. **B,** Palpation of the right levator labii superioris alaeque nasi as the client elevates the upper lip and flares the nostril.

MUSCLES OF FACIAL EXPRESSION—SEATED—*cont'd*

Levator Labii Superioris

☑ATTACHMENTS

☐ Maxilla

to the

☐ fascia and muscular tissue of the upper lip (Figure 13-42, *A*)

☑ACTIONS

☐ Elevates the upper lip
☐ Everts the upper lip

Palpation Steps

1. Gently place palpating finger(s) approximately ½ inch (1 cm) lateral to the center of the upper lip, at its superior margin.
2. Ask the client to elevate the upper lip to show you the upper gum, and feel for the contraction of the levator labii superioris (see Figure 13-42, *B*).
3. Once felt, palpate the entire muscle toward the eye as the client alternately contracts and relaxes it. Note: It can be difficult to distinguish the levator labii superioris from the nearby levator labii superioris alaeque nasi (medially) and zygomaticus minor (laterally), both of which contract with elevation of the upper lip.

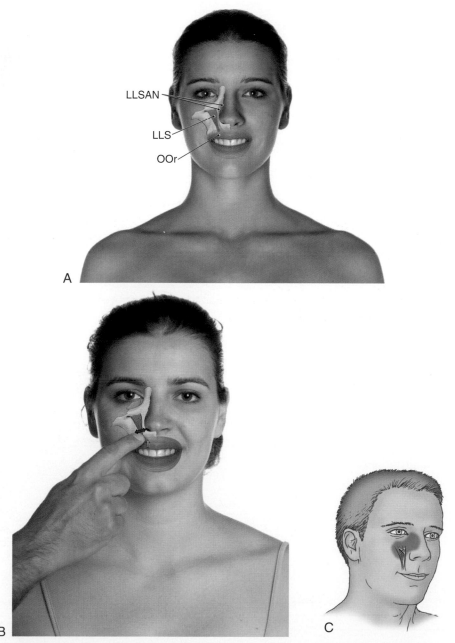

LLSAN

LLS

OOr

A

B

C

Figure 13-42 A, Anterior view of the right levator labii superioris *(LLS).* The orbicularis oris *(OOr)* and levator labii superioris alaeque nasi *(LLSAN)* have been ghosted in. **B,** Palpation of the right levator labii superioris as the client elevates her upper lip. **C,** Anterolateral view illustrating a common levator labii superioris trigger point (TrP) and its corresponding referral zone.

13

MUSCLES OF FACIAL EXPRESSION—SEATED—*cont'd*

TRIGGER POINTS

1. Trigger points (TrPs) in the levator labii superioris (see Figure 13-42, *C*) often result from or are perpetuated by acute or chronic overuse of the muscle (e.g., habitual smiling).
2. TrPs in the levator labii superioris may produce allergy symptoms (sneezing, itchy eyes) and apparent sinus pain.
3. The referral patterns of levator labii superioris TrPs must be distinguished from the referral patterns of TrPs in the other muscles of facial expression, SCM, temporalis, masseter, and frontalis.
4. TrPs in the levator labii superioris are often incorrectly assessed as sinusitis, a cold, or headache.
5. Associated TrPs often occur in the other muscles of facial expression, muscles of mastication (temporalis, masseter, and the lateral and medial pterygoids), SCM, and upper trapezius.

Zygomaticus Minor

☑ ATTACHMENTS

☐ Zygomatic bone

to the

☐ fascia and muscular tissue of the upper lip (Figure 13-43, *A*)

☑ ACTIONS

☐ Everts the upper lip
☐ Elevates the upper lip

Palpation Steps

1. Gently place palpating finger(s) approximately ½ to ¾ inch (1 to 2 cm) lateral to the center of the upper lip, at its superior margin.
2. Ask the client to elevate the upper lip to show you the upper gum, and feel for the contraction of the zygomaticus minor (see Figure 13-43, *B*).
3. Once felt, palpate the entire muscle toward the zygomatic bone as the client alternately contracts and relaxes it. Note: It can be difficult to distinguish the zygomaticus minor from the nearby levator labii superioris (medially), which contracts with elevation of the upper lip, and the nearby zygomaticus major (laterally), which contracts with elevation of the corner of the mouth.

13

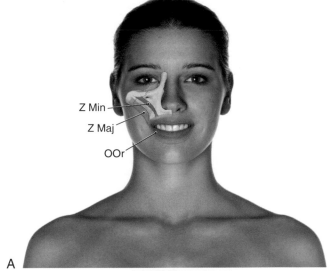

A

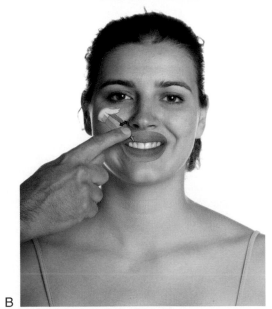

B

Figure 13-43 A, Anterior view of the right zygomaticus minor *(Z Min)*. The orbicularis oris *(OOr)* and zygomaticus major *(Z Maj)* have been ghosted in. **B,** Palpation of the right zygomaticus minor as the client elevates her upper lip. The zygomaticus major has been ghosted in.

MUSCLES OF FACIAL EXPRESSION—SEATED—*cont'd*

Zygomaticus Major

☑ ATTACHMENTS

☐ Zygomatic bone

to the

☐ fascia at the corner (angle) of the mouth* (Figure 13-44, A)

☑ ACTIONS

☐ Elevates the corner of the mouth
☐ Draws the corner of the mouth laterally

Palpation Steps

1. Gently place palpating finger(s) immediately superolateral to the corner of the mouth.
2. Ask the client to smile by drawing the corner of the mouth both superiorly and laterally, and feel for the contraction of the zygomaticus major (see Figure 13-44, *B*).
3. Once felt, palpate the entire muscle toward the zygomatic bone as the client alternately contracts and relaxes it. Note: It can be difficult to distinguish the zygomaticus major from the nearby levator anguli oris, which also elevates the corner of the mouth. Also, be sure to distinguish the zygomaticus major from the nearby zygomaticus minor, which contracts with elevation of the upper lip.

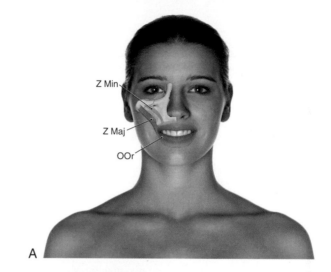

Z Min
Z Maj
OOr

A

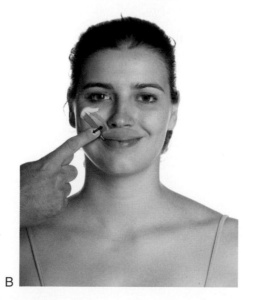

B

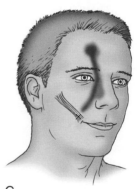

C

Figure 13-44 A, Anterior view of the right zygomaticus major *(Z Maj).* The orbicularis oris *(OOr)* and zygomaticus minor *(Z Min)* have been ghosted in. **B,** Palpation of the right zygomaticus major as the client smiles. The zygomaticus minor has been ghosted in. **C,** Anterolateral view illustrating a common zygomaticus major trigger point (TrP) and its corresponding referral zone.

13

---

*The term *modiolus* is used to describe the fascia at the corner of the mouth that is the common attachment for the zygomaticus major, levator anguli oris, risorius, depressor anguli oris, buccinator, and orbicularis oris. The modiolus can be easily palpated. Wearing either a glove or a finger cot, place the index finger of your palpating hand inside the client's mouth just lateral to the corner of the mouth, and your thumb outside the client's mouth in a similar location. Compress the skin and mucosa of the cheek just lateral to the corner of the mouth between your index finger and thumb, and feel for the modiolus.

MUSCLES OF FACIAL EXPRESSION—SEATED—*cont'd*

TRIGGER POINTS

1. Trigger points (TrPs) in the zygomaticus major (see Figure 13-44, *C*) often result from or are perpetuated by acute or chronic overuse of the muscle (e.g., habitual smiling).
2. TrPs in the zygomaticus major may produce allergy symptoms (sneezing, itchy eyes) and apparent sinus pain.
3. The referral patterns of zygomaticus major TrPs must be distinguished from the referral patterns of TrPs in the other muscles of facial expression, SCM, temporalis, masseter, and frontalis.

4. TrPs in the zygomaticus major are often incorrectly assessed as sinusitis, a cold, or headache.
5. Associated TrPs often occur in the other muscles of facial expression, muscles of mastication (temporalis, masseter, and the lateral and medial pterygoids), SCM, and upper trapezius.

Levator Anguli Oris

☑ ATTACHMENTS

☐ Maxilla

to the

☐ fascia at the corner (angle) of the mouth (Figure 13-45, *A*)

☑ ACTIONS

Elevates the corner of the mouth

Palpation Steps

1. Gently place palpating finger(s) immediately superior to the corner of the mouth.
2. Ask the client to elevate the corner of the mouth directly superiorly as if to show you the canine tooth (making what could be described as a Dracula-like expression), and feel for the contraction of the levator anguli oris (see Figure 13-45, *B*).
3. Once felt, palpate the entire muscle as the client alternately contracts and relaxes it. Note: The most superior aspect of this muscle is deep to the zygomaticus minor and levator labii superioris and can be difficult to palpate and discern from these muscles. Furthermore, try to distinguish the levator anguli oris from the zygomaticus major, which also elevates the corner of the mouth.

13

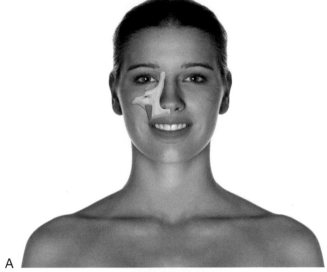

A

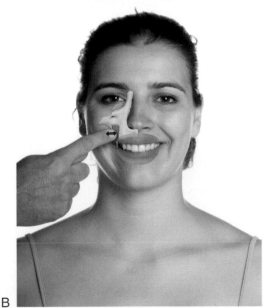

B

Figure 13-45 A, Anterior view of the right levator anguli oris. The orbicularis oris has been ghosted in. **B,** Palpation of the right levator anguli oris as the client elevates the corner of the mouth (making a Dracula-like expression).

MUSCLES OF FACIAL EXPRESSION—SEATED—*cont'd*

Risorius

✅ATTACHMENTS

- ☐ Fascia superficial to the masseter

  to the

- ☐ fascia at the corner (angle) of the mouth (Figure 13-46, *A*)

✅ACTIONS

- ☐ Draws the corner of the mouth laterally

Palpation Steps

1. Gently place palpating finger(s) immediately lateral to the corner of the mouth.
2. Ask the client to draw the corner of the mouth directly laterally, and feel for the contraction of the risorius (see Figure 13-46, *B*).
3. Once felt, palpate the entire muscle as the client alternately contracts and relaxes it. Note: Make sure that you are not palpating too far superiorly on the zygomaticus major, which can also draw the corner of the mouth laterally.

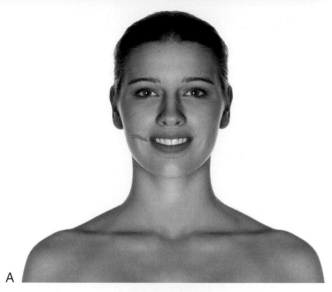

A

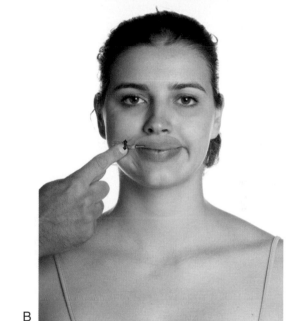

B

Figure 13-46 A, Anterior view of the right risorius. The orbicularis oris has been ghosted in. **B,** Palpation of the right risorius as the client draws the corner of the mouth laterally.

13

MUSCLES OF FACIAL EXPRESSION—SEATED—*cont'd*

Depressor Anguli Oris

✅ ATTACHMENTS

☐ Mandible

to the

☐ fascia at the corner (angle) of the mouth (Figure 13-47, *A*)

✅ ACTIONS

☐ Depresses the corner of the mouth
☐ Draws the corner of the mouth laterally

Palpation Steps

1. Gently place palpating finger(s) inferior and slightly lateral to the corner of the mouth.
2. Ask the client to frown by depressing and drawing the corner of the mouth laterally and feel for the contraction of the depressor anguli oris (see Figure 13-47, *B*).
3. Once felt, palpate the entire muscle as the client alternately contracts and relaxes it. Note: It can be very difficult to distinguish the depressor anguli oris from the nearby depressor labii inferioris, because both muscles engage with depressing and drawing laterally the lower lip/corner of the mouth.

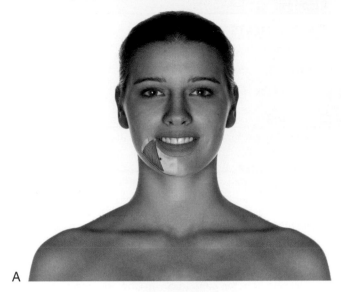

A

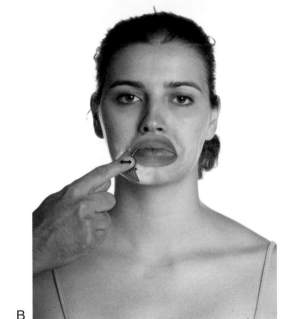

B

Figure 13-47 A, Anterior view of the right depressor anguli oris. The orbicularis oris has been ghosted in. **B,** Palpation of the right depressor anguli oris as the client frowns. The orbicularis oris has been ghosted in.

13

MUSCLES OF FACIAL EXPRESSION—SEATED—*cont'd*

Depressor Labii Inferioris

☑ ATTACHMENTS

☐ Mandible

to the

☐ fascia of the lower lip (Figure 13-48, *A*)

☑ ACTIONS

☐ Depresses the lower lip
☐ Everts the lower lip
☐ Draws the lower lip laterally

Palpation Steps

1. Gently place palpating finger(s) inferior to the lower lip and slightly lateral to the midline.
2. Ask the client to depress and draw the lower lip laterally, and feel for the contraction of the depressor labii inferioris (see Figure 13-48, *B*).
3. Once felt, palpate the entire muscle as the client alternately contracts and relaxes it. Note: It can be very difficult to distinguish the depressor labii inferioris from the nearby depressor anguli oris, because both muscles engage with depressing and drawing laterally the lower lip/corner of the mouth.

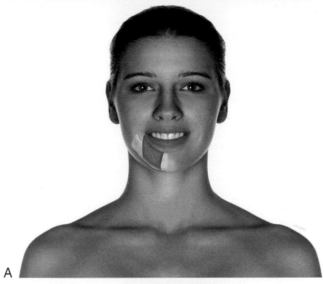

A

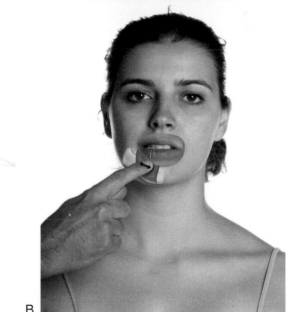

B

Figure 13-48 A, Anterior view of the right depressor labii inferioris. The orbicularis oris has been ghosted in. **B,** Palpation of the right depressor labii inferioris as the client depresses and draws the lower lip laterally. The orbicularis oris has been ghosted in.

13

MUSCLES OF FACIAL EXPRESSION—SEATED—*cont'd*

Mentalis

☑ ATTACHMENTS

☐ Mandible

to the

☐ fascia and skin of the chin (Figure 13-49, A)

☑ ACTIONS

☐ Elevates the lower lip
☐ Protracts the lower lip
☐ Everts the lower lip
☐ Wrinkles the skin of the chin

Palpation Steps

1. Gently place palpating finger(s) approximately 1 inch (2.5 cm) inferior to the lower lip and slightly lateral to the midline.
2. Ask the client to depress and stick out the lower lip as if pouting, and feel for the contraction of the mentalis (see Figure 13-49, *B*).
3. Once felt, palpate the entire muscle as the client alternately contracts and relaxes it. Note: The inferior aspect of the mentalis is superficial and easy to palpate. The superior aspect of the mentalis is more challenging to palpate and discern, because it is deep to the depressor labii inferioris.

13

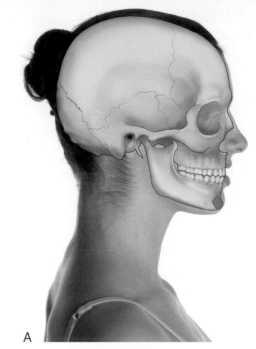

A

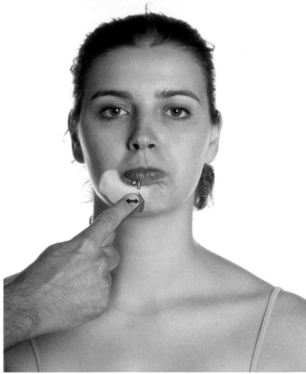

B

Figure 13-49 A, Lateral view of the right mentalis. **B,** Palpation of the right mentalis as the client sticks out the lower lip as if pouting.

MUSCLES OF FACIAL EXPRESSION—SEATED—cont'd

Buccinator

☑ATTACHMENTS

☐ Maxilla and the mandible

to the

☐ fascia at the corner of the mouth and the muscular tissue of the lips (Figure 13-50, *A*)

☑ACTIONS

☐ Compresses the cheek against the teeth

Palpation Steps

1. Gently place palpating finger(s) lateral and slightly superior to the corner of the mouth.
2. Ask the client to take in a deep breath, purse the lips, and press the lips against the teeth as if expelling air while playing the trumpet, and feel for the contraction of the buccinator (see Figure 13-50, *B*).
3. Once felt, palpate the entire muscle as the client alternately contracts and relaxes it. Note: Much of the buccinator is deep to the masseter and other muscles of facial expression, making its palpation and discernment more difficult.

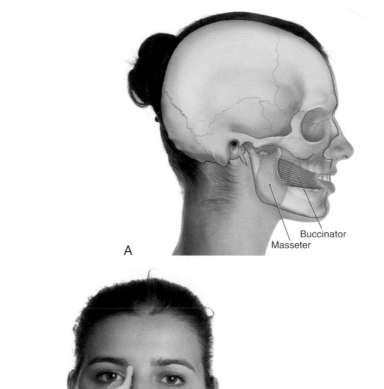

A

Buccinator
Masseter

13

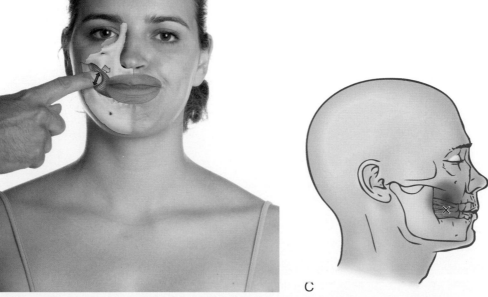

B

C

Figure 13-50 A, Lateral view of the right *buccinator*. The *masseter* has been ghosted in. **B,** Palpation of the right buccinator: after the client takes in a deep breath, the client purses the lips and presses the lips against the teeth as if playing the trumpet. **C,** Lateral view illustrating a common buccinator trigger point (TrP) and its corresponding referral zone.

MUSCLES OF FACIAL EXPRESSION—SEATED—*cont'd*

TRIGGER POINTS

1. Trigger points (TrPs) in the buccinator (see Figure 13-50, *C*) often result from or are perpetuated by acute or chronic overuse of the muscle (e.g., playing a brass or woodwind instrument or repeatedly blowing up balloons) or poor-fitting dental appliances (e.g., braces, night guards).
2. TrPs in the buccinator tend to produce a deep aching in the jaw and difficulty chewing and swallowing.
3. The referral patterns of buccinator TrPs must be distinguished from the referral patterns of TrPs in the other muscles of facial expression, the temporalis, and the masseter.
4. TrPs in the buccinator are often incorrectly assessed as a headache or TMJ dysfunction.
5. Associated TrPs often occur in the other muscles of facial expression, muscles of mastication (temporalis, masseter, and lateral and medial pterygoids), SCM, and upper trapezius.

Orbicularis Oris

☑ ATTACHMENTS

☐ The orbicularis oris encircles the mouth (Figure 13-51, *A*).

☑ ACTIONS

☐ Closes the mouth
☐ Protracts the lips

Palpation Steps

1. Wearing a finger cot or glove, gently place palpating finger(s) on the tissue of the lips.
2. Ask the client to pucker up the lips, and feel for the contraction of the orbicularis oris (see Figure 13-51, *B*).
3. Once felt, palpate the entire muscle as the client alternately contracts and relaxes it. Note: Be careful to distinguish the inferior aspect of the orbicularis oris from the mentalis, because both muscles elevate and protract the lower lip.

13

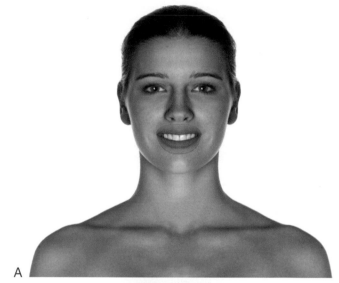

A

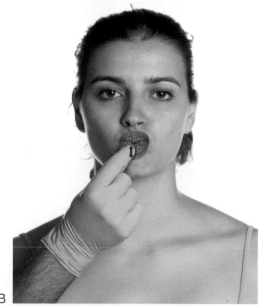

B

Figure 13-51 A, Anterior view of the orbicularis oris (bilaterally). **B,** Palpation of the orbicularis oris on the right side as the client puckers the lips.

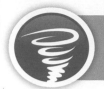

WHIRLWIND TOUR

Muscles of the Head

The following *Whirlwind Tour* is an abbreviated set of palpation protocols for the muscles of this chapter. Once you have read and become comfortable with each of the protocols presented thus far, this *Whirlwind Tour* allows you to quickly and efficiently run through the palpations protocols for all the muscles of the chapter.

For all palpations of the muscles of the head, the client is supine; you are seated at the head of the table.

Scalp Muscle(s)

1. **Occipitofrontalis:** First place palpating hands over the frontal bone, then over the occipital bone, each time feeling for the contraction of the occipitofrontalis as the client contracts the muscle by elevating the eyebrows. Once felt, palpate the entire muscle. Note: This muscle is often palpated just as well when it is relaxed.
2. **Detour to other scalp muscles (temporoparietalis and auricularis anterior, superior, and posterior):** For the temporoparietalis, palpate approximately 1 to 2 inches (2.5 to 5 cm) superior and slightly anterior to the ear; feel for the contraction of the temporoparietalis as the client elevates the ear. For the auricularis anterior, superior, and posterior, palpate immediately anterior, superior, and posterior to the ear, respectively, as the client tries to move the ear in that direction. Note: Most people are unable to control the contraction of these muscles, so they must usually be palpated when relaxed.

Muscles of Mastication

3. **Temporalis:** Place palpating fingers over the temporal fossa and feel for the contraction of the temporalis as the client elevates the mandible at the TMJs by clenching the teeth. Once felt, palpate the entire muscle as the client alternately contracts and relaxes it.
4. **Masseter:** Place palpating fingers between the zygomatic arch and the angle of the mandible, and feel for the contraction of the masseter as the client elevates the mandible at the TMJs by clenching the teeth. Once felt, palpate from the zygomatic arch to the angle of the mandible as the client alternately contracts and relaxes the muscle.
5. **Lateral pterygoid:** Wearing a finger cot or glove, run a palpating finger along the external surface of the upper teeth until you reach the back molars. Then press posteriorly and superiorly and feel for a little pocket. Palpate here for the lateral pterygoid between the condyle of the mandible and the gum above the upper teeth. To contract the lateral pterygoid, ask the client to either protract or slowly and carefully contralaterally deviate the mandible at the TMJs.
6. **Medial pterygoid:** Curl palpating fingers around the angle of the mandible to the internal surface and palpate for the contraction of the medial pterygoid's inferior attachment as the client elevates the mandible at the TMJs by clenching the teeth. Once felt, try to palpate it as superiorly as possible. Note: The medial pterygoid can be palpated inside the mouth. Wearing a finger cot or glove, run an index finger along the internal surfaces of the bottom teeth until you reach the back molars. Then press posterolaterally against the inside wall of the mouth, and feel for the contraction of the medial pterygoid as the client protracts the mandible at the TMJs.

Muscles of Facial Expression of the Eye

7. **Orbicularis oculi:** Gently place palpating fingers on the tissue around the client's eye. Ask the client to somewhat forcefully close the eye as if to squint, and feel for the contraction of the orbicularis oculi. Once felt, palpate the entire muscle as the client alternately contracts and relaxes it.
8. **Levator palpebrae superioris:** Gently place palpating fingers on the client's upper eyelid. Ask the client to elevate the upper eyelid, and feel for the contraction of the levator palpebrae superioris. Once felt, palpate as much of the muscle as possible as the client alternately contracts and relaxes it.
9. **Corrugator supercilii:** Gently place palpating fingers on the medial portion of the client's eyebrow. Ask the client to frown, bringing the eyebrows down, and feel for the contraction of the corrugator supercilii. Once felt, palpate the entire muscle as the client alternately contracts and relaxes it.

Muscles of Facial Expression of the Nose

10. **Procerus:** Gently place palpating fingers on the bridge of the client's nose. Ask the client to make a look of disdain, bringing the eyebrows down and/or wrinkling the skin of the nose upward, and feel for the contraction of the procerus. Once felt, palpate the entire muscle as the client alternately contracts and relaxes it.
11. **Nasalis:** Gently place palpating fingers on the inferolateral aspect of the client's nose. Ask the client to flare the nostril (as when taking in a deep breath), and feel for the contraction of the alar part of the nasalis. Then place the palpating fingers on the superolateral aspect of the client's nose and ask the client to constrict the nostril (as if pulling the middle of the nose down toward the mouth) and feel for the contraction of the transverse part of the nasalis. Once felt, palpate the entire muscle as the client alternately contracts and relaxes it.
12. **Depressor septi nasi:** Gently place palpating fingers directly inferior to the client's nose. Ask the client to constrict the nostril (as if pulling the middle of the nose down toward the mouth), and feel for the contraction of the depressor septi nasi. Once felt, palpate the entire muscle as the client alternately contracts and relaxes it.

13

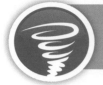

Muscles of the Head—*cont'd*

Muscles of Facial Expression of the Mouth

13. **Levator labii superioris alaeque nasi:** Gently place palpating fingers just lateral to the client's nose. Ask the client to either elevate the upper lip to show you the upper gum or flare the nostril, and feel for the contraction of the levator labii superioris alaeque nasi. Once felt, palpate the entire muscle as the client alternately contracts and relaxes it.

14. **Levator labii superioris:** Gently place palpating fingers approximately ½ inch (1 cm) lateral to the center of the upper lip at its superior margin. Ask the client to elevate the upper lip to show you the upper gum, and feel for the contraction of the levator labii superioris. Once felt, palpate the entire muscle toward the eye as the client alternately contracts and relaxes it.

15. **Zygomaticus minor:** Gently place palpating fingers approximately ½ to ¾ inch (1 to 2 cm) lateral to the center of the upper lip at its superior margin. Ask the client to elevate the upper lip to show you the upper gum, and feel for the contraction of the zygomaticus minor. Once felt, palpate the entire muscle toward the zygomatic bone as the client alternately contracts and relaxes it.

16. **Zygomaticus major:** Gently place palpating fingers immediately superolateral to the corner of the mouth. Ask the client to smile by drawing the corner of the mouth both superiorly and laterally, and feel for the contraction of the zygomaticus major. Once felt, palpate the entire muscle toward the zygomatic bone as the client alternately contracts and relaxes it.

17. **Levator anguli oris:** Gently place palpating fingers immediately superior to the corner of the mouth. Ask the client to elevate the corner of the mouth directly superiorly as if to show you the canine tooth (making what could be described as a Dracula-like expression), and feel for the contraction of the levator anguli oris. Once felt, palpate the entire muscle as the client alternately contracts and relaxes it.

18. **Risorius:** Gently place palpating fingers immediately lateral to the corner of the mouth. Ask the client to draw the corner of the mouth directly laterally, and feel for the contraction of the risorius. Once felt, palpate the entire muscle as the client alternately contracts and relaxes it.

19. **Depressor anguli oris:** Gently place palpating fingers inferior and slightly lateral to the corner of the mouth. Ask the client to depress and draw the corner of the mouth laterally, and feel for the contraction of the depressor anguli oris. Once felt, palpate the entire muscle as the client alternately contracts and relaxes it.

20. **Depressor labii inferioris:** Gently place palpating fingers inferior to the lower lip and slightly lateral to the midline. Ask the client to depress and draw the lower lip laterally, and feel for the contraction of the depressor labii inferioris. Once felt, palpate the entire muscle as the client alternately contracts and relaxes it.

21. **Mentalis:** Gently place palpating fingers approximately 1 inch (2.5 cm) inferior to the lower lip and slightly lateral to the midline. Ask the client to depress and stick out the lower lip as if pouting, and feel for the contraction of the mentalis. Once felt, palpate the entire muscle as the client alternately contracts and relaxes it.

22. **Buccinator:** Gently place palpating finger(s) lateral and slightly superior to the corner of the mouth. Ask the client to take in a deep breath, purse the lips, and press the lips against the teeth as if playing a trumpet, and feel for the contraction of the buccinator. Once felt, palpate the entire muscle as the client alternately contracts and relaxes it.

23. **Orbicularis oris:** Wearing a finger cot or glove, place palpating finger(s) on the tissue of the lips. Ask the client to pucker up the lips, and feel for the contraction of the orbicularis oris. Once felt, palpate the entire muscle as the client alternately contracts and relaxes it.

13

Review Questions

1. List the attachments of the lateral pterygoid.
2. List the attachments of the masseter.
3. What are the actions of the occipitofrontalis?
4. What are the actions of the medial pterygoid?
5. What is the *Palpation Key* for the temporalis?
6. In which muscles does the ability to move the ear make palpation easier?
7. How can a therapist access the inferior attachment of the temporalis?
8. What action of the masseter is the most advantageous for palpation? How can we best describe this action for a client in simple terms?
9. Describe the placement of the palpatory finger to begin assessing the lateral pterygoid.
10. Asking the client to take a deep breath, purse the lips, and press the lips against the teeth as if expelling air while playing the trumpet is the method of engaging which muscle for palpation?
11. Describe the method of palpating the nasalis.
12. TrPs in which muscles can mimic allergy symptoms (sneezing, itchy eyes) and sinus pain, and often result from habitual smiling?
13. In what way do referral patterns between the temporalis/masseter and the medial/lateral pterygoids differ?
14. A client using his hand to laterally deviate the jaw to the left side would be performing the stretch for which muscle(s)?
15. Describe how to stretch the pterygoid muscles both as a group and individually.
16. Describe some of the difficulties in palpating the muscles of facial expression and how to minimize their impact.

CASE STUDY

Over the past 6 months, a 60-year-old male client has been experiencing ringing in the ears, pain and a "popping" sensation in the TMJs, and a feeling of pressure deep to the right ear. He also has pain while chewing food or talking for long periods of time that registers a five out of ten on the pain scale. At rest it is two out of ten.

Prior treatment by another massage therapist failed to reduce the pain or other symptoms. Upon request of the client at discharge from the previous therapist, copies of session notes were given. The client presents them at intake, and you see that the other therapist mentions several times that the medial and lateral pterygoids are tight and "spasmed," but the extraoral techniques failed to produce the desired muscular release.

History shows no prior injury to the area, but he did have two root canals shortly before the symptoms began. There is no evidence of teeth grinding or infectious process. Physical examination reveals bilateral tightness and tenderness over the temporal fossas and the TMJs and general discomfort all along the mandible.

1. What specific muscles deserve further specific examination?
2. Discuss the considerations for intraoral and extraoral treatment of the muscles of mastication?
3. What home care advice would you give this client?

13

CHAPTER 14

Tour #4 **Palpation of the Muscles of the Arm**

Overview

This chapter is a palpation tour of the muscles of the arm. The tour begins with the deltoid, then covers the muscles of the anterior arm, and finishes with palpation of the posterior arm. Palpation for each of the muscles is shown in the seated position, but alternate palpation positions are also described. The major muscles of the region are each given a separate layout; there are also a number of detours to other muscles of the region. Trigger point (TrP) information and stretching, both therapist-assisted and self-care stretching, are given for each of the muscles covered in this chapter. The chapter closes with an advanced *Whirlwind Tour* that describes the sequential palpation of all of the muscles of the chapter.

Chapter Outline

Deltoid—Seated
Biceps Brachii—Seated
Brachialis—Seated
    Detour to the Brachioradialis
Coracobrachialis—Seated
    Detour to the Humeral Attachments of the Subscapularis, Latissimus Dorsi, and Teres Major
Triceps Brachii—Seated
    Detour to the Anconeus
Whirlwind Tour: Muscles of the Arm

Chapter Objectives

After completing this chapter, the student/therapist should be able to perform the following for each of the muscles covered in this chapter:
1. State the attachments.
2. State the actions.
3. Describe the starting position for palpation.
4. Describe and explain the purpose of each of the palpation steps.
5. Palpate each muscle.
6. State the "Palpation Key."
7. Describe alternate palpation positions.
8. State the locations of the most common TrP(s).
9. Describe the TrP referral zones.
10. State the most common factors that create and/or perpetuate TrPs.
11. State the symptoms most commonly caused by TrPs.
12. Describe and perform the therapist-assisted and self-care stretches.

e Go to http://evolve.elsevier.com/Muscolino/palpation for video demonstrations of the muscle palpations presented in this chapter.

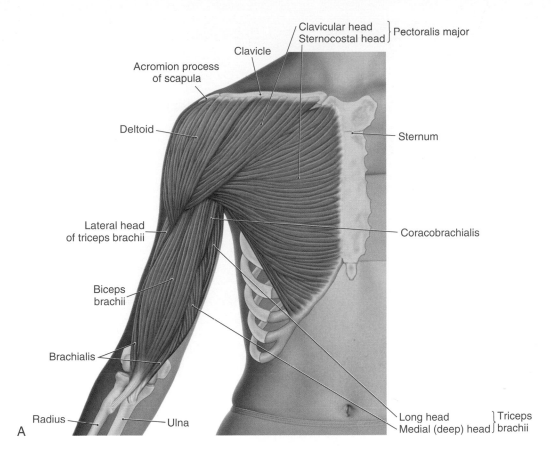

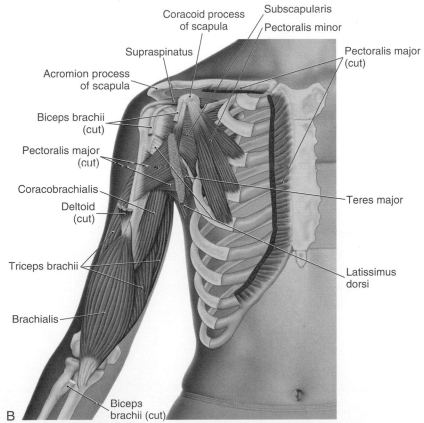

Figure 14-1 Anterior views of the right arm region. **A,** Superficial view. **B,** Deep view with the pectoralis major and deltoid cut and/or removed.

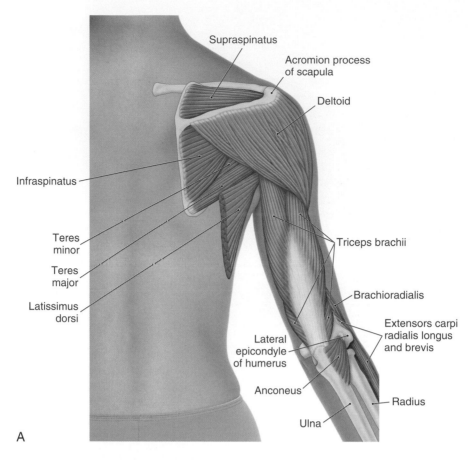

A

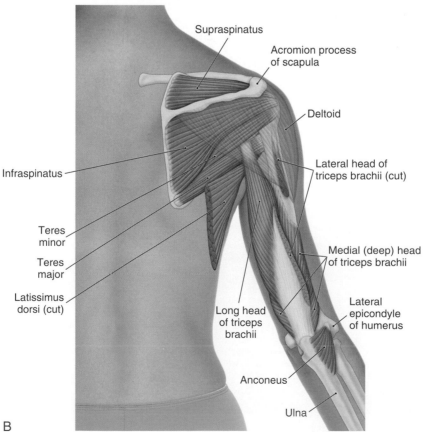

B

Figure 14-2 Posterior views of the right arm region. **A,** Superficial view. **B,** Deep view with the deltoid ghosted in.

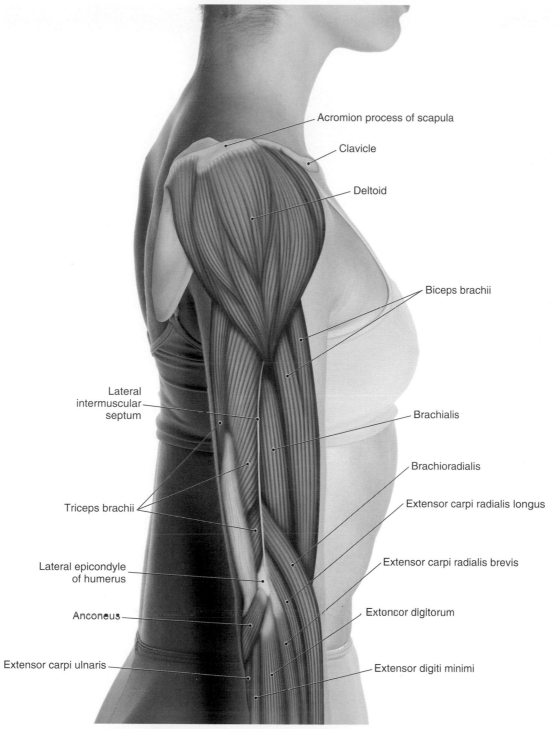

Acromion process of scapula

Clavicle

Deltoid

Biceps brachii

Lateral intermuscular septum

Brachialis

Brachioradialis

Triceps brachii

Extensor carpi radialis longus

Extensor carpi radialis brevis

Lateral epicondyle of humerus

Anconeus

Extensor digitorum

Extensor carpi ulnaris

Extensor digiti minimi

14

Figure 14-3 Lateral view of the right arm region.

14

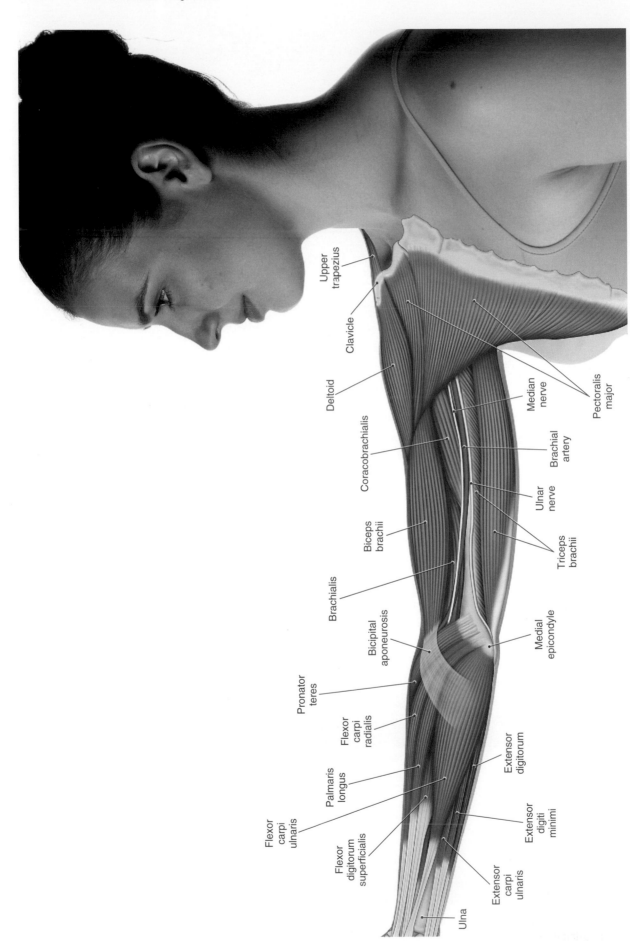

Upper trapezius

Clavicle

Deltoid

Coracobrachialis

Biceps brachii

Brachialis

Bicipital aponeurosis

Pronator teres

Flexor carpi radialis

Palmaris longus

Flexor carpi ulnaris

Flexor digitorum superficialis

Ulna

Extensor carpi ulnaris

Extensor digiti minimi

Extensor digitorum

Median nerve

Pectoralis major

Brachial artery

Ulnar nerve

Triceps brachii

Medial epicondyle

Figure 14-4 Medial view of the right arm region.

DELTOID—SEATED

☑ ATTACHMENTS

☐ Lateral ⅓ of the clavicle and the acromion process and spine of the scapula

to the

☐ deltoid tuberosity of the humerus

☑ ACTIONS

Entire deltoid:

☐ Abducts the arm at the glenohumeral (GH) joint
☐ Downwardly rotates the scapula at the scapulocostal and GH joints

The anterior deltoid also:

☐ Flexes the arm at the GH joint
☐ Medially rotates the arm at the GH joint
☐ Horizontally flexes the arm at the GH joint
☐ Adducts the arm at the GH joint (lowest fibers)

The posterior deltoid also:

☐ Extends the arm at the GH joint
☐ Laterally rotates the arm at the GH joint
☐ Horizontally extends the arm at the GH joint
☐ Adducts the arm at the GH joint (lowest fibers)

Starting Position (Figure 14-6):

■ Client seated
■ Therapist standing behind the client
■ Palpating hand placed on the lateral arm immediately distal to the acromion process of the scapula

■ Support hand placed on the distal arm, just proximal to the elbow joint

Palpation Steps

1. To palpate the entire deltoid, resist the client from abducting the arm at the GH joint and feel for the contraction of the deltoid.
2. Continue palpating the deltoid toward its distal attachment by strumming perpendicular to its fibers (Figure 14-7).
3. To isolate the anterior deltoid, place palpating hand just inferior to the lateral clavicle, resist the client from horizontally flexing the arm at the GH joint, and feel for the contraction of the anterior deltoid; palpate to the distal attachment while strumming perpendicular to its fibers (Figure 14-8, *A*).
4. To isolate the posterior deltoid, place palpating hand just inferior to the spine of the scapula, resist the client from horizontally extending the arm at the GH joint, and feel for the contraction of the posterior deltoid; palpate to the distal attachment by strumming perpendicular to its fibers (see Figure 14-8, *B*).
5. Once the entire deltoid has been located, have the client relax it and palpate to assess its baseline tone.

14

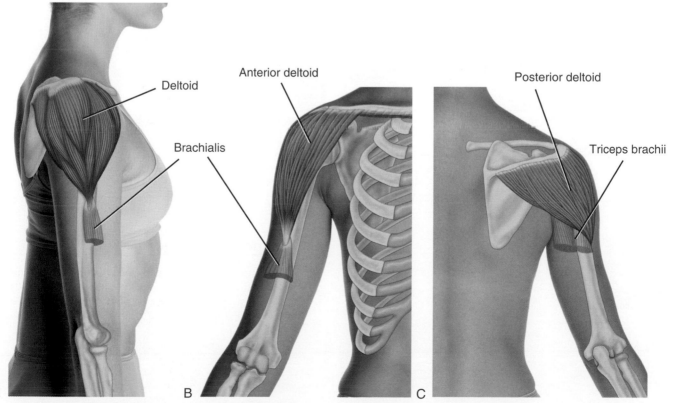

Figure 14-5 The right deltoid. **A,** Lateral view. The proximal end of the brachialis has been ghosted in. **B,** Anterior view. The proximal ends of the pectoralis major and brachialis have been ghosted in. **C,** Posterior view. The proximal end of the triceps brachii has been ghosted in.

DELTOID—SEATED—*cont'd*

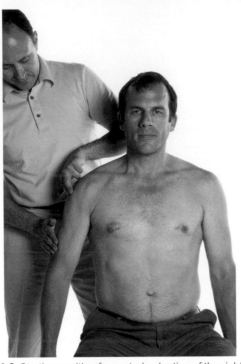

Figure 14-6 Starting position for seated palpation of the right deltoid.

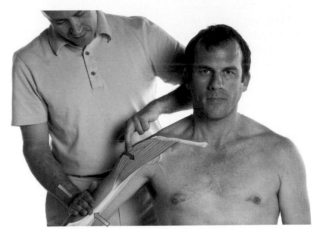

Figure 14-7 Close-up strumming of the right middle deltoid as the client abducts the arm against resistance.

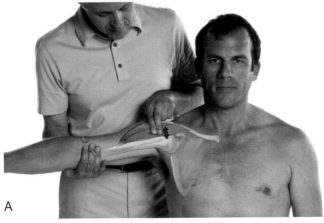

A

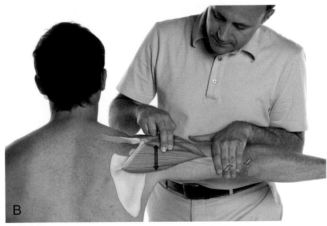

B

Figure 14-8 Palpation of the anterior and posterior deltoid. **A,** Palpation of the anterior deltoid as the client horizontally flexes the arm against resistance. **B,** Palpation of the posterior deltoid as the client horizontally extends the arm against resistance.

Palpation Key:
Resist abduction for the entire muscle.

Alternate Palpation Position—Supine

The anterior deltoid can be palpated with the client supine. See Palpation of the Anterior Deltoid in Tour #1 (p. 160).

The posterior deltoid can be palpated with the client prone. See Palpation of the Posterior Deltoid in Tour #1 (p. 147).

DELTOID—SEATED—*cont'd*

PALPATION NOTES

1. The posterior deltoid attaches on the spine of the scapula much further medially than most people realize. The attachment extends nearly to the root of the spine of the scapula.
2. When horizontally flexing the arm at the glenohumeral (GH) joint to palpate the anterior deltoid, the clavicular head of the pectoralis major also contracts. It is usually not difficult to discern the border between these two muscles, because there is usually a visible and palpable groove located between them.
3. Because the scapula sits in an oblique plane that is approximately 30 degrees off the frontal plane toward the sagittal plane, the motion caused by the entire deltoid is not necessarily pure abduction but also has a component of flexion.

TRIGGER POINTS

1. Trigger points (TrPs) in the deltoid often result from or are perpetuated by acute overuse, chronic overuse (e.g., holding the arm up in abduction for prolonged periods), direct trauma (e.g., impact during sports), injections, and TrPs in the supraspinatus or infraspinatus.
2. TrPs in the deltoid may produce weakness when performing abduction of the arm at the GH joint.
3. The referral patterns of deltoid TrPs must be distinguished from the referral patterns of TrPs in the scalenes, supraspinatus, infraspinatus, teres minor, teres major, subscapularis, pectoralis major and minor, coracobrachialis, biceps brachii, and triceps brachii.
4. TrPs in the deltoid are often incorrectly assessed as a rotator cuff tear, bicipital tendinitis, subdeltoid/subacromial bursitis, GH or acromioclavicular joint arthritis, or C5 nerve compression.
5. Associated TrPs often occur in the clavicular head of the pectoralis major, supraspinatus, biceps brachii, teres major, infraspinatus, triceps brachii, and latissimus dorsi.

14

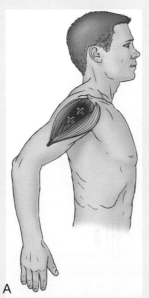
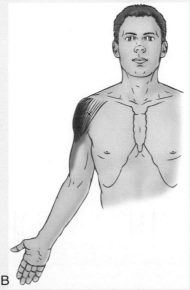
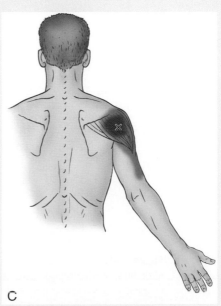

Figure 14-9 Common deltoid trigger points (TrPs) and their corresponding referral zones. **A,** Middle deltoid. **B,** Anterior deltoid. **C,** Posterior deltoid.

DELTOID—SEATED—*cont'd*

STRETCHING THE DELTOID

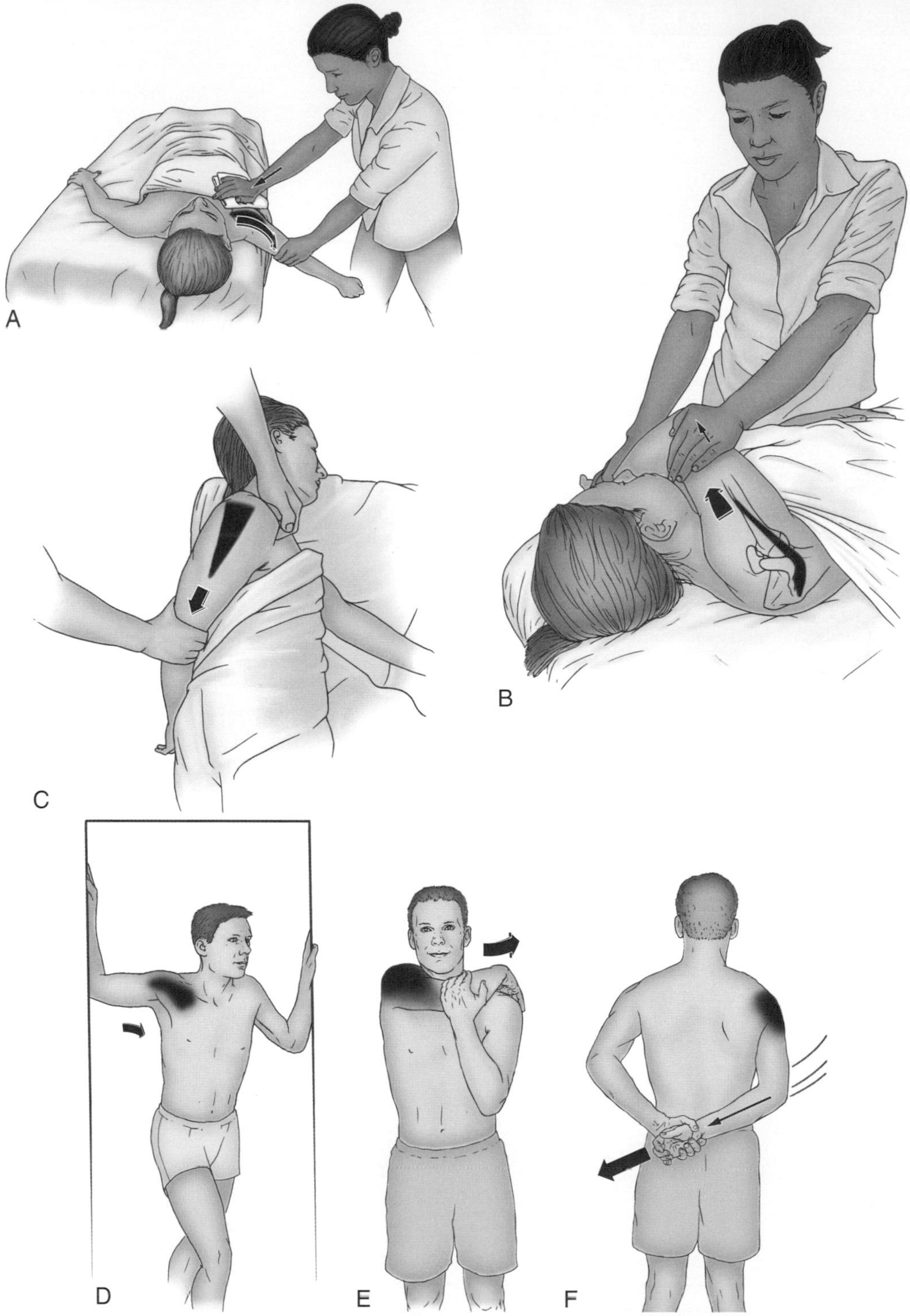

Figure 14-10 Stretching the three functional parts of the right deltoid. **A, B,** and **C,** Therapist-assisted stretching of the anterior, posterior, and middle deltoid respectfully. **A,** The arm is abducted to 90 degrees and horizontally extended. Note that the client's trunk/shoulder girdle is stabilized by the therapist's right hand; a cushion is used for comfort. **B,** The client's right arm is horizontally flexed, keeping the trunk facing forward. **C,** With the client side-lying, the client's arm is extended and dropped into adduction behind the body. **D, E,** and **F,** Self-care stretching of the anterior, posterior, and middle deltoid respectfully. **D,** The client presses the forearm against a doorframe and leans in by stepping in with the same-side foot. **E,** The client pulls the arm across the front of the body. **F,** The client pulls the arm behind the body. Note: See also Figure 11-50, *B* for another middle deltoid stretch.

BICEPS BRACHII—SEATED

✅ ATTACHMENTS

☐ Supraglenoid tubercle (long head) and coracoid process (short head) of the scapula

to the

☐ radial tuberosity and the deep fascia overlying the common flexor tendon

✅ ACTIONS

☐ Flexes the forearm at the elbow joint
☐ Supinates the forearm at the radioulnar joints
☐ Flexes the arm at the glenohumeral (GH) joint
☐ Long head abducts the arm at the GH joint
☐ Short head adducts the arm at the GH joint

Starting Position (Figure 14-12):

■ Client seated with the arm relaxed and the forearm fully supinated and resting on the client's thigh
■ Therapist seated to the side and facing the client
■ Palpating hand placed in the middle of the anterior arm
■ Support hand placed on the client's anterior distal forearm, just proximal to the wrist joint

Palpation Steps

1. With mild to moderate force, resist the client from flexing the forearm at the elbow joint, and feel for the contraction of the biceps brachii (Figure 14-13).
2. Strumming perpendicular to the fibers, first palpate to the distal tendon on the radius; then palpate toward the proximal attachments as far as possible.
3. Once the biceps brachii has been located, have the client relax it and palpate to assess its baseline tone.

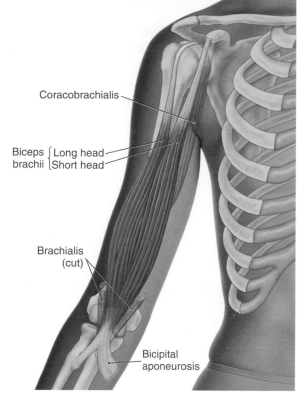

Figure 14-11 Anterior view of the right biceps brachii. The coracobrachialis and distal end of the brachialis have been ghosted in.

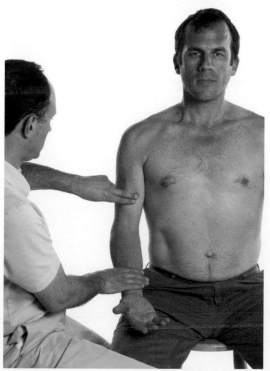

Figure 14-12 Starting position for seated palpation of the right biceps brachii.

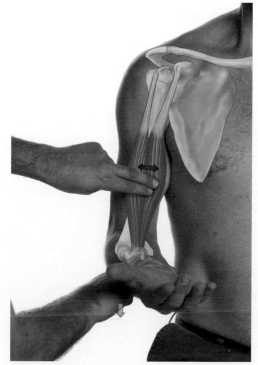

Figure 14-13 Palpation of the right biceps brachii as the client flexes the forearm at the elbow joint against resistance.

14

BICEPS BRACHII—SEATED—cont'd

PALPATION NOTES

1. Because the biceps brachii is a flexor and supinator of the forearm, it is best to resist the client's forearm flexion when the forearm is fully supinated.
2. It is important that the client's arm is fully relaxed and hanging vertically. Otherwise, flexors of the arm at the GH joint will have to contract to hold it in flexion, and the contractions of these muscles will make it more difficult to discern the biceps brachii from other muscles in the proximal arm.
3. In addition to palpating the biceps brachii when it is contracted, it is easy to palpate it when it is relaxed. When relaxed, the biceps brachii can usually be gently pinched away from the underlying muscles. Also, with the arm muscles relaxed, feel for the groove between the biceps brachii and the brachialis on the lateral side of the arm (Figure 14-14, *A*).
4. The biceps brachii is not as wide as most people think. It does not cover the entire anterior arm. Much of the

anterolateral arm is composed of the brachialis muscle. See Figure 14-1.
5. The distal aponeurosis of the biceps brachii that attaches into soft tissue overlying the common flexor tendon (near the medial epicondyle of the humerus) can often be palpated and discerned from adjacent soft tissue.
6. The proximal attachment of the biceps brachii on the coracoid process of the scapula can be palpated through the axilla by reaching deep to the pectoralis major and anterior deltoid. To do this, the pectoralis major and anterior deltoid must be slackened and relaxed; this can be accomplished by passively flexing the arm and supporting it in this position (see Figure 14-14, *B*) and slowly reaching toward the coracoid process with the palpating fingers. The proximal tendon of the long head of the biceps brachii can also be accessed in this manner albeit not as far proximally (see Figure 14-14, *B*); the supraglenoid tubercle attachment on the scapula is usually not palpable.

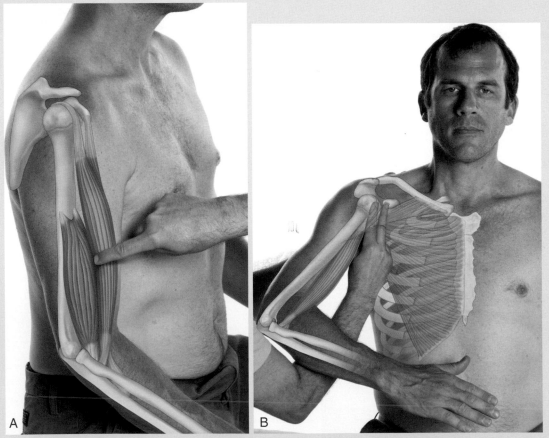

Figure 14-14 Palpation of the lateral border and proximal tendons of the right biceps brachii. **A,** Palpation of the border between the biceps brachii and the brachialis when they are relaxed. **B,** Palpation of the proximal tendons in the axilla deep to the pectoralis major (ghosted in) and anterior deltoid (not shown).

BICEPS BRACHII—SEATED—*cont'd*

TRIGGER POINTS

1. Trigger points (TrPs) in the biceps brachii often result from or are perpetuated by acute or chronic overuse of the muscle (e.g., lifting a heavy object with the forearm fully supinated at the radioulnar joints, prolonged use of a manual screwdriver) or TrPs in the infraspinatus.
2. TrPs in the biceps brachii may produce a pain that is superficial and dull, or restrict elbow joint extension.
3. The referral patterns of biceps brachii TrPs must be distinguished from the referral patterns of TrPs in the deltoid, coracobrachialis, brachialis, supinator, pectoralis major and minor, subclavius, infraspinatus, subscapularis, and scalenes.
4. TrPs in the biceps brachii are often incorrectly assessed as bicipital tendinitis, subdeltoid/subacromial bursitis, GH joint arthritis, or C5 nerve compression.
5. Associated TrPs often occur in the brachialis, coracobrachialis, supinator, triceps brachii, anterior deltoid, supraspinatus, upper trapezius, and coracobrachialis.

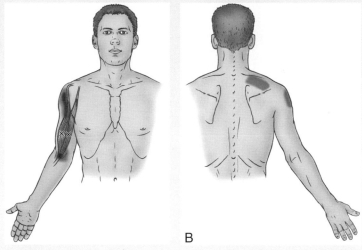

A   B

Figure 14-15 A, Anterior view illustrating common biceps brachii trigger points (TrPs) and their corresponding referral zone. **B,** Posterior view showing the remainder of the referral zone.

14

Palpation Key:
Resist forearm flexion with the forearm fully supinated.

Alternate Palpation Position—Supine

The biceps brachii can also be easily palpated with the client supine. Follow the seated directions.

BICEPS BRACHII—SEATED—*cont'd*

STRETCHING THE BICEPS BRACHII

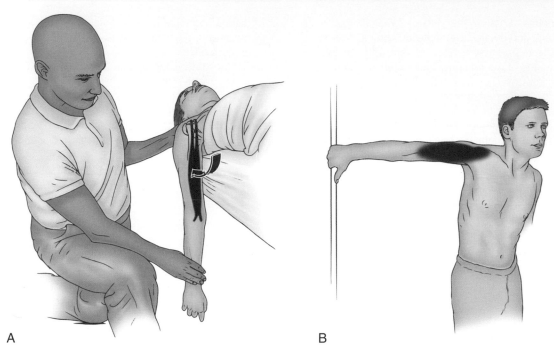

A   B

Figure 14-16 Stretching the right biceps brachii. The elbow joint is fully extended with the forearm fully pronated. **A,** Therapist-assisted stretch. The therapist contacts the client's forearm to bring the arm back into further extension. Note that the therapist stabilizes the client's shoulder girdle with the other hand. **B,** Self-care stretch. The client holds onto a doorframe and leans away.

14

BRACHIALIS—SEATED

☑ ATTACHMENTS

☐ Distal ½ of the anterior shaft of the humerus (beginning just distal to the deltoid tuberosity)

to the

☐ tuberosity and coronoid process of the ulna

☑ ACTIONS

☐ Flexes the forearm at the elbow joint

Starting Position (Figure 14-18)

■ Client seated with the arm relaxed and the forearm fully pronated and resting on the client's thigh
■ Therapist seated to the side and facing the client
■ Palpating hand placed on the anterolateral arm (immediately posterior to the biceps brachii)
■ Supporting hand placed on the client's anterior distal forearm, just proximal to the wrist joint

Palpation Steps

1. With gentle force, resist the client from flexing the forearm at the elbow joint (with the forearm fully pronated), and feel for the contraction of the brachialis (Figure 14-19).
2. Strumming perpendicular to the fibers, palpate the lateral side of the brachialis to its proximal attachment and then to its distal attachment.
3. The preceding two steps can also be used to palpate the anterior aspect of the brachialis through the relaxed biceps brachii, as the brachialis is contracting.
4. Once the brachialis has been located, have the client relax it and palpate to assess its baseline tone.

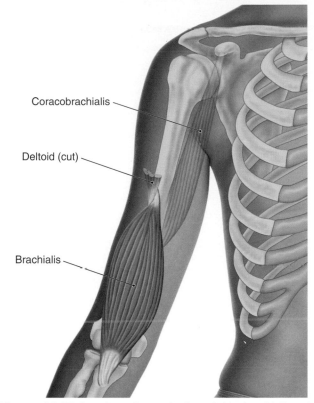

Figure 14-17 Anterior view of the right brachialis; the coracobrachialis and distal end of the deltoid have been ghosted in.

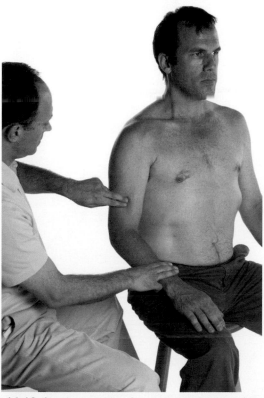

Figure 14-18 Starting position for seated palpation of the right brachialis.

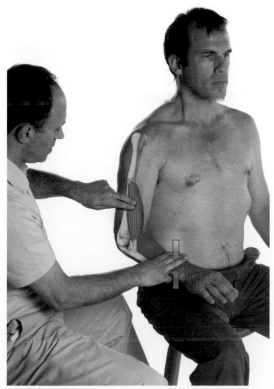

Figure 14-19 Palpation of the right brachialis as the client is gently resisted from flexing the forearm at the elbow joint with the forearm in a fully pronated position.

14

BRACHIALIS—SEATED—*cont'd*

PALPATION NOTES

1. The brachialis can flex the forearm at the elbow joint whether the forearm is pronated or supinated. The reason that it is important to palpate the brachialis (the lateral or anterior aspect) with the forearm pronated is that it relaxes the biceps brachii via reciprocal inhibition (the biceps brachii is a supinator of the forearm). However, resistance to the client's forearm flexion must be gentle, or reciprocal inhibition will be overridden and the biceps brachii will be recruited to contract, making palpation of the brachialis more difficult.
2. The proximal attachment of the brachialis is located around the deltoid tuberosity of the humerus; therefore this landmark is useful to help locate the brachialis.
3. The anterior aspect of the brachialis does not have to be palpated through the biceps brachii; rather, it can also be palpated directly. Passively flex the client's fully supinated forearm approximately 45 degrees to relax and slacken the biceps brachii. Locate the border between these two muscles and push the biceps brachii medially out of the way. Now palpate posteriorly toward the shaft of the humerus to palpate directly the anterior aspect of the brachialis (Figure 14-20).
4. The medial aspect of the brachialis is partially superficial and palpable in the distal half of the medial arm. Palpation here must be done prudently due to the presence of the brachial artery and the median and ulnar nerves (see Figure 14-4).
5. It is difficult to palpate the brachialis all the way to its ulnar attachment.

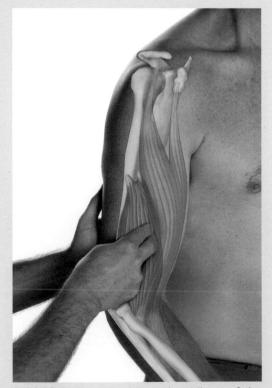

Figure 14-20 Pushing the biceps brachii out of the way medially to access the anterior aspect of the right brachialis.

Alternate Palpation Position—Supine

The brachialis can also be easily palpated with the client supine. Follow the seated directions.

TRIGGER POINTS

1. Trigger points (TrPs) in the brachialis often result from or are perpetuated by acute or chronic overuse of the muscle (e.g., heavy lifting, especially with forearms fully pronated) or prolonged shortening of the muscle (e.g., sleeping with elbow joint fully flexed).
2. TrPs in the brachialis may produce soreness of the thumb or radial nerve entrapment.
3. The referral patterns of brachialis TrPs must be distinguished from the referral patterns of TrPs in the brachioradialis, subclavius, extensor carpi radialis longus, pronator teres, supinator, adductor pollicis, opponens pollicis, and scalenes.
4. TrPs in the brachialis are often incorrectly assessed as bicipital tendinitis, supraspinatus tendinitis, C5 or C6 nerve compression, or carpal tunnel syndrome.
5. Associated TrPs often occur in the biceps brachii, brachioradialis, supinator, and adductor pollicis.

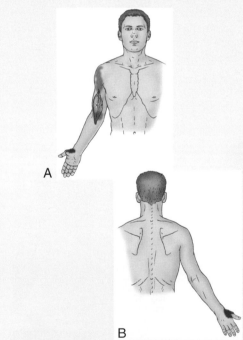

Figure 14-21 A, Anterior view illustrating common brachialis trigger points (TrPs) and their corresponding referral zone. **B,** Posterior view showing the remainder of the referral zone.

Palpation Key:
Gently resist forearm flexion with the forearm fully pronated.

BRACHIALIS—SEATED—*cont'd*

STRETCHING THE BRACHIALIS

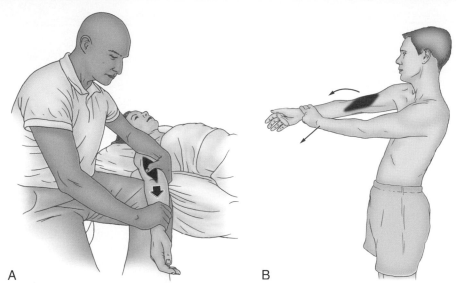

A   B

Figure 14-22 Stretching the right brachialis. The client's elbow joint is fully extended with the forearm in a position that is halfway between full supination and full pronation. **A,** Therapist-assisted stretch. The therapist's knee is used as a pivot under the elbow joint to maximize extension of the elbow joint. **B,** Self-care stretch. The client's other hand is used to pull the elbow joint into full extension.

 DETOUR

Brachioradialis:

The three major flexors of the forearm at the elbow joint—the biceps brachii, brachialis, and brachioradialis—are all palpated by resisting flexion of the forearm at the elbow joint. The difference is that the biceps brachii is palpated with the forearm in full supination; the brachialis is palpated with the forearm in full pronation; and the brachioradialis is palpated with the forearm in a position that is halfway between full supination and full pronation.

14

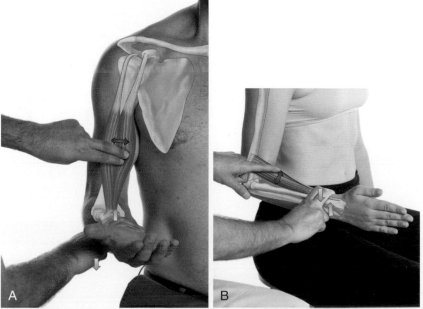

A   B

Figure 14-23 Palpation of the right biceps brachii and brachioradialis. **A,** Palpation of the biceps brachii with the client's forearm in full supination. **B,** Palpation of the brachioradialis with the client's forearm positioned halfway between full supination and full pronation.

CORACOBRACHIALIS—SEATED

✅ ATTACHMENTS

☐ Coracoid process of the scapula

to the

☐ middle ⅓ of the medial shaft of the humerus

✅ ACTIONS

☐ Flexes the arm at the glenohumeral (GH) joint
☐ Adducts the arm at the GH joint
☐ Horizontally flexes the arm at the GH joint

Starting Position (Figure 14-25)

■ Client seated with the arm abducted to 90 degrees and laterally rotated at the GH joint, and the forearm flexed at the elbow joint approximately 90 degrees
■ Therapist seated or standing in front of the client
■ Palpating hand placed on the medial aspect of the proximal half of the client's arm
■ Support hand placed on the distal end of the client's arm, just proximal to the elbow joint

Palpation Steps

1. Resist the client's horizontal flexion of the arm at the GH joint, and feel for the contraction of the coracobrachialis (Figure 14-26).
2. Strumming perpendicular to the fibers, palpate from attachment to attachment.
3. Once the coracobrachialis has been located, have the client relax it and palpate to assess its baseline tone.

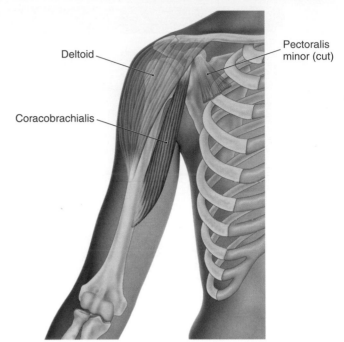

Figure 14-24 Anterior view of the right coracobrachialis. The deltoid and proximal end of the pectoralis minor have been ghosted in.

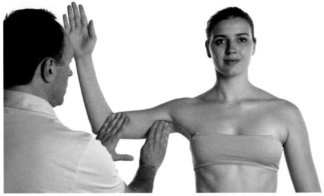

Figure 14-25 Starting position for seated palpation of the right coracobrachialis.

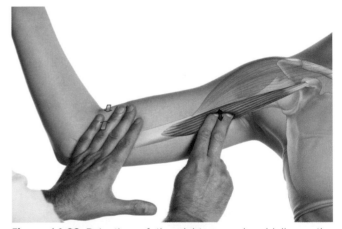

Figure 14-26 Palpation of the right coracobrachialis as the client horizontally flexes the arm at the glenohumeral (GH) joint against resistance. Note: The deltoid has been ghosted in.

🖐 PALPATION NOTES

1. To easily discern the coracobrachialis from the short head of the biceps brachii, it is important for the forearm to be passively flexed 90 degrees or more so that the biceps brachii stays relaxed.
2. If there is doubt as to whether you are on the coracobrachialis or the short head of the biceps brachii, resist the client from performing flexion of the forearm at the elbow joint. This will cause the short head of the biceps brachii

to contract, but not the coracobrachialis. Where these two muscles overlap, the coracobrachialis is deep (posterior) to the short head of the biceps brachii.
3. Palpation of the coracobrachialis must be done prudently because of the presence of the brachial artery and the median, ulnar, and musculocutaneous nerves (see Figure 14-4).

CORACOBRACHIALIS—SEATED—*cont'd*

TRIGGER POINTS

1. Trigger points (TrPs) in the coracobrachialis often result from or are perpetuated by acute or chronic overuse of the muscle (e.g., lifting heavy objects in front of the body) or TrPs in synergistic muscles.
2. TrPs in the coracobrachialis may produce severe pain, restricted (GH joint motion (abduction and extension), and entrapment of the musculocutaneous nerve.
3. The referral patterns of coracobrachialis TrPs must be distinguished from the referral patterns of TrPs in the biceps brachii, triceps brachii, scalenes, supraspinatus, infraspinatus, anterior deltoid, pectoralis major and minor, extensor carpi radialis longus, extensor digitorum, extensor indicis, and second dorsal interosseus manus.
4. TrPs in the coracobrachialis are often incorrectly assessed as carpal tunnel syndrome, subdeltoid/subacromial bursitis, acromioclavicular joint arthritis, supraspinatus tendinitis, or C5, C6, or C7 nerve compression.
5. Associated TrPs often occur in the anterior deltoid, biceps brachii, pectoralis major, and triceps brachii long head.

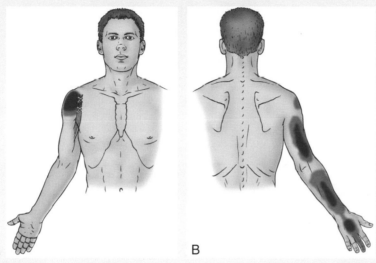

A   B

Figure 14-27 A, Anterior view illustrating common coracobrachialis trigger points (TrPs) and their corresponding referral zone. **B,** Posterior view showing the remainder of the referral zone.

14

Alternate Palpation Position—Supine

The coracobrachialis can be palpated with the client supine. Follow the seated directions.

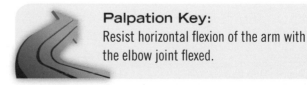

Palpation Key:
Resist horizontal flexion of the arm with the elbow joint flexed.

CORACOBRACHIALIS—SEATED—*cont'd*

STRETCHING THE CORACOBRACHIALIS

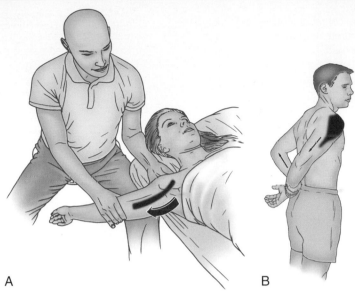

A   B

Figure 14-28 Stretching the right coracobrachialis. **A,** Therapist-assisted stretch. The client's arm is brought back into extension and abduction. Note that the therapist's left hand stabilizes the client's shoulder girdle. **B,** Self-care stretch. The client's arm is extended and adducted behind the body.

DETOUR

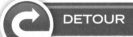

Humeral Attachments of the Subscapularis, Latissimus Dorsi, and Teres Major:

If the humeral attachment of the coracobrachialis has been found, the humeral attachments of the latissimus dorsi, teres major, and subscapularis are close by. The latissimus dorsi and teres major are on the medial lip of the bicipital groove, proximal to the humeral attachment of the coracobrachialis.

Just proximal to the bicipital groove attachments of these two muscles is the humeral attachment of the subscapularis on the lesser tubercle of the humerus. To locate all three of these muscular attachments, palpate more proximally into the axilla against the humerus while resisting extension and adduction of the arm for the latissimus dorsi and teres major; then palpate further proximally onto the lesser tubercle while resisting medial rotation of the arm for the subscapularis.

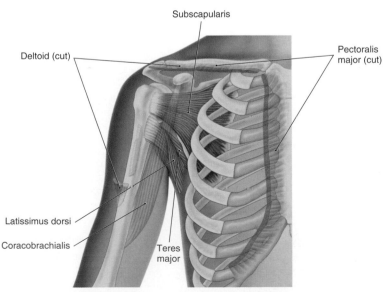

Figure 14-29 The humeral attachments of the right latissimus dorsi, teres major, and subscapularis are shown. The coracobrachialis and cut ends of the pectoralis major and deltoid are ghosted in.

TRICEPS BRACHII—SEATED

☑ ATTACHMENTS

☐ Infraglenoid tubercle of the scapula (long head) and the posterior shaft of the humerus (lateral and medial heads)

to the

☐ olecranon process of the ulna

☑ ACTIONS

Entire Muscle

☐ Extends the forearm at the elbow joint
  Long head also:
☐ Adducts the arm at the glenohumeral (GH joint)
☐ Extends the arm at the GH joint

Starting Position (Figure 14-31)

■ Client seated with the arm relaxed and hanging vertically, and the posterior forearm resting on the client's or therapist's thigh
■ Therapist seated in front of or to the side of the client
■ Palpating hand placed on the posterior surface of the arm

Palpation Steps

1. Ask the client to extend the forearm at the elbow joint by pressing the forearm against the thigh, and feel for the contraction of the triceps brachii (Figure 14-32).
2. Palpate from attachment to attachment while strumming perpendicular to the fibers.
3. Once the triceps brachii has been located, have the client relax it and palpate to assess its baseline tone.

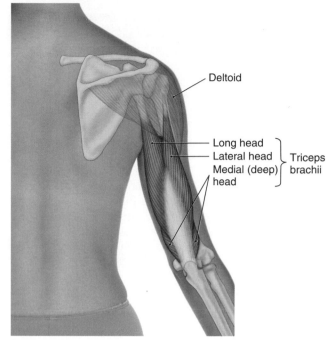

Figure 14-30 Posterior view of the right triceps brachii. The deltoid has been ghosted in.

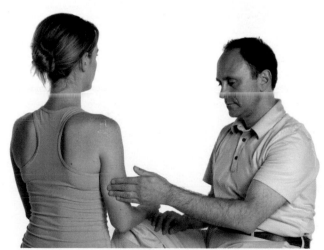

Figure 14-31 Starting position for seated palpation of the right triceps brachii.

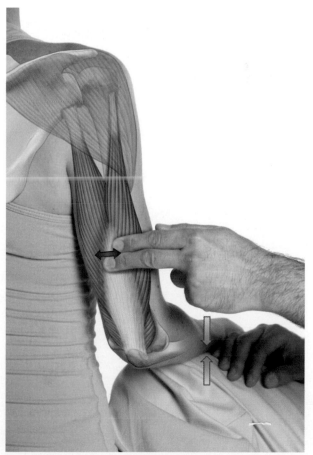

Figure 14-32 Palpation of the belly of the right triceps brachii as the client extends the forearm against resistance.

14

TRICEPS BRACHII—SEATED—*cont'd*

Alternate Palpation Position—Prone

PALPATION NOTES

1. The proximal attachment of the triceps brachii on the scapula can be difficult to palpate and discern, because it is deep to the posterior deltoid and teres minor muscles (Figure 14-33). To palpate it, follow the triceps brachii proximally with baby steps as the client alternately contracts and relaxes the triceps brachii (extending the forearm at the elbow joint by pressing the forearm against the thigh and then relaxing it). It is important that the musculature across the GH joint stays relaxed. If the posterior deltoid and teres minor can be slackened by holding the client's GH joint in a small degree of passive extension and lateral rotation, greater access to the triceps brachii is usually allowed.

2. The lateral and medial borders of the triceps brachii can be discerned from the brachialis by asking the client to alternately perform forearm extension against resistance (by pressing the forearm against the thigh) and forearm flexion against resistance (you provide the resistance to forearm flexion with your support hand). The triceps brachii contraction will be felt with forearm extension; the brachialis contraction will be felt with forearm flexion.

3. Resistance of GH joint adduction and/or extension can be used to engage the long head of the triceps brachii and discern it from the lateral and medial heads.

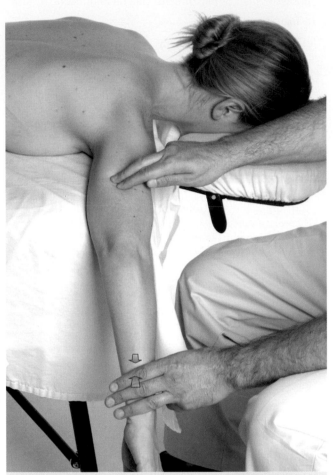

Figure 14-34 The triceps brachii can be easily palpated with the client prone. Position the client prone with the arm abducted 90 degrees at the glenohumeral (GH) joint and resting on the table, and the forearm flexed 90 degrees at the elbow joint and hanging off the table. In this position, ask the client to extend the forearm at the elbow joint against gravity and feel for the contraction of the triceps brachii (added resistance to forearm extension with your support hand can be given).

Palpation Key:
Client presses the forearm against the thigh.

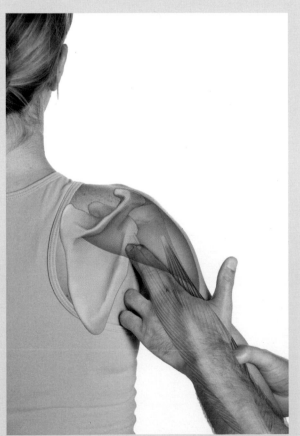

Figure 14-33 Palpation of the proximal scapular attachment of the triceps brachii deep to the posterior deltoid (ghosted in) and teres minor (not shown).

14

TRICEPS BRACHII—SEATED—*cont'd*

TRIGGER POINTS

1. Trigger points (TrPs) in the triceps brachii often result from or are perpetuated by acute or chronic overuse of the muscle (e.g., using the backhand stroke in tennis, doing push-ups, shifting gears manually when driving, using crutches).
2. TrPs in the triceps brachii may produce vague diffuse pain in its referral zone and radial nerve entrapment (resulting in paresthesia of the posterior distal forearm and posterior hand).
3. The referral patterns of triceps brachii TrPs must be distinguished from the referral patterns of TrPs in the anconeus, extensor carpi radialis longus, brachioradialis, extensor digitorum, supinator, scalenes, pectoralis minor, supraspinatus, infraspinatus, teres minor, teres major, subscapularis, deltoid, coracobrachialis, latissimus dorsi, flexor digitorum superficialis, flexor digitorum profundus, abductor digiti minimi manus, and first dorsal interosseus manus.
4. TrPs in the triceps brachii are often incorrectly assessed as lateral or medial epicondylitis/epicondylosis, olecranon bursitis, thoracic outlet syndrome, cubital tunnel syndrome, C7 nerve compression, or elbow joint arthritis.
5. Associated TrPs often occur in the biceps brachii, brachialis, brachioradialis, anconeus, supinator, extensor carpi radialis longus, latissimus dorsi, teres major, teres minor, and serratus posterior superior.

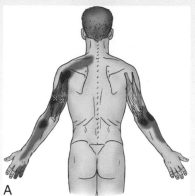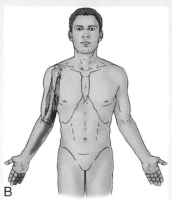

Figure 14-35 Common triceps brachii trigger points (TrPs) and their corresponding referral zones. **A,** Posterior view showing long and lateral head TrPs on the left and a medial head TrP and an attachment TrP on the right. **B,** Anterior view of another medial head TrP.

14

STRETCHING THE TRICEPS BRACHII

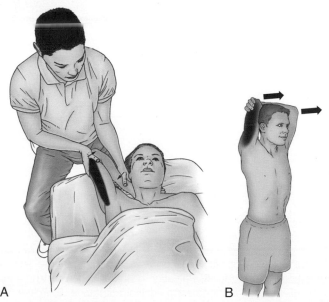

Figure 14-36 Stretching the right triceps brachii. The arm is abducted to 180 degrees with the forearm fully flexed at the elbow joint. **A,** Therapist-assisted stretch. The therapist increases the stretch while maintaining the elbow joint flexion. **B,** Self-care stretch. The client pulls his arm behind his head while maintaining the elbow joint flexion.

DETOUR

Anconeus:

The anconeus is superficial and easily palpated on the posterior side of the proximal forearm. It attaches from the lateral epicondyle of the humerus to the posterior proximal ulna (Figure 14-37, *A*) and extends the forearm at the elbow joint. To palpate the anconeus, first place your palpating finger directly between the olecranon process of the ulna and the lateral epicondyle of the humerus. Then palpate the anconeus toward its distal attachment as you strum perpendicular to its fibers while the client performs extension of the forearm at the elbow joint against resistance (see Figure 14-37, *B*).

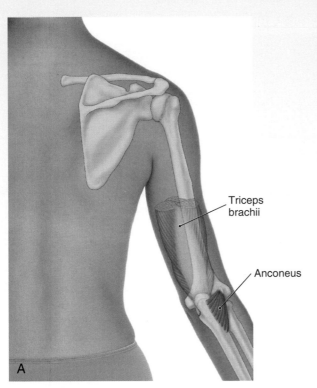

Triceps brachii

Anconeus

A

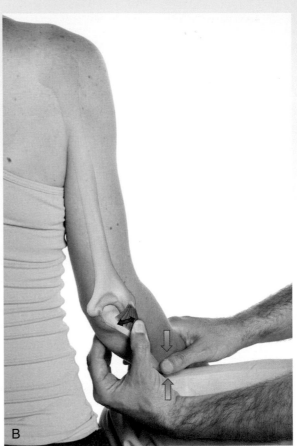

B

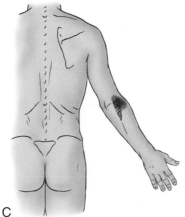

C

Figure 14-37 The right anconeus. **A,** Posterior view of the anconeus. The distal end of the triceps brachii has been ghosted in. **B,** Palpation of the anconeus, strumming perpendicular to the fibers as the client extends the forearm against resistance. **C,** Posterior view illustrating a common anconeus trigger point (TrP) and its corresponding referral zone. Note: A TrP in the anconeus might be incorrectly assessed as tennis elbow.

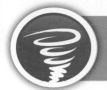

Muscles of the Arm

The following *Whirlwind Tour* is an abbreviated set of palpation protocols for the muscles of this chapter. Once you have read and become comfortable with each of the protocols presented thus far, this *Whirlwind Tour* allows you to quickly and efficiently run through the palpations protocols for all the muscles of the chapter.

CLIENT SEATED

1. **Deltoid:** The client is seated; you are standing behind the client. To palpate the entire deltoid, palpate proximally on the lateral arm immediately distal to the acromion process of the scapula, and feel for the contraction of the deltoid as the client abducts the arm at the GH joint (resistance may be added if needed). Palpate the deltoid toward its distal attachment by strumming perpendicular to the fibers as the client alternately contracts and relaxes the muscle. To isolate the anterior deltoid, resist the client's horizontal flexion of the arm at the GH joint, and feel for its contraction. Strum perpendicular to the fibers from attachment to attachment. To isolate the posterior deltoid, resist the client's horizontal extension of the arm at the GH joint and feel for its contraction. Strum perpendicular to the fibers from attachment to attachment.

2. **Biceps brachii:** The client is seated; you are seated to the side and facing the client. Palpate in the middle of the anterior arm, and feel for the contraction as you resist the client's forearm flexion at the elbow joint with the forearm in full supination. (Note: Be sure that the support hand that gives resistance is on the distal forearm and not on the client's hand.) Once felt, continue palpating to the distal tendon and then continue palpating proximally as far as possible while strumming perpendicular to the fibers as the client alternately contracts and relaxes the muscle. The proximal tendons can be palpated in the axilla, deep to the pectoralis major and anterior deltoid. The short head's tendon can be palpated all the way to the coracoid process; the supraglenoid tubercle attachment of the long head cannot usually be palpated. (Note: To distinguish the short head from the coracobrachialis, the short head of the biceps brachii contracts with elbow joint flexion; the coracobrachialis does not.) To distinguish the lateral border of the biceps brachii from the brachialis, ask the client to gently alternately flex the forearm with the forearm supinated and then pronated. The biceps brachii contraction is more easily felt when the forearm is fully supinated; the brachialis contraction is more easily felt when the forearm is fully pronated.

3. **Brachialis:** The client is seated; you are seated to the side and facing the client. Feel for the contraction of the brachialis in the anterolateral arm as the client flexes the forearm at the elbow joint with the forearm fully pronated. If resistance is given, apply only a gentle force to the client's forearm flexion. Once felt, continue palpating the brachialis in the anterolateral arm, both proximally toward the deltoid tuberosity and distally as far as possible. Then palpate the brachialis deep to the biceps brachii as the client flexes the forearm, with the forearm fully pronated, against gentle resistance. To distinguish the border between the brachialis and biceps brachii in the anterolateral arm, ask the client to gently alternately flex the forearm with it pronated and then supinated. The brachialis contraction is more easily felt when the forearm is fully pronated; the biceps brachii contraction is more easily felt when the forearm is fully supinated. To distinguish the border between the brachialis and the triceps brachii, have the client alternately flex and extend the forearm against moderate to strong resistance; the brachialis contraction is felt with forearm flexion; the triceps brachii contraction is felt with forearm extension.

4. **Coracobrachialis:** Have the client seated with the arm abducted 90 degrees and laterally rotated at the GH joint, and the forearm flexed at the elbow joint approximately 90 degrees; you are seated or standing in front of the client. Place palpating hand on the medial aspect of the proximal half of the client's arm, and feel for the contraction of the coracobrachialis as you resist the client's horizontal flexion of the arm at the GH joint. Once felt, strum perpendicular to the fibers from attachment to attachment. Note: To distinguish the coracobrachialis from the short head of the biceps brachii, use flexion of the forearm at the elbow joint; the biceps brachii short head contracts with elbow joint flexion; the coracobrachialis does not.

5. **Triceps brachii:** The client is seated with the arm relaxed and hanging vertically, and the posterior forearm resting on the client's or therapist's thigh; you are seated facing the client. Place palpating hand on the posterior arm, and feel for the contraction of the triceps brachii as the client extends the forearm against the resistance of the thigh. Once felt, palpate to the olecranon process attachment and then as far proximally as possible while strumming perpendicular to the fibers as the client alternately contracts and relaxes the muscle. Following the long head to its scapular attachment deep to the deltoid and teres minor is challenging but can be done if the deltoid is sufficiently relaxed. To distinguish the border between the triceps brachii and the brachialis, have the client alternately extend and flex the forearm against moderate to strong resistance; the triceps brachii contraction is felt with forearm extension; the brachialis contraction is felt with forearm flexion.

14

Review Questions

1. What are the attachments of the deltoid?
2. What are the attachments of the anconeus?
3. List the actions of the coracobrachialis.
4. List the actions of the triceps brachii.
5. When palpating the deltoid, what joint action causes the entire muscle to contract?
6. Describe the positioning for palpation of the entire biceps brachii.
7. What positioning is advantageous during palpation of the brachialis to discriminate it from more superficial musculature?
8. What is the correct method of engaging the brachioradialis during palpation?
9. Palpation of the coracobrachialis must be done with care due to the presence of what adjacent structures?
10. Palpation of the proximal attachment of the triceps brachii on the scapula is aided by what positioning and joint action?
11. Between what two anatomic structures is palpation of the anconeus conducted?
12. Name two incorrect assessments often given in the case of deltoid TrPs.
13. TrPs in the triceps brachii may produce entrapment of which nerve?
14. Describe a stretch for the entire biceps brachii.
15. Describe stretches for all parts of the left deltoid.
16. Explain the difference in methods for palpating the brachialis and the biceps brachii.
17. When palpating the triceps brachii, describe how to distinguish the medial and lateral heads from the long head.

CASE STUDY

A semi-regular client comes in on a Saturday for her quarterly massage session complaining of pain in the right forearm. She is right-handed, 32 years of age, and in excellent physical shape. She has an active lifestyle that includes full-time employment as a vehicle mechanic, daily yoga, regular exercise, and playing on a recreational soccer team as their goalkeeper.

For the past week at work, she has been engaged in repetitive work as a recall forced repairs of large numbers of vehicles as quickly as possible. This included extensive time spent with manual tools tightening and loosening bolts. Beginning on Wednesday, she began to notice soreness in the right posterior proximal forearm that radiated to her elbow with the pain registering a three out of ten on the pain scale. The pain increased over the next day, and during her soccer game Thursday night, the pain went from a dull soreness to a sharp pain when throwing the ball into play. From there on through the game the pain worsened to an eight out of ten on the pain scale. After the game, she applied ice and consumed a glass of wine. Physical exam and palpation reveals tenderness and swelling in the area of complaint.

1. What activity of the client likely caused the initial injury, and how had that been exacerbated over time?
2. What assessments would you perform to evaluate the muscle and joints affected?
3. How would you treat this client?

CHAPTER 15

Tour #5

Palpation of the Muscles of the Forearm

Overview

This chapter is a palpation tour of the muscles of the forearm. The tour begins with the muscles of the anterior forearm from superficial to deep, then describes palpation of the radial group, and finishes with palpation of the muscles of the posterior forearm from superficial to deep. Palpation for each of the muscles is shown in the seated position, but alternate palpation positions are also described. The major muscles or muscle groups of the region are each given a separate layout; there is also a detour to the pronator quadratus. Trigger point (TrP) information and stretching, both therapist-assisted and self-care stretching, are given for each of the muscles covered in this chapter. The chapter closes with an advanced *Whirlwind Tour* that describes the sequential palpation of all of the muscles of the chapter.

Chapter Outline

Chapter Objectives

After completing this chapter, the student/therapist should be able to perform the following for each of the muscles covered in this chapter:

1. State the attachments.
2. State the actions.
3. Describe the starting position for palpation.
4. Describe and explain the purpose of each of the palpation steps.
5. Palpate each muscle.
6. State the "Palpation Key."
7. Describe alternate palpation positions.
8. State the locations of the most common TrP(s).
9. Describe the TrP referral zones.
10. State the most common factors that create and/or perpetuate TrPs.
11. State the symptoms most commonly caused by TrPs.
12. Describe and perform the therapist-assisted and self-care stretches.

e Go to http://evolve.elsevier.com/Muscolino/palpation for video demonstrations of the muscle palpations presented in this chapter.

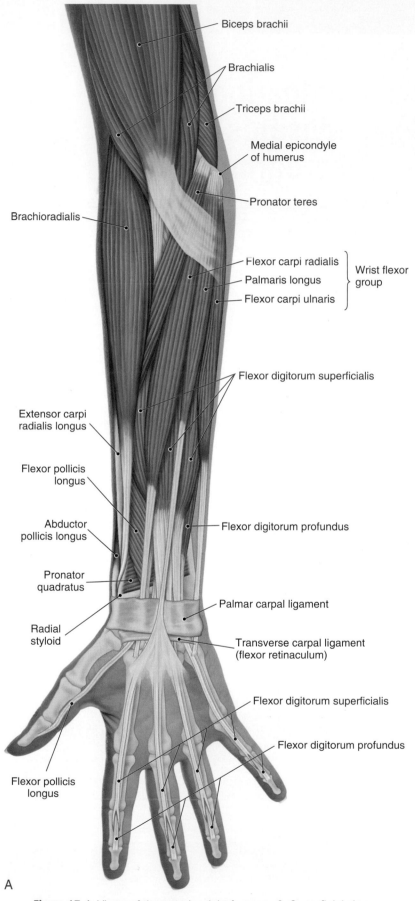

Figure 15-1 Views of the anterior right forearm. **A,** Superficial view.

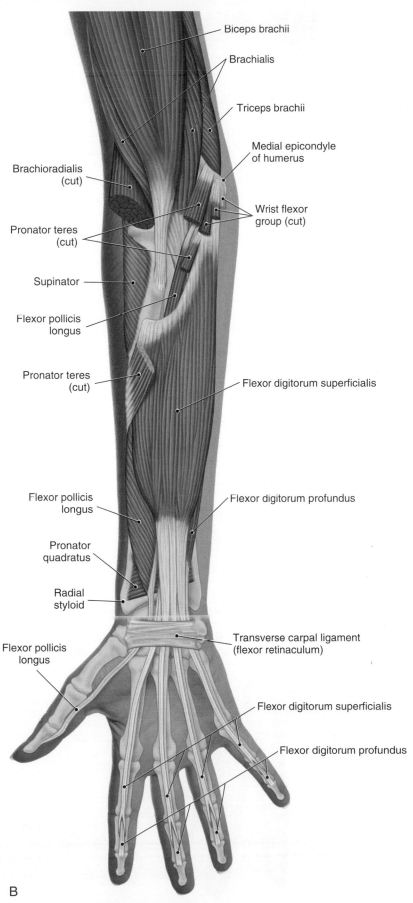

Biceps brachii

Brachialis

Triceps brachii

Medial epicondyle
of humerus

Brachioradialis
(cut)

Wrist flexor
group (cut)

Pronator teres
(cut)

Supinator

Flexor pollicis
longus

Pronator teres
(cut)

Flexor digitorum superficialis

Flexor pollicis
longus

Flexor digitorum profundus

Pronator
quadratus

Radial
styloid

Transverse carpal ligament
(flexor retinaculum)

Flexor pollicis
longus

Flexor digitorum superficialis

Flexor digitorum profundus

15

B

Figure 15-1, cont'd B, Intermediate view.

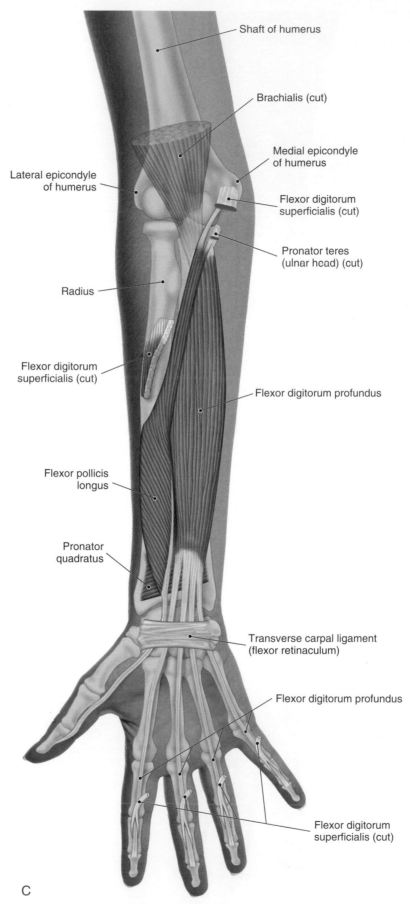

Shaft of humerus

Brachialis (cut)

Medial epicondyle of humerus

Lateral epicondyle of humerus

Flexor digitorum superficialis (cut)

Pronator teres (ulnar head) (cut)

Radius

Flexor digitorum superficialis (cut)

Flexor digitorum profundus

Flexor pollicis longus

Pronator quadratus

Transverse carpal ligament (flexor retinaculum)

Flexor digitorum profundus

Flexor digitorum superficialis (cut)

C

Figure 15-1, cont'd C, Deep view.

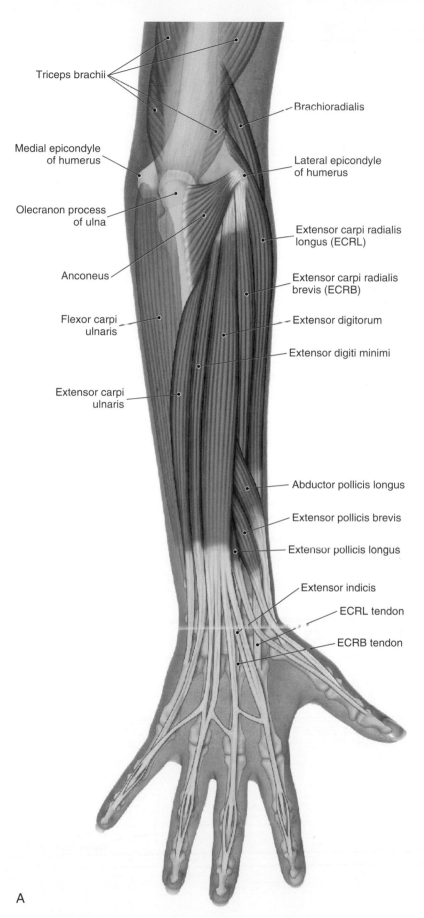

Figure 15-2 Views of the posterior right forearm. **A,** Superficial view.

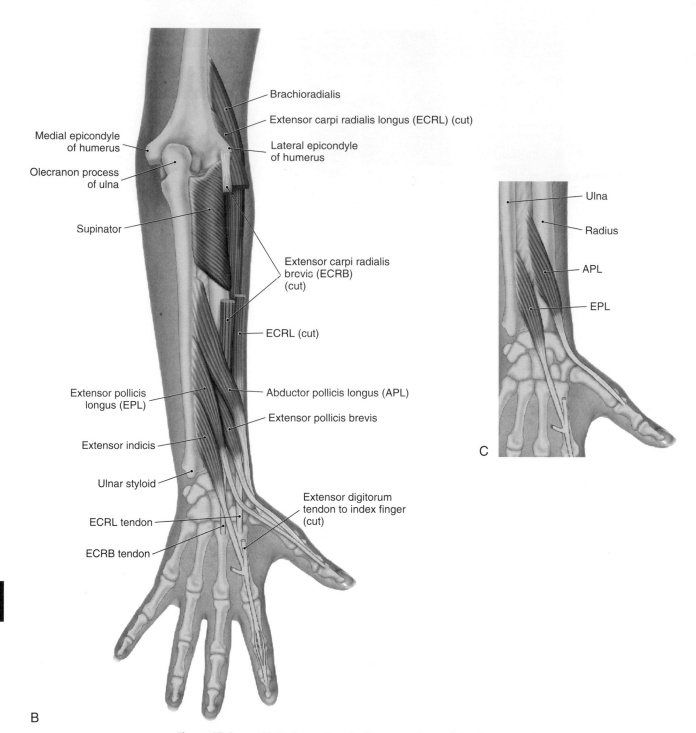

Figure 15-2, cont'd B, Deep view. **C,** Close-up of two of the deep muscles.

15

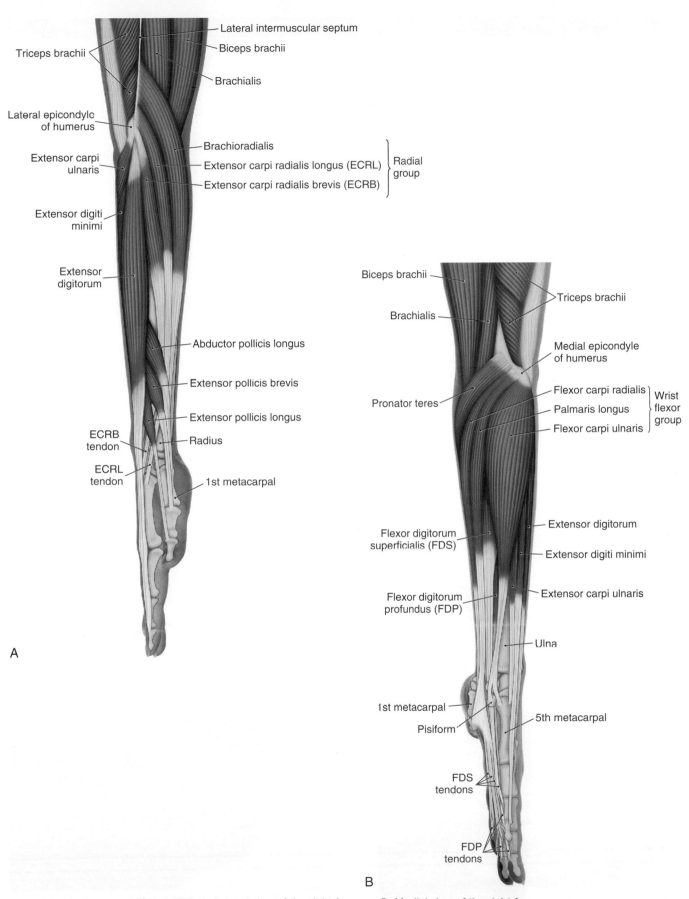

Figure 15-3 A, Lateral view of the right forearm. **B,** Medial view of the right forearm.

BRACHIORADIALIS—SEATED

☑ ATTACHMENTS

☐ Proximal ⅔ of the lateral supracondylar ridge of the humerus

to the

☐ styloid process of the radius

☑ ACTIONS

☐ Flexes the forearm at the elbow joint
☐ Pronates the supinated forearm at the radioulnar joints to a position halfway between full pronation and supination
☐ Supinates the pronated forearm at the radioulnar joints to a position halfway between full pronation and supination

Starting Position (Figure 15-5)

■ Client seated with the arm relaxed and the forearm flexed at the elbow joint and in a position that is halfway between full pronation and full supination, and resting on the client's thigh
■ Therapist seated to the side and facing the client
■ Palpating hand placed on the proximal anterolateral forearm
■ Support hand placed on the client's anterior distal forearm, just proximal to the wrist joint

Palpation Steps

1. With moderate force, resist the client from flexing the forearm at the elbow joint, and feel for the contraction of the brachioradialis (Figure 15-6).
2. Strumming perpendicular to the fibers, palpate from attachment to attachment.
3. Once the brachioradialis has been located, have the client relax it and palpate to assess its baseline tone.

15

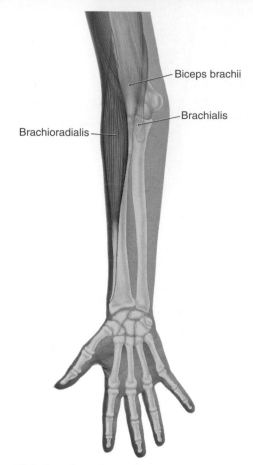

Biceps brachii

Brachialis

Brachioradialis

Figure 15-4 Anterior view of the right brachioradialis. The biceps brachii and brachialis have been ghosted in.

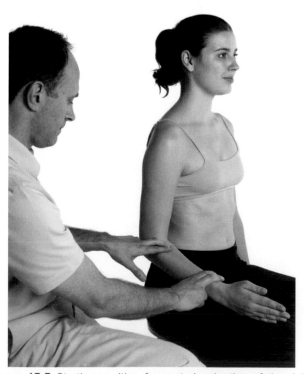

Figure 15-5 Starting position for seated palpation of the right brachioradialis.

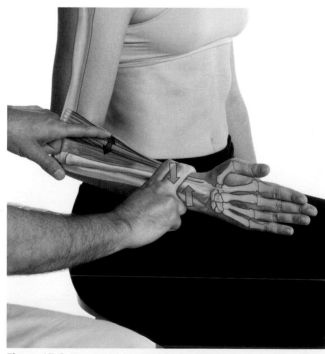

Figure 15-6 Palpation of the right brachioradialis as the client's forearm flexion at the elbow joint is resisted while the forearm is positioned halfway between full pronation and full supination. Note: The extensor carpi radialis longus (ECRL) has been ghosted in.

BRACHIORADIALIS—SEATED—*cont'd*

PALPATION NOTES

1. The brachioradialis is superficial for its entire path except where the abductor pollicis longus and extensor pollicis brevis cross superficial to it in the distal forearm.

2. The three major flexors of the elbow joint are the biceps brachii, the brachialis, and the brachioradialis. They are all palpated by resisting flexion of the forearm at the elbow joint; the difference is the position of the forearm. For palpation of the biceps brachii, the forearm is fully supinated; for the brachialis, the forearm is fully pronated; for the brachioradialis, the forearm is halfway between full pronation and full supination (Figure 15-7).

3. The "key" to recall the palpation position for the brachioradialis is to think of the position of the upper extremity when hitchhiking: the forearm is flexed and halfway between full pronation and full supination. However, the thumb should be relaxed; if it is extended as in hitchhiking, the abductor pollicis longus and extensor pollicis brevis will contract, making it more difficult to palpate the distal end of the brachioradialis.

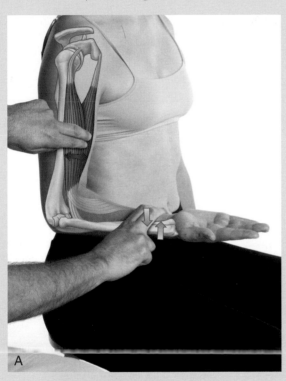

A

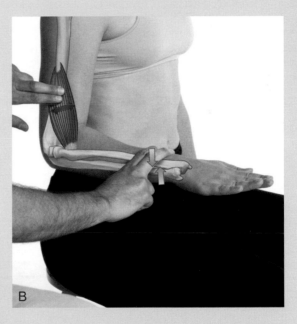

B

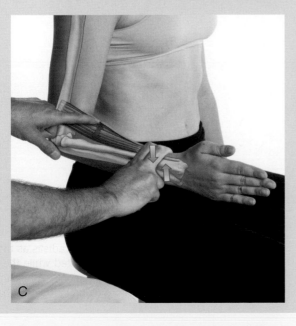

C

Figure 15-7 Palpation of the three major elbow joint flexors as forearm flexion at the elbow joint is resisted. Note that the difference between the three palpations lies in the degree of pronation or supination of the forearm at the radioulnar joints. **A,** Palpation of the biceps brachii with the forearm fully supinated. **B,** Palpation of the brachialis with the forearm fully pronated. **C,** Palpation of the brachioradialis with the forearm halfway between full supination and full pronation.

15

TRIGGER POINTS

1. Trigger points (TrPs) in the brachioradialis often result from or are perpetuated by acute or chronic overuse of the muscle (e.g., lifting objects with the forearm halfway between full pronation and full supination, digging with a shovel, extensive handshaking).
2. TrPs in the brachioradialis may produce weakness of forearm flexion at the elbow joint and limited forearm pronation when coupled with forearm extension.
3. The referral patterns of brachioradialis TrPs must be distinguished from the referral patterns of TrPs in the supinator, extensor carpi radialis longus (ECRL) and brevis, extensor digitorum, subclavius, scalenes, supraspinatus, coracobrachialis, brachialis, triceps brachii, and first dorsal interosseus manus.
4. TrPs in the brachioradialis are often incorrectly assessed as lateral epicondylitis/epicondylosis, C5 or C6 nerve compression, or de Quervain stenosing tenosynovitis.
5. Associated TrPs often occur in the ECRL and brevis, extensor digitorum, extensor digiti minimi, supinator, and triceps brachii.

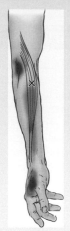

Figure 15-8 Right lateral view illustrating a common brachioradialis trigger point (TrP) and its corresponding referral zone.

STRETCHING THE BRACHIORADIALIS

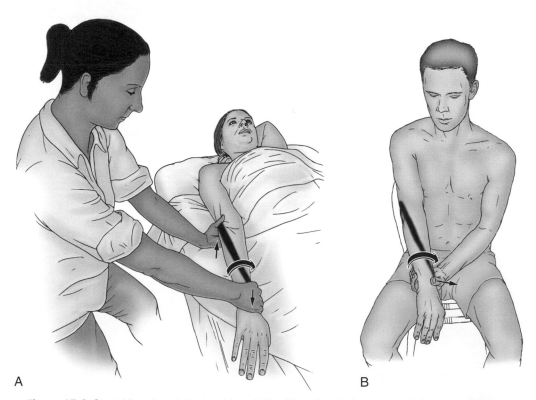

A

B

Figure 15-9 Stretching the right brachioradialis. The client's forearm is fully extended and pronated. **A,** Therapist-assisted stretch. Note that the therapist stabilizes the client's arm with the other hand. **B,** Self-care stretch.

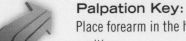

Palpation Key:
Place forearm in the hitchhiking position.

PRONATOR TERES—SEATED

☑ ATTACHMENTS

- ☐ Medial epicondyle of the humerus (via the common flexor tendon), the medial supracondylar ridge of the humerus, and the coronoid process of the ulna

  to the

- ☐ middle ⅓ of the lateral radius

☑ ACTIONS

- ☐ Pronates the forearm at the radioulnar joints
- ☐ Flexes the forearm at the elbow joint

Starting Position (Figure 15-11)

- ■ Client seated with the arm relaxed and the forearm flexed at the elbow joint and in a position that is halfway between full pronation and full supination, and resting on the client's thigh
- ■ Therapist seated facing the client
- ■ Palpating hand placed on the proximal anterior forearm
- ■ Support hand placed on the client's anterior distal forearm, just proximal to the wrist joint

Palpation Steps

1. With moderate force, resist the client from pronating the forearm at the radioulnar joints, and feel for the contraction of the pronator teres (Figure 15-12).
2. Strumming perpendicular to the fibers, palpate from attachment to attachment. Be sure to strum across the entire muscle belly.
3. Once the pronator teres has been located, have the client relax it and palpate to assess its baseline tone.

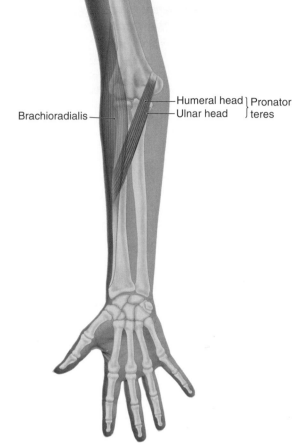

Brachioradialis —
Humeral head ⎤ Pronator
Ulnar head ⎦ teres

Figure 15-10 Anterior view of the right pronator teres. The brachioradialis is ghosted in.

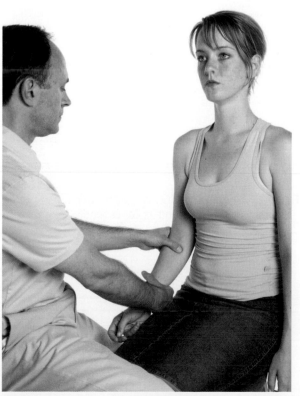

Figure 15-11 Starting position for seated palpation of the right pronator teres.

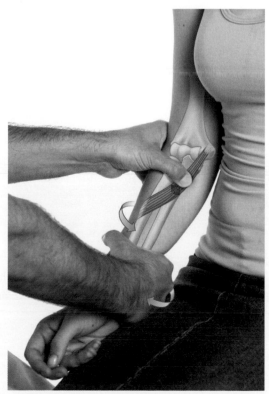

Figure 15-12 Palpation of the right pronator teres as the client pronates the forearm at the radioulnar joints against resistance.

15

PRONATOR TERES—SEATED —cont'd

PALPATION NOTES

1. When resisting the client's forearm pronation, a gentle but firm grasp is needed by the support hand. Otherwise only the client's skin is held and the underlying forearm bones are allowed to move. This results in unsuccessful resistance to forearm pronation and is uncomfortable for the client.
2. The belly of the pronator teres is superficial and should be easily palpable.
3. The distal end of the pronator teres runs deep to the brachioradialis and can be challenging to palpate. To palpate the distal attachment on the radius, passively flex the client's elbow joint to slacken the brachioradialis; then push the brachioradialis laterally and press deep to it, feeling for the pronator teres attachment on the radius (Figure 15-13).
4. Most of the pronator teres can be palpated if the client is resisted from pronating the forearm with the forearm starting in anatomic position. However, in this position, the brachioradialis may be recruited for pronation, blocking our ability to palpate the distal attachment of the pronator teres. To better palpate the distal attachment of the pronator teres through the brachioradialis, relax the brachioradialis by having the client begin with the forearm halfway between full pronation and full supination.
5. The pronator teres can also be palpated by resisting the client's forearm flexion at the elbow joint. However, this causes every elbow joint flexor to contract, which makes it difficult to discern the pronator teres from adjacent muscles.
6. It is difficult to discern the humeral head of the pronator teres from its ulnar head.
7. The median nerve runs between the humeral and ulnar heads of the pronator teres; therefore, deep work should be done prudently.

15

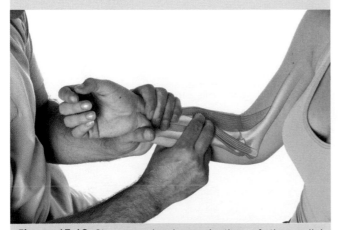

Figure 15-13 Close-up showing palpation of the radial attachment of the right pronator teres by slackening and pushing the brachioradialis out of the way (see Palpation Note #3).

Alternate Palpation Position—Supine

The pronator teres can also be palpated with the client supine. Follow the palpation steps indicated for the seated palpation.

TRIGGER POINTS

1. Trigger points (TrPs) in the pronator teres often result from or are perpetuated by acute or chronic overuse of the muscle (e.g., using a screwdriver, hitting a forehand in tennis with poor form).
2. TrPs in the pronator teres may entrap the median nerve.
3. The referral patterns of pronator teres TrPs must be distinguished from the referral patterns of TrPs in the flexor carpi radialis (FCR), brachialis, subscapularis, supraspinatus, infraspinatus, subclavius, scalenes, and adductor pollicis.
4. TrPs in the pronator teres are often incorrectly assessed as medial epicondylitis/epicondylosis, thoracic outlet syndrome, carpal tunnel syndrome, or wrist joint dysfunction.
5. Associated TrPs often occur in the biceps brachii, brachialis, and pronator quadratus.

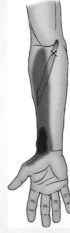

Figure 15-14 Anterior view illustrating a common pronator teres trigger point (TrP) and its corresponding referral zone.

PRONATOR TERES—SEATED —*cont'd*

STRETCHING THE PRONATOR TERES

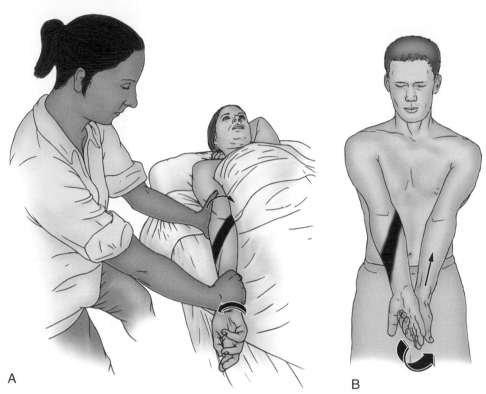

A   B

Figure 15-15 Stretching the right pronator teres. The client's forearm is fully extended and supinated. **A,** Therapist-assisted stretch. Note that the therapist stabilizes the client's arm with the other hand. **B,** Self-care stretch.

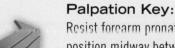

Palpation Key:
Resist forearm pronation from a position midway between pronation and supination.

15

WRIST FLEXOR GROUP—SEATED

The wrist flexor group is composed of the flexor carpi radialis (FCR), palmaris longus (PL), and flexor carpi ulnaris (FCU).

☑ ATTACHMENTS

- ☐ Proximal attachments:
  - ☐ All three wrist flexors attach to the medial epicondyle of the humerus via the common flexor tendon.
  - ☐ The FCU also attaches to the proximal ⅔ of the ulna.
- ☐ Distal attachments:
  - ☐ The FCR attaches to the radial side of the anterior hand at the bases of the second and third metacarpals.
  - ☐ The PL attaches into the palmar aponeurosis of the palm of the hand.
  - ☐ The FCU attaches to the ulnar side of the anterior hand at the base of the fifth metacarpal, the pisiform, and the hook of the hamate.

☑ ACTIONS

- ☐ All three wrist flexors flex the hand at the wrist joint.
- ☐ The FCR also radially deviates the hand at the wrist joint.
- ☐ The FCU also ulnar deviates the hand at the wrist joint.

Starting Position (Figure 15-17)

- ■ Client seated with the arm relaxed and the forearm flexed at the elbow joint and fully supinated, and resting on the client's thigh
- ■ Therapist seated to the side and facing the client
- ■ Palpating hand placed on the distal anterior forearm (after visualizing the distal tendons)
- ■ Support hand placed on the client's hand, just proximal to the fingers

Palpation Steps

1. Resist the client from flexing the hand at the wrist joint, and look for the distal tendons of all three wrist flexors to become visible (Be sure that you do not contact the fingers when offering resistance because that causes finger flexor muscles to be engaged also, making it more difficult to discern the muscles of the wrist flexor group.) (Figure 15-18).
2. If all three wrist flexors do not become visible, they should be palpable while strumming perpendicularly across them.
3. Continue palpating the FCR proximally to the medial epicondyle while strumming across its fibers. Repeat this for the other two wrist flexors.
4. Once the wrist flexors have been located, have the client relax them and palpate to assess their baseline tone.

15

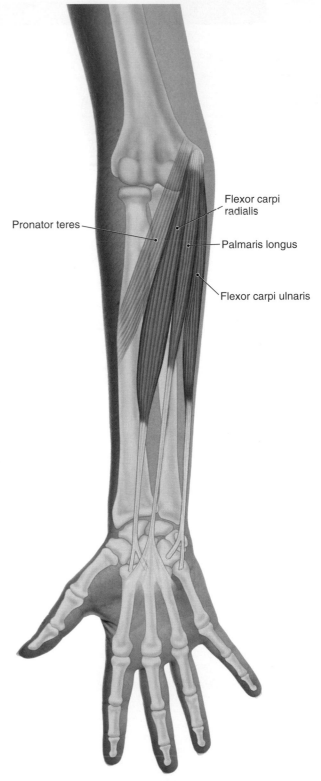

Pronator teres
Flexor carpi radialis
Palmaris longus
Flexor carpi ulnaris

Figure 15-16 Anterior view of the right wrist flexor group of muscles. The pronator teres has been ghosted in.

WRIST FLEXOR GROUP—SEATED—*cont'd*

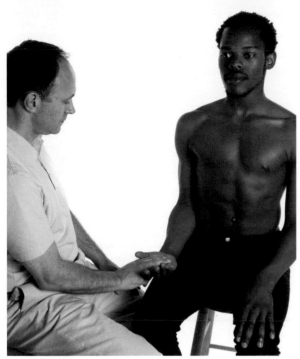

Figure 15-17 Starting position for seated palpation of the right wrist flexor group.

PALPATION NOTES

1. The palmaris longus (PL) is often missing (unilaterally or bilaterally).
2. The distal tendon of the flexor carpi radialis (FCR) is much closer to the PL's distal tendon near the wrist than is the flexor carpi ulnaris' (FCU's) distal tendon.
3. All wrist flexors contract with wrist joint flexion, so to engage and isolate only one muscle in the group, which is especially important because their muscle bellies merge proximally, a different action must be used. Resist radial deviation of the hand at the wrist joint to engage the FCR (Figure 15-19, *A*), and resist ulnar deviation of the hand at the wrist joint to engage the FCU (see Figure 15-19, *B*). The PL stays relaxed and soft when both radial and ulnar deviations are done (if the client starts in anatomic position).
4. The PL can often be made visible and palpable by asking the client to cup the hand (see Figure 15-19, *C*).
5. It is especially important to not cross the finger joints when resisting the client's wrist joint flexion, because doing so would engage the flexor muscles of the fingers (flexors digitorum superficialis and profundus and flexor pollicis longus). This would make distinguishing the superficial wrist flexor muscles from these deeper muscles difficult.
6. Another method to engage and palpate the FCU is to ask the client to actively perform abduction of the little finger at the metacarpophalangeal (MCP) joint. This will require the FCU to contract to stabilize the pisiform (Figure 15-20).

Continued

15

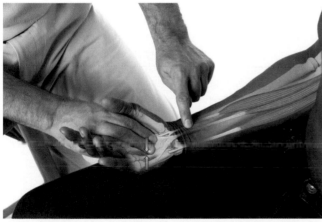

Figure 15-18 All three muscles of the right wrist flexor group are engaged with flexion of the hand against resistance. The distal tendons are often visible, as seen here; the tendon of the flexor carpi radialis (FCR) is being palpated.

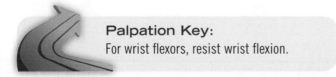

Palpation Key:
For wrist flexors, resist wrist flexion.

WRIST FLEXOR GROUP—SEATED—*cont'd*

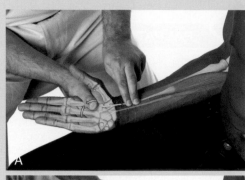

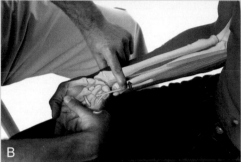

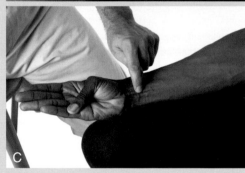

Figure 15-19 Palpation of the muscles of the right wrist flexor group. **A,** Palpation of the flexor carpi radialis (FCR) as the client radially deviates the hand against resistance. The palmaris longus (PL) has been ghosted in. **B,** Palpation of the flexor carpi ulnaris (FCU) as the client ulnar deviates the hand against resistance. (The PL has been ghosted in.) **C,** The PL is engaged when the client cups his hand.

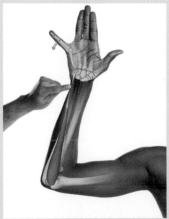

Figure 15-20 Abduction of the little finger at the metacarpophalangeal (MCP) joint causes the flexor carpi ulnaris (FCU) to engage as a stabilizer of the pisiform bone.

Alternate Palpation Position—Supine

The wrist flexor muscles can also be palpated with the client supine. Follow the palpation steps indicated for the seated palpation.

TRIGGER POINTS

1. Trigger points (TrPs) in the wrist flexors often result from or are perpetuated by acute or chronic overuse of the muscle (e.g., gripping objects, painting, playing tennis), trauma to the forearm/wrist/hand, or TrPs in the pectoralis minor (for the FCR and FCU), triceps brachii (for the PL), latissimus dorsi, and serratus posterior superior (for the FCU).

2. TrPs in the PL usually produce a sharp needlelike referral pain, which is different in quality than the usual deeper aching pain typical of TrPs; they also typically result in tenderness in the palm when gripping and handling objects (e.g., gardening and power tools). TrPs in the FCU may cause entrapment of the ulnar nerve.

3. The referral pattern of a TrP in a wrist flexor must be distinguished from the referral patterns of TrPs in the other wrist flexors, pronator teres, subclavius, subscapularis, infraspinatus, latissimus dorsi, brachialis, and opponens pollicis.

4. TrPs in the wrist flexors are often incorrectly assessed as medial epicondylitis/epicondylosis, pathologic cervical disk, thoracic outlet syndrome, carpal tunnel syndrome, wrist joint dysfunction (for the FCR and FCU), or ulnar nerve compression (for the FCU).

5. Associated TrPs often occur in the other wrist joint flexors, flexor digitorum superficialis, and flexor digitorum profundus.

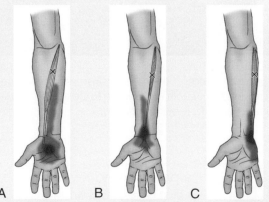

Figure 15-21 Common trigger points (TrPs) and their corresponding referral zones for the muscles of the wrist flexor group. **A,** Flexor carpi radialis (FCR). **B,** Palmaris longus (PL). **C,** Flexor carpi ulnaris (FCU).

15

WRIST FLEXOR GROUP—SEATED—*cont'd*

STRETCHING THE WRIST FLEXOR GROUP

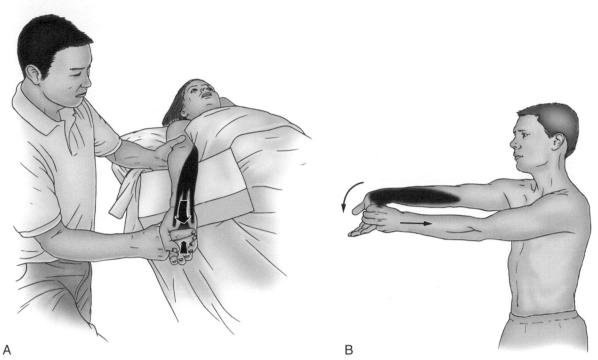

A   B

Figure 15-22 Stretching the right wrist flexor group. The hand is extended at the wrist joint with the forearm fully extended at the elbow joint. Note that the fingers are not extended. If ulnar deviation is added to the extension, the stretch of the flexor carpi radialis (FCR) is enhanced (but the flexor carpi ulnaris [FCU] slackens). If radial deviation is added to the extension, the stretch of the FCU is enhanced (but the FCR slackens). **A,** Therapist-assisted stretch. Note that the therapist stabilizes the client's arm with the other hand and that a cushion is placed under the client's forearm to help maintain extension at the elbow joint. **B,** Self-care stretch.

15

FLEXORS DIGITORUM SUPERFICIALIS AND PROFUNDUS—SEATED

Flexor Digitorum Superficialis

☑ ATTACHMENTS

☐ Medial epicondyle of the humerus (via the common flexor tendon) and the coronoid process of the ulna, and the proximal ½ of the anterior shaft of the radius

to the

☐ anterior surfaces of the middle phalanges of fingers two through five

☑ ACTIONS

☐ Flexes fingers two through five at the metacarpophalangeal (MCP) and proximal interphalangeal (IP) joints
☐ Flexes the hand at the wrist joint
☐ Flexes the forearm at the elbow joint

Flexor Digitorum Profundus

☑ ATTACHMENTS

☐ Proximal ½ of the anterior surface of the ulna (and the interosseus membrane)

to the

☐ anterior surfaces of the distal phalanges of fingers two through five

☑ ACTIONS

☐ Flexes fingers two through five at the MCP and the proximal and distal IP joints
☐ Flexes the hand at the wrist joint

Starting Position (Figure 15-24)

■ Client seated with the arm relaxed and the forearm flexed at the elbow joint and fully supinated, and resting on the client's thigh
■ Therapist seated to the side and facing the client
■ Begin palpating the flexor digitorum superficialis by placing your palpating fingers on the proximal medial forearm (slightly anterior and distal to the medial epicondyle of the humerus)

Palpation Steps

1. For the flexor digitorum superficialis, ask the client to flex the proximal phalanges of fingers two through five at the MCP joints, and feel for the contraction of the flexor digitorum superficialis (Figure 15-25, *A*). If resistance is added with your support hand, be sure to isolate your pressure against the proximal phalanges (i.e., do not cross the proximal IP joints to contact either the middle or distal phalanges).
2. Palpate the flexor digitorum superficialis while strumming perpendicular to the fibers from the proximal attachment at the medial epicondyle of the humerus to the distal tendons at the anterior wrist.
3. For the flexor digitorum profundus, begin palpation more medially and posteriorly on the forearm against the shaft of the ulna. Ask the client to flex the distal phalanges of fingers two through five at the IP joints, and feel for the contraction of the flexor digitorum profundus (see Figure 15-25, *B*).
4. Palpate the flexor digitorum profundus as far distally as possible while strumming perpendicular to the fibers.
5. Once the flexors digitorum superficialis and profundus have been located, have the client relax them and palpate to assess their baseline tone.

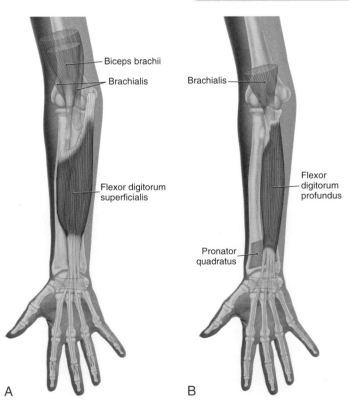

A   B

Figure 15-23 Anterior views of the right flexors digitorum superficialis and profundus. **A,** Anterior view of the right flexor digitorum superficialis. The distal ends of the biceps brachii and brachialis have been ghosted in. **B,** Anterior view of the right flexor digitorum profundus. The pronator quadratus and distal end of the brachialis have been ghosted in.

15

FLEXORS DIGITORUM SUPERFICIALIS AND PROFUNDUS—SEATED—*cont'd*

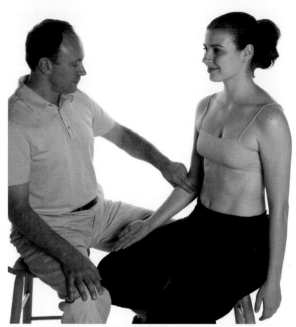

Figure 15-24 Starting position for seated palpation of the right flexor digitorum superficialis.

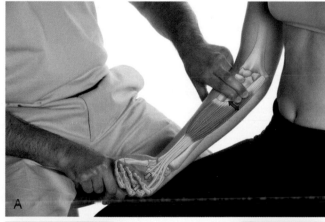

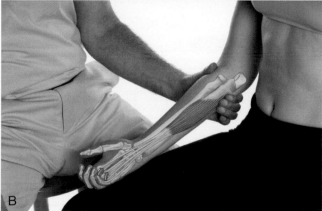

Figure 15-25 Palpation of the flexors digitorum superficialis and profundus. **A,** Palpation of the right flexor digitorum superficialis, starting distal and anterior to the medial epicondyle of the humerus. **B,** Palpation of the right flexor digitorum profundus, starting against the shaft of the ulna. Note the difference in the type of finger flexion that is performed by the client against resistance.

PALPATION NOTES

1. Although most clients are able to isolate flexion of the fingers at the MCP joints for the flexor digitorum superficialis palpation, it is usually difficult for them to isolate flexion of the fingers at the distal IP joints for the ideal palpation of the flexor digitorum profundus. However, even if the proximal IP joints flex somewhat with this palpation, it is usually still possible to discern the flexor digitorum profundus.
2. To palpate the flexor digitorum profundus, it is important to use the medial border of the shaft of the ulna as a landmark. Once this landmark has been found, drop just off it anteriorly and you will be on the flexor digitorum profundus. (You will actually be palpating through the ulnar head of the flexor carpi ulnaris [FCU], but the FCU is very thin here and does not obstruct palpation of the flexor digitorum profundus.)
3. Once the flexors digitorum superficialis and profundus split distally to form separate tendons, isolating flexion of an individual finger allows for individual palpation of the tendons. For example, have the client flex only the index finger and feel for the tendon to that finger to tense and the associated muscle belly fibers to contract. This can be done for the flexor digitorum superficialis and the flexor digitorum profundus.

Alternate Palpation Position—Supine

The two flexor digitorum muscles can also be palpated with the client supine. Follow the palpation steps indicated for the seated palpation.

15

Palpation Key:
Flex MCP joints for the flexor digitorum superficialis.
Flex distal IP joints and palpate against the shaft of the ulna for the flexor digitorum profundus.

FLEXORS DIGITORUM SUPERFICIALIS AND PROFUNDUS—SEATED—*cont'd*

TRIGGER POINTS

1. Trigger points (TrPs) in the flexors digitorum superficialis and profundus often result from or are perpetuated by acute or chronic overuse of the muscle (e.g., repetitive or forceful gripping of a steering wheel, tennis racquet, golf club, or gardening or work tools).
2. TrPs in the flexors digitorum superficialis and profundus may produce sharp referral pain that is felt not only throughout the anterior aspect of the finger that it flexes, but also phantom pain that is felt beyond the tip of the finger, entrapment of the median and/or ulnar nerve, and restriction of extension of the finger joints and wrist joint.
3. The referral patterns of flexors digitorum superficialis and profundus TrPs must be distinguished from the referral patterns of TrPs in the triceps brachii, subclavius, pectoralis minor, latissimus dorsi, and first dorsal interosseus manus.
4. TrPs in the flexors digitorum superficialis and profundus are often incorrectly assessed as a pathologic cervical disc, thoracic outlet syndrome, carpal tunnel syndrome, pronator teres syndrome, or joint dysfunction or arthritis of the MCP and IP joints.
5. Associated TrPs often occur in the flexor carpi radialis (FCR), flexor carpi ulnaris (FCU), pectoralis minor, and scalenes.

6. Note: No distinction has been made between TrPs within the flexor digitorum superficialis and the flexor digitorum profundus.

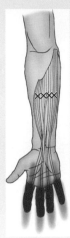

Figure 15-26 Anterior view illustrating common flexor digitorum superficialis and flexor digitorum profundus trigger points (TrPs) and their corresponding referral zones.

STRETCHING THE FLEXORS DIGITORUM SUPERFICIALIS AND PROFUNDUS

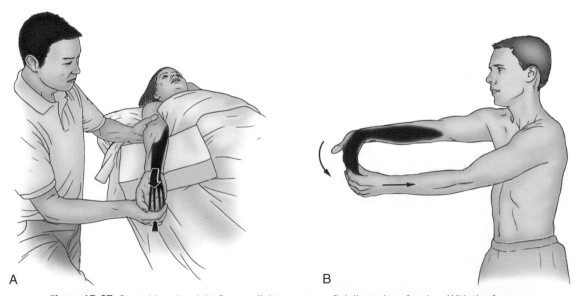

A   B

Figure 15-27 Stretching the right flexors digitorum superficialis and profundus. With the forearm and hand fully extended, the fingers are fully extended at the metacarpophalangeal (MCP) and interphalangeal (IP) joints. **A,** Therapist-assisted stretch. Note that the therapist stabilizes the client's arm with the other hand and that a cushion is placed under the client's forearm to help maintain extension at the elbow joint. **B,** Self-care stretch.

15

FLEXOR POLLICIS LONGUS—SEATED

✅ ATTACHMENTS

- ☐ Anterior surface of the distal radius and the interosseus membrane, the coronoid process of the ulna, and the medial epicondyle of the humerus

  to the

- ☐ anterior surface of the base of the distal phalanx of the thumb

✅ ACTIONS

- ☐ Flexes the thumb at the carpometacarpal (CMC), metacarpophalangeal (MCP), and interphalangeal (IP) joints
- ☐ Flexes the hand at the wrist joint
- ☐ Flexes the forearm at the elbow joint

Starting Position (Figure 15-29)

- ■ Client seated with the arm relaxed and the forearm flexed at the elbow joint and fully supinated, and resting on the client's thigh
- ■ Therapist seated to the side and facing the client
- ■ Palpating fingers placed on the distal anterior forearm (near the tendon of the flexor carpi radialis)

Palpation Steps

1. Ask the client to flex the distal phalanx of the thumb at the IP joint, and feel for the contraction of the flexor pollicis longus near the wrist (Figure 15-30).
2. Continue palpating the flexor pollicis longus as far proximal as possible while the client alternately contracts and relaxes it by flexing the thumb at the IP joint. Because this muscle is so deep, it is usually not helpful to try to strum perpendicular to its fibers.
3. Once the flexor pollicis longus has been located, have the client relax it and palpate to assess its baseline tone.

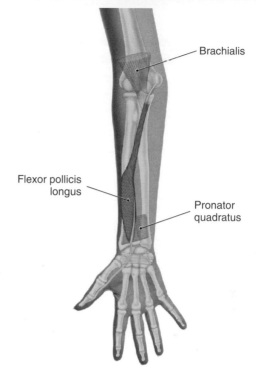

Figure 15-28 Anterior view of the right flexor pollicis longus. The pronator quadratus and distal end of the brachialis have been ghosted in.

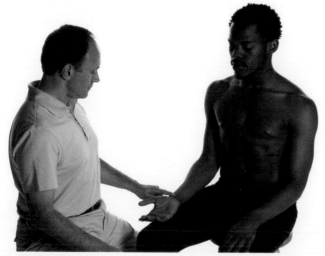

Figure 15-29 Starting position for seated palpation of the right flexor pollicis longus.

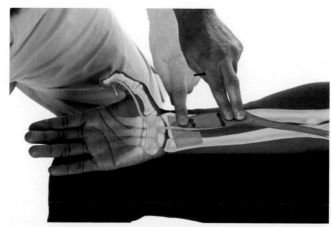

Figure 15-30 Palpation of the belly of the right flexor pollicis longus as the thumb flexes at the interphalangeal (IP) joint. The pronator quadratus has been ghosted in.

15

FLEXOR POLLICIS LONGUS—SEATED—*cont'd*

PALPATION NOTES

1. The flexor pollicis longus is often missing the ulnar and humeral attachments proximally. In these individuals, the muscle usually stops approximately halfway up the forearm. Furthermore, when present, the humeroulnar head is usually small and therefore difficult to palpate.
2. Even though this muscle is deep, it is usually not necessary to use much pressure to feel its contraction when the client flexes the thumb at the IP joint.
3. The radial artery is near the flexor pollicis longus, so if you feel a pulse, move off the artery.
4. It is best to palpate the flexor pollicis longus by asking the client to isolate flexion of the thumb at the IP joint. If the client also flexes the thumb at the CMC and/or MCP joints, other muscles of the thumb will be engaged, lessening the strength of the flexor pollicis longus contraction. Furthermore, these other muscles are located in the thenar eminence of the hand, and their contraction makes it more difficult to palpate and discern the distal tendon of the flexor pollicis longus.

Palpation Key:
Think of clicking a lighter with your thumb.

Alternate Palpation Position—Supine

The flexor pollicis longus can also be palpated with the client supine. Follow the palpation steps indicated for the seated palpation.

TRIGGER POINTS

1. Trigger points (TrPs) in the flexor pollicis longus often result from or are perpetuated by acute or chronic overuse of the muscle (e.g., repetitive or forceful gripping of a steering wheel, tennis racquet, golf club, or gardening or work tools).
2. TrPs in the flexor pollicis longus may produce sharp referral pain that is felt not only throughout the anterior aspect of the thumb but also beyond the tip of the thumb (phantom pain). In addition, extension of the thumb joints and wrist joint may be restricted.
3. The referral patterns of flexor pollicis longus TrPs must be distinguished from the referral patterns of TrPs in the opponens pollicis, adductor pollicis, brachialis, and subclavius.
4. TrPs in the flexor pollicis longus are often incorrectly assessed as medial epicondylitis/epicondylosis, carpal tunnel syndrome, thoracic outlet syndrome, pathologic cervical disc, thoracic outlet syndrome, or osteoarthritis of the thumb.
5. Associated TrPs often occur in the flexor digitorum superficialis and flexor digitorum profundus.

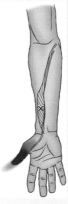

Figure 15-31 Anterior view illustrating a common flexor pollicis longus trigger point (TrP) and its corresponding referral zone.

15

FLEXOR POLLICIS LONGUS—SEATED—*cont'd*

STRETCHING THE FLEXOR POLLICIS LONGUS

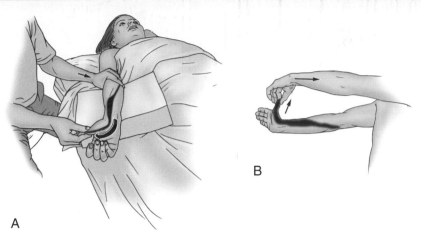

Figure 15-32 Stretching the right flexor pollicis longus. The client's thumb is extended with the hand fully extended and the forearm fully extended and supinated. **A,** Therapist-assisted stretch. Note that the therapist stabilizes the client's arm with the other hand and that a cushion is placed under the client's forearm to help maintain extension at the elbow joint. **B,** Self-care stretch.

 DETOUR

Pronator Quadratus:

The pronator quadratus (Figure 15-33, *A*) is deep and difficult to palpate and discern. It attaches from the distal anterior ulna to the distal anterior radius, and pronates the forearm at the radioulnar joints. Palpate with firm pressure in the anterior distal forearm on the radial side while resisting the client's forearm pronation at the radioulnar joints; be sure to apply resistance to the client's forearm, not the hand (Figure 15-33, *B*). If you are successful in feeling the pronator quadratus, follow it toward its ulnar attachment. Note: The median and ulnar nerves and the radial and ulnar arteries are all located in the anterior wrist; therefore, prudence must be exercised when palpating deeply here.

Trigger Points

1. The same factors that create and/or perpetuate trigger points (TrPs) in the pronator teres are likely to create and/or perpetuate TrPs in the pronator quadratus.
2. TrPs in the pronator quadratus are associated with TrPs in the pronator teres.
3. TrP referral patterns have not been established for the pronator quadratus.

15

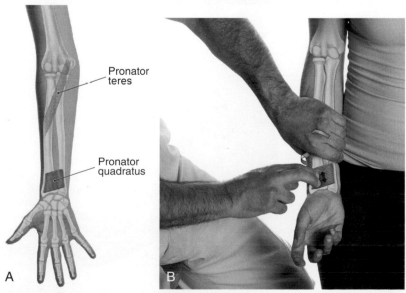

Pronator teres

Pronator quadratus

Figure 15-33 A, Anterior view of the right pronator quadratus. The pronator teres has been ghosted in. **B,** View of the pronator quadratus being palpated as pronation of the forearm at the radioulnar joints is resisted.

RADIAL GROUP—SEATED

The radial group is composed of the brachioradialis, the extensor carpi radialis longus (ECRL), and the extensor carpi radialis brevis (ECRB). Palpation of the brachioradialis has already been covered in this chapter (see p. 292). Here we discuss palpation of the other two radial group muscles.

☑ ATTACHMENTS

ECRL
☐ Distal ⅓ of the lateral supracondylar ridge of the humerus

   to the

☐ radial side of the posterior hand at the base of the second metacarpal

ECRB
☐ Lateral epicondyle of the humerus (via the common extensor tendon)

   to the

☐ radial side of the posterior hand at the base of the third metacarpal

☑ ACTIONS

Both extensor carpi radialis muscles:
☐ Radially deviate (abduct) the hand at the wrist joint
☐ Extend the hand at the wrist joint
☐ Flex the forearm at the elbow joint

Starting Position (Figure 15-35)
■ Client seated with the arm relaxed and the forearm flexed at the elbow joint and in a position that is halfway between full pronation and full supination, and resting on the client's thigh
■ Therapist seated to the side and facing the client
■ The radial group is pinched with the palpating fingers

Palpation Steps
1. The radial group of muscles can usually be pinched and separated from the rest of the musculature of the forearm. Pinch the radial group of muscles between your thumb on one side and your index finger (or index and middle fingers) on the other side, and gently pull the musculature away from the forearm (see Figure 15-35).
2. Move your palpating fingers onto the ECRL and ECRB (posterior to the brachioradialis), and feel for their contraction as the client radially deviates the hand at the wrist joint (Figure 15-36, *A*). Resistance to radial deviation can be added with your support hand if desired.
3. Continue palpating the extensor carpi radialis muscles toward their distal attachments while strumming perpendicularly across them.
4. Once the ECRL and ECRB have been located, have the client relax them and palpate to assess their baseline tone.

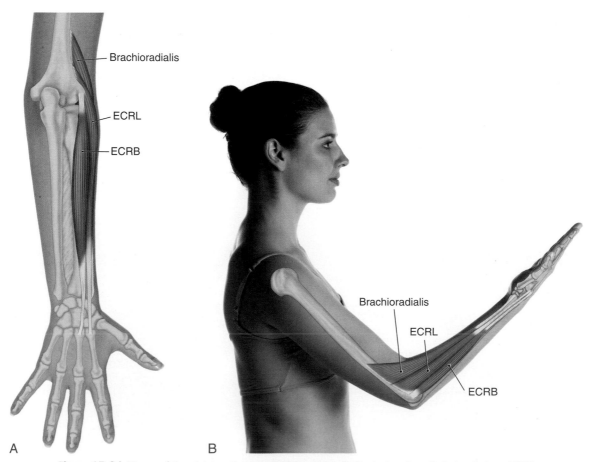

A   B

Figure 15-34 Views of the right radial group of muscles. **A,** Posterior view. **B,** Lateral view. *ECRL,* Extensor carpi radialis longus; *ECRB,* extensor carpi radialis brevis.

RADIAL GROUP—SEATED—cont'd

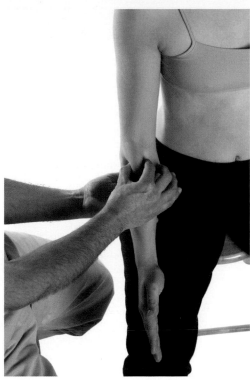

Figure 15-35 The right radial group of muscles is being pinched between the thumb and index finger of the therapist.

Palpation Key:
Pinch the radial group away from the forearm.

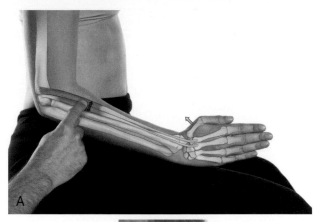

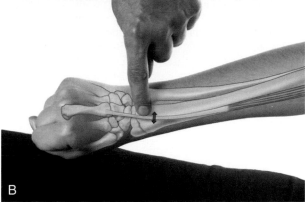

Figure 15-36 Palpation of the right extensors carpi radialis longus and brevis. **A,** Palpation of the extensors carpi radialis longus and brevis as the client radially deviates the hand at the wrist joint. **B,** Palpation of the distal tendon of the extensor carpi radialis brevis (ECRB) as it engages to stabilize the hand from flexing at the wrist joint when the hand makes a fist (see Palpation Note #5).

PALPATION NOTES

1. The brachioradialis is the most anterior of the three muscles of the radial group; the extensor carpi radialis brevis (ERCB) is the most posterior; the extensor carpi radialis longus (ERCL) is in the middle.
2. Immediately posterior to the radial group (i.e., posterior to the ECRB) is the extensor digitorum.
3. To distinguish the border between the ECRB and extensor digitorum, have the client alternately perform radial deviation of the hand at the wrist joint and extension of the fingers at the MCP and IP joints. The ECRB contracts with radial deviation of the hand, and the extensor digitorum contracts with finger extension.
4. To distinguish the border between the ECRL and brachioradialis, have the client alternately perform radial deviation

of the hand at the wrist joint and flexion of the forearm at the elbow joint. The ECRL contracts with radial deviation of the hand, and the brachioradialis contracts with forearm flexion.
5. Distinguishing between the bellies of the two extensor carpi radialis muscles is challenging. One way is by location. Another method is to ask the client to perform gentle to moderate flexion of the fingers (i.e., make a fist). This tends to engage the ERCB to stabilize the wrist joint from flexing (because of the pull of the finger flexor muscles), but not the ECRL. Flexion of the fingers usually causes palpable and often visible tensing of the distal tendon of the ECRB (see Figure 15-36, *B*).

Alternate Palpation Position—Supine

The extensor carpi radialis muscles can also be palpated with the client supine. Follow the palpation steps indicated for the seated palpation.

15

RADIAL GROUP—SEATED—*cont'd*

TRIGGER POINTS

1. Trigger points (TrPs) in the ECRL and ECRB often result from or are perpetuated by acute or chronic overuse of the muscle (e.g., forceful or repetitive gripping of the hand, hitting a one-handed backhand in tennis) and TrPs in the scalenes or supraspinatus.

2. TrPs in the extensors carpi radialis may produce a weak or painful grip (e.g., when shaking hands), restricted ulnar deviation of the hand at the wrist joint, and entrapment of the radial nerve (the ECRB only).

3. The referral patterns of extensors carpi radialis TrPs must be distinguished from the referral patterns of TrPs in the brachioradialis, extensor digitorum, extensor indicis, supinator, triceps brachii, subclavius, scalenes, supraspinatus, infraspinatus, subscapularis, coracobrachialis, brachialis, latissimus dorsi, adductor pollicis, and first dorsal interosseus manus.

4. TrPs in the extensors carpi radialis are often incorrectly assessed as lateral epicondylitis/epicondylosis, C7 or C8 nerve compression, carpal tunnel syndrome, wrist joint dysfunction or arthritis, or de Quervain stenosing tenosynovitis.

5. Associated TrPs of the extensors carpi radialis often occur in the brachioradialis, extensor digitorum, supinator, scalenes, and supraspinatus.

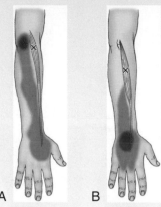

A   B

Figure 15-37 Posterior views illustrating common extensor carpi radialis longus and brevis trigger points (TrPs) and their corresponding referral zones. **A,** Extensor carpi radialis longus (ERCL). **B,** Extensor carpi radialis brevis (ECRB).

STRETCHING THE RADIAL GROUP

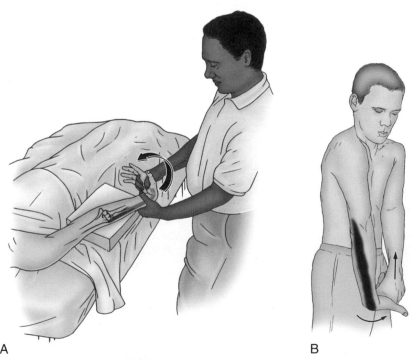

A   B

Figure 15-38 Stretching the right extensors carpi radialis longus and brevis. The client's hand is flexed and ulnar deviated. **A,** Therapist-assisted stretch. Note that the therapist stabilizes the client's forearm with the other hand and that a cushion is placed under the client's forearm to help maintain extension at the elbow joint. **B,** Self-care stretch. Note: See Figure 15-9, for a stretch of the brachioradialis of the radial group.

EXTENSOR DIGITORUM AND EXTENSOR DIGITI MINIMI—SEATED

☑ ATTACHMENTS

Extensor digitorum

☐ Lateral epicondyle of the humerus (via the common extensor tendon)

to the

☐ posterior surfaces of the middle and distal phalanges of fingers two through five

Extensor digiti minimi

☐ Lateral epicondyle of the humerus (via the common extensor tendon)

to the

☐ posterior surfaces of the middle and distal phalanges of the little finger (by attaching into the distal tendon of the extensor digitorum to the little finger)

☑ ACTIONS

Extensor digitorum

☐ Extends fingers two through five at the metacarpophalangeal (MCP) and interphalangeal (IP) joints
☐ Extends the hand at the wrist joint
☐ Extends the forearm at the elbow joint

Extensor digiti minimi

☐ Extends the little finger (#5) at the MCP and IP joints
☐ Extends the hand at the wrist joint
☐ Extends the forearm at the elbow joint

Starting Position (Figure 15-40)

■ Client seated with the arm relaxed, and the forearm flexed at the elbow joint, fully pronated at the radioulnar joints, and resting on the client's thigh
■ Therapist seated facing the client
■ Palpating fingers placed on the middle of the posterior proximal forearm
■ Support hand placed on the posterior side of the client's fingers (if resistance is given)

Palpation Steps

1. Ask the client to fully extend fingers two through five at the MCP and IP joints, and feel for the contraction of the extensor digitorum and extensor digiti minimi (Figure 15-41). Resistance can be given to finger extension with your supporting hand if desired. (Be sure that the client is not attempting to extend the hand at the wrist joint, or all muscles in the posterior forearm will contract.)
2. Continue palpating toward the distal attachments while strumming perpendicular to the fibers of these two muscles.
3. The distal tendons of the finger extensors can often be seen on the posterior surface of the hand. If not visible, they are usually easily palpable while strumming perpendicular to them.
4. Once the extensor digitorum and extensor digiti minimi have been located, have the client relax them and palpate to assess their baseline tone.

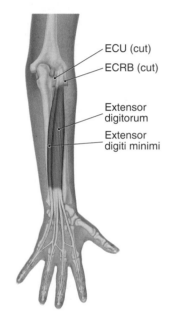

ECU (cut)
ECRB (cut)

Extensor digitorum
Extensor digiti minimi

Figure 15-39 Posterior view of the right extensor digitorum and extensor digiti minimi. The proximal ends of the extensor carpi ulnaris (ECU) and extensor carpi radialis brevis (ECRB) have been cut and ghosted in.

15

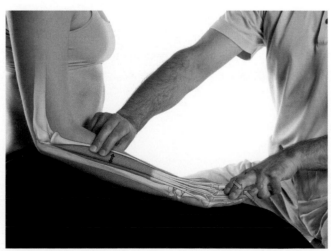

Figure 15-41 Palpation of the right extensor digitorum and extensor digiti minimi as the client extends fingers two through five against resistance.

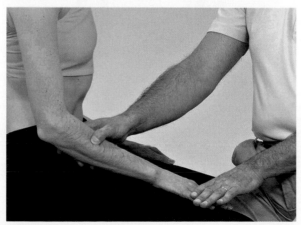

Figure 15-40 Starting position for seated palpation of the right extensor digitorum and extensor digiti minimi.

EXTENSOR DIGITORUM AND EXTENSOR DIGITI MINIMI—SEATED—*cont'd*

PALPATION NOTES

1. If the client is asked to extend one finger at a time, the tendon and associated muscle belly fibers of the extensor digitorum that go to that finger can be separately palpated.
2. Distinguishing between the extensor digitorum and the extensor carpi radialis brevis (ERCB) is accomplished by asking the client to radially deviate the hand at the wrist joint. This engages the ECRB but not the extensor digitorum. Or have the client extend the fingers; this engages the extensor digitorum but not the ECRB.
3. Distinguishing between the extensor digiti minimi and the extensor carpi ulnaris (ECU) is accomplished by asking the client to ulnar deviate the hand at the wrist joint. This engages the ECU but not the extensor digiti minimi. Or have the client extend the fingers; this engages the extensor digiti minimi but not the ECU.
4. Distinguishing between the extensor digitorum fibers that go to the little finger and the extensor digiti minimi (i.e., locating the border between these two muscles) is extremely difficult, because they are next to each other and they are both engaged with the same action (extension of the little finger).

Alternate Palpation Position—Supine

The extensor digitorum and extensor digiti minimi can also be palpated with the client supine. Follow the palpation steps indicated for the seated palpation.

Palpation Key:
Extend the fingers and palpate in the middle of the posterior forearm.

TRIGGER POINTS

1. Trigger points (TrPs) in the extensor digitorum and extensor digiti minimi often result from or are perpetuated by acute or chronic overuse of the muscle (e.g., repetitive finger movements, such as typing or playing piano), keeping the muscle in a chronically lengthened state (e.g., sleeping with the fingers in flexion), or TrPs in the scalenes.
2. TrPs in the extensor digitorum and extensor digiti minimi may produce stiffness of the fingers (i.e., decreased flexion).
3. The referral patterns of extensor digitorum and extensor digiti minimi TrPs must be distinguished from the referral patterns of TrPs in the extensor indicis, dorsal interossei manus, scalenes, subclavius, latissimus dorsi, coracobrachialis, and triceps brachii.
4. TrPs in the extensor digitorum and extensor digiti minimi are often incorrectly assessed as lateral epicondylitis/epicondylosis, arthritis of the fingers, C7 or C6 nerve compression, or carpal joint dysfunction.
5. Associated TrPs often occur in the extensor carpi radialis longus (ECRL), extensor carpi radialis brevis (ECRB), supinator, brachioradialis, and extensor carpi ulnaris.
6. Note: A TrP in the extensor digitorum or extensor digiti minimi usually results in referral of pain into the dorsum of the hand and the finger that is controlled by those muscle fibers. TrPs occur most commonly in the fibers of the middle and ring fingers.

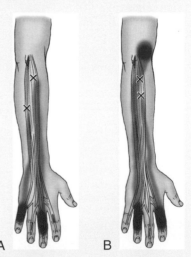

Figure 15-42 Posterior views illustrating common extensor digitorum and extensor digiti minimi trigger points (TrPs) and their corresponding referral zones. **A,** A TrP in the extensor digiti minimi referring into the little finger, and a TrP in the extensor digitorum referring into the middle finger. **B,** TrPs in the extensor digitorum referring into the index and ring fingers.

15

EXTENSOR DIGITORUM AND EXTENSOR DIGITI MINIMI—SEATED—*cont'd*

STRETCHING THE EXTENSOR DIGITORUM AND EXTENSOR DIGITI MINIMI

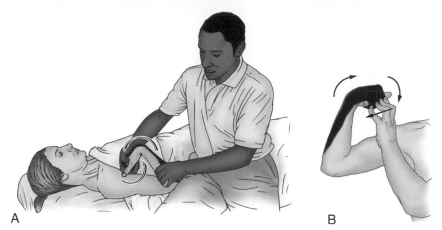

Figure 15-43 Stretching the right extensors digitorum and digiti minimi. With the forearm and hand fully flexed, the client's fingers two through five are fully flexed at the metacarpophalangeal (MCP) and interphalangeal (IP) joints. **A,** Therapist-assisted stretch. The therapist flexes the client's hand and fingers with one hand and flexes the client's forearm with the other. **B,** Self-care stretch.

EXTENSOR CARPI ULNARIS—SEATED

☑ ATTACHMENTS

☐ Lateral epicondyle of the humerus (via the common extensor tendon) and the middle ⅓ of the posterior ulna

to the

☐ ulnar side of the posterior hand at the base of the fifth metacarpal

☑ ACTIONS

☐ Extends the hand at the wrist joint
☐ Ulnar deviates the hand at the wrist joint
☐ Extends the forearm at the elbow joint

Starting Position (Figure 15-45)

■ Client seated with the arm relaxed, and the forearm flexed at the elbow joint, fully pronated at the radioulnar joints, and resting on the client's thigh
■ Therapist seated facing the client
■ Palpating fingers placed immediately posterior to the shaft of the ulna
■ Support hand placed on the ulnar side of the hand, proximal to the fingers (if resistance is given)

Palpation Steps

1. Ask the client to ulnar deviate the hand at the wrist joint, and feel for the contraction of the extensor carpi ulnaris (Figure 15-46). Resistance can be given with your support hand if desired.

2. Palpate proximally toward the lateral epicondyle and distally toward the fifth metacarpal while strumming perpendicular to the fibers as the client alternately contracts and relaxes the muscle.
3. Once the extensor carpi ulnaris has been located, have the client relax it and palpate to assess its baseline tone.

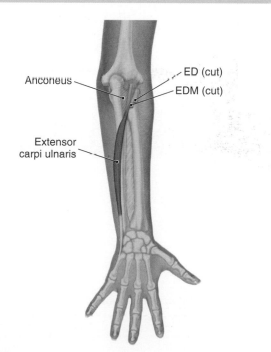

Figure 15-44 Posterior view of the right extensor carpi ulnaris. The anconeus has been ghosted in. The proximal tendons of the extensor digitorum and extensor digiti minimi have been cut and ghosted in.

15

EXTENSOR CARPI ULNARIS—SEATED—*cont'd*

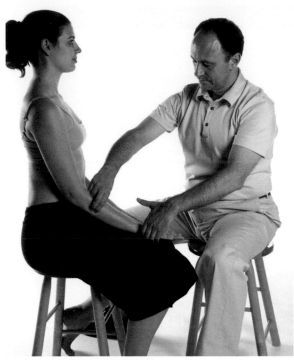

Figure 15-45 Starting position for seated palpation of the right extensor carpi ulnaris.

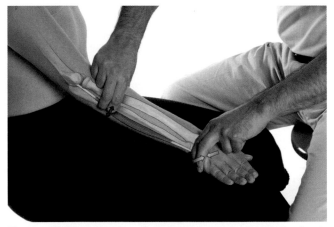

Figure 15-46 Palpation of the right extensor carpi ulnaris immediately posterior to the shaft of the ulna as the client ulnar deviates the hand at the wrist joint against resistance.

PALPATION NOTES

1. The extensor carpi ulnaris is all the way on the ulnar side of the posterior forearm, directly adjacent to the shaft of the ulna.
2. When having the client perform ulnar deviation of the hand at the wrist joint, make sure that the client's fingers are relaxed. If the fingers are extended, the extensor digitorum and extensor digiti minimi will be engaged, making it difficult to discern the extensor carpi ulnaris from these muscles.
3. Distinguishing between the extensor carpi ulnaris and the extensor digiti minimi is accomplished by asking the client to extend the little finger. This engages the extensor digiti minimi but not the extensor carpi ulnaris. Or have the client ulnar deviate the hand at the wrist joint; this engages the extensor carpi ulnaris but not the extensor digiti minimi.

Alternate Palpation Position—Supine

The extensor carpi ulnaris can also be palpated with the client supine. Follow the palpation steps indicated for the seated palpation.

Palpation Key:
Palpate immediately posterior to the shaft of the ulna.

15

EXTENSOR CARPI ULNARIS—SEATED—*cont'd*

TRIGGER POINTS

1. Trigger points (TrPs) in the extensor carpi ulnaris often result from or are perpetuated by acute or chronic overuse of the muscle (e.g., holding the hands in ulnar deviation when typing), direct trauma, and TrPs in the scalenes or serratus posterior superior.
2. The referral patterns of extensor carpi ulnaris TrPs must be distinguished from the referral patterns of TrPs in the extensor carpi radialis brevis (ECRB), extensor indicis, supinator, scalenes, subscapularis, and coracobrachialis.
3. TrPs in the extensor carpi ulnaris are often incorrectly assessed as wrist joint dysfunction or arthritis, carpal tunnel syndrome, or C7 or C8 nerve compression.
4. Associated TrPs often occur in the extensor digitorum, extensor digiti minimi, scalenes, and serratus posterior superior.
5. Note: Because the extensor carpi ulnaris does not have to support a weight against gravity as often as the radial deviators of the hand (extensors carpi radialis longus and brevis), it usually does not develop trigger points as often as they do.

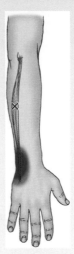

Figure 15-47 Posterior view illustrating a common extensor carpi ulnaris trigger point (TrP) and its corresponding referral zone.

STRETCHING THE EXTENSOR CARPI ULNARIS

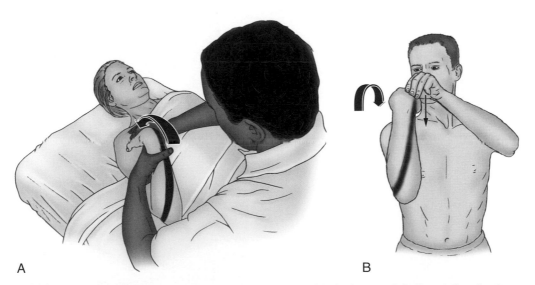

A   B

Figure 15-48 Stretching the right extensor carpi ulnaris. With the forearm fully flexed, the client's hand is flexed and radially deviated. **A,** Therapist-assisted stretch. The therapist uses one hand to flex the client's hand at the wrist joint and the other hand to flex the client's forearm at the elbow joint. **B,** Self-care stretch.

15

SUPINATOR—SEATED

☑ ATTACHMENTS

☐ Lateral epicondyle of the humerus and the supinator crest of the ulna

to the

☐ proximal ⅓ of the radius (posterior, lateral, and anterior sides)

☑ ACTION

☐ Supinates the forearm at the radioulnar joints

Starting Position (Figure 15-50):

■ Client seated with the arm relaxed, and the forearm flexed at the elbow joint, in a position that is halfway between full pronation and full supination, and resting on the client's thigh
■ Therapist seated facing the client
■ Palpating fingers pinch the radial group of muscles away from the forearm
■ Support hand placed on the client's distal forearm, just proximal to the wrist joint

Palpation Steps:

1. The radial group of muscles can usually be pinched and separated from the rest of the musculature of the forearm. Pinch the radial group of muscles between your thumb on one side and your index and middle fingers on the other side, and gently pull them away from the forearm.

2. Gently but firmly sink in (between the extensor carpi radialis brevis [ECRB] of the radial group and the extensor digitorum) toward the supinator attachment on the radius; ask the client to supinate the forearm against resistance, and feel for the contraction of the supinator (Figure 15-51).
3. Continue palpating the supinator (through the more superficial musculature) toward its proximal attachment, and feel for its contraction as the client alternately contracts and relaxes the supinator.
4. Once the supinator has been located, have the client relax it and palpate to assess its baseline tone.

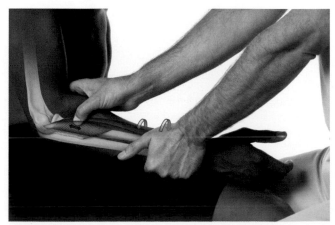

Figure 15-50 Starting position for seated palpation of the right supinator.

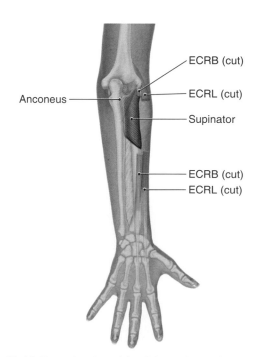

ECRB (cut)
ECRL (cut)
Anconeus
Supinator
ECRB (cut)
ECRL (cut)

Figure 15-49 Posterior view of the right supinator. The anconeus has been ghosted in. The extensor carpi radialis longus (ECRL) and extensor carpi radialis brevis (ECRB) have been cut and ghosted in.

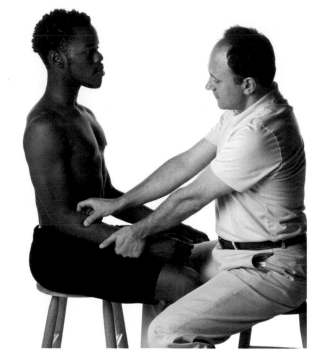

Figure 15-51 Palpation of the right supinator against the radius between the radial group of muscles and the extensor digitorum.

15

SUPINATOR—SEATED—*cont'd*

 PALPATION NOTES

1. When resisting the client's forearm supination, a gentle but firm grasp is needed by the support hand. Otherwise only the client's skin is held and the underlying forearm bones are allowed to move. This results in unsuccessful resistance to forearm supination and is uncomfortable for the client.

2. The supinator can also be palpated on the anterior/medial side of the brachioradialis. Have the client's brachioradialis slackened by passively flexing the client's elbow joint (20 to 30 degrees). Push the brachioradialis laterally, and then press in deep toward the head and shaft of the radius; you will encounter the supinator (Figure 15-52).

3. The deep branch of the radial nerve runs through the supinator muscle. Be aware of this when pressing in deeply against the supinator.

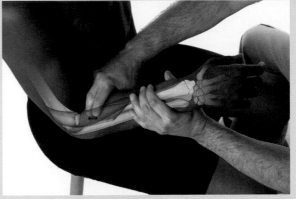

Figure 15-52 Palpation of the right supinator by pushing the brachioradialis laterally and then pressing in toward the radius (see Palpation Note #2).

TRIGGER POINTS

1. Trigger points (TrPs) in the supinator often result from or are perpetuated by acute or chronic overuse of the muscle (e.g., using a screwdriver, turning tight doorknobs, hitting a backhand in tennis with poor form).

2. TrPs in the supinator may produce entrapment of the deep branch of the radial nerve; supinator TrPs are the most common TrPs that cause lateral epicondylar pain.

3. The referral patterns of supinator TrPs must be distinguished from the referral patterns of TrPs in the extensor carpi radialis longus (ECRL), brachioradialis, extensor digitorum, biceps brachii, brachialis, triceps brachii, supraspinatus, infraspinatus, subclavius, scalenes, adductor pollicis, and first dorsal interosseus manus.

4. TrPs in the supinator are often incorrectly assessed as lateral epicondylitis/epicondylosis, C5 or C6 nerve compression, or de Quervain stenosing tenosynovitis.

5. Associated TrPs often occur in the ECRL, extensor carpi radialis brevis (ECRB), extensor digitorum, extensor digiti minimi, triceps brachii, anconeus, brachioradialis, biceps brachii, brachialis, and palmaris longus (PL).

15

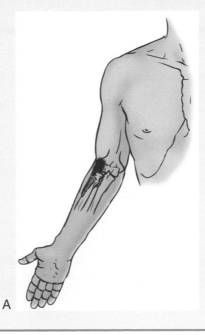

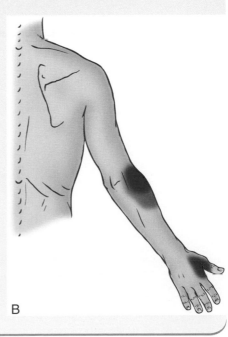

Figure 15-53 A, Anterior view illustrating a common supinator trigger point (TrP) and its corresponding referral zone. **B,** Posterior view showing the remainder of the referral zone.

A   B

SUPINATOR—SEATED—*cont'd*

Alternate Palpation Position—Supine

The supinator can also be palpated with the client supine. Follow the palpation steps indicated for the seated palpation.

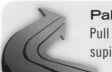

Palpation Key:
Pull radial group away and sink into the supinator against the radius.

STRETCHING THE SUPINATOR

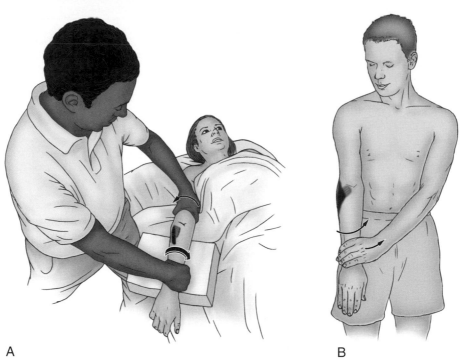

A

B

Figure 15-54 Stretching the right supinator. The client's forearm is fully pronated. Note: It is easy to confuse pronation of the forearm at the radioulnar joints with medial rotation of the arm at the shoulder joint. Be sure that forearm pronation is being done. **A,** Therapist-assisted stretch. The therapist stabilizes the client's arm from medially rotating with the other hand. **B,** Self-care stretch.

DEEP DISTAL FOUR GROUP—SEATED

The deep distal four group is composed of the abductor pollicis longus, extensor pollicis brevis, extensor pollicis longus, and extensor indicis.

☑ ATTACHMENTS

Abductor pollicis longus
☐ Middle ⅓ of the posterior radius, interosseus membrane, and ulna

to the

☐ base of the metacarpal of the thumb

Extensor pollicis brevis
☐ Distal ⅓ of the posterior radius and interosseus membrane

to the

☐ base of the proximal phalanx of the thumb

Extensor pollicis longus
☐ Middle ⅓ of the posterior ulna and interosseus membrane

to the

☐ base of the distal phalanx of the thumb

Extensor indicis
☐ Distal ⅓ of the posterior ulna and interosseus membrane

to the

☐ posterior surfaces of the middle and distal phalanges of the index finger (by attaching into the ulnar side of the distal tendon of the extensor digitorum to the index finger)

☑ ACTIONS

Abductor pollicis longus
☐ Abducts the thumb at the carpometacarpal (CMC) joint
☐ Extends the thumb at the CMC joint
☐ Radially deviates the hand at the wrist joint

Extensor pollicis brevis
☐ Abducts the thumb at the CMC joint
☐ Extends the thumb at the CMC joint and the metacarpophalangeal (MCP) joint
☐ Radially deviates the hand at the wrist joint

Extensor pollicis longus
☐ Extends the thumb at the CMC, MCP, and interphalangeal (IP) joints
☐ Radially deviates the hand at the wrist joint

Extensor indicis
☐ Extends the index finger at the MCP and IP joints
☐ Extends the hand at the wrist joint

Starting Position (Figure 15-56)
■ Client seated with the arm relaxed and the forearm flexed at the elbow joint and fully pronated at the radioulnar joints, and resting on the client's thigh; client's thumb actively extended (Note: Extension of the thumb at the CMC joint is a frontal plane motion away from the palm of the hand.)
■ Therapist seated facing the client
■ Palpating fingers placed on the radial side of the posterior wrist (after visualizing the tendons)

Palpation Steps
1. First visualize the distal tendons of the abductor pollicis longus, extensor pollicis brevis, and extensor pollicis longus as they define the anatomic snuffbox (see Palpation Note #1) by asking the client to actively extend the thumb at the CMC joint (see Figure 15-56). Note that the tendons of the abductor pollicis longus and extensor pollicis brevis are right next to each other and may appear to be one tendon (see Palpation Note #2).
2. Once located, palpate each of these muscles individually back to its proximal attachment while strumming perpendicular to the fibers as the client alternately contracts and relaxes that muscle by extending the thumb (Figure 15-57).
3. To palpate the extensor indicis, first locate its distal tendon on the posterior side of the hand by asking the client to extend the index finger at the MCP and IP joints (Figure 15-58).
4. Continue palpating the extensor indicis proximally while strumming perpendicular to its fibers as the client alternately contracts and relaxes the muscle.
5. Once the muscles of the deep distal four group have been located, have the client relax them and palpate to assess their baseline tone.

15

DEEP DISTAL FOUR GROUP—SEATED—*cont'd*

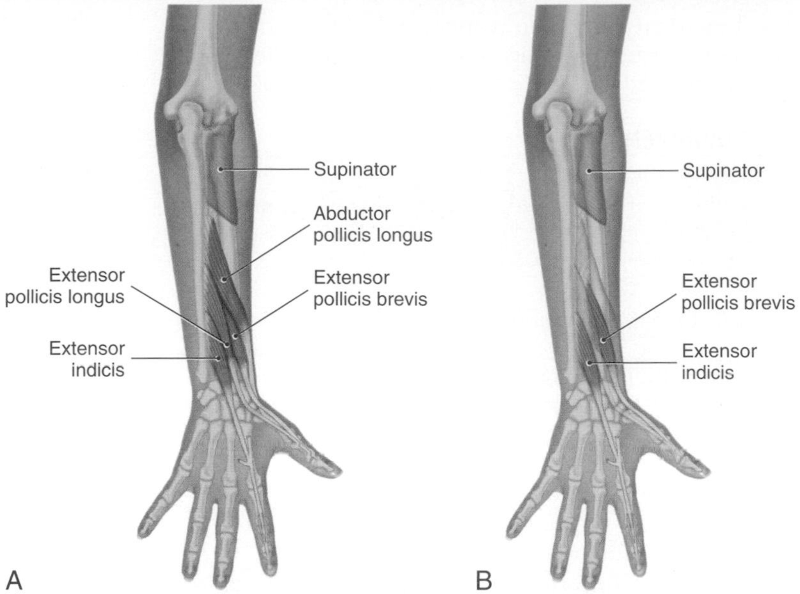

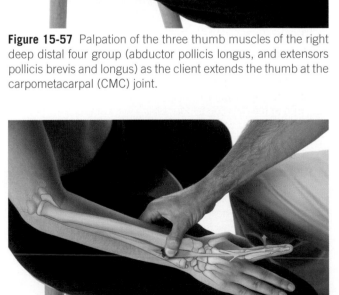

Figure 15-55 Posterior views of the muscles of the right deep distal four group. **A,** All four muscles with the supinator ghosted in. **B,** Same illustration with the abductor pollicis longus and extensor pollicis longus ghosted in.

Supinator
Abductor pollicis longus
Extensor pollicis longus
Extensor pollicis brevis
Extensor indicis

Supinator
Extensor pollicis brevis
Extensor indicis

A   B

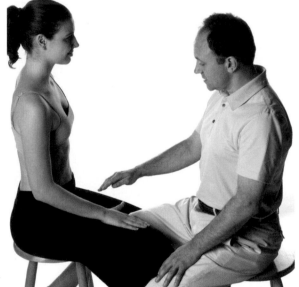

Figure 15-56 Starting position for seated palpation of the right deep distal four muscles. Before beginning their palpation, first visualize the tendons of the anatomic snuffbox by having the client extend the thumb (see Palpation Note #1).

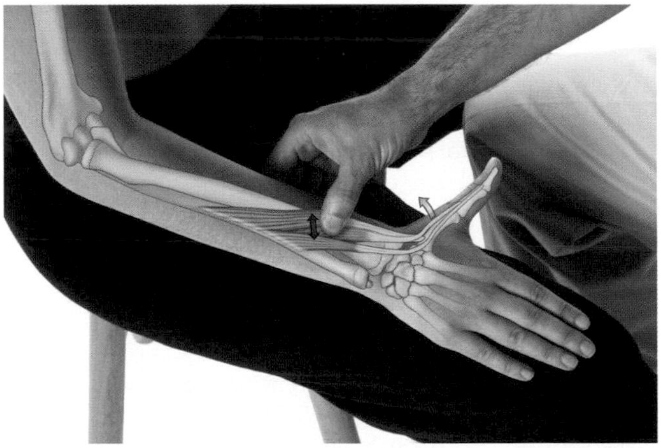

Figure 15-57 Palpation of the three thumb muscles of the right deep distal four group (abductor pollicis longus, and extensors pollicis brevis and longus) as the client extends the thumb at the carpometacarpal (CMC) joint.

Palpation Key:
Extend the thumb (thumb/pollicis muscles).
Extend the index finger (extensor indicis).

Figure 15-58 Palpation of the right extensor indicis of the deep distal four group as the client extends the index finger at the metacarpophalangeal (MCP) joint.

DEEP DISTAL FOUR GROUP—SEATED—*cont'd*

PALPATION NOTES

1. The anatomic snuffbox is a depression that is bordered by the three thumb (pollicis) muscles of the deep distal four group. The abductor pollicis longus and extensor pollicis brevis border the anatomic snuffbox on the radial side; the extensor pollicis longus borders the anatomic snuffbox on the ulnar side.
2. The distal tendons of the abductor pollicis longus and extensor pollicis brevis are extremely close to each other and often appear to be one tendon. If so, these two tendons can be separated by gently placing a fingernail between them. These two tendons run superficial to the distal end of the brachioradialis muscle.
3. To engage the thumb muscles of the deep distal four group and make them more readily visible and palpable, a small amount of thumb abduction at the CMC joint in addition to thumb extension can be done.
4. Even though the muscles of the deep distal four group are deep, they are usually easily palpable through the more superficial muscles.
5. It can be difficult to discern the extensor indicis from the portion of the extensor digitorum that goes to the index finger. Perhaps the best way to distinguish these two muscles from each other is to note the different locations of the bellies and therefore the different directions of fibers. The extensor indicis orients much more transversely across the distal forearm from radial to ulnar to reach its proximal attachment on the ulna; whereas the extensor digitorum is oriented much more longitudinally in the forearm, traveling proximally to the lateral epicondyle of the humerus. In the dorsum of the hand, the distal tendon of the extensor indicis is located to the ulnar side of the distal tendon of the extensor digitorum that goes to the index finger.

Alternate Palpation Position—Supine

The muscles of the deep distal four group can also be palpated with the client supine. Follow the palpation steps indicated for the seated palpation.

TRIGGER POINTS

1. Trigger points (TrPs) in the muscles of the deep distal four group often result from or are perpetuated by acute or chronic overuse of the muscle (e.g., repetitive motions of the index finger or thumb, such as playing a musical instrument or typing).
2. TrPs in the deep distal four group may produce discomfort and difficulty when performing fine motor tasks with the index finger and/or thumb.
3. The referral patterns of extensor indicis TrPs must be distinguished from the referral patterns of TrPs in the extensors carpi radialis brevis and longus, extensor carpi ulnaris, extensor digitorum, coracobrachialis, brachialis, supinator, scalenes, subclavius, and first dorsal interosseus.
4. TrPs in the muscles of the deep distal four group are often incorrectly assessed as wrist joint dysfunction or de Quervain stenosing tenosynovitis.
5. Associated TrPs often occur in the extensor digitorum and extensor digiti minimi.
6. Note: TrP referral patterns have not yet been established for the deep distal four group muscles that go to the thumb. When assessing these muscles for TrPs, look primarily for central TrPs in the middle of the bellies.

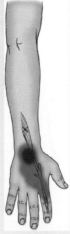

Figure 15-59 Posterior view illustrating a common extensor indicis trigger point (TrP) and its corresponding referral zone.

15

DEEP DISTAL FOUR GROUP—SEATED—*cont'd*

STRETCHING THE DEEP DISTAL FOUR GROUP

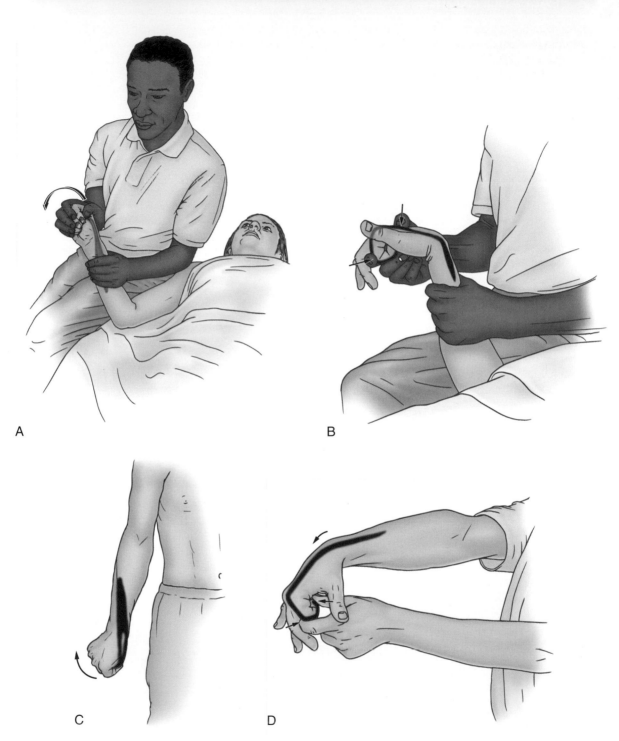

A

B

C

D

Figure 15-60 Stretching the muscles of the right deep distal four group. To stretch the thumb muscles of the group, the client's thumb is flexed and adducted (and cupped under the other fingers) while the hand is ulnar deviated at the wrist joint. To stretch the extensor indicis, the client's index finger is flexed at the metacarpophalangeal (MCP) and interphalangeal (IP) joints while the hand is flexed at the wrist joint. **A** and **B,** Therapist-assisted stretches of the three thumb muscles of the group and the extensor indicis, respectively. Note that the therapist stabilizes the client's forearm with the other hand. **C** and **D,** Self-care stretches of the three thumb muscles of the group and the extensor indicis, respectively.

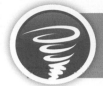

WHIRLWIND TOUR

Muscles of the Forearm

The following *Whirlwind Tour* is an abbreviated set of palpation protocols for the muscles of this chapter. Once you have read and become comfortable with each of the protocols presented thus far, this *Whirlwind Tour* allows you to quickly and efficiently run through the palpations protocols for all the muscles of the chapter.

For all palpations of the muscles of the forearm, the client is seated with the arm relaxed in neutral position, and the forearm is flexed at the elbow joint to 90 degrees and relaxed on the client's thigh. You are seated to the side or directly in front of the client and facing the client.

1. **Brachioradialis:** The client is seated with the arm relaxed; the forearm is flexed and in a position that is halfway between full pronation and full supination and resting on the client's thigh. Resist further flexion of the forearm at the elbow joint; first look for the brachioradialis to become visible, then palpate for it at the proximal anterolateral forearm. Once felt, continue palpating it to its proximal and distal attachments while strumming perpendicular to its fibers as the client alternately contracts and relaxes it. Note: The brachioradialis is superficial and is easily palpable for its entire length except for a small distal portion that is deep to the abductor pollicis longus and the extensor pollicis brevis.

2. **Pronator teres:** The client is seated with the arm relaxed; the forearm is flexed and in a position that is halfway between full pronation and full supination and resting on the client's thigh. Resist further pronation of the forearm and feel for the contraction of the pronator teres in the proximal anterior forearm. Once felt, continue palpating to the proximal attachment on the medial epicondyle and toward its distal attachment on the radius while strumming perpendicular to its fibers as the client alternately contracts and relaxes the muscle. Note: The pronator teres is superficial for its entire course except at its distal attachment on the radius where it is deep to the brachioradialis. To palpate it there, either palpate through the brachioradialis, or if it is possible to slacken the brachioradialis, try to push the brachioradialis out of the way and palpate directly on the radial attachment of the pronator teres.

3. **Wrist flexor group (FCR, PL, FCU):** The client is seated with the arm relaxed; the forearm is flexed, fully supinated, and resting on the client's thigh. Resist the client from flexing the hand at the wrist joint and first look for the three wrist flexor tendons to become visible. The PL is dead center, the FCR is slightly radial to the PL, and the FCU is far to the ulnar side of the wrist. Then palpate them one at a time. Once a tendon is felt, continue palpating it proximally to its proximal attachment on the medial epicondyle while strumming perpendicular to it as the client alternately contracts and relaxes the muscle. Note: To discern these muscles as their bellies merge proximally, ask the client to do radial deviation to contract the FCR and ulnar deviation to contract the FCU; the PL is located between the other two and will stay relaxed with radial and ulnar deviation of the hand.

4. **Flexor digitorum superficialis and flexor digitorum profundus:** The client is seated with the arm relaxed; the forearm is flexed, fully supinated, and resting on the client's thigh. Ask the client to flex the proximal phalanges of fingers two through five at the MCP joints, and feel for the contraction of the flexor digitorum superficialis in the proximal anteromedial forearm, just posterior to the humeral belly of the FCU. (If resistance is given, be sure to isolate pressure against only the proximal phalanges.) Once felt, palpate the flexor digitorum superficialis proximally to the medial epicondyle and distally as far as possible while strumming perpendicular to its fibers as the client alternately contracts and relaxes the muscle. To palpate the flexor digitorum profundus, palpate more medially and posteriorly on the proximal forearm against the shaft of the ulna, and feel for its contraction as the client flexes fingers two through five at the IP joints. Once felt, palpate the flexor digitorum profundus proximally and distally as far as possible while strumming perpendicular to its fibers as the client alternately contracts and relaxes the muscle.

5. **Flexor pollicis longus:** The client is seated with the arm relaxed; the forearm is flexed, fully supinated, and resting on the client's thigh. Place your palpating fingers on the distal anterior forearm (just radial to the tendon of the FCR), and feel for the contraction of the flexor pollicis longus as the client flexes the distal phalanx of the thumb at the IP joint. Once felt, continue palpating the flexor pollicis longus proximally as far as possible as the client alternately contracts and relaxes the muscle. Note: It is usually not helpful to try to strum perpendicular to its fibers.

6. **Detour to pronator quadratus:** The pronator quadratus is deep and difficult to palpate. Palpate with firm pressure in the anterior distal forearm on the radial side while resisting pronation of the forearm at the radioulnar joints. To prevent the more superficial tendons of the wrist and finger flexors from tensing and obscuring the contraction of the pronator quadratus, be sure when resisting the client's forearm pronation that you apply the resistance to the forearm only. If you apply it to the client's hand, these more superficial muscles and their tendons will contract and tense. If you are successful in feeling the pronator quadratus, follow it toward its ulnar attachment.

7. **Radial group (brachioradialis, ECRL, ECRB):** The client is seated with the arm relaxed; the forearm is flexed and in a position that is halfway between full pronation and full supination and resting on the client's thigh. Pinch the radial group of muscles between your thumb and index/middle fingers and lift it away from the forearm, separating it from the rest of the forearm musculature. The brachioradialis is the most anterior; the ECRB is the

15

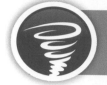

Muscles of the Forearm—*cont'd*

most posterior; and the ECRL is between the other two. Then palpate for the contraction of the ECRL and ECRB as the client radially deviates the hand at the wrist joint (resistance can be added). Once felt, continue palpating the ECRL and ECRB toward their distal attachments while strumming perpendicular to their fibers as the client alternately contracts and relaxes them. Note: The distal tendon of the ECRB can be palpated and often visualized at the wrist if the client is asked to make a fist with the hand in a neutral position or slight extension at the wrist joint.

8. **Extensor digitorum and extensor digiti minimi:** The client is seated with the arm relaxed; the forearm is flexed at the elbow joint, fully pronated at the radioulnar joints, and resting on the client's thigh. Feel for the contraction of the extensor digitorum and extensor digiti minimi in the middle of the posterior forearm as the client fully extends fingers two through five at the MCP and IP joints. Once felt, continue palpating the extensor digitorum and extensor digiti minimi proximally to the lateral epicondyle of the humerus and distally as far as possible while strumming perpendicular to its fibers as the client alternately contracts and relaxes the muscles. The extensor digiti minimi is the most ulnar of the fibers that are felt to contract (discerning the border of the extensor digitorum and extensor digiti minimi is extremely difficult). Note: The distal tendons of the finger extensors can usually be seen on the posterior surface of the hand. If not visible, they are usually easily palpable while strumming perpendicular to them.

9. **Extensor carpi ulnaris:** The client is seated with the arm relaxed; the forearm is flexed at the elbow joint, fully pronated at the radioulnar joints, and resting on the client's thigh. Feel for the contraction of the extensor carpi ulnaris immediately posterior to the shaft of the ulna as the client ulnar deviates the hand at the wrist joint. (Resistance can be given.) Once felt, continue palpating the extensor carpi ulnaris proximally to the lateral epicondyle of the humerus and distally toward the fifth metacarpal while strumming perpendicular to the fibers as the client contracts and relaxes the muscle.

10. **Supinator:** The client is seated with the arm relaxed; the forearm is flexed and in a position that is halfway between full pronation and full supination and resting on the client's thigh. Pinch the radial group of muscles between your thumb and index/middle fingers; lift it away from the forearm, separating it from the rest of the forearm musculature. Slowly and gently but firmly sink in toward the radius between the ECRB and the extensor digitorum, and feel for the contraction of the supinator as the client supinates the forearm against your resistance. Once felt, continue palpating the supinator (through the more superficial musculature) toward its proximal attachment as the client alternately contracts and relaxes the muscle.

11. **Deep distal four group (abductor pollicis longus, extensor pollicis brevis, extensor pollicis longus, extensor indicis):** The client is seated with the arm relaxed; the forearm is flexed, fully pronated, and resting on the client's thigh. First visualize the distal tendons of the abductor pollicis longus, extensor pollicis brevis, and extensor pollicis longus on the radial side of the posterior wrist as they define the anatomic snuffbox, by asking the client to actively extend the thumb at the CMC joint. (Note: The tendons of the abductor pollicis longus and extensor pollicis brevis lie next to each other and may appear to be one tendon.) Then palpate each tendon one at a time while strumming perpendicular to it as the client alternately contracts and relaxes the muscle by doing extension of the thumb at the CMC joint; palpate as far proximally and distally as possible toward the attachments of each muscle. To palpate the extensor indicis, first visually locate its distal tendon on the posterior side of the hand as the client extends the index finger at the MCP and IP joints. Then palpate it distally and proximally while strumming perpendicular to its fibers as the client alternately contracts and relaxes the muscle. Note: The extensor indicis can be discerned from the extensor digitorum by the direction of the fibers. The extensor indicis travels somewhat transversely across the distal forearm to reach its proximal attachment on the distal ulna. The extensor digitorum travels much more longitudinally in the forearm to reach its proximal attachment on the lateral epicondyle of the humerus. On the dorsum of the hand, the distal tendon of the extensor indicis is located to the ulnar side of the distal tendon of the extensor digitorum that goes to the index finger.

15

Review Questions

1. List the attachments of the pronator teres.
2. List the attachments of the extensor carpi radialis brevis.
3. What are the actions of the brachioradialis?
4. What are the actions of the flexor pollicis longus?
5. Though the palpation key for the brachioradialis is placing the forearm in the hitchhiking position, what palpation difficulty does this iconic position pose?
6. What sensitive structure might be impacted by palpation of the proximal pronator teres?
7. What is the alternate method of engaging the flexor carpi ulnaris that does not involve wrist joint flexion?
8. What muscle action can a therapist use to distinguish flexor digitorum superficialis from the flexor digitorum profundus during palpation?
9. What is the importance of a proper grip by the support hand when palpating the supinator?
10. What three muscles make up the anatomic snuffbox and on which side does each reside?
11. By what methods can a therapist discern the extensor digiti minimi from the extensor carpi ulnaris?
12. TrPs in which muscles may produce entrapment the median nerve?
13. TrPs in which muscles may produce entrapment of the radial nerve?
14. Describe a stretch for the flexors digitorum superficialis and profundus.
15. Describe a stretch for the extensor digitorum and extensor digiti minimi.
16. When stretching the wrist flexor group, what positional considerations must be addressed?
17. From anterior to posterior, what is the order of the radial group muscles? How can a therapist clearly discern the posterior border of this group?

CASE STUDY

A 58-year-old man comes to your office with pain and stiffness in his right distal forearm, wrist, and hand. The pain is two out of ten at rest, and varies from six to eight out of ten while at work where his duties include regular lifting of loads in excess of 50 pounds, repeated use of a cutting tool to remove raw products from precision molds, and frequent climbing of ladders. The pain has been present for years, and he is now starting to feel a loss of hand strength on occasion. He stated that he has been evaluated by his physician and was told that he had arthritic changes to the elbow and wrist joints that were consistent with his age and activities.

An examination reveals that the client's ranges of motion at the elbow and wrist joints are normal, and pain is only produced during resisted wrist motions. Gripping activities reproduce his pain as well.

1. What other questions might you ask this client during the interview?
2. What muscles would you expect to be tight and why?
3. What are your treatment plans and recommendations for this client?

15

CHAPTER 16

Tour #6 — Palpation of the Intrinsic Muscles of the Hand

Overview

This chapter is a palpation tour of the intrinsic muscles of the hand. The tour begins with the muscles of the thenar group, then covers the muscles of the hypothenar group, and finishes with palpation of the muscles of the central compartment. Palpation for each of the muscles is shown in the seated position, but alternate palpation positions are also described. The major muscles or muscle groups of the region are each given a separate layout; there is also a detour to the palmaris brevis. Trigger point (TrP) information and stretching, both therapist-assisted and self-care stretching, are given for each of the major muscles covered in this chapter. The chapter closes with an advanced *Whirlwind Tour* that explains the sequential palpation of all of the muscles of the chapter.

Chapter Outline

Thenar Group—Seated
 Abductor Pollicis Brevis (APB)
 Flexor Pollicis Brevis (FPB)
 Opponens Pollicis (OP)
Hypothenar Group—Seated
 Abductor Digiti Minimi Manus (ADMM)
 Flexor Digiti Minimi Manus (FDMM)
 Opponens Digiti Minimi (ODM)
 Detour to the Palmaris Brevis
Adductor Pollicis—Seated
Lumbricals Manus—Seated
Palmar Interossei (PI)—Seated
Dorsal Interossei Manus (DIM)—Seated

Chapter Objectives

After completing this chapter, the student/therapist should be able to perform the following for each of the muscles covered in this chapter:

1. State the attachments.
2. State the actions.
3. Describe the starting position for palpation.
4. Describe and explain the purpose of each of the palpation steps.
5. Palpate each muscle.
6. State the "Palpation Key."
7. Describe alternate palpation positions.
8. State the locations of the most common TrP(s).
9. Describe the TrP referral zones.
10. State the most common factors that create and/or perpetuate TrPs.
11. State the symptoms most commonly caused by TrPs.
12. Describe and perform the therapist-assisted and self-care stretches.

Go to http://evolve.elsevier.com/Muscolino/palpation for video demonstrations of the muscle palpations presented in this chapter.

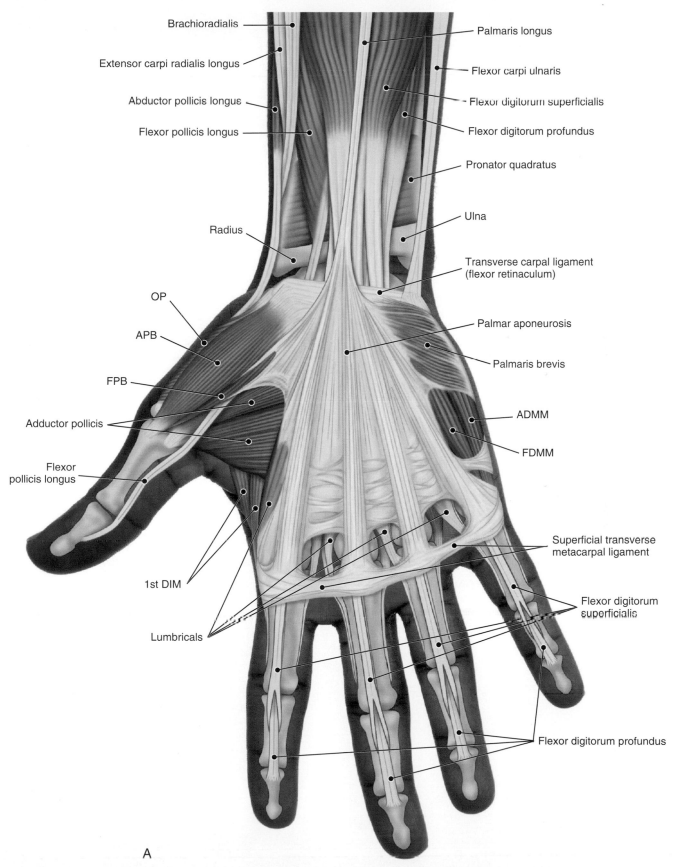

Figure 16-1 Anterior (palmar) views of the musculature of the hand. **A,** Superficial view of the hand with the palmar aponeurosis. *ADMM,* Abductor digiti minimi manus; *APB,* abductor pollicis brevis; *DIM,* dorsal interosseus manus; *FDMM,* flexor digiti minimi manus; *FPB,* flexor pollicis brevis; *ODM,* opponens digiti minimi; *OP,* opponens pollicis; *PI,* palmar interosseus.

16

16

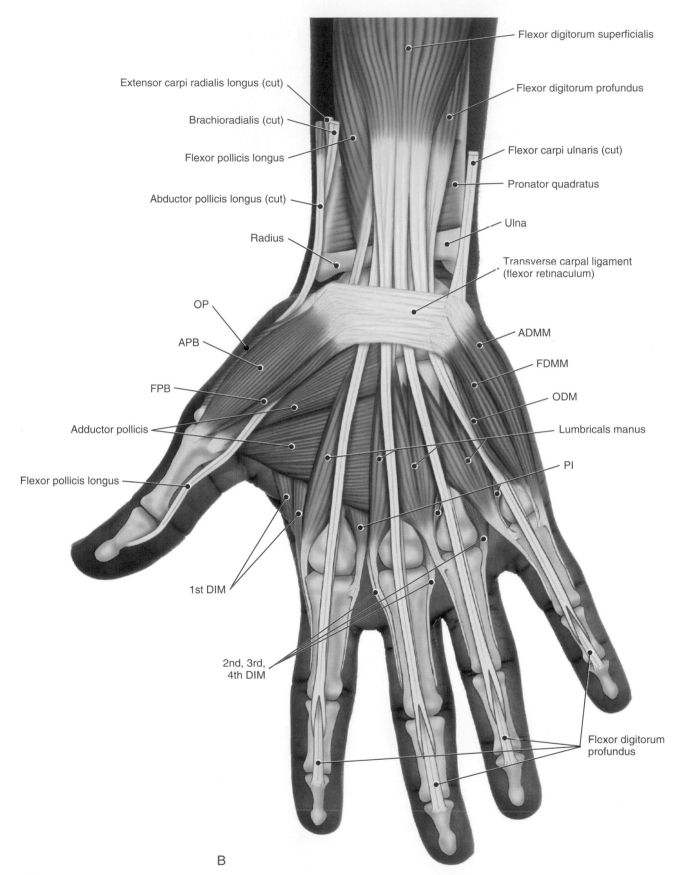

Flexor digitorum superficialis

Extensor carpi radialis longus (cut)

Brachioradialis (cut)

Flexor pollicis longus

Abductor pollicis longus (cut)

Radius

OP

APB

FPB

Adductor pollicis

Flexor pollicis longus

1st DIM

2nd, 3rd, 4th DIM

Flexor digitorum profundus

Flexor carpi ulnaris (cut)

Pronator quadratus

Ulna

Transverse carpal ligament (flexor retinaculum)

ADMM

FDMM

ODM

Lumbricals manus

PI

Flexor digitorum profundus

B

Figure 16-1, cont'd B, Superficial view of the musculature with the palmar aponeurosis removed. *ADMM,* Abductor digiti minimi manus; *APB,* abductor pollicis brevis; *DIM,* dorsal interosseus manus; *FDMM,* flexor digiti minimi manus; *FPB,* flexor pollicis brevis; *ODM,* opponens digiti minimi; *OP,* opponens pollicis; *PI,* palmar interosseus.

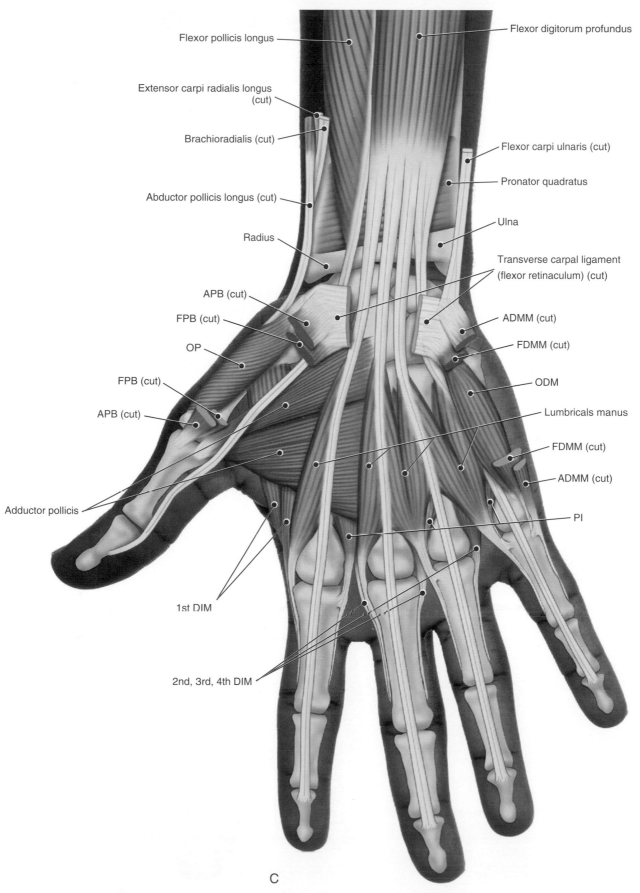

Flexor pollicis longus

Flexor digitorum profundus

Extensor carpi radialis longus (cut)

Brachioradialis (cut)

Flexor carpi ulnaris (cut)

Pronator quadratus

Abductor pollicis longus (cut)

Ulna

Radius

Transverse carpal ligament (flexor retinaculum) (cut)

APB (cut)

ADMM (cut)

FPB (cut)

FDMM (cut)

OP

ODM

FPB (cut)

Lumbricals manus

APB (cut)

FDMM (cut)

ADMM (cut)

Adductor pollicis

PI

1st DIM

2nd, 3rd, 4th DIM

C

Figure 16-1, cont'd C, Intermediate view with the more superficial thenar and hypothenar muscles cut. *ADMM,* Abductor digiti minimi manus; *APB,* abductor pollicis brevis; *DIM,* dorsal interosseus manus; *FDMM,* flexor digiti minimi manus; *FPB,* flexor pollicis brevis; *ODM,* opponens digiti minimi; *OP,* opponens pollicis; *PI,* palmar interosseus.

16

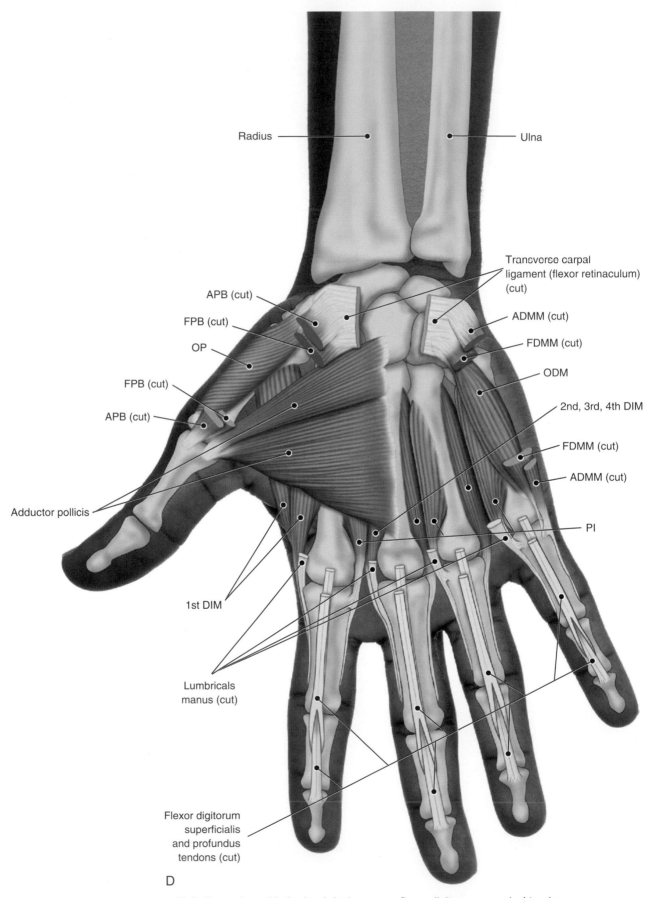

Figure 16-1, cont'd D, Deep view with the lumbricals manus, flexor digitorum muscles' tendons, and all forearm muscles cut and/or removed. *ADMM,* Abductor digiti minimi manus; *APB,* abductor pollicis brevis; *DIM,* dorsal interosseus manus; *FDMM,* flexor digiti minimi manus; *FPB,* flexor pollicis brevis; *ODM,* opponens digiti minimi; *OP,* opponens pollicis; *PI,* palmar interosseus.

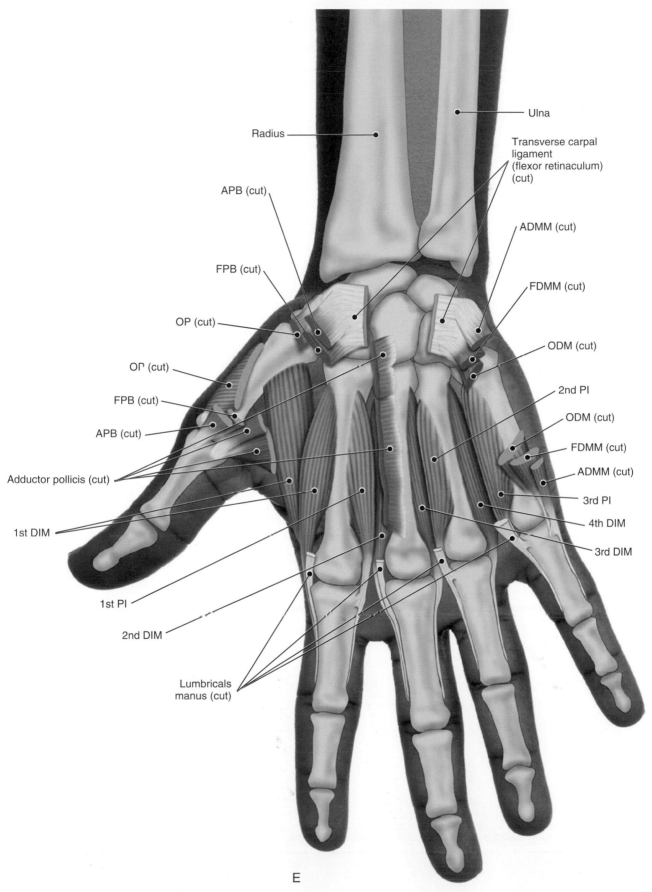

Figure 16-1, cont'd E, Deepest view of the palmar musculature. *ADMM,* Abductor digiti minimi manus; *APB,* abductor pollicis brevis; *DIM,* dorsal interosseus manus; *FDMM,* flexor digiti minimi manus; *FPB,* flexor pollicis brevis; *ODM,* opponens digiti minimi; *OP,* opponens pollicis; *PI,* palmar interosseus.

16

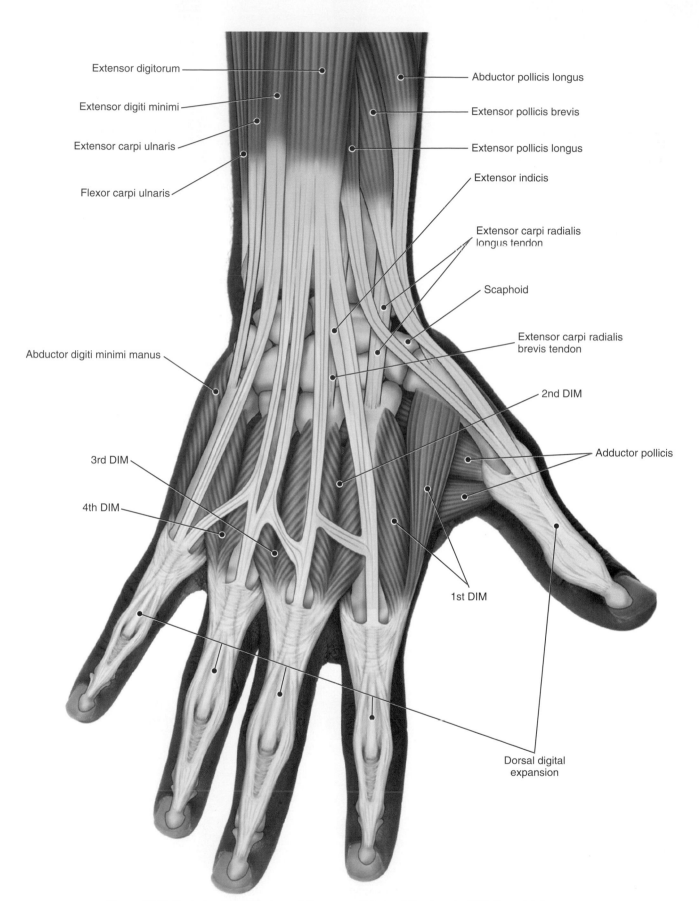

Figure 16-2 Posterior (dorsal) view of the musculature of the hand. *DIM,* Dorsal interosseus manus.

16

THENAR GROUP—SEATED

The thenar group is composed of the abductor pollicis brevis (APB), flexor pollicis brevis (FPB), and the opponens pollicis (OP).

Abductor Pollicis Brevis (APB)

☑ ATTACHMENTS

☐ Tubercles of the scaphoid and trapezium, and the flexor retinaculum

to the

☐ lateral side of the base of the proximal phalanx of the thumb (and the dorsal digital expansion)

☑ ACTIONS

☐ Abducts the thumb at the carpometacarpal (CMC) joint
☐ Extends the thumb at the CMC joint
☐ Flexes the thumb at the metacarpophalangeal (MCP) joint
☐ Extends the thumb at the interphalangeal (IP) joint

Flexor Pollicis Brevis (FPB)

☑ ATTACHMENTS

☐ Palmar side of the trapezium and the flexor retinaculum

to the

☐ lateral side of the base of the proximal phalanx of the thumb

☑ ACTIONS

☐ Flexes the thumb at the CMC joint
☐ Abducts the thumb at the CMC joint
☐ Flexes the thumb at the MCP joint

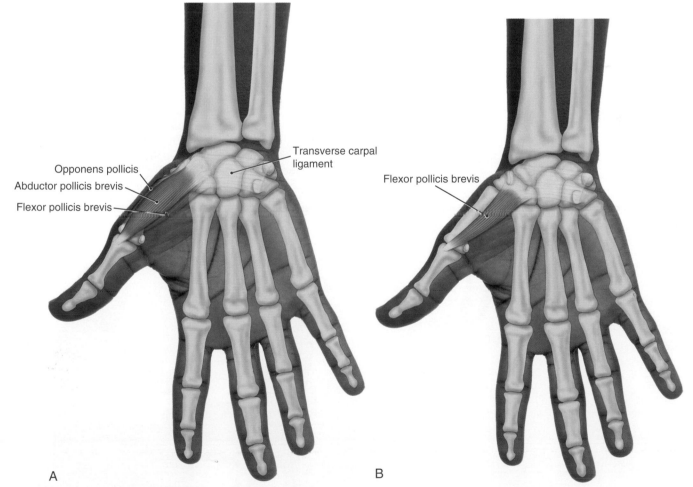

Figure 16-3 Anterior views of the muscles of the right thenar group. **A,** Abductor pollicis brevis (APB). The flexor pollicis brevis (FPB) and opponens pollicis (OP) have been ghosted in. **B,** FPB.

16

THENAR GROUP—SEATED—*cont'd*

Opponens Pollicis (OP)

☑ATTACHMENTS

☐ Tubercle of the trapezium and the flexor retinaculum

  to the

☐ anterior surface and lateral border of the shaft of the first metacarpal (of the thumb)

☑ACTIONS

☐ Opposes (flexes, medially rotates, and abducts) the thumb at the CMC joint

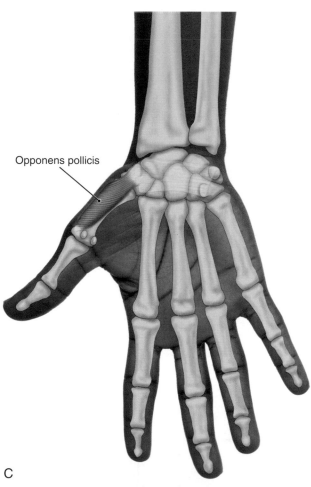

Opponens pollicis

C

Figure 16-3, cont'd C, OP.

Starting Position (Figure 16-4)

■ Client seated

■ Therapist seated facing the client

■ Palpating fingers placed on the lateral side of the thenar eminence of the client

■ Support hand placed on the anterior surface of the proximal phalanx of the client's thumb

Palpation Steps

1. APB: Palpating the lateral side of the thenar eminence, gently to moderately resist thumb abduction at the CMC (saddle) joint and feel for the contraction of the APB. It can be helpful to pinch the muscle between your thumb and index finger, as seen in Figure 16-5, *A*.

2. Once felt, palpate proximally and distally to the attachments of the APB. Also try to discern the medial border of the APB from the FPB.

3. FPB: Now place palpating fingers at the most medial aspect of the thenar eminence, gently to moderately resist thumb flexion at the CMC (saddle) joint, and feel for the contraction of the FPB (see Figure 16-5, *B*).

4. Once the FPB's contraction is felt in the medial thenar eminence, try to palpate it deep to the ABP as the client alternately contracts the muscle against gentle resistance and relaxes it.

5. OP: To palpate the OP, curl your palpating finger(s) around the shaft of the metacarpal of the thumb as seen in Figure 16-5, *C*. Ask the client to oppose the thumb against the little finger, exerting gentle pressure against the pad of the little finger, and feel for the OP to contract.

6. Once the OP's contraction is felt against the metacarpal, attempt to palpate the rest of this muscle deep to the other thenar muscles. It can be very difficult to discern the OP from the other thenar muscles. For this reason, it is usually more effective to palpate for tight spots in this muscle with the thenar musculature relaxed.

7. Once the thenar muscles have been located, have the client relax them and palpate to assess their baseline tone.

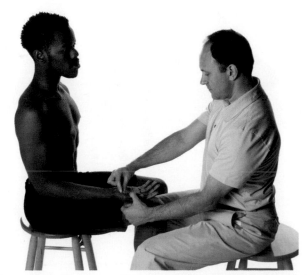

Figure 16-4 Starting position for seated palpation of the right thenar group.

THENAR GROUP—SEATED—*cont'd*

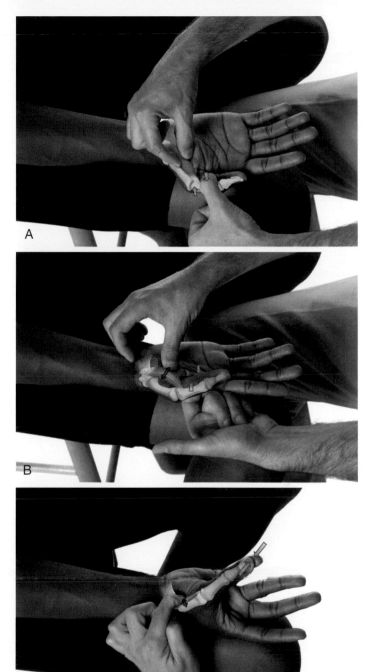

Figure 16-5 Palpation of the right thenar group. **A,** Palpation of the abductor pollicis brevis (APB) as the client abducts the thumb at the carpometacarpal (CMC) joint against resistance. **B,** Palpation of the flexor pollicis brevis (FPB) as the client flexes the thumb at the CMC joint against resistance. **C,** Palpation of the opponens pollicis (OP) by curling around the metacarpal of the thumb as the client opposes the thumb at the CMC joint to the little finger.

Palpation Key:

APB: Palpate the lateral aspect of the thenar eminence.

FPB: Palpate at the most medial aspect of the thenar eminence.

OP: Curl your finger(s) around the shaft of the metacarpal of the thumb.

16

THENAR GROUP—SEATED—*cont'd*

PALPATION NOTES

1. Movements of the thumb at the saddle are unusual in their direction. Flexion and extension occur within the frontal plane along the plane of the palm of the hand; and abduction and adduction occur within the sagittal plane (perpendicular to the plane of the palm of the hand). Furthermore, opposition is a combination of flexion, abduction, and medial rotation. It is important to know these motions so that the client can be asked to do the proper joint actions to engage the correct muscles to contract for palpation.
2. The APB is superficial in the thenar eminence and easily palpable.
3. Only a small part of the FPB is superficial on the medial side of the thenar eminence. The majority of it is deep to the APB.
4. Only a very small part of the OP is accessible superficially in the lateral aspect of the thenar eminence against the shaft of the metacarpal of the thumb. The rest of the OP is deep to the other thenar eminence muscles and difficult to palpate and discern from them.
5. Even though the APB is superficial and easily palpable, sometimes it can be difficult to discern its medial border from the FPB because both of these muscles abduct and flex the thumb at the CMC. So if excessive resistance is given to either joint motion, both muscles are engaged to contract. However, the APB is preferentially contracted with abduction, and the FPB is preferentially contracted with flexion of the thumb. Therefore, to better palpate these muscles and to discern their border, it is important to offer only mild or moderate resistance or both muscles will contract, making it impossible to discern these two muscles from each other.
6. The OP is the most difficult thenar muscle to palpate and discern, because it is mostly deep to other thenar muscles, and because its action of opposition incorporates both abduction and flexion of the thumb at the saddle joint. Therefore, when the OP is engaged to contract, the more superficial APB and FPB tend to contract as well.

TRIGGER POINTS

1. Trigger points (TrPs) in the thenar muscles often result from or are perpetuated by acute or chronic overuse of the muscle (e.g., prolonged pincer gripping such as when writing) or trauma (e.g., falling on an outstretched hand).
2. TrPs in the thenar muscles may produce soreness with use of the thumb (especially when gripping objects with the pincer grip), or weakness and difficulty with fine motor skills of the thumb.
3. The referral patterns of OP TrPs must be distinguished from the referral patterns of TrPs in the adductor pollicis, flexor carpi radialis, pronator teres, brachialis, subscapularis, subclavius, and scalenes.
4. TrPs in the thenar muscles are often incorrectly assessed as carpal tunnel syndrome, de Quervain stenosing tenosynovitis, cervical disc syndrome, or first carpometacarpal (CMC) osteoarthritis.
5. Associated TrPs often occur in the adductor pollicis, first dorsal interosseus manus, APB, and FPB.
6. Note: TrP referral patterns have not yet been established for the APB and FPB; they likely follow the referral patterns for the OP. When assessing these muscles for TrPs, look primarily for central TrPs located in the middle of the bellies.

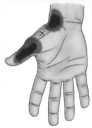

Figure 16-6 Anterior view illustrating a common opponens pollicis (OP) trigger point (TrP) and its corresponding referral zone.

16

THENAR GROUP—SEATED—*cont'd*

STRETCHING THE THENAR GROUP

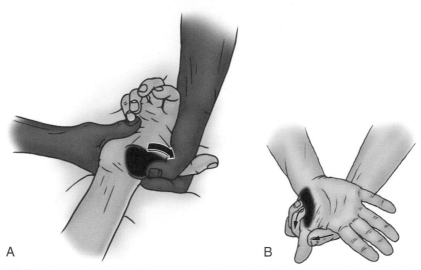

A   B

Figure 16-7 Stretching the right thenar group of muscles. The client's thumb is extended and adducted at the carpometacarpal (CMC) and metacarpophalangeal (MCP) joints. **A,** Therapist-assisted stretch. Note that the therapist uses their other hand to stabilize the client's hand. **B,** Self-care stretch.

Alternate Palpation Position—Supine or Prone

The thenar muscles of the hand can also be easily palpated with the client supine or prone. Follow the palpation steps indicated for the seated palpation.

16

HYPOTHENAR GROUP—SEATED

The hypothenar group is composed of the abductor digiti minimi manus (ADMM), flexor digiti minimi manus (FDMM), and opponens digiti minimi (ODM).

Abductor Digiti Minimi Manus (ADMM)

☑ ATTACHMENTS

☐ Pisiform and the tendon of the flexor carpi ulnaris

   to the

☐ medial side of the base of the proximal phalanx of the little finger (and the dorsal digital expansion)

☑ ACTIONS

☐ Abducts the little finger at the metacarpophalangeal (MCP) and carpometacarpal (CMC) joints
☐ Extends the little finger at the proximal and distal interphalangeal (IP) joints

Flexor Digiti Minimi Manus (FDMM)

☑ ATTACHMENTS

☐ Hook of the hamate and the flexor retinaculum

   to the

☐ anteromedial side of the base of the proximal phalanx of the little finger

☑ ACTIONS

☐ Flexes the little finger at the MCP and CMC joints

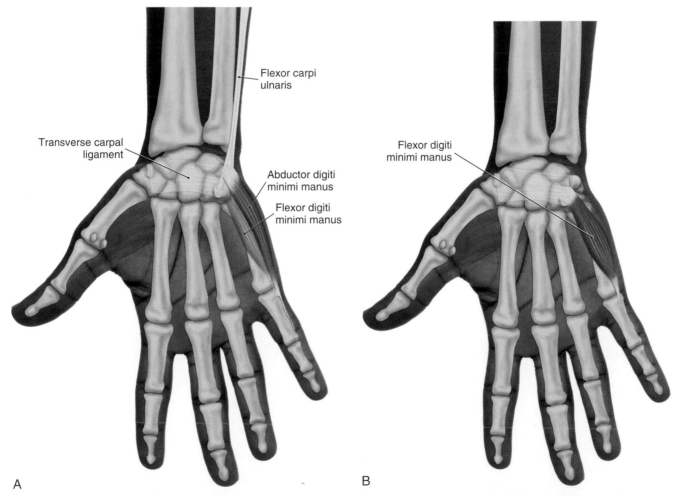

Flexor carpi ulnaris

Transverse carpal ligament

Abductor digiti minimi manus

Flexor digiti minimi manus

Flexor digiti minimi manus

A

B

Figure 16-8 Anterior views of the muscles of the right hypothenar group. **A,** Abductor digiti minimi manus (ADMM). The flexor digiti minimi manus (FDMM) has been ghosted in. **B,** Flexor digiti minimi manus.

16

HYPOTHENAR GROUP—SEATED—*cont'd*

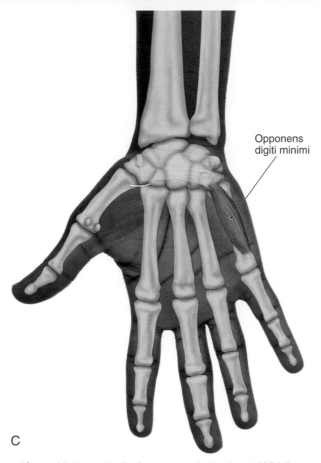

Opponens
digiti minimi

C

Figure 16-8, cont'd C, Opponens digiti minimi (ODM).

Opponens Digiti Minimi (ODM)

✓ ATTACHMENTS

☐ Hook of the hamate and the flexor retinaculum

to the

☐ anterior surface and the medial border of the shaft of the fifth metacarpal

✓ ACTIONS

☐ Opposes (flexes, adducts, laterally rotates) the little finger at the CMC joint

Starting Position (Figure 16-9)

■ Client seated
■ Therapist seated facing the client
■ Palpating fingers placed on the medial side of the hypothenar eminence of the client
■ Support hand placed on the medial surface of the proximal phalanx of the client's little finger

Palpation Steps

1. ADMM: Palpating the medial side of the hypothenar eminence, resist the client from abducting the little finger at the MCP joint and feel for the contraction of the ADMM (Figure 16-10, *A*).
2. Once felt, palpate distally to the medial side of the base of the proximal phalanx, and proximally to the pisiform.

Also try to discern the lateral border of the ADMM from the FDMM.

3. FDMM: Palpating the lateral side of the hypothenar eminence, ask the client to flex the little finger at the MCP joint (but keep the IP joints fully extended) and feel for the contraction of the FDMM. If needed, flexion can be gently resisted by placing a finger of your support hand against the anterior surface of the proximal phalanx of the little finger (see Figure 16-10, *B*).
4. Once felt, palpate distally to the anteromedial surface of the base of the proximal phalanx, and proximally to the hook of the hamate. If not previously done, try to discern the border between the FDMM and the ADMM.
5. ODM: Locate the hook of the hamate and palpate immediately distal to it on the most lateral aspect of the hypothenar eminence, and feel for the contraction of the ODM as the client opposes the little finger against the thumb (see Figure 16-10, *C*).
6. Once felt, palpate distally as far as possible deep to the other muscles of the hypothenar eminence.
7. The most distal attachment of the ODM can usually be palpated by curling your palpating finger around to the anterior side of the shaft of the fifth metacarpal (Note: This is similar to how the OP was palpated against the first metacarpal.) (see Figure 16-10, *D*).
8. Once the hypothenar muscles have been located, have the client relax them and palpate to assess their baseline tone.

16

HYPOTHENAR GROUP—SEATED—*cont'd*

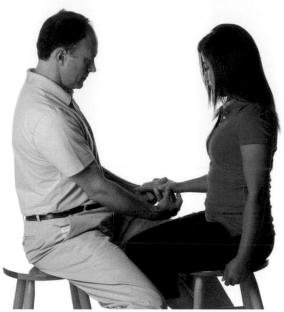

Figure 16-9 Starting position for seated palpation of the right hypothenar group.

Palpation Key:
ADMM: Palpate the medial side of the hypothenar eminence.
FDMM: Flex the little finger at only the MCP joint.
ODM: Find the hook of the hamate and palpate immediately distal to it at the most lateral aspect of the hypothenar eminence.

16

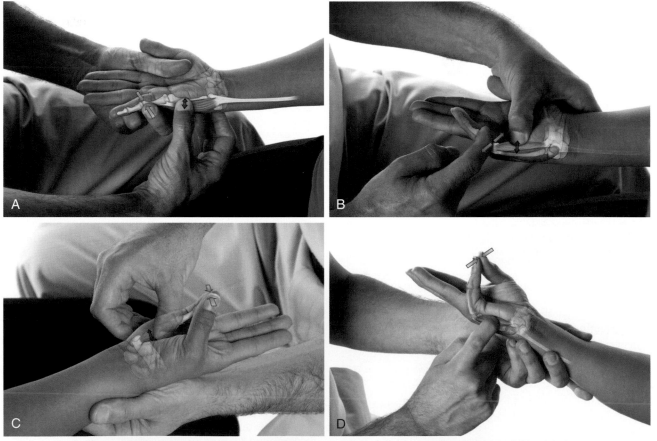

Figure 16-10 Palpation of the right hypothenar group. **A,** Palpation of the abductor digiti minimi manus (ADMM) at the medial side of the hypothenar eminence as the client abducts the little finger against resistance. **B,** Palpation of the flexor digiti minimi manus (FDMM) at the lateral side of the hypothenar eminence as the client flexes the proximal phalanx of the little finger against resistance. **C,** Palpation of the opponens digiti minimi (ODM) at the far lateral side of the hypothenar eminence as the client opposes the little finger against resistance. **D,** Palpation of the ODM against the metacarpal of the little finger as the client opposes the little finger against resistance.

HYPOTHENAR GROUP—SEATED—*cont'd*

PALPATION NOTES

1. The ADMM is wholly superficial in the hypothenar eminence and easily palpable.
2. The majority of the FDMM is superficial on the lateral side of the hypothenar eminence. Its most medial aspect is deep to the ADMM.
3. The majority of the ODM is deep to the other hypothenar muscles. However, its most lateral aspect is superficial on the lateral side of the hypothenar eminence.
4. Sometimes it is difficult to discern the border between the ADMM and the FDMM. When palpating for the ADMM, be sure that the client is not also flexing the little finger. When palpating for the FDMM, be sure that the client is not also abducting the little finger.
5. It is important when palpating for the FDMM that the client only moves the proximal phalanx at the MCP joint. If the IP joints are moved, long finger flexors from the forearm (flexors digitorum superficialis and profundus) will tend to be engaged. For this reason, it is also important that any resistance given is applied only to the proximal phalanx.
6. It is also important when palpating the FDMM that only mild to moderate resistance is given to flexion of the little finger, or the long finger flexors will be engaged.
7. Given the location of the tendons of the long finger flexors next to the ODM, be sure to also discern these structures from each other.
8. The tendons of the long finger flexors to the little finger are located just lateral to the bellies of the FDMM and ODM. To feel the contraction of the tendons of the long finger flexors, have the client flex only the middle and distal phalanges of the little finger at the IP joints. This will engage the long finger flexors but not the FDMM.
9. It can be very difficult to palpate and discern the ODM deep to the FDMM, because flexion of the little finger is a component of opposition of the little finger. For this reason, when opposition of the little finger is done, the FDMM may be engaged, making it difficult to feel the contraction of the deeper ODM.

TRIGGER POINTS

1. Trigger points (TrPs) in the hypothenar muscles often result from or are perpetuated by acute or chronic overuse of the muscle (e.g., prolonged pincer gripping, such as when writing), or trauma (e.g., falling on an outstretched hand).
2. TrPs in the hypothenar muscles may produce weakness or difficulty with fine motor skills of the little finger, or entrapment of the ulnar nerve by the ODM, causing weakness of intrinsic muscles of the hand.
3. The referral patterns of ADMM TrPs must be distinguished from the referral patterns of TrPs in the first dorsal interosseus manus, latissimus dorsi, and triceps brachii.
4. TrPs in the hypothenar muscles are often incorrectly assessed as osteoarthritis of the fingers, cervical disc syndrome, or thoracic outlet syndrome.
5. Associated TrPs often occur in the other hypothenar muscles and the dorsal interossei manus (DIM).
6. Note: TrP referral patterns have not yet been established for the FDMM and ADMM. They likely will follow the referral patterns for the ODM. When assessing these muscles for TrPs, look primarily for central TrPs located in the middle of the bellies.

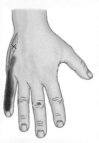

Figure 16-11 Posterior view illustrating a common abductor digiti minimi manus (ADMM) trigger point (TrP) and its corresponding referral zone.

16

Alternate Palpation Position—Supine or Prone

The hypothenar muscles of the hand can also be easily palpated with the client supine or prone. Follow the palpation steps indicated for the seated palpation.

HYPOTHENAR GROUP—SEATED—*cont'd*

STRETCHING THE HYPOTHENAR GROUP

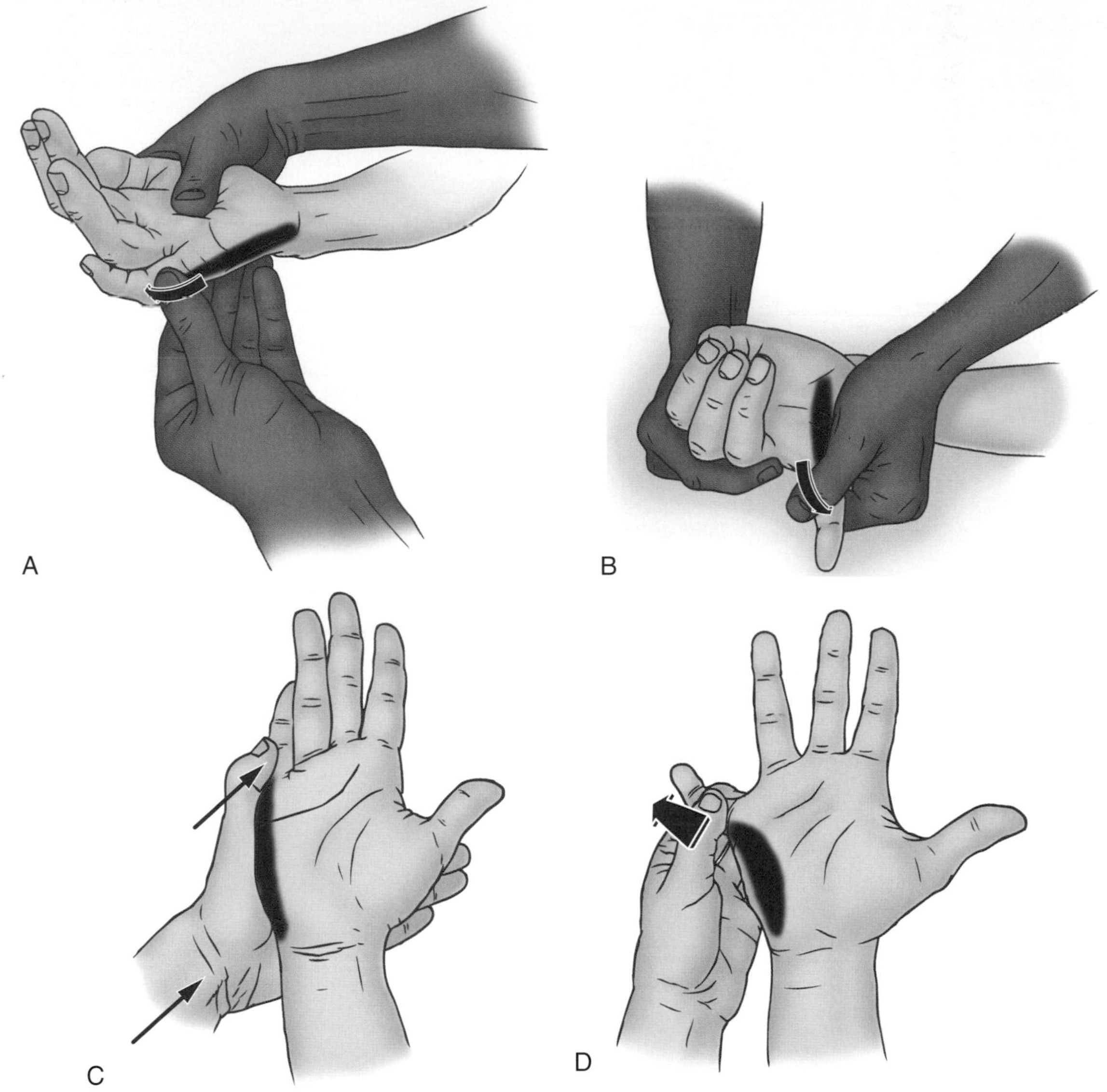

A

B

C

D

Figure 16-12 Stretching the right hypothenar group of muscles. To stretch the abductor digiti minimi manus (ADMM), the client's little finger is extended and adducted. To stretch the flexor digiti minimi manus (FDMM) and opponens digiti minimi (ODM), the client's little finger and its metacarpal are extended and abducted. Therapist-assisted stretches of the ADMM **(A)** and the FDMM and OPD **(B).** Note that the therapist stabilizes the client's hand with the other hand. Self-care stretches of the ADMM **(C)** and the FDMM and OPD **(D).**

16

HYPOTHENAR GROUP—SEATED—*cont'd*

DETOUR

Palmaris Brevis:

The palmaris brevis is located in the dermis of the proximal hand on the medial side, over the hypothenar eminence (Figure 16-13, *A*). This muscle is extremely thin and difficult to discern from adjacent soft tissue. Given that this muscle's action is to wrinkle the skin of the palm, ask the client to do this by cupping the palm of the hand and feel for this muscle's contraction (This will likely also cause the palmaris longus to contract.) (see Figure 16-13, *B*). Note: Be sure that the little finger is either not moved or moved as little as possible, or you will feel the contraction of the hypothenar muscles.

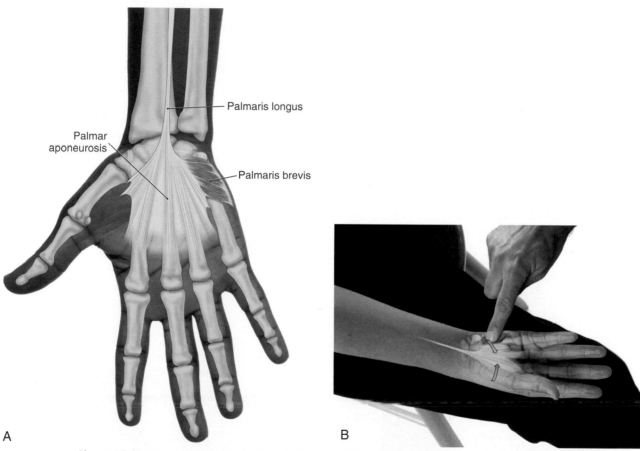

— Palmaris longus

Palmar aponeurosis

— Palmaris brevis

A

B

Figure 16-13 The palmaris brevis. **A,** Anterior view of the right palmaris brevis. **B,** Palpation of the right palmaris brevis.

16

ADDUCTOR POLLICIS—SEATED

☑ ATTACHMENTS

☐ Capitate, anterior base and shaft of the third metacarpal, and the anterior base of the second metacarpal

to the

☐ anteromedial side of the base of the proximal phalanx of the thumb (and the dorsal digital expansion)

☑ ACTIONS

☐ Adducts the thumb at the carpometacarpal (CMC) joint
☐ Flexes the thumb at the CMC joint
☐ Extends the thumb at the interphalangeal (IP) joint

Starting Position (Figure 16-15)

■ Client seated
■ Therapist seated facing the client
■ Palpating fingers placed on the anterior surface of the thumb web of the client's hand
■ Fingers of the support hand placed on the posterior surface of the proximal phalanx of the client's thumb

Palpation Steps

1. Palpating the anterior side of the thumb web of the hand, resist the client from adducting the thumb at the CMC (saddle) joint, and feel for the contraction of the adductor pollicis (Figure 16-16).
2. Once felt, palpate the entire adductor pollicis from the proximal phalanx of the thumb to the third metacarpal and capitate.
3. Once the adductor pollicis muscle has been located, have the client relax it and palpate to assess its baseline tone.

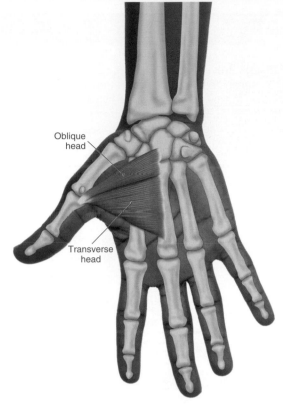

Oblique head

Transverse head

Figure 16-14 Anterior view of the right adductor pollicis.

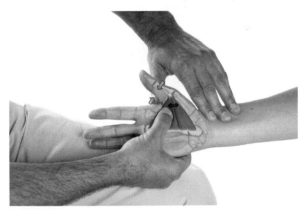

Figure 16-16 Palpation of the right adductor pollicis as the client adducts the thumb against resistance.

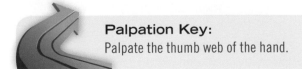

Palpation Key:
Palpate the thumb web of the hand.

Alternate Palpation Position—Supine or Prone

The adductor pollicis of the hand can also be easily palpated with the client supine or prone. Follow the palpation steps indicated for the seated palpation.

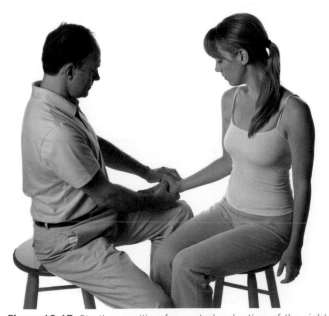

Figure 16-15 Starting position for seated palpation of the right adductor pollicis.

16

ADDUCTOR POLLICIS—SEATED—*cont'd*

PALPATION NOTES

1. Adduction of the thumb at the saddle joint occurs within the sagittal plane and is a motion toward the palm of the hand.
2. When palpating for the adductor pollicis in the thumb web of the hand, note that other muscles are located within the web (see Figure 16-1). The first dorsal interosseus manus is located within the thumb web and is attached to both the first and second metacarpals. The flexor pollicis brevis (FPB) is also located within the thumb web close to the first metacarpal, and the first lumbrical manus is located within the thumb web close to the second metacarpal. Of these other muscles, only the FPB also moves the thumb and might engage when asking the client to move the thumb. To be sure that you are not engaging the FPB, make sure that the client is doing pure adduction of the thumb (i.e., is not flexing the thumb as well).

TRIGGER POINTS

1. Trigger points (TrPs) in the adductor pollicis often result from or are perpetuated by acute or chronic overuse of the muscle (e.g., prolonged pincer gripping, such as when writing) or trauma (e.g., falling on an outstretched hand).
2. TrPs in the adductor pollicis may produce pain in the thumb web, soreness with use of the thumb (especially when gripping objects with the pincer grip), or weakness and difficulty coordinating the thumb for fine motor activities.
3. The referral patterns of adductor pollicis TrPs must be distinguished from the referral patterns of TrPs in the opponens pollicis (OP), supinator, extensor carpi radialis longus, brachioradialis, brachialis, scalenes, pronator teres, and subclavius.
4. TrPs in the adductor pollicis are often incorrectly assessed as de Quervain stenosing tenosynovitis, carpal tunnel syndrome, cervical disc syndrome, thoracic outlet syndrome, or joint dysfunction or osteoarthritis of the first CMC or MCP joint.

5. Associated TrPs often occur in the OP, first dorsal interosseus manus, abductor pollicis brevis (APB), or flexor pollicis brevis (FPB).

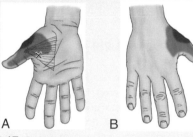

Figure 16-17 A, Anterior view illustrating a common adductor pollicis trigger point (TrP) and its corresponding referral zone. **B,** Posterior view showing the remainder of the referral zone.

STRETCHING THE ADDUCTOR POLLICIS

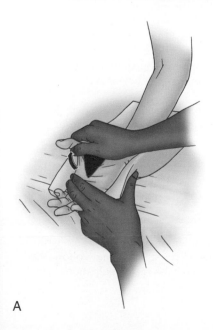

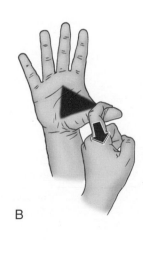

Figure 16-18 Stretching the right adductor pollicis. The client's thumb is abducted and extended. **A,** Therapist-assisted stretch. Note that the therapist uses their other hand to stabilize the client's hand. **B,** Self-care stretch.

16

LUMBRICALS MANUS—SEATED

There are four lumbricals manus muscles, numbered one to four from lateral to medial, respectively.

✅ ATTACHMENTS

☐ Distal tendons of the flexor digitorum profundus

to the

☐ distal tendons of the extensor digitorum (the dorsal digital expansion).
☐ Proximally, each lumbrical manus attaches to a tendon or tendons of the flexor digitorum profundus muscle and is located between metacarpals on the lateral side of the finger to which it attaches distally.
☐ Distally, each lumbrical manus muscle attaches to the lateral side of the distal tendon of the extensor digitorum (dorsal digital expansion) of a finger.
☐ Overall, the lumbricals manus muscles attach to fingers two through five.

✅ ACTIONS

☐ Flex fingers two through five at the metacarpophalangeal (MCP) joints
☐ Extend fingers two through five at the proximal and distal interphalangeal (IP) joints

Starting Position (Figure 16-20)

■ Client seated
■ Therapist seated facing the client
■ Place palpating finger(s) over the anterolateral surface of the shaft of the second metacarpal of the client's hand
■ If resistance is given, place fingers of the support hand on the anterior surface of the proximal phalanx of the finger of the lumbrical manus being palpated (not seen in Figure 16-20)

Palpation Steps

1. First lumbrical manus: Palpating over the anterolateral surface of the shaft of the second metacarpal, ask the client to flex the index finger at the MCP joint while keeping the IP joints completely extended, and feel for the contraction of the first lumbrical manus muscle (Figure 16-21, *A*).
2. Once located, follow the first lumbrical manus proximally and distally from attachment to attachment while the client alternately contracts and relaxes the muscle, as indicated in Step 1.
3. Second lumbrical manus: Follow the same procedure as used for the first lumbrical manus muscle. Palpate over the anterolateral surface of the third metacarpal, and feel for its contraction as the client flexes the third finger at the MCP joint (with the IP joints fully extended) (see Figure 16-21, *B*). Once located, palpate from attachment to attachment.

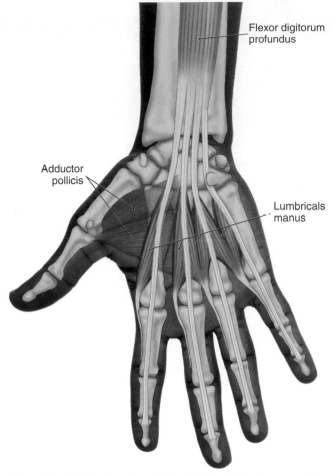

Figure 16-19 Anterior view of the right lumbricals manus. The adductor pollicis has been ghosted in.

4. Third and fourth lumbricals manus: Palpating the third and fourth lumbrical manus muscles is similar to the palpation of the first and second lumbricals manus. The only difference is that the placement of the palpating fingers must be more centered between the adjacent metacarpals because of the broader proximal attachments of these lumbricals. For the third lumbrical manus, palpate between the third and fourth metacarpals. For the fourth lumbrical manus, palpate between the fourth and fifth metacarpals.
5. Once each lumbrical manus has been located, have the client relax it and palpate to assess its baseline tone.

16

LUMBRICALS MANUS—SEATED—*cont'd*

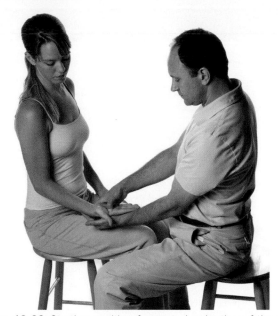

Figure 16-20 Starting position for seated palpation of the right lumbricals manus.

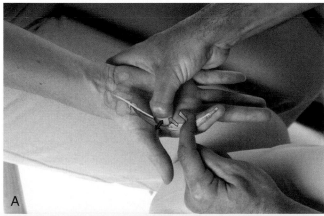

A

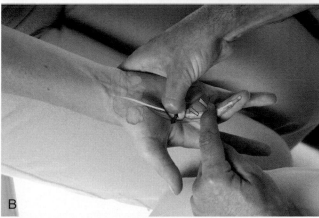

B

Figure 16-21 Palpation of the right lumbricals manus. **A,** Palpation of the first lumbrical manus on the radial side of the metacarpal of the index finger. **B,** Palpation of the second lumbrical manus on the radial side of the metacarpal of the middle finger.

 PALPATION NOTES

1. The lumbricals manus muscles are actually quite superficial in the hand (for the most part, they are only deep to the palmar fascia) and therefore fairly easy to palpate.
2. To engage a lumbrical manus muscle, be sure that the middle and distal phalanges stay completely extended at the IP joints when the proximal phalanx of the finger is flexed at the MCP joint. Otherwise, the long flexors of the fingers (flexor digitorum superficialis [FDS] and flexor digitorum profundus [FDP]) will tend to be engaged, making it more difficult to palpate and discern the lumbricals manus.
3. To be sure that you are palpating the lumbrical manus muscle and not the tendon of either the FDS or the FDP, ask the client to flex the finger at the proximal and distal IP joints. If what you are palpating engages with this motion, you are on the tendon of one or both of the long finger flexors (FDS or FDP). If what you are palpating does not engage, then you are on the lumbrical manus muscle to that finger.
4. Because the dorsal interosseus manus and palmar interosseus muscles can also flex the MCP joint of a finger and extend the IP joints of a finger, it is important that the client does not also abduct or adduct the finger at the MCP joint when flexing it. Otherwise, an interosseus muscle to that finger will also be engaged, making it difficult to palpate and discern the lumbrical manus muscle that is being palpated.
5. Perhaps the most difficult lumbrical manus muscle to palpate and discern is the fourth, because it lies adjacent to the flexor digiti minimi manus (FDMM), which also engages with flexion of the little finger at the MCP joint.

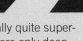 16

Alternate Palpation Position—Supine or Prone

The lumbricals manus of the hand can also be easily palpated with the client supine or prone. Follow the palpation steps indicated for the seated palpation.

 Palpation Key:
Flex the MCP joint, but keep the IP joints extended.

LUMBRICALS MANUS—SEATED—*cont'd*

TRIGGER POINTS

1. Trigger points (TrPs) in the lumbricals manus often result from or are perpetuated by acute or chronic overuse of the muscle (e.g., typing, prolonged pincer gripping, such as when writing) or altered biomechanics of the fingers (often due to arthritic changes).

2. TrPs in a lumbrical manus muscle generally produce pain along the radial side of the finger to which it attaches. Lumbricals manus TrPs may also produce weakness or difficulty with fine motor skills of the fingers.

3. The referral patterns of lumbricals manus TrPs must be distinguished from the referral patterns of TrPs in the palmar or dorsal interossei muscles of the hand, extensor digitorum, extensor digiti minimi, flexors digitorum superficialis and profundus, pectoralis minor, scalenes, latissimus dorsi, subclavius, and triceps brachii.

4. TrPs in the lumbricals manus are often incorrectly assessed as osteoarthritis of the fingers, cervical disc syndrome, thoracic outlet syndrome, or carpal tunnel syndrome.

5. Associated TrPs often occur in the palmar interossei (PI), the dorsal interossei manus (DIM), and the thenar muscles of the thumb.

6. Note: Pain referral patterns from TrPs in the lumbricals manus muscles are not distinguished from the referral patterns of the PI and DIM muscles of the hand.

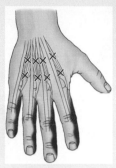

Figure 16-22 Posterior (dorsal) view illustrating common lumbricals manus trigger points (TrPs) and their corresponding referral zone. Note: These TrPs are located and therefore palpated anteriorly.

STRETCHING THE LUMBRICALS MANUS

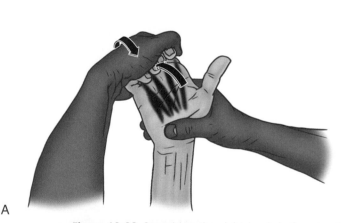

A

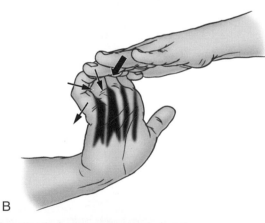

B

Figure 16-23 Stretching the right lumbricals manus. The client's fingers are extended at the metacarpophalangeal (MCP) joints and flexed at the interphalangeal (IP) joints. **A,** Therapist-assisted stretch. Note that the therapist uses their other hand to stabilize the client's hand. **B,** Self-care stretch.

16

PALMAR INTEROSSEI (PI)—SEATED

There are three PI muscles, numbered one to three from lateral to medial, respectively.

☑ATTACHMENTS

☐ From the "middle finger side" of the anterior surface of the metacarpals of fingers two, four, and five

to the

☐ base of the proximal phalanx on the middle finger side of fingers two, four, and five (and the dorsal digital expansion)

☑ACTIONS

☐ Adduct fingers two, four, and five at the metacarpophalangeal (MCP) joints
☐ Flex fingers two, four, and five at the MCP joints
☐ Extend fingers two, four, and five at the proximal and distal interphalangeal (IP) joints

Starting Position (Figure 16-25)

■ Client seated with a pencil or highlighter placed between the index and middle fingers
■ Therapist seated facing the client
■ Palpating finger(s) placed on the palm of the client's hand, between the second and third metacarpals

Palpation Steps

1. First PI: Palpating in the palm against the second metacarpal between the second and third metacarpals, ask the client to squeeze the highlighter between the index and middle fingers, and feel for the contraction of the first PI muscle (Figure 16-26, *A*).
2. Once felt, try to follow the first PI proximally and distally from attachment to attachment while the client alternately contracts and relaxes the muscle as indicated in Step 1.
3. Second PI: Follow the same procedure as used for the first PI muscle. Palpate in the palm against the fourth metacarpal between the fourth and third metacarpals, and feel for the contraction of the second PI as the client squeezes the highlighter between the ring and middle fingers. Once located, palpate from attachment to attachment (see Figure 16-26, *B*).

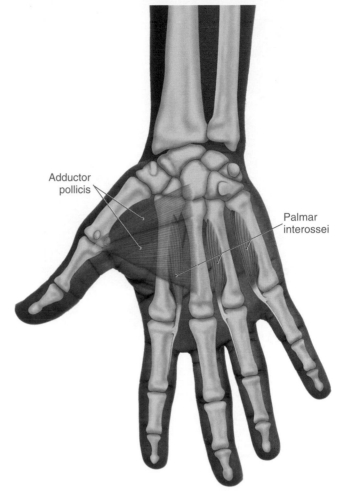

Figure 16-24 Anterior view of the right palmar interossei (PI). The adductor pollicis has been ghosted in.

4. Third PI: Following the same procedure, palpate in the palm against the fifth metacarpal between the fifth and fourth metacarpals, and feel for the contraction of the third PI as the client squeezes the highlighter between the little and ring fingers. Once located, palpate from attachment to attachment (see Figure 16-26, *C*).
5. Once each PI has been located, have the client relax it and palpate to assess its baseline tone.

16

PALMAR INTEROSSEI (PI)—SEATED—*cont'd*

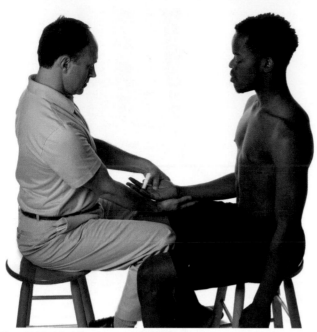

Figure 16-25 Starting position for seated palpation of the right palmar interossei (PI).

Palpation Key:
Squeeze a pencil or highlighter between two fingers.

PALPATION NOTES

1. Adduction of the index, ring, and little fingers is a frontal plane motion that is toward the middle finger.
2. The PI are deep within the palm of the hand, but can be fairly easily palpated and discerned.
3. Squeezing a pencil or highlighter between the index and middle fingers requires adduction of the index finger, thereby engaging the first PI. Similarly, squeezing the pencil or highlighter can be used to engage the other two PI.
4. To isolate a PI, it is important that the client does not attempt to flex the finger at the MCP or IP joints when squeezing (adducting), or the lumbricals and/or long finger flexors (flexors digitorum superficialis and profundus) will be engaged, making it more difficult to palpate and discern the PI muscle.
5. Careful palpation must be done to discern a PI muscle from the nearby long finger flexor tendons to that finger, because they may engage with adduction of the finger. To determine if you are palpating a long finger flexor tendon, ask the client to flex the finger at the IP joints, being sure to keep the MCP joint completely extended. If what you are palpating tenses, then it is a long finger flexor.

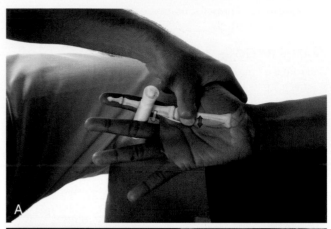

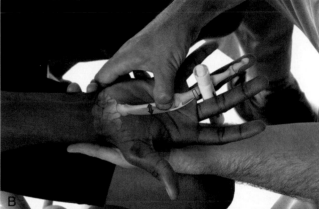

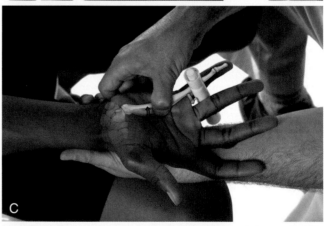

Figure 16-26 Palpation of the right palmar interossei (PI). **A,** Palpation of the first PI as the client adducts the index finger against resistance (provided by a highlighter). **B,** Palpation of the second PI as the client adducts the ring finger against resistance. **C,** Palpation of the third PI as the client adducts the little finger against resistance.

16

PALMAR INTEROSSEI (PI)—SEATED—*cont'd*

Alternate Palpation Position—Supine or Prone

The PI can also be easily palpated with the client supine or prone. Follow the palpation steps indicated for the seated palpation.

TRIGGER POINTS

1. Trigger points (TrPs) in the PI often result from or are perpetuated by acute or chronic overuse of the muscle (e.g., prolonged regular gripping, such as holding a tennis racquet or tool; or pincer gripping, such as when writing) or altered biomechanics of the fingers (often due to arthritic changes).
2. TrPs in a PI muscle usually produce pain along the side of the finger where it attaches. PI TrPs may also produce weakness or difficulty with fine motor skills of the associated finger, entrapment of the median or ulnar nerve, or restriction of finger abduction at the MCP joint.
3. The referral patterns of PI TrPs must be distinguished from the referral patterns of TrPs in the lumbricals manus, extensor digitorum, extensor digiti minimi, flexors digitorum superficialis and profundus, scalenes, pectoralis minor, subclavius, latissimus dorsi, and triceps brachii.
4. TrPs in the PI are often incorrectly assessed as osteoarthritis or joint dysfunction of the fingers, cervical disc syndrome, thoracic outlet syndrome, or carpal tunnel syndrome.
5. Associated TrPs often occur in the dorsal interossei manus (DIM), lumbricals manus, thenar muscles, and adductor pollicis.
6. Note: Pain referral patterns from TrPs in the PI muscles are not distinguished from the referral patterns of the lumbricals manus muscles (and DIM muscles).

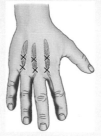

Figure 16-27 Posterior view illustrating common palmar interossei (PI) trigger points (TrPs) and their corresponding referral zones. Note: These TrPs are located and therefore palpated anteriorly.

STRETCHING THE PALMER INTEROSSEI

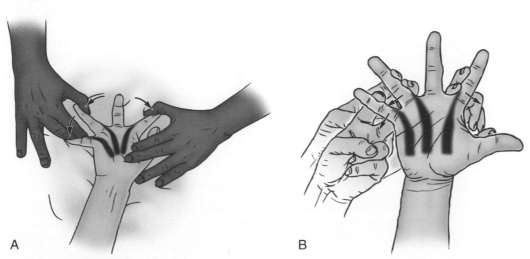

A   B

Figure 16-28 Stretching the three palmar interossei (PI) muscles of the right hand. The client's index, ring, and little fingers are abducted away from the middle finger. **A,** Therapist-assisted stretch. Note that the client's hand is stabilized down against the table. **B,** Self-care stretch.

16

DORSAL INTEROSSEI MANUS (DIM)—SEATED

There are four dorsal interossei manus (DIM) muscles, numbered one to four from lateral to medial, respectively.

☑ATTACHMENTS

- ☐ Proximally, DIM muscles attach to both sides of adjacent metacarpals of fingers one through five.
- ☐ Distally, each one attaches to one side of the proximal phalanx of a finger (on the side away from the center of the third finger), and to the tendon of the extensor digitorum (dorsal digital expansion) to that finger.

☑ACTIONS

- ☐ Abduct fingers two through four at the metacarpophalangeal (MCP) joints
- ☐ Flex fingers two through four at the MCP joints
- ☐ Extend fingers two through four at the proximal and distal interphalangeal (IP) joints

Starting Position (Figure 16-30)

- ■ Client seated
- ■ Therapist seated facing the client
- ■ Palpating finger(s) placed on the dorsal side of the client's hand, between the fourth and fifth metacarpals
- ■ Fingers of the support hand placed on the medial side of the proximal phalanx of the fourth finger

Palpation Steps

1. Fourth DIM: Palpating on the dorsal side of the hand between the fourth and fifth metacarpals, ask the client to abduct the ring finger against your resistance, and feel for the contraction of the fourth DIM (Figure 16-31, *A*).
2. Once felt, try to follow the fourth DIM proximally and distally from attachment to attachment while the client alternately contracts and relaxes the muscle as indicated in Step 1.
3. Third DIM: Following the same procedure, palpate between the third and fourth metacarpals while resisting ulnar abduction of the middle finger, and feel for the contraction of the third DIM (see Figure 16-31, *B*). Once felt, palpate from attachment to attachment as the client alternately contracts and relaxes the muscle.
4. Second DIM: Following the same procedure, palpate between the third and second metacarpals while resisting radial abduction of the middle finger, and feel for the contraction of the second DIM (see Figure 16-31, *C*). Once felt, palpate from attachment to attachment as the client alternately contracts and relaxes the muscle.

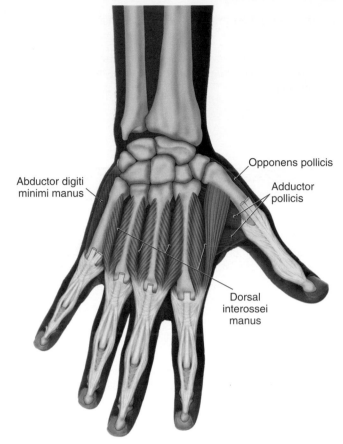

Figure 16-29 Posterior view of the right dorsal interossei manus (DIM). The adductor pollicis, opponens pollicis (OP), and abductor digiti minimi manus (ADMM) have been ghosted in.

5. First DIM: Palpate in the thumb web of the hand on the dorsal side, especially against the second metacarpal, and feel for the contraction of the first DIM as the client abducts the index finger. Resistance may be added if needed (see Figure 16-31, *D*). Once felt, palpate from attachment to attachment as the client alternately contracts and relaxes the muscle.
6. Once each DIM has been located, have the client relax it and palpate to assess its baseline tone.

16

DORSAL INTEROSSEI MANUS (DIM)—SEATED—*cont'd*

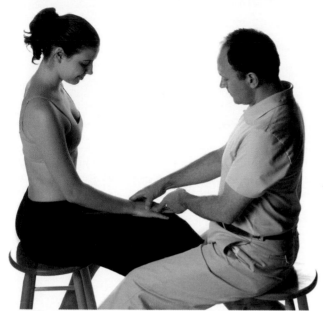

Figure 16-30 Starting position for seated palpation of the right dorsal interossei manus (DIM).

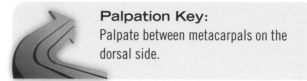

Palpation Key:
Palpate between metacarpals on the dorsal side.

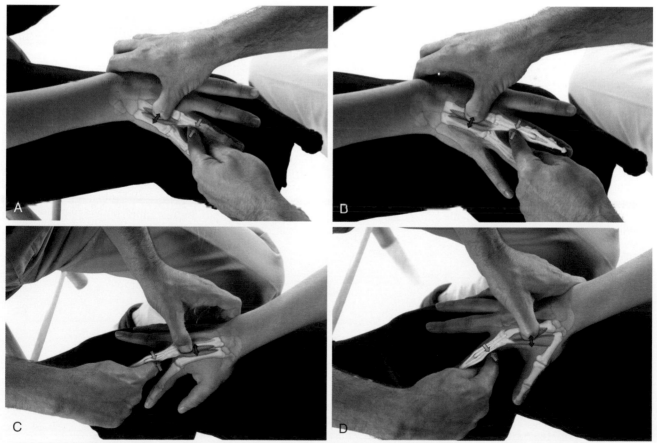

Figure 16-31 Palpation of the right dorsal interossei manus (DIM). **A,** Palpation of the fourth DIM as the client abducts the ring finger against resistance. **B,** Palpation of the third DIM as the client ulnar abducts the middle finger against resistance. **C,** Palpation of the second DIM as the client radially abducts the middle finger against resistance. **D,** Palpation of the first DIM as the client abducts the index finger against resistance.

16

DORSAL INTEROSSEI MANUS (DIM)—SEATED—*cont'd*

PALPATION NOTES

1. Finger abduction is a frontal plane motion away from an imaginary line through the center of the middle finger when it is in anatomic position.
2. The middle finger abducts in two directions, ulnar abduction when moving medially (in the ulnar direction) and radial abduction when moving laterally (in the radial direction).
3. Many people have difficulty isolating abduction motions of their fingers.
4. The DIM muscles are superficial and easy to palpate between the metacarpal bones on the dorsal side of the hand. The only musculoskeletal structures located superficial to them are the extensor tendons of the fingers (extensor digitorum, extensor digiti minimi, and extensor indicis). To be sure that these other muscles are not contracting, resulting in a tensing of their tendons (which might make palpation and discernment of the DIM more difficult), make sure that the client is not also extending the finger as it is abducted.

Alternate Palpation Position—Supine or Prone

The DIM can also be easily palpated with the client supine or prone. Follow the palpation steps indicated for the seated palpation.

TRIGGER POINTS

1. Trigger points (TrPs) in the DIM often result from or are perpetuated by acute or chronic overuse of the muscle (e.g., typing, prolonged pincer gripping, such as when writing) or altered biomechanics of the fingers (often due to arthritic changes).
2. TrPs in a DIM usually produce pain along the side of the finger where it attaches, weakness or difficulty with fine motor skills of the finger, or entrapment of the median or ulnar nerve.
3. The referral patterns of DIM TrPs must be distinguished from the referral patterns of TrPs in the lumbricals manus, adductor pollicis, brachioradialis, supinator, scalenes, extensor digitorum, flexors digitorum superficialis and profundus, coracobrachialis, brachialis, triceps brachii, subclavius, pectoralis minor, and latissimus dorsi.
4. TrPs in the DIM are often incorrectly assessed as osteoarthritis or joint dysfunction of the fingers, cervical disc syndrome, thoracic outlet syndrome, or carpal tunnel syndrome.
5. Associated TrPs often occur in the palmar interossei (PI), lumbricals manus, thenar muscles, and adductor pollicis.
6. Note: Pain referral patterns from TrPs in the DIM are not distinguished from the referral patterns of the lumbricals manus muscles (and PI muscles).

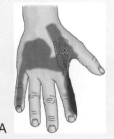
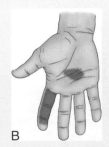
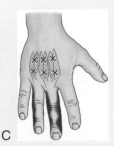

A   B   C

Figure 16-32 Common dorsal interossei manus (DIM) trigger points (TrPs) and their corresponding referral zones. **A,** First DIM TrP and its referral zone; **B,** Remainder of first DIM TrP referral zone. **C,** TrPs and their corresponding referral zones for the second, third, and fourth DIM muscles.

16

DORSAL INTEROSSEI MANUS (DIM)—SEATED—*cont'd*

STRETCHING THE DORSAL INTEROSSEI MANUS

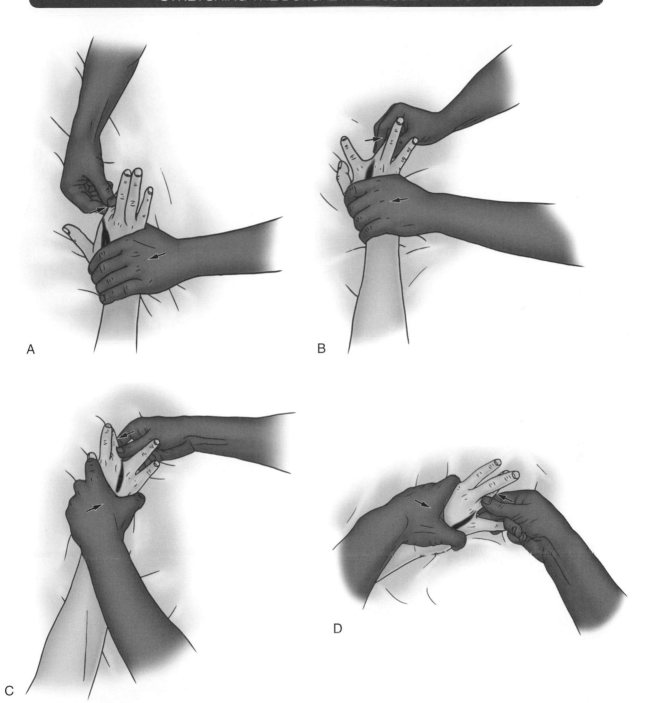

Figure 16-33 Stretching the four dorsal interossei manus (DIM) muscles of the right hand. The first DIM is stretched by adducting the index finger toward the middle finger. The second DIM is stretched by ulnar abducting the middle finger toward the ring finger. The third DIM is stretched by radially abducting the middle finger toward the index finger. The fourth DIM is stretched by adducting the ring finger toward the middle finger. **A, B, C,** and **D,** Therapist-assisted stretches of the first, second, third, and fourth DIM, respectively. Note that the therapist uses their other hand to stabilize the client's hand.

16

DORSAL INTEROSSEI MANUS (DIM)—SEATED—*cont'd*

STRETCHING THE DORSAL INTEROSSEI MANUS—*cont'd*

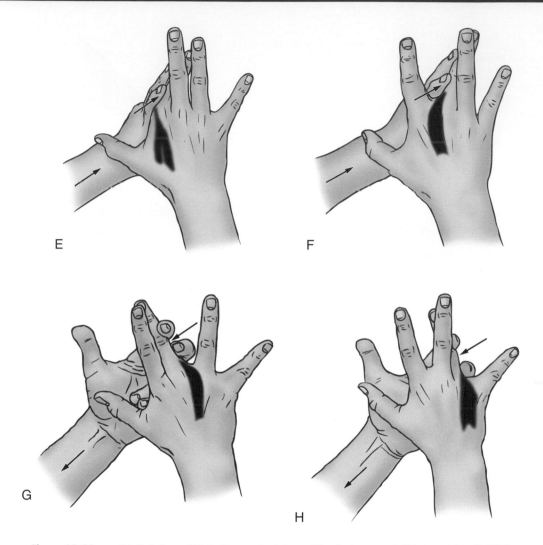

E

F

G

H

Figure 16-33, cont'd E, F, G, and **H,** Self-care stretches of the first, second, third, and fourth DIM, respectively.

Intrinsic Muscles of the Hand

The following *Whirlwind Tour* is an abbreviated set of palpation protocols for the muscles of this chapter. Once you have read and become comfortable with each of the protocols presented thus far, this *Whirlwind Tour* allows you to quickly and efficiently run through the palpations protocols for all the muscles of the chapter.

For all palpations of the intrinsic muscles of the hand, the client is seated and the therapist is seated, facing the client.

Thenar Group

1. **APB:** Palpate on the lateral side of the thenar eminence and feel for the APB as the client abducts the thumb at the CMC joint against gentle resistance. Palpate from the tubercles of the scaphoid and trapezium to the lateral side of the base of the proximal phalanx of the thumb.
2. **FPB:** Now move over to the medial side of the thenar eminence and feel for the FPB as the client flexes the thumb at the CMC joint against gentle resistance. Palpate from attachment to attachment (palmar surface of the trapezium to the lateral side of the base of the proximal phalanx of the thumb) as best as possible, including the part of the muscle that is deep to the APB.
3. **OP:** Now move over to the shaft of the metacarpal of the thumb. Curl your palpating fingers around from posterior to anterior on the lateral shaft, and feel for the contraction of the OP against the metacarpal as the client gently opposes the thumb against the pad of the little finger. Once felt, try to palpate the rest of this muscle deep to the other two thenar muscles. Because it can be very challenging to feel and discern the contraction of the OP from the contraction of other thenar muscles, it is often advisable to palpate this muscle when the thenar muscles are relaxed.

Hypothenar Group

4. **ADMM:** Palpate on the medial side of the hypothenar eminence, and feel for the ADMM as the client abducts the little finger at the MCP joint against resistance. Palpate from the pisiform to the medial side of the base of the proximal phalanx of the little finger.
5. **FDMM:** Now palpate on the lateral side of the hypothenar eminence, and feel for the FDMM as the client flexes the little finger at the MCP joint (with the IP joints extended). Add resistance only if needed. Palpate from the hook of

the hamate to the anteromedial side of the base of the proximal phalanx of the little finger.
6. **ODM:** Locate the hook of the hamate and then palpate immediately distal to it on the most lateral aspect of the hypothenar eminence. Feel for the contraction of the ODM as the client opposes the little finger against the thumb. Once felt, palpate it deep to the other hypothenar muscles as far as possible. Note: The distal attachment of the ODM can be palpated by curling the palpating the fingers around to the anterior surface of the shaft of the fifth metacarpal.
7. **Detour to the palmaris brevis:** Palpate gently over the proximal hypothenar eminence while asking the client to wrinkle the skin of the hand by cupping the palm. This muscle is difficult to palpate and discern.

Central Compartment Muscles

8. **Adductor pollicis:** Palpate the thumb web of the hand from the anterior side while resisting the client from adducting the thumb, and feel for the contraction of the adductor pollicis. Once felt, palpate from the base of the proximal phalanx of the thumb to the third metacarpal and capitate.
9. **Lumbricals manus:** For the first and second lumbricals manus, palpate on the anterolateral surface of the metacarpal of the index and middle fingers, respectively. For the third and fourth lumbricals manus, palpate between metacarpals on the lateral side of the ring and little fingers, respectively. Ask the client to flex the finger at the MCP joint while keeping the IP joints extended, and feel for the contraction of the muscle. Once felt, palpate each one from attachment to attachment as the client alternately contracts and relaxes the muscle.
10. **PI:** For PI one, two, and three, palpate on the middle finger side of the metacarpal of fingers two, four, and five, respectively, as the client adducts each of the these fingers at the MCP joint by squeezing a pencil or highlighter. Once each one is felt, follow from attachment to attachment as the client alternately contracts and relaxes the muscle.
11. **DIM:** On the dorsal side of the hand, palpate between metacarpals on the side of the finger (fingers two, three, and four) that is away from the center of the middle finger while the client abducts the finger at the MCP joint. Once each DIM is felt, palpate from attachment to attachment.

16

Review Questions

1. List the attachments of the OP.
2. List the attachments of the FDMM.
3. What are the actions of the lumbricals manus?
4. What are the actions of the DIM?
5. When palpating the FDMM, where should resistance be given and why?
6. Palmaris brevis palpation can difficult for what reasons? Is there anything that can be of help for a clear palpation?
7. Pure adduction of the thumb without any flexion is necessary for a clear palpation of what muscle?
8. What important limitations must a therapist place on motion of the finger when attempting to palpate the lumbricals manus?
9. Placing a pen or highlighter between the index and middle fingers and then asking the client to squeeze is a method of engaging what muscle?
10. What piece of information about the middle finger is important in regards to the DIM?
11. TrPs in the ODM may entrap what nerve?
12. TrPs in the intrinsic muscles of the hands are most commonly brought on by what single factor?
13. What is the positioning for stretching the lumbricals manus?
14. What steps are necessary for completely stretching the right DIM?
15. Explain the difficulties a therapist faces when palpating the thenar eminence group of muscles.
16. Using logical reasoning and general anatomy knowledge, how can we know which fingers have PI and which fingers have DIM muscles attached to them?

CASE STUDY

A 38-year-old semi-professional cyclist arrives for a massage complaining of weakness and cramping in the left hand. This is accompanied by clumsiness in the same hand that is affecting her ability to perform tasks at work. A magnetic resonance imaging (MRI) scan showed no lesion or injury. She explains during intake that she completed a 10-day, 400-mile ride only 1 week ago and that the problem began during day 3 of the trip.

Exam and palpation of the left hand reveals diminished sensation in the fourth and fifth fingers with normal sensation in all other areas of the hand. There are TrPs in the ADMM, FDMM, and all three PI.

1. Based upon the information given, what would be your assessment of the cause of the client's symptoms?
2. What would your treatment plan include in terms of treatment and self-care?

16

CHAPTER 17

Tour #7 Palpation of the Trunk Muscles

Overview

This chapter is a palpation tour of the muscles of the trunk. The tour begins with palpation of the posterior trunk muscles and then addresses the muscles of the anterolateral and anterior trunk. Palpation of the posterior trunk muscles is shown in the prone position (except the interspinales, which are shown seated); palpation of the anterolateral musculature is shown with the client side lying; and anterior trunk muscle palpation is shown in the supine position, except the iliopsoas, which is demonstrated with the client seated. Alternate palpation positions are also described. The major muscles or muscle groups of the region are each given a separate layout, and there are also a few detours to other muscles of the region. Trigger point (TrP) information and stretching, both therapist-assisted and self-care stretching, are given for each of the muscles covered in this chapter. The chapter closes with an advanced *Whirlwind Tour* that explains the sequential palpation of all of the muscles of the chapter.

Chapter Outline

Latissimus Dorsi—Prone
    Detour to the Serratus Posterior Inferior
    Detour to the Trapezius and Rhomboids
Erector Spinae Group—Prone
Transversospinalis (TS) Group—Prone
Quadratus Lumborum (QL)—Prone
Interspinales—Seated
    Detour to the Intertransversarii and Levatores Costarum
External and Internal Intercostals—Side Lying
    Detour to the Subcostales and Transversus Thoracis
    Detour to the Other Muscles of the Anterior Chest
Rectus Abdominis—Supine
External and Internal Abdominal Obliques—Supine
    Detour to the Transversus Abdominis
Diaphragm—Supine
Iliopsoas—Seated
    Detour to the Iliopsoas Distal Belly and Tendon
    Detour to the Psoas Minor
Whirlwind Tour: Muscles of the Trunk

Chapter Objectives

After completing this chapter, the student/therapist should be able to perform the following for each of the muscles covered in this chapter:
1. State the attachments.
2. State the actions.
3. Describe the starting position for palpation.
4. Describe and explain the purpose of each of the palpation steps.
5. Palpate each muscle.
6. State the "Palpation Key."
7. Describe alternate palpation positions.
8. State the locations of the most common TrP(s).
9. Describe the TrP referral zones.
10. State the most common factors that create and/or perpetuate TrPs.
11. State the symptoms most commonly caused by TrPs.
12. Describe and perform the therapist-assisted and self-care stretches.

📀 Go to http://evolve.elsevier.com/Muscolino/palpation for video demonstrations of the muscle palpations presented in this chapter.

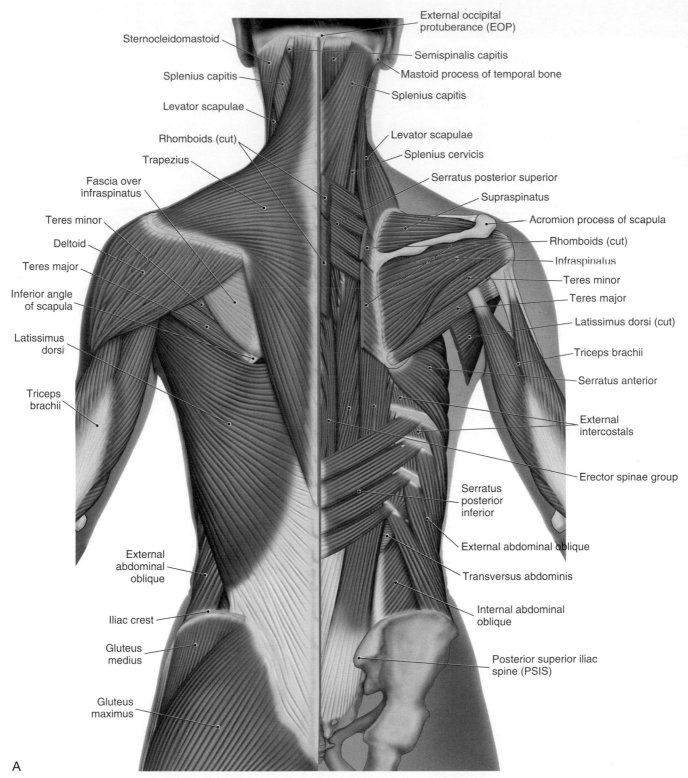

Sternocleidomastoid
Splenius capitis
Levator scapulae
Rhomboids (cut)
Trapezius
Fascia over infraspinatus
Teres minor
Deltoid
Teres major
Inferior angle of scapula
Latissimus dorsi
Triceps brachii
External abdominal oblique
Iliac crest
Gluteus medius
Gluteus maximus

External occipital protuberance (EOP)
Semispinalis capitis
Mastoid process of temporal bone
Splenius capitis
Levator scapulae
Splenius cervicis
Serratus posterior superior
Supraspinatus
Acromion process of scapula
Rhomboids (cut)
Infraspinatus
Teres minor
Teres major
Latissimus dorsi (cut)
Triceps brachii
Serratus anterior
External intercostals
Erector spinae group
Serratus posterior inferior
External abdominal oblique
Transversus abdominis
Internal abdominal oblique
Posterior superior iliac spine (PSIS)

A

Figure 17-1 Posterior views of the muscles of the trunk. **A,** Superficial view on the left and an intermediate view on the right.

17

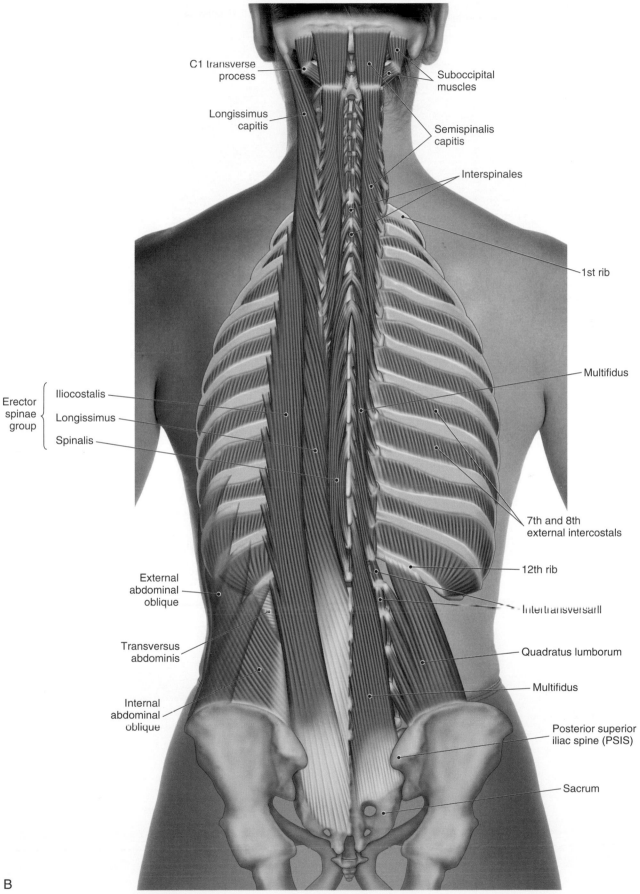

C1 transverse process

Longissimus capitis

Suboccipital muscles

Semispinalis capitis

Interspinales

1st rib

Multifidus

Erector spinae group
Iliocostalis
Longissimus
Spinalis

7th and 8th external intercostals

12th rib

Intertransversarii

External abdominal oblique

Transversus abdominis

Quadratus lumborum

Multifidus

Internal abdominal oblique

Posterior superior iliac spine (PSIS)

Sacrum

B

Figure 17-1, cont'd B, Two deeper views, the right side deeper than the left.

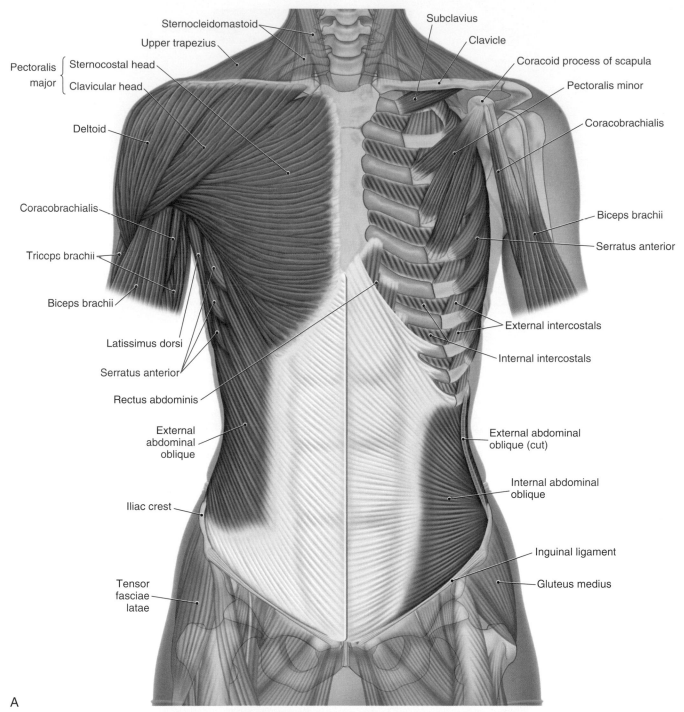

Figure 17-2 Anterior views of the muscles of the trunk. **A,** Superficial view on the right and an intermediate view on the left.

17

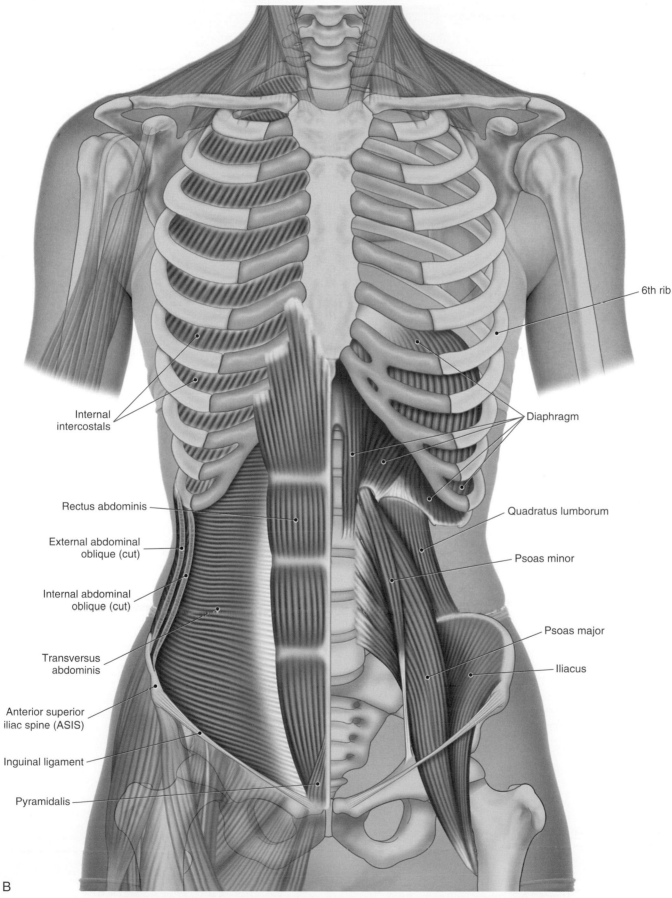

6th rib

Internal
intercostals

Diaphragm

Rectus abdominis

Quadratus lumborum

External abdominal
oblique (cut)

Psoas minor

Internal abdominal
oblique (cut)

Psoas major

Transversus
abdominis

Iliacus

Anterior superior
iliac spine (ASIS)

Inguinal ligament

Pyramidalis

B

Figure 17-2, cont'd B, Deeper views with the posterior abdominal wall seen on the left.

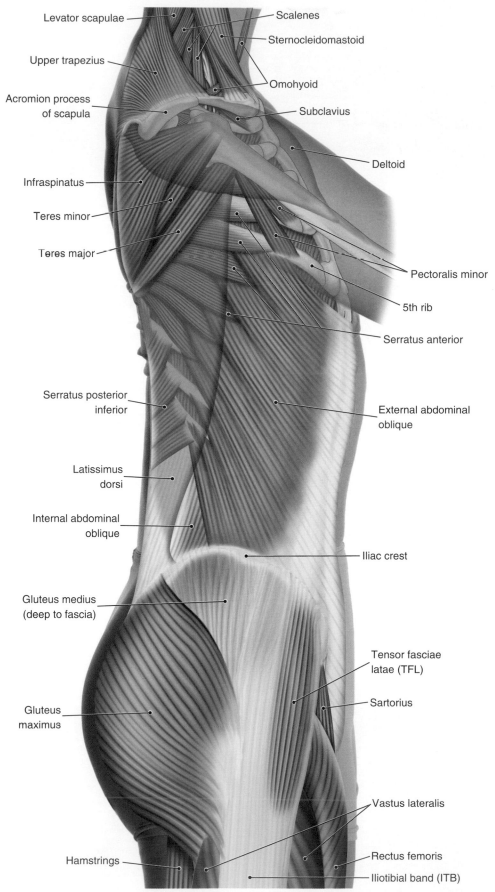

Figure 17-3 Lateral view of the trunk. The latissimus dorsi and deltoid have been ghosted in.

LATISSIMUS DORSI—PRONE

☑ ATTACHMENTS

☐ Spinous processes of T7-L5, posterior sacrum, and the posterior iliac crest (all via the thoracolumbar fascia)

to the

☐ lowest three to four ribs and the inferior angle of the scapula

to the

☐ medial lip of the bicipital groove of the humerus

☑ ACTIONS

☐ Extends the arm at the glenohumeral (GH) joint
☐ Adducts the arm at the GH joint
☐ Medially rotates the arm at the GH joint
☐ Anteriorly tilts the pelvis at the lumbosacral (LS) joint
☐ Depresses the scapula (shoulder girdle) at the scapulocostal joint (via its attachment to the scapula)

Starting Position (Figure 17-5)
■ Client prone with the arm relaxed at the side
■ Therapist seated to the side of the client
■ Palpating fingers placed on the posterior axillary fold of tissue
■ Support hand placed on the posterior aspect of the client's arm (just proximal to the elbow joint)

Palpation Steps
1. Ask the client to extend the arm at the GH joint and feel for the contraction of the latissimus dorsi in the posterior axillary fold of tissue (Figure 17-6, *A*).
2. Palpate toward its inferior attachment as the client alternately contracts and relaxes the latissimus dorsi.
3. Beginning again at the posterior axillary fold of tissue; while strumming perpendicular, palpate the distal tendon into the axilla all the way to the humerus (see Figure 17-6, *B*).
4. Once the latissimus dorsi has been located, have the client relax it, and palpate to assess its baseline tone.

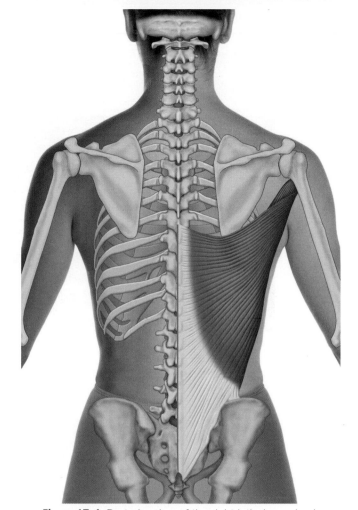

Figure 17-4 Posterior view of the right latissimus dorsi.

Palpation Key:
Palpate the posterior axillary fold of tissue.

17

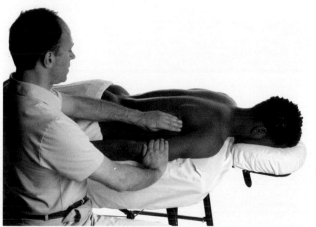

Figure 17-5 Starting position for prone palpation of the right latissimus dorsi.

LATISSIMUS DORSI—PRONE—*cont'd*

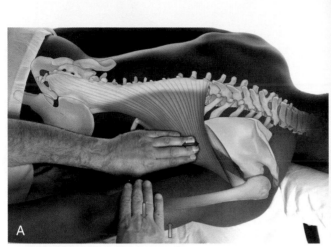
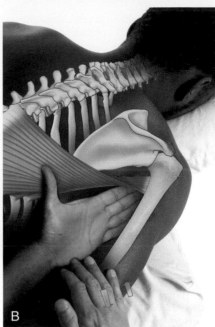

Figure 17-6 Palpation of the right latissimus dorsi as the client extends the arm against resistance. **A,** Palpation of the latissimus dorsi in the posterior axillary fold. **B,** Palpation of the humeral attachment at the medial lip of the bicipital groove of the humerus.

PALPATION NOTES

1. The posterior axillary fold of tissue is composed of the latissimus dorsi and teres major. If the client moves the arm away from body wall and you gently grasp the posterior fold of tissue in your palpating fingers, you are holding the latissimus dorsi and teres major (Figure 17-7).
2. Even though the distal tendon of the latissimus dorsi is up in the axilla, it is quite easy to follow to the humerus. At the humerus, the tendon of the latissimus dorsi is anterior to the tendon of the teres major (see Figure 17-6, *B*).
3. The teres major is located directly next to (medial to) the latissimus dorsi within the posterior axillary fold of tissue. The teres major also attaches onto the medial lip of the bicipital groove of the humerus and has the same three actions upon the arm at the GH joint. Distinguishing between these two muscles within the posterior axillary fold of tissue can be challenging. Feel for the rounded contour of the teres major, close to the scapula, medial to the latissimus dorsi. For palpation of the teres major, see Tour #1.

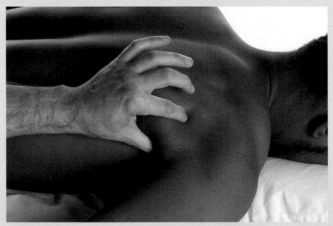

Figure 17-7 The posterior axillary fold, which contains the latissimus dorsi and teres major, is being pinched.

LATISSIMUS DORSI—PRONE—*cont'd*

Alternate Palpation Position—Standing

The latissimus dorsi can be easily palpated with the client standing. The client stands with the arm on the shoulder of the therapist, who is standing to the front and side of the client. Ask the client to push his arm down onto your shoulder in the direction of extension and adduction of the arm at the GH joint, and feel for the contraction of the latissimus dorsi. In this position, it is especially easy to follow the latissimus dorsi to its humeral attachment.

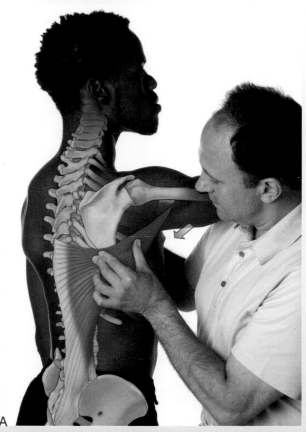

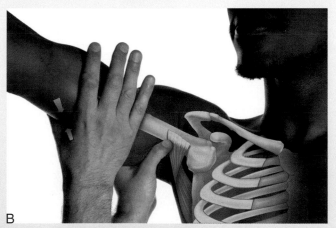

Figure 17-8 Standing palpation of the right latissimus dorsi. **A,** The starting position in which the client has his distal arm (just proximal to the elbow joint) on the shoulder of the therapist. **B,** Shows palpation of the humeral attachment as the client tries to move the arm obliquely toward extension and adduction against resistance.

17

LATISSIMUS DORSI—PRONE—*cont'd*

TRIGGER POINTS

1. Trigger points (TrPs) in the latissimus dorsi often result from or are perpetuated by acute or chronic overuse of the muscle (e.g., rowing, pushing the hand down on a surface to move the body, any activity that requires a forceful motion of pulling the arms down from overhead), overstretching the muscle by hanging from a hand or from both hands, compression of the muscle (e.g., wearing a tight bra) resulting in irritation and ischemia, and TrPs in the serratus posterior superior.

2. TrPs in the latissimus dorsi tend to produce a constant aching pain at rest as well as with contraction of the muscle, difficulty sleeping on the affected side due to pressure on the TrP(s), and joint dysfunction of the vertebrae to which it is attached.

3. The referral patterns of latissimus dorsi TrPs must be distinguished from the referral patterns of TrPs in the scalenes, infraspinatus, subscapularis, erector spinae/transversospinalis of the thoracic region, serratus anterior, serratus posterior superior, rectus abdominis, rhomboids, lower trapezius, teres major, deltoid, and pectoralis minor.

4. TrPs in the latissimus dorsi are often incorrectly assessed as cervical disc syndrome, thoracic outlet syndrome (causing ulnar nerve compression), entrapment of the suprascapular nerve, or bicipital tendinitis.

5. Associated TrPs often occur in the teres major, triceps brachii long head, lower trapezius, erector spinae of the thoracic region, flexor carpi ulnaris, and serratus posterior superior.

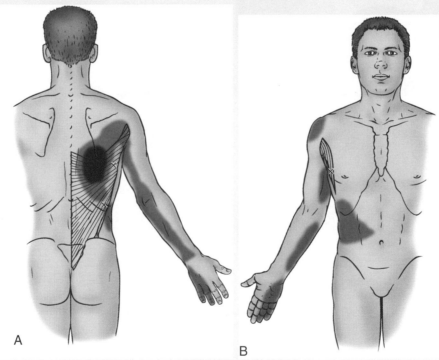

A   B

Figure 17-9 A, Posterior view illustrating common latissimus dorsi trigger points (TrPs) and their corresponding referral zones. **B,** Anterior view showing another common latissimus dorsi TrP and its referral zone.

17

LATISSIMUS DORSI—PRONE—*cont'd*

STRETCHING THE LATISSIMUS DORSI

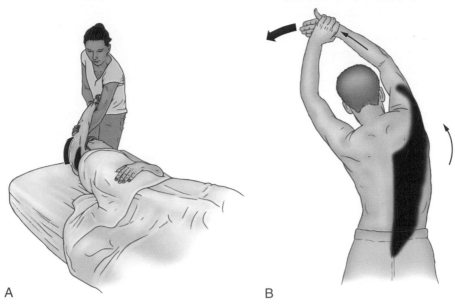

A   B

Figure 17-10 Stretching the right latissimus dorsi. The client's arm is flexed, laterally rotated, and horizontally flexed across their body. **A,** Therapist-assisted stretch. **B,** Self-care stretch. Note that the client is also left laterally flexing the trunk. See Figure 11-43 for another self-care stretch of the latissimus dorsi.

DETOUR

Serratus Posterior Inferior:
The serratus posterior inferior (SPI) is a thin respiratory muscle that attaches from the spinous processes of T11-L2 to ribs nine to twelve; its action is to depress ribs nine to twelve. It is located deep to and has the same general direction of fibers as the latissimus dorsi, therefore it can be difficult to palpate and discern the SPI. This muscle may be hypertrophied and easier to palpate in clients who have a chronic obstructive pulmonary disorder. If palpation is attempted, place palpating fingers over the lateral aspect of the muscle (lateral to the erector spinae), ask the client to exhale, and feel for its contraction while strumming perpendicular to its fibers.

Trigger Points:
1. Trigger points (TrPs) in the SPI often result from or are perpetuated by acute or chronic overuse of the muscle (e.g., in clients who have labored breathing due to chronic obstructive respiratory diseases, such as asthma, bronchitis, and emphysema) or trauma (e.g., back strain).
2. TrPs in the SPI tend to produce an aching pain in the lower posterior ribcage and joint dysfunction of T11-L2.
3. The referral patterns of SPI TrPs must be distinguished from the referral patterns of TrPs in the intercostal muscles, latissimus dorsi, and rectus abdominis.
4. TrPs in the SPI are often incorrectly assessed as kidney disease or rib joint dysfunction.
5. Associated TrPs likely occur in the latissimus dorsi and the erector spinae or transversospinalis (TS) muscles of the trunk.

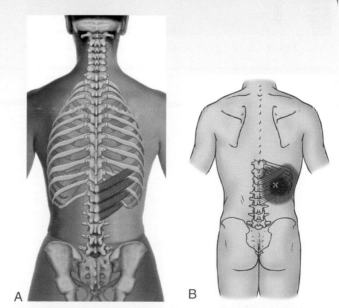

A   B

Figure 17-11 The right serratus posterior inferior (SPI). **A,** Posterior view of the right SPI. **B,** Posterior view showing a common SPI trigger point (TrP) and its corresponding referral zone.

17

LATISSIMUS DORSI—PRONE—*cont'd*

DETOUR

Trapezius and Rhomboids:

The trapezius and rhomboids were palpated in the palpation tour of the shoulder girdle (Tour #1 in Chapter 11). However, they may also be palpated in this palpation tour of the trunk.

For palpation of the trapezius, have the client prone, and ask her to abduct the arm at the GH joint to 90 degrees with the elbow joint extended and to slightly retract the scapula at the scapulocostal joint by pinching the shoulder blade toward the spine. Adding gentle resistance to the client's arm abduction with your support hand might be helpful (Figure 17-12).

For palpation of the rhomboids, have the client prone with the hand in the small of the back. Then ask him to lift the hand up away from the small of the back and feel for the contraction of the rhomboids (Figure 17-13).

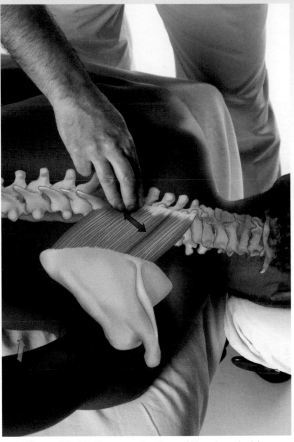

Figure 17-13 Prone palpation of the rhomboids.

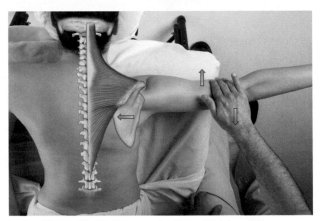

Figure 17-12 Prone palpation of the trapezius.

ERECTOR SPINAE GROUP—PRONE

✔ ATTACHMENTS

☐ Running parallel with the spine; attaching onto the pelvis, spine, ribcage, and head

✔ ACTIONS

☐ Extends the trunk, neck, and head at the spinal joints
☐ Laterally flexes the trunk, neck, and head at the spinal joints
☐ Ipsilaterally rotates the trunk, neck, and head at the spinal joints
☐ Anteriorly tilts the pelvis at the lumbosacral (LS) joint
☐ Elevates the pelvis at the LS joint

Starting Position (Figure 17-15)

■ Client prone
■ Therapist standing to the side of the client
■ Palpating hand placed just lateral to the lumbar spine

Palpation Steps

1. Ask the client to extend the trunk, neck, and head, and feel for the contraction of the erector spinae musculature in the lumbar region (Figure 17-16).
2. Palpate to the inferior attachment on the pelvis and then toward the superior attachment as far as possible while strumming perpendicular to the fibers.
3. Once the erector spinae has been located, have the client relax it, and palpate to assess its baseline tone.

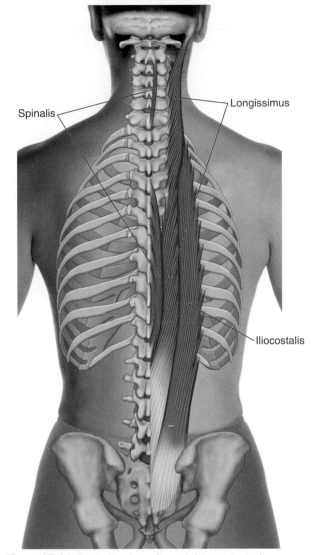

Figure 17-14 Posterior view of the right erector spinae group.

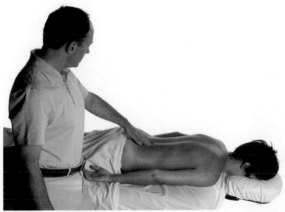

Figure 17-15 Starting position for prone palpation of the right erector spinae group.

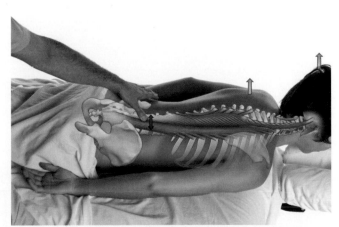

Figure 17-16 Palpation of the right erector spinae group as the client extends the head, neck, and trunk.

17

ERECTOR SPINAE GROUP—PRONE—*cont'd*

PALPATION NOTES

1. Even though the erector spinae group is not superficial, it is so thick and massive that it is usually easy to palpate.
2. The erector spinae group is easiest to palpate in the lumbar region.
3. In the thoracic region, the erector spinae spreads out. Most of its fibers are lateral to the laminar groove in the interscapular region and easy to palpate. However, some of its fibers run so far lateral that they are located deep to the scapula. To allow for direct access to these fibers, have the client hang the forearm/arm off the table, causing the scapula to protract.

4. There is very little erector spinae musculature in the cervical region. The only appreciable presence of erector spinae in the neck is the longissimus capitis, which attaches far lateral onto the mastoid process of the temporal bone. It is difficult to discern the longissimus capitis from adjacent musculature.
5. When palpating the erector spinae, keep in mind that the fibers are vertically oriented.
6. The erector spinae group is composed of three muscles: the iliocostalis, longissimus, and spinalis. It may be challenging to discern the border between the iliocostalis and longissimus; it is usually more difficult to discern the border between the longissimus and the spinalis.

TRIGGER POINTS

1. Trigger points (TrPs) in the erector spinae group often result from or are perpetuated by acute or chronic overuse of the muscle (e.g., prolonged standing posture that is stooped or inclined forward; lifting objects, especially with the spine flexed and/or rotated), prolonged immobility (e.g., long car rides), scoliosis (often caused by inequality of lower extremity length or pelvic asymmetry), prolonged sitting, poor seated posture, or carrying a wallet in a back pocket.
2. TrPs in the erector spinae group tend to produce restricted range of motion of the trunk at the spinal joints (specifically restricted flexion and/or contralateral lateral flexion), increased lumbar lordosis, or decreased thoracic kyphosis.
3. The referral patterns of erector spinae group TrPs must be distinguished from the referral patterns of TrPs in the serratus anterior, serratus posterior superior and inferior, rectus abdominis, rhomboids, levator scapulae, scalenes, infraspinatus, latissimus dorsi, quadratus lumborum (QL), psoas major, gluteus maximus, gluteus medius, gluteus minimus, intercostals, and piriformis.

4. TrPs in the erector spinae group are often incorrectly assessed as spinal joint dysfunction, osteoarthritis, pathologic disc conditions, facet syndrome, angina pectoris, pathologic conditions of the lung or abdominal viscera, sacroiliac joint dysfunction, or sciatica.
5. Associated TrPs often occur in the latissimus dorsi, QL, psoas major, transversospinalis (TS) group, and serratus posterior superior and inferior.
6. Notes: 1) TrPs can develop at any segmental level; the TrPs shown are examples. 2) TrPs are most likely to develop within the longissimus and iliocostalis; patterns of TrPs and TrP referral zones for the spinalis have not yet been identified. 3) Erector spinae TrPs in the thoracic region usually refer pain both superiorly and inferiorly, whereas erector spinae TrPs in the lumbar region usually refer pain only inferiorly (usually into the buttock). 4) Generally, erector spinae TrPs refer pain more laterally and in a more diffuse pattern than TS TrPs. 5) Erector spinae TrPs can also refer pain to the anterior thoracic and abdominal wall, usually at the same segmental level.

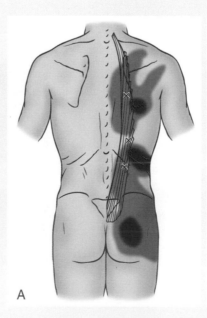
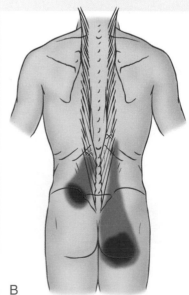

Figure 17-17 Erector spinae (iliocostalis and longissimus) trigger points (TrPs). **A,** Posterior view showing common iliocostalis TrPs and their referral zones. **B,** Posterior view showing common longissimus TrPs and their referral zones.

A   B

ERECTOR SPINAE GROUP—PRONE—*cont'd*

STRETCHING THE ERECTOR SPINAE GROUP

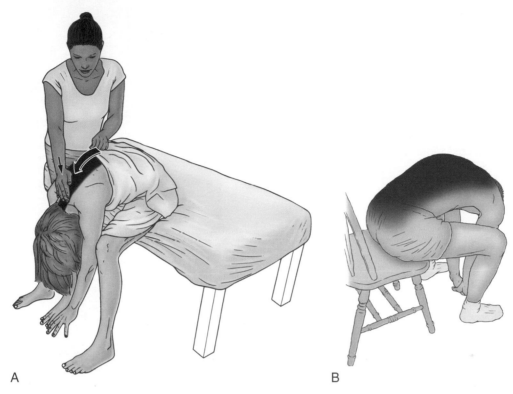

A   B

Figure 17-18 Stretching the bilateral erector spinae groups. The client's trunk and neck are flexed al the spinal joints. The stretch for one side can be enhanced by adding lateral flexion to the opposite side. **A,** Therapist-assisted stretch. Note that the therapist's other hand holds and secures the draping. **B,** Self-care stretch. Note: For both the therapist-assisted and self-care stretch, when returning back to the seated position, it is best for the client to place the forearms on the thighs, using them to push herself/himself back up.

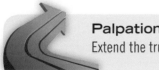

Palpation Key:
Extend the trunk from prone position.

17

TRANSVERSOSPINALIS (TS) GROUP—PRONE

☑ATTACHMENTS
- ☐ Located in the laminar groove, attaching onto the pelvis, spine, and head
- ☐ Generally, each individual transversospinalis (TS) muscle attaches from a transverse process inferiorly

  to a

- ☐ spinous process superiorly

☑ACTIONS
- ☐ Extends the trunk, neck, and head at the spinal joints
- ☐ Laterally flexes the trunk, neck, and head at the spinal joints
- ☐ Contralaterally rotates the trunk and neck at the spinal joints
- ☐ Anteriorly tilts the pelvis at the lumbosacral (LS) joint
- ☐ Elevates the pelvis at the LS joint

Starting Position (Figure 17-20)
- ■ Client prone
- ■ Therapist standing to the side of the client
- ■ Palpating fingers placed just lateral to the spinous processes of the lumbar spine within the laminar groove

Palpation Steps
1. With palpating finger(s) over the laminar groove of the lumbar spine, ask the client to slightly extend and rotate the lower trunk to the opposite side of the body (contralaterally rotate) at the spinal joints. Feel for the contraction of the TS musculature of the lumbar spine, particularly the multifidus group (Figure 17-21).
2. Once located, try to strum perpendicular to the direction of fibers, and feel for the multifidus deep to the erector spinae.
3. Repeat this procedure superiorly up the spine.
4. To palpate the semispinalis group in the cervical region, have the client prone with the hand in the small of the back (Palpation Note #1). Place palpating fingers over the laminar groove of the cervical spine, and ask the client to slightly extend the head and neck at the spinal joints, feeling for the contraction of the semispinalis deep to the upper trapezius (Figure 17-22).
5. Once located, follow the semispinalis up to the attachment on the head while strumming perpendicular to the direction of fibers.
6. Once the TS musculature has been located, have the client relax it, and palpate to assess its baseline tone.

17

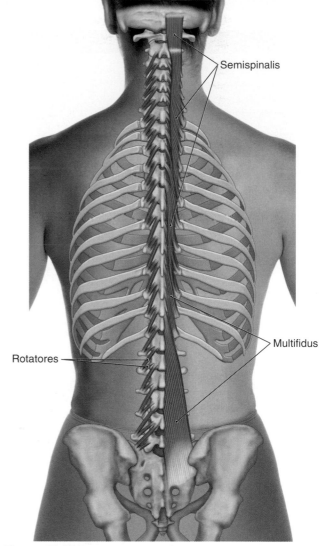

Figure 17-19 Posterior view of the transversospinalis (TS) group. The semispinalis and multifidus are seen on the right; the rotators are seen on the left.

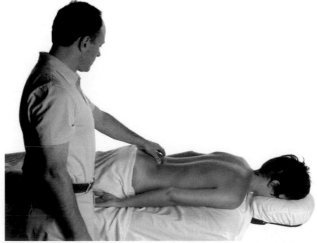

Figure 17-20 Starting position for prone palpation of the right transversospinalis (TS) group.

TRANSVERSOSPINALIS (TS) GROUP—PRONE—*cont'd*

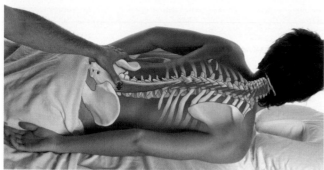

Figure 17-21 Palpation of the right lumbar multifidus as the client extends and contralaterally (left) rotates the trunk.

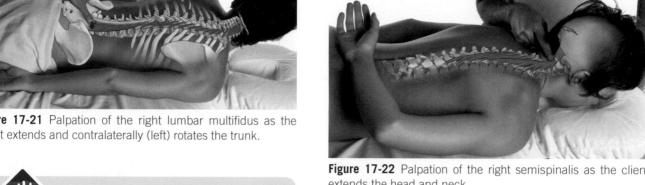

Figure 17-22 Palpation of the right semispinalis as the client extends the head and neck.

PALPATION NOTES

1. The TS group is composed of three subgroups: the semispinalis, multifidus, and rotatores. Each subgroup is then composed of smaller individual muscles. The rotatores attach to a vertebra one to two levels above, the multifidus attach to a vertebra three to four levels above, and the semispinales attach to a vertebra five levels above or more.
2. The TS musculature is located deep within the laminar groove of the spine. Although it is quite massive and bulky in the low back (The multifidus is the largest muscle of the lumbar spine.) and neck (The semispinalis is the largest muscle of the posterior cervical spine.), it can be difficult to clearly discern the TS musculature from more superficial and adjacent musculature.
3. The laminar groove lies within the spinal column between the transverse processes laterally and the spinous processes medially. The TS musculature is located within the laminar groove (except the semispinalis of the neck, which is also located lateral to the laminar groove).
4. When asking the client to extend the trunk to engage the TS of the trunk, the more superficial erector spinae will likely contract at the same time, making it more difficult to discern the TS musculature. Asking the client to also contralaterally rotate is important, because it not only engages the TS musculature but also reciprocally inhibits the erector spinae musculature.
5. When palpating the semispinalis in the cervical region, the client's hand is placed in the small of the back, because this reciprocally inhibits and relaxes the more superficial upper trapezius (placing the hand in the small of the back requires extension and adduction of the arm at the glenohumeral [GH] joint, which requires the coupled action of downward rotation of the scapula at the scapulocostal joint; scapular downward rotation reciprocally inhibits scapular upward rotators; the upper trapezius is a scapular upward rotator).
6. The multifidus is considered by many to be one of the two most important muscles of core/lumbosacral stabilization (the other being the transversus abdominis).

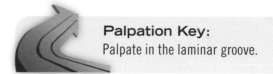

Palpation Key:
Palpate in the laminar groove.

Alternate Palpation Position—Supine

The semispinalis of the neck can also be palpated with the client supine (see Tour #2, Semispinalis Capitis Palpation). In the supine position it is more awkward, but the client can still be asked to place the hand in the small of the back.

17

TRANSVERSOSPINALIS (TS) GROUP—PRONE—*cont'd*

TRIGGER POINTS

1. Trigger points (TrPs) in the TS group often result from or are perpetuated by acute or chronic overuse of the muscle (e.g., prolonged standing posture that is stooped or inclined forward; lifting objects, especially with the spine flexed and/or rotated), prolonged immobility (e.g., long car rides), prolonged sitting, poor seated posture, scoliosis (often caused by inequality of lower extremity length or pelvic asymmetry), or carrying a wallet in a back pocket.

2. TrPs in the TS group tend to produce deep pain, restricted range of motion of the trunk at the spinal joints (specifically restricted flexion, extension beyond anatomic position, contralateral lateral flexion, and ipsilateral rotation), increased lumbar lordosis, or decreased thoracic kyphosis.

3. The referral patterns of TS group TrPs must be distinguished from the referral patterns of TrPs in the erector spinae group, rectus abdominis, quadratus lumborum (QL), psoas major, gluteus maximus, gluteus medius, piriformis, and pelvic floor muscles.

4. TrPs in the TS group are often incorrectly assessed as spinal joint dysfunction, osteoarthritis, pathologic disc conditions, facet syndrome, angina pectoris, pathologic conditions of the lung or abdominal viscera, sacroiliac joint dysfunction, or sciatica.

5. Associated TrPs often occur in the psoas major and erector spinae group.

6. Notes: 1) TrPs can develop at any segmental level; the TrPs shown are examples. 2) Semispinalis TrPs generally refer in the same pattern as longissimus TrPs of the erector spinae group (see Figure 17-17, *B*). 3) Generally, rotator TrPs refer pain more medially (usually directly over the spine and slightly lateral to the spine) and in a more circumscribed manner than multifidus TrPs. 4) TS TrPs in the lumbar region can also refer pain to the anterior abdominal wall, usually at the same segmental level.

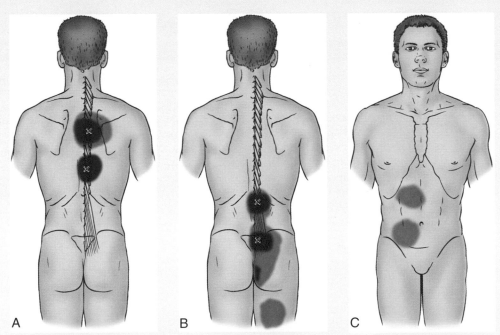

A   B   C

Figure 17-23 Transversospinalis (multifidus and rotatores) trigger points (TrPs). **A,** Posterior view showing thoracic TS TrPs and their corresponding referral zones. **B,** Posterior view showing lumbar TS TrPs and their corresponding referral zones. **C,** The remainder of the lumbar TrP referral zones.

17

TRANSVERSOSPINALIS (TS) GROUP—PRONE—*cont'd*

STRETCHING THE TRANSVERSOSPINALIS GROUP

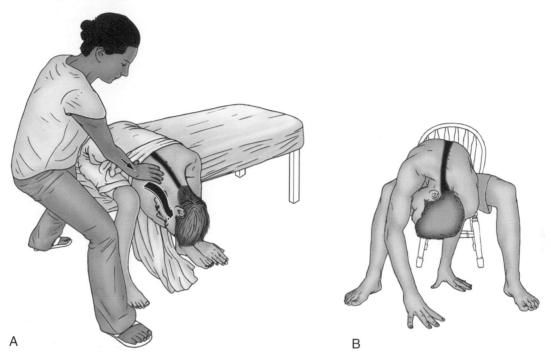

A   B

Figure 17-24 Stretching the right transversospinalis (TS) group. The client's trunk and neck are flexed and ipsilaterally (right) rotated at the spinal joints. This stretch is particularly effective for the multifidus and rotatores of the TS group. Note: The semispinalis can also be effectively stretched with the stretch shown in Figure 17-18. **A,** Therapist-assisted stretch. Note: The therapist's other hand holds and secures the draping. **B,** Self-care stretch. Note: For both the therapist-assisted and self-care stretch, when returning back to the seated position, it is best for the client to place the forearms on the thighs, using them to push herself/himself back up.

17

QUADRATUS LUMBORUM (QL)—PRONE

☑ ATTACHMENTS

- ☐ Inferomedial border of the twelfth rib and the transverse processes of L1-L4

  to the

- ☐ posteromedial iliac crest

☑ ACTIONS

- ☐ Elevates the pelvis at the lumbosacral (LS) joint
- ☐ Anteriorly tilts the pelvis at the LS joint
- ☐ Extends the trunk at the spinal joints
- ☐ Laterally flexes the trunk at the spinal joints
- ☐ Depresses the twelfth rib at the costovertebral joint

Starting Position (Figure 17-26)

- ◼ Client prone
- ◼ Therapist standing to the side of the client
- ◼ Palpating hand placed just lateral to the lateral border of the erector spinae in the lumbar region
- ◼ Support hand sometimes placed directly on the palpation hand for support (not shown)

Palpation Steps

1. First locate the lateral border of the erector spinae musculature (To do so, ask the client to raise the head and upper trunk from the table.); then place palpating fingers just lateral to the lateral border of the erector spinae.
2. Direct palpating pressure medially, deep to the erector spinae musculature, and feel for the quadratus lumborum (QL).
3. To engage the QL and to be certain that you are on it, ask the client to elevate the pelvis on that side at the LS joint (Note: This involves moving the pelvis along the plane of the table toward the head; in other words, the pelvis should not lift up in the air, away from the table.) and feel for its contraction (Figure 17-27).
4. Once located, palpate medially and superiorly toward the twelfth rib, medially and inferiorly toward the iliac crest, and directly medially toward the transverse processes of the lumbar spine (Figure 17-28).
5. Once the QL has been located, have the client relax it, and palpate to assess its baseline tone.

17

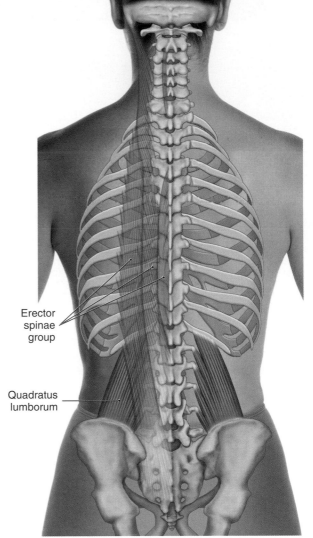

Erector spinae group

Quadratus lumborum

Figure 17-25 Posterior view of the right quadratus lumborum (QL). The left QL and ghosted left erector spinae group have been drawn in as well.

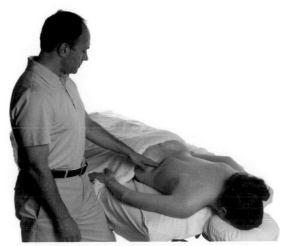

Figure 17-26 Starting position for prone palpation of the right quadratus lumborum (QL).

QUADRATUS LUMBORUM (QL)——PRONE—*cont'd*

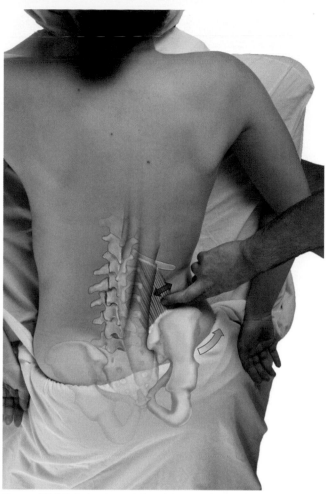

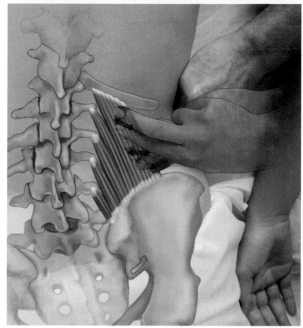

Figure 17-28 Once the quadratus lumborum (QL) has been located, palpate in all three directions toward the rib, transverse process, and iliac attachments.

Figure 17-27 Palpation of the right quadratus lumborum (QL) as the client elevates the right side of the pelvis. The outline of the right erector spinae group has been ghosted in.

Alternate Palpation Position—Side Lying

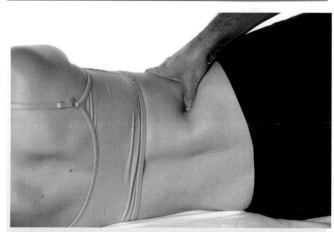

Figure 17-29 The quadratus lumborum (QL) can be easily palpated with the client side lying. As with the prone palpation, be sure that your palpating fingers are first located lateral to the erector spinae musculature. In this position, press down toward the table to access the belly and attachments of the QL.

PALPATION NOTES

1. The QL cannot be palpated through the erector spinae musculature because the erector spinae is so thick. To successfully palpate the QL, you must be lateral to the erector spinae, and then press in firmly with a medial direction to your pressure.
2. The client in Figure 17-28 has a lot of the QL accessible lateral to the erector spinae musculature. However, the amount of exposure of the QL lateral to the erector spinae varies. In some individuals, the erector spinae is wider and/or the QL is narrower, causing very little of the QL to be accessible lateral to the erector spinae musculature.
3. Whenever pressing deeply to palpate a muscle, always press in firmly but slowly! Ask the client to take in a deep breath, and then slowly press in as the client exhales. This procedure may be repeated two to three times, each time pressing in slightly deeper to access the QL.
4. The rib and iliac crest attachments of the QL are usually the easiest to palpate; the transverse processes attachment is usually the most challenging to palpate.

17

QUADRATUS LUMBORUM (QL)——PRONE—*cont'd*

TRIGGER POINTS

1. Trigger points (TrPs) in the quadratus QL often result from or are perpetuated by acute or chronic overuse of the muscle (e.g., repeated lifting of heavy objects or bending the trunk into flexion), a sudden overload while stretching the muscle (e.g., when bending the spine into flexion, especially combined with contralateral lateral flexion and/or rotation to either side), joint dysfunction of the thoracolumbar spine, an asymmetrically short lower extremity, or carrying a wallet in a back pocket.

2. TrPs in the QL tend to produce a low back ache that is usually felt deeply, occasional sharp stabs of pain (The pain may be felt at rest, but is usually most severe when sitting or standing.), difficulty sleeping (due to referred tenderness to the greater trochanter), difficulty turning over in bed or getting up out of bed or a chair, strong pain when coughing or sneezing, decreased spinal flexion and contralateral lateral flexion, an ipsilaterally elevated pelvis,

and a scoliosis with convexity to the opposite side. Pain may also refer to the groin, and even into the scrotum and testicle of a male.

3. The referral patterns of QL TrPs must be distinguished from the referral patterns of TrPs in the erector spinae and transversospinalis (TS) groups of the trunk, iliopsoas, gluteus maximus, medius, and minimus, piriformis and other deep lateral rotators of the hip joint, and tensor fasciae latae.

4. TrPs in the QL are often incorrectly assessed as sacroiliac joint dysfunction, lumbar disc syndrome, sciatica, or trochanteric bursitis.

5. Associated TrPs often occur in the contralateral QL and the ipsilateral erector spinae group or TS group of the trunk; gluteus minimus, medius, and maximus; iliopsoas; piriformis and other deep lateral rotators of the hip joint; and the external abdominal oblique.

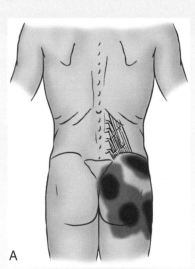

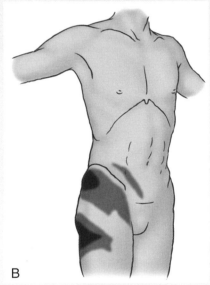

A   B

Figure 17-30 A, Posterior view of common quadratus lumborum (QL) trigger points (TrPs) and their corresponding referral zones. **B,** Anterolateral view showing the remainder of the referral zones.

17

QUADRATUS LUMBORUM (QL)——PRONE—*cont'd*

STRETCHING THE QUADRATUS LUMBORUM

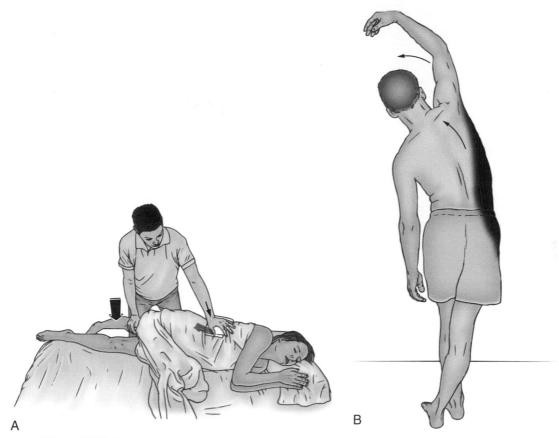

A

B

Figure 17-31 Stretching the right quadratus lumborum (QL). **A,** Therapist-assisted stretch. The therapist contacts the client's distal lateral thigh (not the leg). Note that the client's thorax is stabilized by the therapist's left hand; a cushion is used for comfort. **B,** Self-care stretch. The client places the left foot in front of the right and then left laterally flexes the trunk with the arm raised overhead and brought to the left side. See Figure 18-18 for another stretch of the QL.

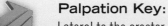

Palpation Key:
Lateral to the erector spinae, and press in medially.

17

INTERSPINALES—SEATED

☑ ATTACHMENTS

☐ From a spinous process

to the

☐ spinous process immediately superior (in the lumbar and cervical regions)

☑ ACTIONS

☐ Extends the neck and trunk at the spinal joints

Starting Position (Figure 17-33)

■ Client seated
■ Therapist seated behind the client
■ Palpating finger placed between two spinous processes in the lumbar region (Figures 17-33 and 17-34 show two interspinales muscles being palpated, hence two palpating fingers are seen contacting the client.)
■ Stabilizing hand placed on the upper trunk of the client

Palpation Steps

1. With palpating finger between two adjacent spinous processes of the lumbar spine, ask the client to slightly flex forward, and feel for the interspinous muscle between the spinous processes.
2. From this position of flexion, ask the client to extend back to anatomic position, and feel for the contraction of the interspinalis muscle. If desired, resistance can be given to the client's trunk extension with your support hand (see Figure 17-34).
3. This procedure can be repeated for other interspinales muscles between other spinous processes.
4. Once the interspinales muscles have been located, have the client relax them, and palpate to assess their baseline tone.

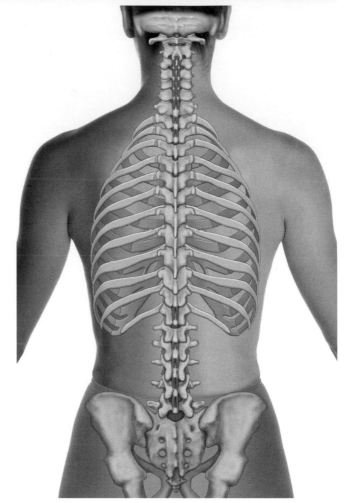

Figure 17-32 Posterior view of the right and left interspinales.

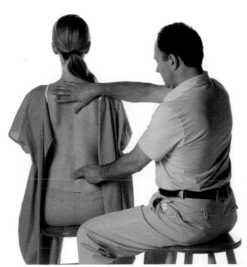

Figure 17-33 Starting position for seated palpation of the interspinales.

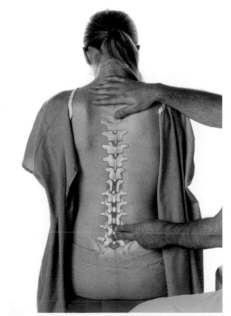

Figure 17-34 Palpation of the interspinales as the client extends the trunk back to anatomic position from a position of slight flexion.

17

INTERSPINALES—SEATED—*cont'd*

PALPATION NOTES

1. Note that the interspinales are generally located in the lumbar and cervical regions only. More specifically, they are usually located between C2 and T2, T11 and T12, and L1 and L5. However, variations exist and they are often found in other locations—most often in the upper or lower thoracic spine.
2. Flexing the lumbar spine opens up the spaces between spinous processes, making access to the interspinales muscles easier. However, if the client flexes too far, more superficial soft tissues in this region become stretched and taut, restricting access to the interspinales muscles.
3. Because of the lordotic curve of the lumbar and cervical spinal regions, the interspinales can be difficult to palpate and discern. Generally, lumbar interspinales are easier to palpate than cervical interspinales.

Alternate Palpation Position—Prone

The interspinales can also be palpated with the client prone. It is helpful to place a roll under the client's abdomen to help open up the spaces between the spinous processes in the lumbar region.

TRIGGER POINTS

Note: The patterns of trigger points (TrPs) and TrP referral zones for the interspinales have not been discerned and mapped out.

STRETCHING THE INTERSPINALES

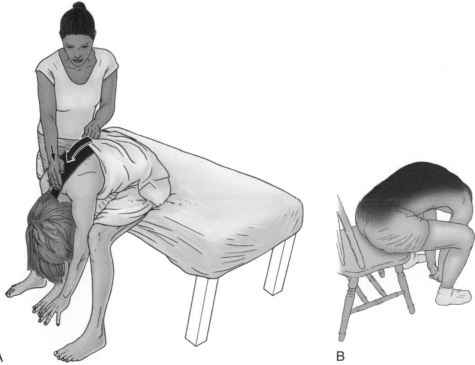

A   B

Figure 17-35 Stretching the bilateral interspinales. **A,** Therapist-assisted stretch. Note that the therapist's other hand holds and secures the draping. **B,** Self-care stretch. Note: For both the therapist-assisted and self-care stretch, when returning back to the seated position, it is best for the client to place the forearms on the thighs, using them to push herself/himself back up.

17

INTERSPINALES—SEATED—*cont'd*

DETOUR

Intertransversarii and Levatores Costarum:
Muscles called *intertransversarii* are located between adjacent transverse processes of the lumbar and cervical regions of the spine. They laterally flex the trunk and neck at the spinal joints. These muscles are very small and very deep, making palpation and discernment of them relative to adjacent soft tissues nearly impossible.

Muscles called *levatores costarum* are located in the thoracic region of the spine between the transverse processes of C7-T11 and ribs one to twelve. Their action is to elevate the ribs. Levatores costarum are also quite small and deep, making their palpation and discernment extremely challenging. If their palpation is attempted, have the client prone, and place palpating fingers between the mass of the erector spinae musculature and the angles of the ribs while asking the client to slowly and deeply breathe in and out; try to feel for their contraction as the client inhales.

Note: The patterns of trigger points (TrPs) and TrP referral zones for the intertransversarii and levatores costarum have not been discerned and mapped out.

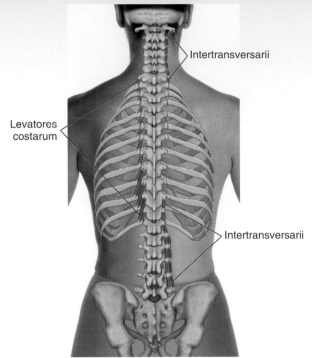

Figure 17-36 Posterior view showing the intertransversarii on the right and the levatores costarum on the left.

Palpation Key:
Palpate between spinous processes.

EXTERNAL AND INTERNAL INTERCOSTALS—SIDE LYING

☑ ATTACHMENTS

☐ From a rib

to the

☐ rib immediately superior (within an intercostal space)

☑ ACTIONS

☐ The intercostal muscles can elevate and depress the ribs at the sternocostal and costospinal joints for breathing (The upper intercostals are generally more active with elevation for inhalation; the lower intercostals are generally more active with depression for exhalation.)

☐ Both external and internal intercostals laterally flex the trunk at the spinal joints

☐ The external intercostals contralaterally rotate the trunk at the spinal joints

☐ The internal intercostals ipsilaterally rotate the trunk at the spinal joints

Starting Position (Figure 17-38)

■ Client side lying

■ Therapist standing behind the client

■ Palpating finger(s) placed in an intercostal space (between two ribs) in the lateral trunk (Two levels of intercostals are seen being palpated in Figures 17-38 and 17-39.)

Palpation Steps

1. To locate an intercostal space, feel for the hard texture of the ribs in the lateral trunk, and then drop your palpating fingers into the intercostal space between them (see Figure 17-39).

2. Once located, palpate in the intercostal space as far anteriorly and posteriorly as possible.

3. Once the intercostals have been located, make sure that the client is breathing lightly so that they are relaxed, and palpate to assess their baseline tone.

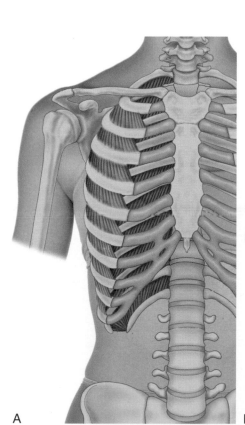
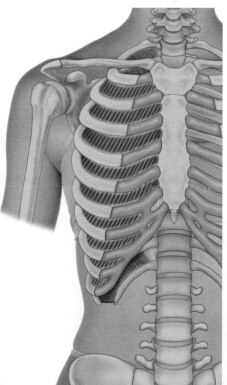
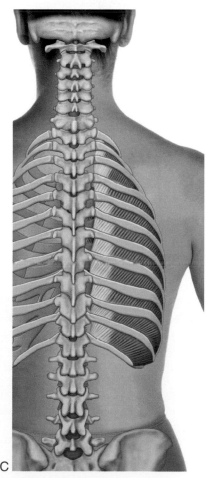

A   B   C

Figure 17-37 Views of the right intercostals. **A,** Anterior view of the right external intercostals. **B** and **C,** Anterior and posterior views of the right internal intercostals, respectively.

17

EXTERNAL AND INTERNAL INTERCOSTALS—SIDE LYING—*cont'd*

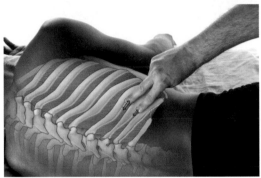

Figure 17-38 Starting position for side lying palpation of the right external and internal intercostal muscles.

Figure 17-39 Palpation of right intercostal muscles between the ribs in the lateral trunk.

Palpation Key:
First locate in an intercostal space that is not deep to other musculature.

PALPATION NOTES

1. If you ask the client to take in a deep breath, the ribs move apart slightly, increasing the size of the intercostal space and allowing better access to the intercostal muscles.
2. Discerning an external intercostal muscle from its underlying internal intercostal muscle (or vice versa) is extremely difficult.
3. All muscles of the trunk (except for the subcostales and the transversus thoracis) are located superficial to the intercostals, making their palpation more challenging. In some cases, these more superficial muscles are thin enough and loose enough to allow palpation of the deeper intercostals. But in others, these more superficial muscles are either too thick or too tight to allow discernment of the underlying intercostal muscles.
4. Only the internal intercostals are located in the spaces between the costal cartilages. Fibers of the external intercostals are located farther posteriorly to the spine.

Alternate Palpation Position—Prone or Supine

Given that the intercostal muscles are located posteriorly, anteriorly, and laterally in the trunk, they can also be palpated with the client prone or supine.

TRIGGER POINTS

1. Trigger points (TrPs) in the intercostals often result from or are perpetuated by acute or chronic overuse of the muscle (e.g., excessive exercise requiring prolonged forceful breathing, chronic coughing, retching, or trunk rotation), trauma (physical trauma or from thoracic surgery), rib fracture or joint dysfunction, herpes zoster, and heart and lung conditions within the thoracic cavity.
2. TrPs in the intercostals tend to produce local pain that spreads anteriorly from the site of the TrP or to adjacent intercostal spaces if more severe, decreased range of motion of the trunk in contralateral lateral flexion and/or rotation in either direction, restricted and often painful range of motion of the arm (due to fascial pulls on the ribcage), pain and therefore difficulty when breathing in deeply, coughing, and sneezing, or difficulty lying on and thereby causing pressure on the TrPs.
3. The referral patterns of intercostal TrPs must be distinguished from the referral patterns of TrPs in the pectoralis major and minor, serratus anterior, serratus posterior inferior (SPI), subclavius, erector spinae and transversospinalis (TS) muscles of the trunk, rectus abdominis, external abdominal oblique, levator scapulae, scalenes, rhomboids, and latissimus dorsi.
4. TrPs in the intercostals are often incorrectly assessed as rib joint dysfunction, costochondritis, myocardial infarction (or other intrathoracic conditions), or herpes zoster.
5. Associated TrPs often occur in the other accessory muscles of respiration and the pectoralis major.
6. Notes: 1) Generally, there is no distinction of pain referral patterns for the external versus the internal intercostals. 2) Intercostal TrPs tend to be located anterolaterally or posterolaterally (or between the costal cartilages far anteriorly).

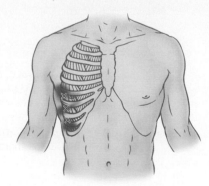

Figure 17-40 Anterior view showing common intercostal muscle trigger points (TrPs) and their corresponding referral zones.

EXTERNAL AND INTERNAL INTERCOSTALS—SIDE LYING—*cont'd*

STRETCHING THE INTERCOSTALS

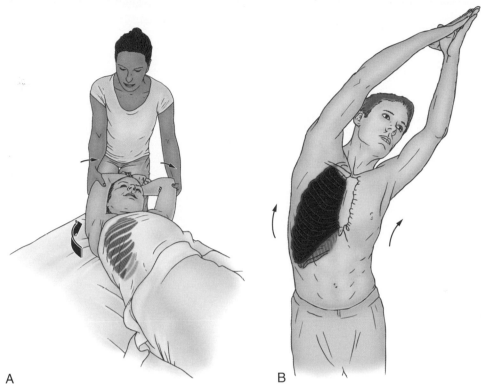

A

B

Figure 17-41 Stretching the right intercostal muscles. The client's trunk is laterally flexed to the opposite (left) side. It is important to isolate the bending to the thoracic region as much as possible. **A,** Therapist-assisted stretch. **B,** Self-care stretch.

DETOUR

Subcostales and Transversus Thoracis:
The subcostales and transversus thoracis are deep to the rib cage and extremely challenging if not impossible to palpate and discern from adjacent musculature.

The subcostales (seen on the right side in Figure 17-42, *A*) attach from ribs ten to twelve to ribs eight to ten; their action is to depress ribs eight to ten. To palpate the subcostales, palpate just lateral to the lateral border of the erector spinae in the posterior intercostal spaces between ribs eight to twelve.

The transversus thoracis (seen on the right side in Figure 17-42, *B*) attaches from the internal surfaces of the sternum, xiphoid process, and adjacent costal cartilages to the internal surfaces of costal cartilages two to six; its action is to depress ribs two to six. To palpate the transversus thoracis, either palpate just lateral to the xiphoid process of the sternum or in the anteromedial intercostal spaces between ribs two to six, just lateral to the sternum.

Note: The patterns of trigger points (TrPs) and TrP referral zones for the subcostales and transversus thoracis have not been discerned and mapped out.

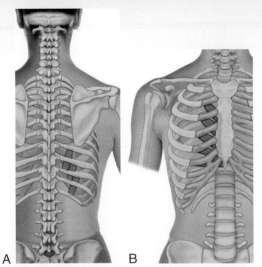

A

B

Figures 17-42 The subcostales and transversus thoracis are deep to the ribcage and extremely challenging to palpate and discern from adjacent musculature.

17

EXTERNAL AND INTERNAL INTERCOSTALS—SIDE LYING—*cont'd*

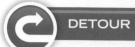

DETOUR

Other Muscles of the Anterior Chest:

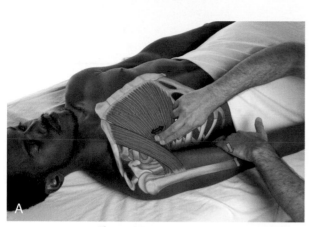

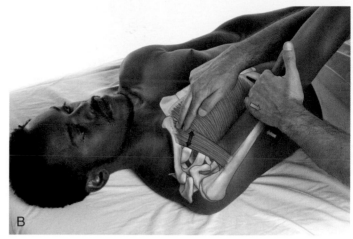

Figure 17-43 Palpation of the right pectoralis major. **A,** Palpation of the sternocostal head as the client adducts the arm against resistance. **B,** Palpation of the clavicular head as the client flexes and adducts the arm against resistance.

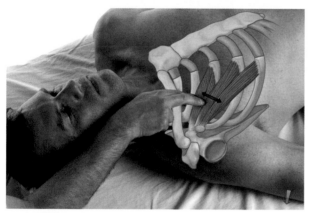

Figure 17-44 Palpation of the right pectoralis minor. The client is supine with his hand under his low back (not well visualized in this figure). Feel for the contraction of the pectoralis minor as the client presses the hand and forearm down against the table.

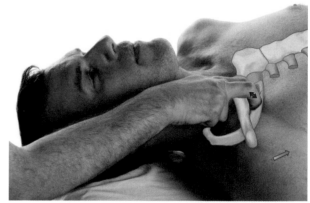

Figure 17-45 Palpation of the right subclavius. Ask the client to depress the clavicle at the sternoclavicular joint (i.e., to depress the shoulder girdle [scapula and clavicle]), and feel for the contraction of the subclavius.

17

RECTUS ABDOMINIS—SUPINE

☑ ATTACHMENTS

- ☐ Crest and symphysis of the pubic bone

  to the

- ☐ xiphoid process of the sternum and the costal cartilages of ribs five to seven

☑ ACTIONS

- ☐ Flexes the trunk at the spinal joints
- ☐ Laterally flexes the trunk at the spinal joints
- ☐ Posteriorly tilts the pelvis at the (lumbosacral) LS joint

Starting Position (Figure 17-47)

- ■ Client supine with a small roll under the knees
- ■ Therapist standing to the side of the client
- ■ Palpating hand placed just off center of the midline of the abdomen

Palpation Steps

1. Ask the client to slightly flex the trunk at the spinal joints (slightly curl the trunk upward), and feel for the contraction of the rectus abdominis (Figure 17-48).
2. With the rectus abdominis contracted, strum laterally (perpendicularly) across its fibers to locate its medial and lateral borders.
3. Continue palpating to the superior attachment and then to the inferior attachment while strumming perpendicularly across the fibers.
4. Once the rectus abdominis has been located, have the client relax it, and palpate to assess its baseline tone.

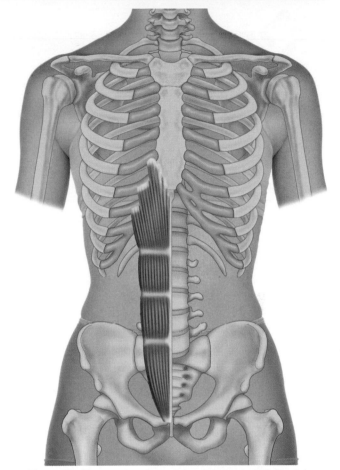

Figure 17-46 Anterior view of the right rectus abdominis.

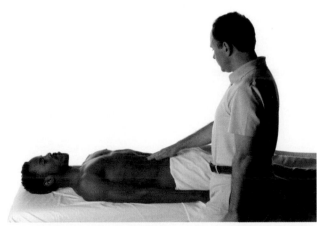

Figure 17-47 Starting position for supine palpation of the right rectus abdominis.

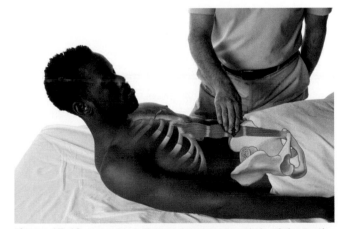

Figure 17-48 Palpation of the right rectus abdominis as the client flexes the trunk against gravity. Palpation should be done perpendicular to the fibers as shown.

17

RECTUS ABDOMINIS—SUPINE—*cont'd*

PALPATION NOTES

1. The rectus abdominis is superficial, and in a well-developed individual it can be visualized. Because of the tendinous inscriptions of the muscle, four separate boxes can usually be seen. For this reason, the rectus abdominis is often called the *six-pack muscle;* perhaps *four-pack muscle* (or *eight-pack* for the two sides of it bilaterally) would be more appropriate.
2. Inexperienced therapists are often apprehensive about palpating all the way to the inferior attachment on the pubic bone because they are afraid of accidentally passing the pubic bone and contacting the client's genitals. To increase certainty when palpating toward the pubic bone, it is helpful to press gently into the abdomen with the rectus abdominis relaxed, feeling for the softness of the abdominal wall. This way, when the pubic bone (and hence the inferior attachment of the rectus abdominis) is reached, the hard feel of the pubic bone is easily distinguished from the softness of the abdominal wall. Carrying out this palpation with the ulnar side of the hand pressing into the client at a 45-degree angle oriented inferiorly is very effective for locating the pubic bone.
3. In the midline of the anterior abdominal wall, the rectus abdominis is the only muscle present. The other three anterior abdominal wall muscles are located lateral to the rectus abdominis.

TRIGGER POINTS

1. Trigger points (TrPs) in the rectus abdominis often result from or are perpetuated by acute or chronic overuse of the muscle (e.g., excessive exercise doing crunches/curl-ups, straining at stool if constipated, chronic coughing, prolonged forceful abdominal breathing), direct trauma (physical trauma or from surgical incisions), visceral disease (e.g., gastrointestinal disease), or emotional stress (resulting in guarding, which tightens the abdominal wall).
2. TrPs in the rectus abdominis may produce pain felt over the lower aspect of the heart (if upper left–sided TrPs), diffuse abdominal discomfort, and visceral symptoms, such as heartburn, indigestion, abdominal cramping, nausea, and even diarrhea or vomiting. They may also entrap an anterior branch of a spinal nerve, resulting in lower abdominal and pelvic pain.
3. The referral patterns of rectus abdominis TrPs must be distinguished from the referral patterns of TrPs in the erector spinae, transversospinalis (TS), external and internal abdominal obliques, transversus abdominis (TA), intercostals, pectoralis major, and serratus posterior inferior (SPI).
4. TrPs in the rectus abdominis are often incorrectly assessed as a multitude of visceral diseases (e.g., peptic ulcer, hiatal hernia, appendicitis, intestinal disease, urinary tract disease, cholecystitis, and gynecologic diseases, such as dysmenorrhea) or sacroiliac and/or lumbar joint dysfunction.
5. Associated TrPs often occur in the other muscles of the anterior abdominal wall (contralateral rectus abdominis and ipsilateral and contralateral TA and external and internal abdominal obliques) and hip joint adductor muscles.
6. Note: The rectus abdominis pattern of pain that refers to the back of the trunk often crosses the midline of the body, so it is felt on both ipsilateral and contralateral sides of the back.

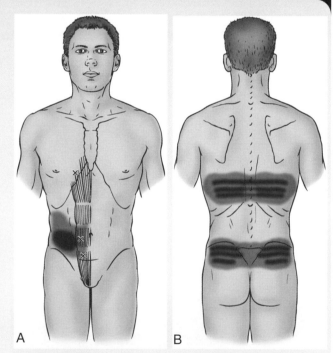

Figure 17-49 A, Anterior view showing common rectus abdominis trigger points (TrPs) and their corresponding referral zone. **B,** Posterior view showing the remainder of the referral zone. Note that posteriorly the referral zones may cross the midline to the contralateral side of the body.

RECTUS ABDOMINIS—SUPINE—*cont'd*

STRETCHING THE RECTUS ABDOMINIS

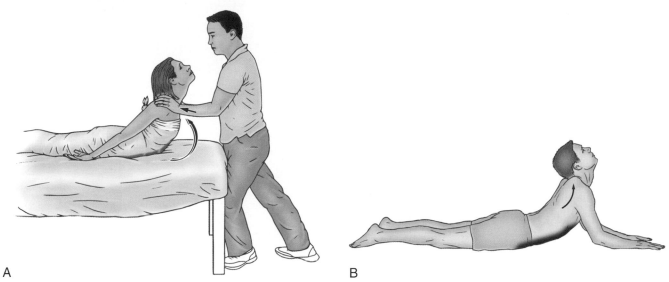

A   B

Figure 17-50 Stretching the bilateral rectus abdominis muscles. The trunk is brought into extension. The stretch of one side muscle can be enhanced by adding lateral flexion to the opposite side. **A,** Therapist-assisted stretch. Note that the draping is tied/knotted at the back of the client. **B,** Self-care stretch. The client lies prone and uses his forearms to help push his trunk into extension.

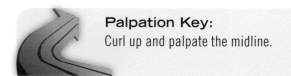

Palpation Key:
Curl up and palpate the midline.

EXTERNAL AND INTERNAL ABDOMINAL OBLIQUES—SUPINE

External Abdominal Oblique

☑ ATTACHMENTS

- ☐ Abdominal aponeurosis, pubic bone, inguinal ligament, and the anterior iliac crest

  to the

- ☐ lower eight ribs (Figure 17-51, *A*)

☑ ACTIONS

- ☐ Flexes the trunk at the spinal joints
- ☐ Laterally flexes the trunk at the spinal joints
- ☐ Contralaterally rotates the trunk at the spinal joints
- ☐ Posteriorly tilts the pelvis at the lumbosacral (LS) joint
- ☐ Elevates the pelvis at the LS joint
- ☐ Ipsilaterally rotates the pelvis at the LS joint
- ☐ Compresses the abdominal contents

Internal Abdominal Oblique

☑ ATTACHMENTS

- ☐ Inguinal ligament, iliac crest, and thoracolumbar fascia

  to the

- ☐ lower three ribs and abdominal aponeurosis (see Figure 17-51, *B*)

☑ ACTIONS

- ☐ Flexes the trunk at the spinal joints
- ☐ Laterally flexes the trunk at the spinal joints
- ☐ Ipsilaterally rotates the trunk at the spinal joints
- ☐ Posteriorly tilts the pelvis at the LS joint
- ☐ Elevates the pelvis at the LS joint
- ☐ Contralaterally rotates the pelvis at the LS joint
- ☐ Compresses the abdominal contents

Starting Position (Figure 17-52)

- ◼ Client supine with a small roll under the knees
- ◼ Therapist standing to the side of the client
- ◼ Palpating hand placed on the anterolateral abdominal wall

Palpation Steps

1. With palpating hand on the anterolateral abdominal wall between the iliac crest and the lower ribs (Be sure that you are lateral to the rectus abdominis.), ask the client to rotate the trunk to the opposite side of the body (contralateral rotation) and feel for the contraction of the external abdominal oblique (Figure 17-53, *A*).
2. Try to feel for the diagonal orientation of the external abdominal oblique fibers by strumming perpendicular to them.
3. Continue palpating the external abdominal oblique toward its superior and inferior attachments.
4. Repeat the same procedure for the internal abdominal oblique, asking the client to instead flex and ipsilaterally rotate the trunk at the spinal joints (see Figure 17-53, *B*).
5. Once the external abdominal and internal abdominal obliques have been located, have the client relax them, and palpate to assess their baseline tone.

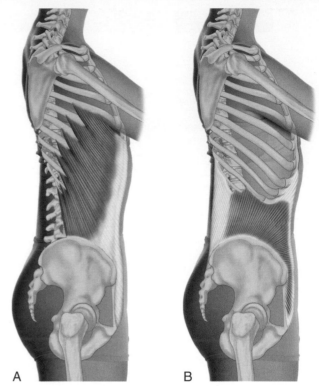

A   B

Figure 17-51 The right abdominal obliques. **A,** Lateral view of the right external abdominal oblique. **B,** Lateral view of the right internal abdominal oblique.

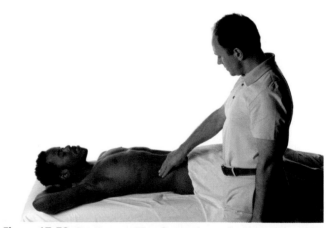

Figure 17-52 Starting position for supine palpation of the right external and internal abdominal obliques.

17

EXTERNAL AND INTERNAL ABDOMINAL OBLIQUES—SUPINE—*cont'd*

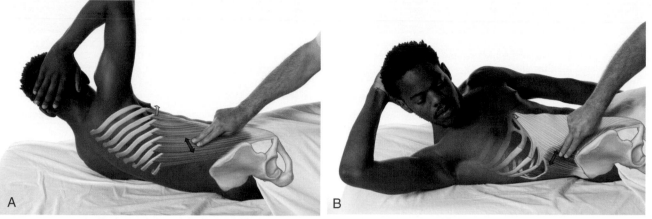

Figure 17-53 Palpation of he right external and internal abdominal obliques. **A,** Palpation of the right external abdominal oblique as the client flexes and contralaterally (left) rotates the trunk against gravity. **B,** Palpation of the right internal abdominal oblique as the client flexes and ipsilaterally (right) rotates the trunk against gravity.

PALPATION NOTES

1. When asking the client to contralaterally rotate (to isolate the external abdominal oblique) and ipsilaterally rotate (to isolate the internal abdominal oblique), try to have the client do as little flexion as possible, or both abdominal obliques on that side will contract.
2. The fiber direction of the external abdominal oblique is similar to the orientation of a coat pocket.
3. Feeling the fiber direction of each of the abdominal obliques and distinguishing between the external and internal abdominal obliques on one side can be challenging.
4. Technically, the inguinal ligament is not an attachment of the external abdominal oblique; rather it is part of its aponeurosis.

Alternate Palpation Position—Side Lying or Prone

Given that the abdominal obliques are also located in the lateral trunk and even attach as far posterior as the thoracolumbar fascia (which attaches into the spine), they can be palpated with the client side lying or even prone.

Palpation Key:

Flex and contralaterally rotate for the external abdominal oblique.
Flex and ipsilaterally rotate for the internal abdominal oblique.

17

EXTERNAL AND INTERNAL ABDOMINAL OBLIQUES—SUPINE—*cont'd*

TRIGGER POINTS

1. Trigger points (TrPs) in the abdominal obliques often result from or are perpetuated by acute or chronic overuse of the muscle (e.g., excessive exercise doing crunches/curl-ups, straining at stool if constipated, chronic coughing, prolonged forceful abdominal breathing, prolonged posture of rotation of the trunk), direct trauma (physical trauma or from surgical incisions), visceral disease (e.g., gastrointestinal disease), or emotional stress (resulting in guarding causing tightening of the abdominal wall).

2. TrPs in the abdominal obliques tend to produce pain in the chest (especially the more superior TrPs), abdomen, pelvis, and groin (especially the more inferior TrPs); and visceral symptoms, such as heartburn, indigestion, abdominal cramping, nausea, and even diarrhea or vomiting.

3. The referral patterns of abdominal obliques TrPs must be distinguished from the referral patterns of TrPs in the rectus abdominis, transversus abdominis (TA), intercostals, and pectoralis major.

4. TrPs in the abdominal obliques are often incorrectly assessed as a multitude of visceral diseases (e.g., peptic ulcer, hiatal hernia, appendicitis, intestinal disease, urinary tract disease, cholecystitis, and gynecologic diseases, such as dysmenorrhea).

5. Associated TrPs often occur in the other muscles of the anterior abdominal wall (contralateral abdominal obliques, and ipsilateral and contralateral TA and rectus abdominis) and hip joint adductor muscles.

6. Notes: 1) For the most part, the external and internal abdominal obliques are next to each other, superficial and deep, and their referral pain patterns have not been discerned from each other. Therefore they are discussed together. (The only exception to this is the presence of TrPs in the upper region of the external abdominal oblique where it does not overlie the internal abdominal oblique.) 2) The abdominal obliques' pattern of referral pain often crosses the midline of the body and is felt on both the ipsilateral and contralateral sides of the body.

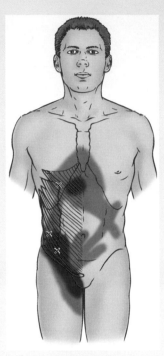

Figure 17-54 Anterior view showing common right-sided external and internal abdominal oblique trigger points (TrPs) and their corresponding referral zones. The upper TrP pictured here is an external abdominal oblique TrP. The lower ones can be in the external or internal abdominal oblique muscles. Note that the referral zones can cross the midline to the contralateral side of the body.

EXTERNAL AND INTERNAL ABDOMINAL OBLIQUES—SUPINE—*cont'd*

STRETCHING THE ABDOMINAL OBLIQUES

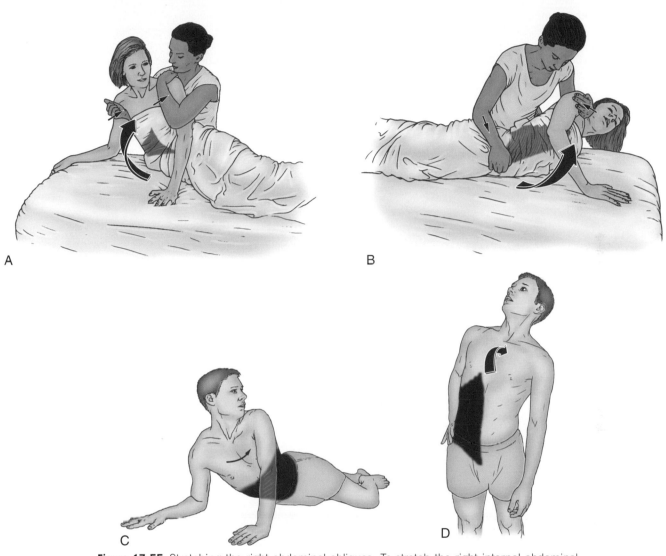

A   B

C   D

Figure 17-55 Stretching the right abdominal obliques. To stretch the right internal abdominal oblique, the client's trunk is extended, left laterally flexed and left (contralaterally) rotated. To stretch the right external abdominal oblique, the client's trunk is extended, left laterally flexed and right (ipsilaterally) rotated. **A** and **B,** Therapist-assisted stretching of the internal abdominal oblique and external abdominal oblique respectively. **C** and **D,** Self-care stretching of the internal abdominal oblique and external abdominal oblique respectively.

17

EXTERNAL AND INTERNAL ABDOMINAL OBLIQUES—SUPINE—*cont'd*

DETOUR

Transversus Abdominis:

The transversus abdominis (TA) attaches from the inguinal ligament, iliac crest, thoracolumbar fascia, and costal cartilages of ribs seven to twelve *to the* abdominal aponeurosis. It acts like a corset, compressing the abdominal contents within the abdominal cavity. It is considered by many to be one of the two most important muscles of core/lumbosacral stabilization (the other being the multifidus). Palpate the client's anterolateral abdominal wall, and ask the client to compress the abdominal contents by forcefully breathing out; feel for the contraction of the TA. The TA is deep to the external and internal abdominal obliques and extremely difficult to discern from these muscles, because they also contract when compressing the abdominal contents.

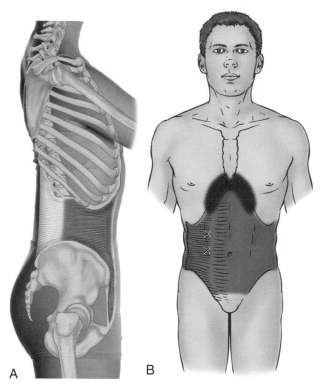

A   B

Figure 17-56 Views of the transversus abdominis (TA). **A,** Lateral view of the right TA. **B,** Anterior view showing common right-sided TA trigger points (TrPs) and their corresponding referral zone. Note: The referral zone can cross the midline to the contralateral side of the body.

DIAPHRAGM—SUPINE

☑ ATTACHMENTS

☐ Internal surfaces of the lower six ribs, the xiphoid process of the sternum, and the anterior surfaces of L1-L3

to the

☐ central tendon (dome) of the diaphragm (located in the center of the muscle)

☑ ACTIONS

☐ Increases the volume of the thoracic cavity, allowing the lungs to expand for inspiration

Starting Position (Figure 17-58)
■ Client supine with a roll under the knees to flex the thighs at the hip joint
■ Therapist seated to the side of the client
■ Palpating fingers curled under the inferior margin of the anterior ribcage

Palpation Steps
1. With your palpating fingers curled around the inferior margin of the anterior ribcage, ask the client to take in a deep breath and then slowly exhale. As the client exhales, curl your fingertips under (inferior and then deep to) the ribcage, and feel for the diaphragm on the internal surface of the ribcage (Figure 17-59).
2. Repeat this procedure anteriorly and posteriorly as far as possible on both sides of the ribcage.
3. Assessment of the diaphragm should only be made when it is totally relaxed, which occurs at the end of the exhalation.

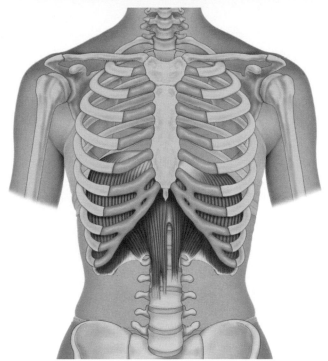

Figure 17-57 Anterior view of the diaphragm.

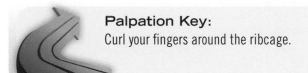

Palpation Key:
Curl your fingers around the ribcage.

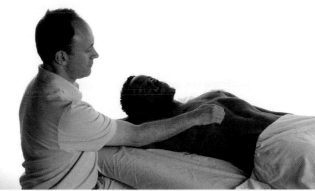

Figure 17-58 Starting position for supine palpation of the diaphragm.

17

DIAPHRAGM—SUPINE—*cont'd*

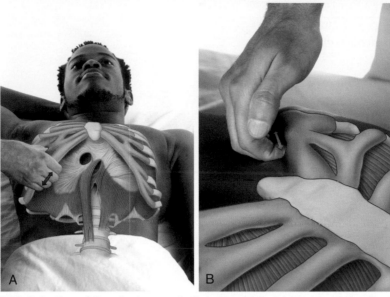

Figure 17-59 Palpation of the diaphragm. **A,** Palpation of the right side of the diaphragm as the client slowly exhales. **B,** Close-up showing palpation of the diaphragm by curling the fingers around the ribcage so that the finger pads are oriented against the muscle.

PALPATION NOTES

1. By placing a roll under the client's knees, the thighs are passively flexed at the hip joints, causing the pelvis to passively posteriorly tilt, slackening the anterior abdominal wall and allowing better access to the diaphragm.
2. As with any muscle palpation that is fairly deep, it is important to use gentle but firm pressure and to sink *slowly* into the tissue.

3. Successful palpation of the diaphragm requires a relaxed and slackened abdominal wall. For this reason, the diaphragm is easiest to palpate anteriorly because the anterior abdominal wall is easiest to relax and slacken. As the lateral abdominal wall is reached, the diaphragm becomes increasingly harder to palpate. It is extremely difficult if not impossible to palpate the diaphragm through the posterior abdominal wall.

Alternate Palpation Positions—Side Lying or Seated

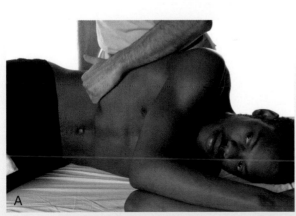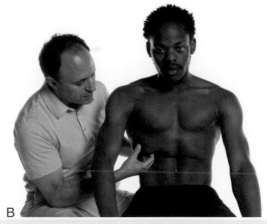

Figure 17-60 The diaphragm can also be palpated with the client side lying or seated. If the client is side lying, have the client's trunk flexed and the thighs passively flexed at the hip joints. This allows for relaxation and slackening of the anterior abdominal wall, allowing better access to the diaphragm. Similarly, if the client is seated, have the client's trunk slightly flexed to slacken the anterior abdominal wall, allowing better access to the diaphragm.

DIAPHRAGM—SUPINE—*cont'd*

TRIGGER POINTS

1. Trigger points (TrPs) in the diaphragm often result from or are perpetuated by acute or chronic overuse of the muscle (e.g., vigorous exercise leading to excessive forceful breathing, chronic hiccups) or chronic coughing.

2. TrPs in the diaphragm tend to produce pain upon exertion (especially at deep exhalation) at the anterolateral ribcage, often described as a "stitch in the side" or shortness of breath.

3. The referral patterns of diaphragm TrPs must be distinguished from the referral patterns of TrPs in the external abdominal oblique, subclavius, and pectoralis minor.

4. TrPs in the diaphragm are often incorrectly assessed as peptic ulcer, gallbladder disease, gastroesophageal reflux, or hiatal hernia.

5. Associated TrPs often occur in the intercostal muscles, rectus abdominis, and external and internal abdominal obliques.

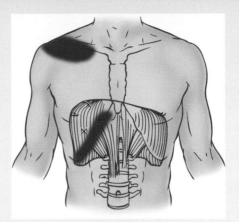

Figure 17-61 Anterior view showing common diaphragm trigger points (TrPs) and their corresponding referral zones.

STRETCHING THE DIAPHRAGM

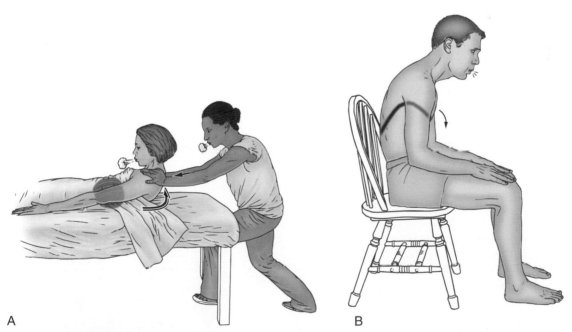

A   B

Figure 17-62 Stretching the diaphragm. The client's trunk is flexed as the client breathes out forcefully, expelling as much air from the lungs a possible. **A,** Therapist-assisted stretch. Note: To facilitate the client's breathing, the therapist breathes with the client. **B,** Self-care stretch.

17

ILIOPSOAS—SEATED

☑ ATTACHMENTS

- ☐ Anterolaterally (bodies, discs, and transverse processes) on vertebrae T12-L5 (psoas major) and the internal surface of the ilium (iliacus)

to the

- ☐ lesser trochanter of the femur

☑ ACTIONS

- ☐ The psoas major flexes the trunk (lower lumbar spine) at the spinal joints.
- ☐ The psoas major extends the trunk (upper lumbar spine) at the spinal joints.
- ☐ The psoas major laterally flexes the trunk at the spinal joints.
- ☐ The psoas major contralaterally rotates the trunk at the spinal joints.
- ☐ Both the psoas major and iliacus flex the thigh at the hip joint
- ☐ Both the psoas major and iliacus laterally rotate the thigh at the hip joint.
- ☐ Both the psoas major and iliacus anteriorly tilt the pelvis at the hip joint.

Starting Position (Figure 17-64)

- ■ Client seated with the trunk slightly flexed
- ■ Therapist seated to the side and slightly to the front of the client
- ■ Palpating hand placed anterolaterally on the client's abdominal wall, approximately halfway between the umbilicus and the anterior superior iliac spine (ASIS); ensure placement is lateral to the lateral border of the rectus abdominis
- ■ Fingers of support hand placed over fingers of palpating hand to increase strength and stability of palpating fingers (not shown in Figure 17-64)

Palpation Steps

1. Ask the client to take in a deep but relaxed breath; as the client exhales, slowly (but firmly) sink in toward the belly of the psoas major by pressing diagonally (posteromedially) in toward the spine. You may need to repeat this procedure two to three times before arriving at the psoas major belly at the spine.
2. To confirm that you are on the psoas major, ask the client to gently flex the thigh at the hip joint by lifting the foot slightly off the floor, and feel for the contraction of the psoas major (Figure 17-65).
3. Strum perpendicularly across the fibers to feel for the width of the muscle.
4. Continue palpating the psoas major toward its superior vertebral attachment and inferiorly as far as possible within the abdominopelvic cavity.
5. To palpate the iliacus, curl your fingers around the iliac crest with your finger pads oriented toward the internal surface of the ilium, and feel for the iliacus (Figure 17-66). To engage the iliacus, ask the client to flex the thigh at the hip joint by lifting the foot slightly off the floor.
6. Once the iliopsoas major has been located, have the client relax it, and palpate to assess its baseline tone.

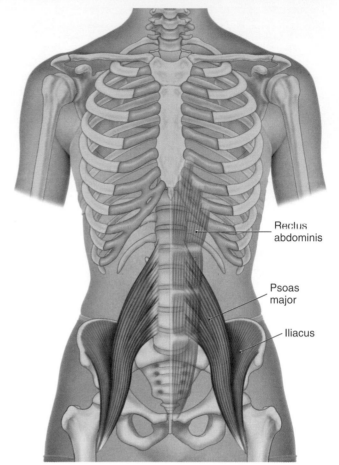

Figure 17-63 Anterior view of the right iliopsoas. The left iliopsoas and ghosted left rectus abdominis have been drawn in as well.

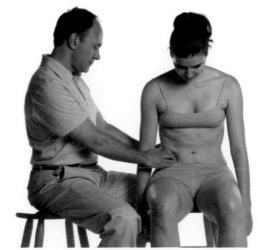

Figure 17-64 Starting position for seated palpation of the right iliopsoas.

ILIOPSOAS—SEATED—*cont'd*

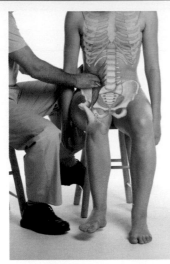

Figure 17-65 Palpation of the right psoas major as the client gently flexes the thigh at the hip joint by lifting her foot up slightly from the floor.

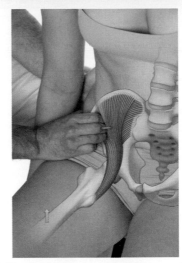

Figure 17-66 The right iliacus is palpated by curling the fingers around the iliac crest so that the finger pads are oriented against the muscle.

PALPATION NOTES

1. The iliopsoas is composed of the psoas major muscle and the iliacus muscle.
2. The client's trunk begins in slight flexion to slacken and thereby relax the muscles of the anterior abdominal wall, allowing easier entry and discernment of the psoas major and iliacus.
3. Before beginning the palpation procedure, have the client demonstrate how he/she will lift the foot off the floor (flexing the thigh at the hip joint) so that no time will be wasted once you are palpating into the abdomen and ready for this step.
4. Only the fibers of the iliacus closest to the iliac crest are palpable; the rest are too deep to be accessed.
5. Be careful when palpating deep into the abdominal cavity for the belly of the psoas major; major blood vessels (aorta and iliac arteries) are located nearby. If you feel a pulse under your fingers, move your palpating fingers off the artery.
6. Palpating the distal belly and tendon of the iliopsoas is most easily done with the client supine (Figure 17-68).
7. Be careful when palpating the iliopsoas in the proximal anterior thigh because the femoral nerve, artery, and vein are located over the iliopsoas and pectineus in this region (see Figure 17-2). If you feel a pulse under your fingers, either gently move the artery out of the way or slightly move your palpating fingers off the artery. Similarly, if you are pressing on the femoral nerve and the client feels shooting pain into the thigh, move your palpating fingers off the nerve.
8. The abdominal belly of the psoas major can also be palpated with the client supine. In this position, it is extremely important to have rolls under the client's knees so that the pelvis posteriorly tilts, allowing the anterior abdominal wall to slacken. The psoas major can also be palpated with the client side lying or ¾ side lying (half way between side lying and supine). The advantage to this position is that abdominal belly fat tends to fall out of the way of the therapist's palpating fingers.

Alternate Palpation Position—Supine or Side Lying

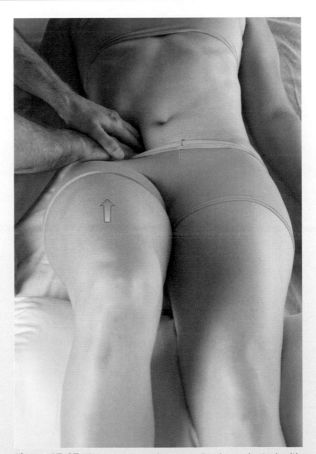

Figure 17-67 The psoas major can also be palpated with the client supine or side lying. The disadvantage of supine palpation position is that when the client flexes the thigh at the hip joint, the muscles of the abdominal wall may contract to stabilize the pelvis. This can interfere with feeling the psoas major, located deep to these muscles. This may also occur to some degree with the side lying palpation position.

17

ILIOPSOAS—SEATED—*cont'd*

DETOUR

Iliopsoas Distal Belly and Tendon:

With the client supine, first locate the sartorius (by asking the client to laterally rotate and flex the thigh at the hip joint); then drop off the sartorius medially onto the iliopsoas distal belly/tendon. To confirm your location, ask the client to flex the trunk by doing a gentle/small curl-up of the trunk, and feel for the tensing of the psoas major belly and tendon; the psoas major is the more medial portion of the iliopsoas. No other muscle in the anterior thigh is a mover of trunk flexion. However, the curl-up must be gentle or moderate in strength because a strong abdominal curl-up might cause other hip flexor muscles

to contract as stabilizers of the pelvis, preventing it from posteriorly tilting (hip flexors are anterior tilters of the pelvis) (Figure 17-68, *A*). Now passively hold the client's thigh into flexion and follow the belly/tendon distally to the lesser trochanter by asking the client to alternately contract and relax the psoas major by gently initiating a curling up of the trunk and then relaxing (Figure 17-68, *B*). The texture of the distal belly/tendon hardens only when the muscle contracts, whereas the lesser trochanter is palpably hard regardless of whether the muscle is contracted. Note: Be aware of the presence of the femoral nerve, artery, and vein in this region (see Palpation Note #7).

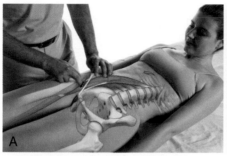
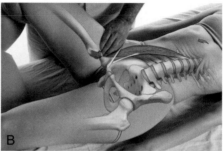

Figure 17-68 Palpation of the distal belly and tendon of the psoas major in the proximal thigh as the client flexes (curls) the trunk at the spinal joints against gravity. **A,** Palpation of the distal belly immediately distal to the inguinal ligament; the sartorius has been ghosted in. **B,** Palpation of the distal tendon and its femoral attachment at the lesser trochanter.

TRIGGER POINTS

1. Trigger points (TrPs) in the iliopsoas often result from or are perpetuated by acute or chronic overuse of the muscle (e.g., excessive exercise doing curl-ups/crunches, excessive running, or excessive kicking when playing soccer), prolonged shortening of the muscle (e.g., sitting with the hip joints flexed, sleeping in fetal position, having an excessive lumbar lordosis), an asymmetrically short lower extremity, or carrying a wallet in a back pocket.

2. TrPs in the iliopsoas tend to produce decreased extension of the thigh at the hip joint or pain in a characteristic vertical pattern along the lumbar spine that is worst when standing and relieved when lying down (pain is also often relieved when the hip joint is passively flexed). TrPs in the psoas major may entrap the femoral nerve or genitofemoral nerve as they exit the abdominal cavity into the pelvis (causing possible altered sensation into the thigh).

3. The referral patterns of iliopsoas TrPs must be distinguished from the referral patterns of TrPs in the quadratus lumborum (QL), erector spinae or transversospinalis (TS) of the trunk, piriformis, gluteus medius and maximus, sartorius, pectineus, adductors longus and brevis, and rectus abdominis.

4. TrPs in the iliopsoas are often incorrectly assessed as lower thoracic, lumbar, or sacroiliac joint dysfunction, or appendicitis.

5. Associated TrPs often occur in the erector spinae and TS muscles of the trunk, QL, rectus abdominis, hamstrings, tensor fasciae latae, rectus femoris, pectineus, and contralateral iliopsoas.

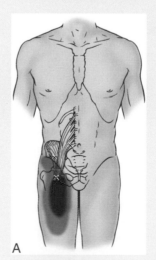
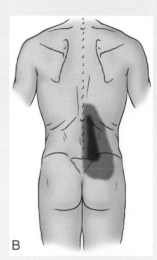

Figure 17-69 A, Anterior view showing common iliopsoas trigger points (TrPs) and their corresponding referral zone. **B,** Posterior view showing the remainder of the referral zone.

17

ILIOPSOAS—SEATED—*cont'd*

STRETCHING THE ILIOPSOAS

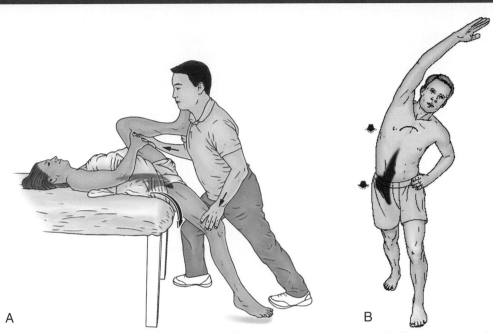

A   B

Figure 17-70 Stretching the right iliopsoas. The client's thigh is extended. **A,** Therapist-assisted stretch. Note: The therapist stabilizes the client's pelvis by holding the client's left thigh into flexion. **B,** Self-care stretch. The client lunges forward with the pelvis and trunk, creating an extension force across the right hip joint. Note: For both the therapist-assisted and self-care stretches, if the client's trunk is laterally flexed to the opposite side (not seen in Figure 17-70, *A*), the stretch to the psoas major increases.

17

ILIOPSOAS—SEATED—*cont'd*

DETOUR

Psoas Minor:

The psoas minor is a small muscle that attaches from the anterolateral bodies of T12 and L1 to the pubic bone. It flexes the trunk at the spinal joints and posteriorly tilts the pelvis at the lumbosacral (LS) joint.

Given that the psoas major also does these actions and that the psoas minor sits directly on the belly of the psoas major, it can be very difficult to discern the psoas minor from the psoas major by engaging the psoas minor with trunk flexion. Furthermore, trunk flexion will likely engage the more superficial abdominal obliques, blocking palpation of the psoas minor.

If psoas minor palpation is attempted, first locate the psoas major, and then feel for a small band of muscle that sits anteriorly on it. To then discern these two muscles from each other, feel for a band of musculature on the psoas major that does not contract with flexion of the thigh at the hip joint.

The psoas minor can be stretched with the same stretch used for the rectus abdominis (see Figure 17-50). TrPs and TrP referral zones for the psoas minor have not been clearly mapped out and separated from TrPs in the belly of the psoas major. Note: The psoas minor is often absent.

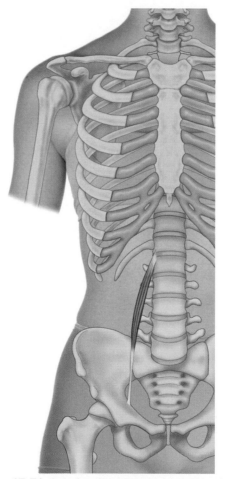

Figure 17-71 Anterior view of the right psoas minor.

Palpation Key:

Psoas major: Press in diagonally toward the spine, slowly but firmly.

Iliacus: Curl your fingers around the iliac crest.

WHIRLWIND TOUR

Muscles of the Trunk

The following *Whirlwind Tour* is an abbreviated set of palpation protocols for the muscles of this chapter. Once you have read and become comfortable with each of the protocols presented thus far, this *Whirlwind Tour* allows you to quickly and efficiently run through the palpations protocols for all the muscles of the chapter.

Client Prone

1. **Latissimus dorsi:** The client is prone with the arm relaxed on the table at the side of the body; you are sitting or standing to the side of the client. Feel for the contraction of the latissimus dorsi at the posterior aspect of the axillary fold as the client extends the arm against resistance. Once felt, continue palpating the latissimus dorsi toward the spinal and pelvic attachment as the client alternately contracts and relaxes the muscle. Then palpate to the humeral attachment in the axilla while strumming perpendicular to the muscle as the client alternately contracts and relaxes the muscle. Note: It can be challenging to discern the latissimus dorsi from the teres major. At the humeral attachment, the latissimus dorsi attachment is located anterior to the teres major attachment, and therefore much easier to palpate directly and feel.

2. **Erector spinae group:** The client is prone; you are standing to the side of the client. Feel for the contraction of the erector spinae group just lateral to the lumbar spine as the client extends the trunk, neck, and head at the spinal joints by lifting the trunk slightly up into the air. Once felt, palpate transversely across the erector spinae to determine its width. Now palpate it to its inferior attachment, and then palpate it as far superior as possible while strumming perpendicular to its fibers as the client alternately contracts and relaxes the muscle. Note: It is usually difficult to palpate and discern the erector spinae musculature in the neck.

3. **Transversospinalis (TS) group:** The client is prone; you are standing to the side of the client. Feel for the contraction of the TS musculature within the laminar groove of the lumbar spine as the client slightly extends and contralaterally rotates the trunk at the spinal joints. (Note: It is primarily the multifidus that is present at this level.) Once located, try to strum perpendicular to the direction of fibers, and feel for the multifidus deep to the erector spinae. Repeat this procedure superiorly up the spine. To palpate the semispinalis group (primarily the semispinalis cervicis and capitis) in the cervical region, have the client prone with the hand in the small of the back. Place your palpating fingers over the laminar groove of the cervical spine, and ask the client to slightly extend the neck at the spinal joints, feeling for the contraction of the semispinalis deep to the upper trapezius. Once located, follow the semispinalis up to the attachment on the head while strumming perpendicular to the direction of fibers as the client alternately contracts and relaxes the muscle.

4. **Quadratus lumborum (QL):** The client is prone; you are standing to the side of the client. Locate the lateral border of the erector spinae group in the lumbar region. Once located, palpate immediately lateral to that. Sink into the tissue slowly but firmly with a direction to your pressure that is anterior and medial toward the QL. To engage the QL and to be certain that you are on it, ask the client to elevate the pelvis at the lumbosacral (LS) joint. (Note: Elevation of the pelvis involves moving the pelvis along the plane of the table toward the head.) Once felt, palpate the QL superomedially to the twelfth rib, inferomedially to the iliac crest, and directly medially toward the transverse processes as the client alternately contracts and relaxes the muscle.

Client Seated

5. **Interspinales:** The client is seated with the trunk slightly flexed at the spinal joints; you are standing or seated behind the client. Place your palpating finger in the interspinous space between two adjacent vertebrae in the lumbar spine, and feel for the interspinous muscle located there. Then ask the client to extend back to anatomic position, and feel for the contraction of the interspinalis muscle. If desired, resistance can be given. Repeat this procedure for other interspinalis muscles. Note: The vertebrae must be flexed to allow access to the interspinalis muscle. However, if the vertebrae are flexed too much, all soft tissues between the vertebrae become taut, and it is not possible to palpate into the interspinous space.

Client Side Lying

6. **External and internal intercostals:** The client is side lying; you are standing behind the client. Intercostal muscles are located between ribs in the anterior, posterior, and lateral trunk. However, it is usually easiest to palpate them laterally, so look to locate them there first. Place your palpating fingers in an intercostal space in the lateral trunk, and feel for the intercostal musculature. Once felt, continue palpating the intercostal musculature at that level as far anteriorly and posteriorly as possible. Repeat this procedure for the other levels of intercostal muscles.

Client Supine with a Small Roll under the Knees

7. **Rectus abdominis:** The client is supine with a small roll under the knees; you are standing to the side of the client. Place your palpating fingers on the anterior abdomen, just lateral to the midline, and feel for the contraction of the rectus abdominis as the client slightly flexes the trunk at the spinal joints. Once felt, strum across the rectus abdominis to determine its width. Then continue palpating to its superior and inferior attachments while strumming perpendicularly to its fibers as the client alternately contracts and relaxes the

17

Muscles of the Trunk—*cont'd*

muscle. Note: It is easiest to locate the inferior attachment on the pubic bone when the rectus abdominis is relaxed.

8. **Anterolateral abdominal wall muscles (external abdominal oblique, internal abdominal oblique, and transversus abdominis [TA]):** The client is supine with a small roll under the knees; you are standing to the side of the client. Place your palpating hand on the anterolateral abdominal wall (lateral to the rectus abdominis), and feel for the contraction of the external abdominal oblique as the client slightly flexes and contralaterally rotates the trunk at the spinal joints. Once a muscle contraction is felt, try to feel for the orientation of the external abdominal oblique's fibers by strumming perpendicular to them; then continue palpating the external abdominal oblique superiorly and inferiorly toward its attachments. Repeat the same procedure for the deeper internal abdominal oblique by asking the client to instead slightly flex and ipsilaterally rotate the trunk at the spinal joints, and feel for their fiber direction running perpendicular in orientation to the fibers of the external abdominal oblique. If successful, strum perpendicular to the internal abdominal oblique's fibers, and palpate from attachment to attachment. To palpate the TA deep to the abdominal obliques, ask the client to compress the abdominal contents (but keep in mind that this can also engage the external and internal abdominal obliques). Note: It can be very difficult to discern the muscles of the anterolateral abdominal wall from each other because both abdominal obliques contract with flexion of the trunk at the spinal joints, and all of them contract with compression of the abdominal contents.

9. **Diaphragm:** The client is supine with a small roll under the knees; you are seated or standing to the side of the client. First curl your palpating fingers under the inferior margin of the client's anterior ribcage with your finger pads oriented toward the muscle. Then ask the client to take in a deep breath and slowly exhale. As the client exhales, reach in and feel for the diaphragm. Repeat this procedure as far anteriorly and posteriorly as possible on both sides of the ribcage.

Client Seated

10. **Iliopsoas (psoas major and iliacus):** The client is seated with the trunk slightly flexed; you are seated diagonally in front of the client. Place your palpating fingers on the client's anterolateral abdominal wall, halfway between the umbilicus and anterior superior iliac spine (ASIS). (Make sure you are lateral to the lateral border of the rectus abdominis.) Ask the client to take in a slow deep breath, and firmly but slowly sink in toward the spine as the client slowly exhales. (Repeat this step once or twice if necessary until you reach the psoas major.) Once you believe that you have reached the psoas major, confirm by asking the client to flex the thigh at the hip joint by gently lifting the foot from the floor a small amount. Once felt, strum perpendicularly across the fibers to feel its width. Then continue palpating to its superior attachment and as far inferiorly as possible while strumming across the muscle as the client alternately contracts and relaxes it. To palpate the iliacus, curl your palpating fingers around the iliac crest toward the iliacus on the internal ilium, and feel for its contraction as the client once again gently lifts the foot from the floor a small amount. Once felt, palpate as much of the iliacus as possible.

11. **Psoas minor:** To feel the psoas minor, first locate the belly of the psoas major, and then feel for a band of muscle that sits anteriorly on the psoas major's belly. The psoas minor will not contract with flexion of the thigh at the hip joint (i.e., lifting the foot from the floor).

Review Questions

1. List the attachments of the diaphragm.
2. List the attachments of the interspinales.
3. What are the actions of the internal abdominal obliques?
4. What are the actions of the erector spinae group?
5. What muscle might pose a challenge when palpating the latissimus dorsi? What is the reason for this challenge, and is there any helpful information that can be used to conduct a clear palpation?
6. Describe palpation of the erector spinae group in the thoracic region and any specific client positioning that could aid its palpation.
7. What muscle of the TS group can be found outside of the laminar groove?
8. What palpatory difficulties, if any, are presented by the QL?
9. When palpating the inferior attachment of the rectus abdominis, what steps can be taken to ease any apprehension on the part of the therapist?
10. At which point during respiration should the diaphragm be assessed?
11. What sensitive structures must a therapist be cautious about when palpating the psoas major and the iliacus?
12. Sacroiliac joint dysfunction, lumbar disc syndrome, sciatica, and trochanteric bursitis are often incorrect assessments for TrPs in what muscle?
13. TrPs in what muscle may entrap an anterior branch of a spinal nerve resulting in lower abdominal and pelvic pain?
14. Describe the positioning for a stretch of the left TS group?
15. Describe a stretch for the internal and external abdominal obliques. Be specific as to which side for each muscle the stretch is intended.
16. Explain a probable scenario for the formation of TrPs in the serratus posterior inferior (SPI).
17. What is the rationale for passive flexion of the thighs at the hip joints during the palpation of abdominal musculature?

CASE STUDY

A regular client, a 56-year-old woman, arrives for a massage session and complains of recent-onset pain in her mid and lower back that also extends around the body to cross the lower ribs. She is also experiencing intermittent pain in her groin and upper inner thigh area. This client's history to date has been unremarkable with no recent trauma, but she reports that she is just beginning to recover from a lower respiratory infection. She is a non-smoker, walks several miles daily, and leads an otherwise healthy lifestyle.

Her pain began approximately 5 days ago and has increased in intensity from a three out of ten to a seven out of ten. The condition is exacerbated by rotation of the trunk, carrying heavy objects at work (she estimates anything over 15 pounds [7 kg]), coughing, and changing positions while lying in bed. Warm showers and non-steroidal anti-inflammatory medications have only produced mild short-term relief.

1. Describe the type of exam and any assessments you would make for this client.
2. What muscles or muscle groups do you suspect may be involved and why?
3. What type(s) of treatment might you perform or recommend?

17

CHAPTER 18

Tour #8   Palpation of the Pelvic Muscles

Overview

This chapter is a palpation tour of the muscles of the pelvis. The tour begins with the gluteal muscles and then covers the piriformis, quadratus femoris, and other "deep lateral rotators" of the thigh at the hip joint. Palpation for each of the muscles is shown in the prone position, except for the gluteus medius, which is described in side lying position. Alternate palpation positions are also described. The major muscles of the region are each given a separate layout; there are also a few detours to other muscles of the region. Trigger point (TrP) information and stretching, both therapist-assisted and self-care stretching, are given for each of the major muscles covered in this chapter (as well as the gluteus minimus). The chapter closes with an advanced *Whirlwind Tour* that explains the sequential palpation of all of the muscles of the chapter.

Chapter Outline

Gluteus Maximus
Gluteus Medius
         Detour to the Gluteus Minimus
Piriformis
Quadratus Femoris
         Detour to the Other Deep Lateral Rotators
Whirlwind Tour: Muscles of the Pelvis

Chapter Objectives

After completing this chapter, the student/therapist should be able to perform the following for each of the muscles covered in this chapter:
1. State the attachments.
2. State the actions.
3. Describe the starting position for palpation.
4. Describe and explain the purpose of each of the palpation steps.
5. Palpate each muscle.
6. State the "Palpation Key."
7. Describe alternate palpation positions.
8. State the locations of the most common TrP(s).
9. Describe the TrP referral zones.
10. State the most common factors that create and/or perpetuate TrPs.
11. State the symptoms most commonly caused by TrPs.
12. Describe and perform the therapist-assisted and self-care stretches.

e Go to http://evolve.elsevier.com/Muscolino/palpation for video demonstrations of the muscle palpations presented in this chapter.

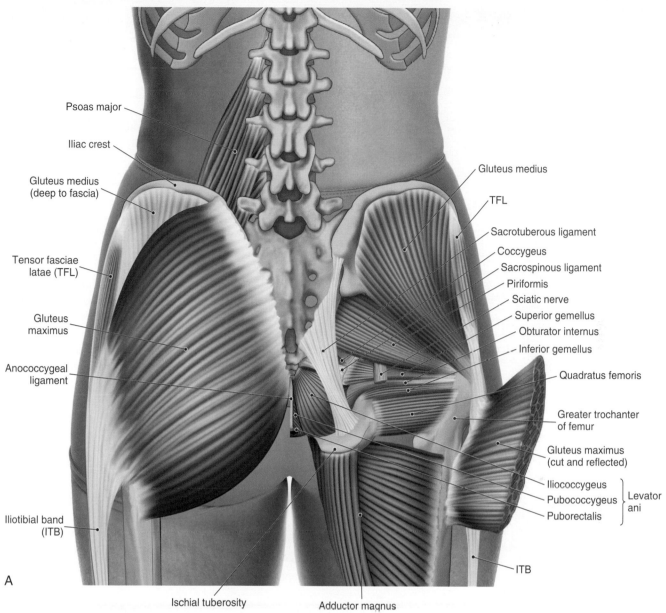

Psoas major

Iliac crest

Gluteus medius
(deep to fascia)

Tensor fasciae
latae (TFL)

Gluteus
maximus

Anococcygeal
ligament

Iliotibial band
(ITB)

Gluteus medius

TFL

Sacrotuberous ligament

Coccygeus

Sacrospinous ligament

Piriformis

Sciatic nerve

Superior gemellus

Obturator internus

Inferior gemellus

Quadratus femoris

Greater trochanter
of femur

Gluteus maximus
(cut and reflected)

Iliococcygeus

Pubococcygeus

Puborectalis

Levator
ani

ITB

A

Ischial tuberosity

Adductor magnus

Figure 18-1 Posterior views of the muscles of the pelvis. **A,** Superficial view on the left and an intermediate view on the right.

18

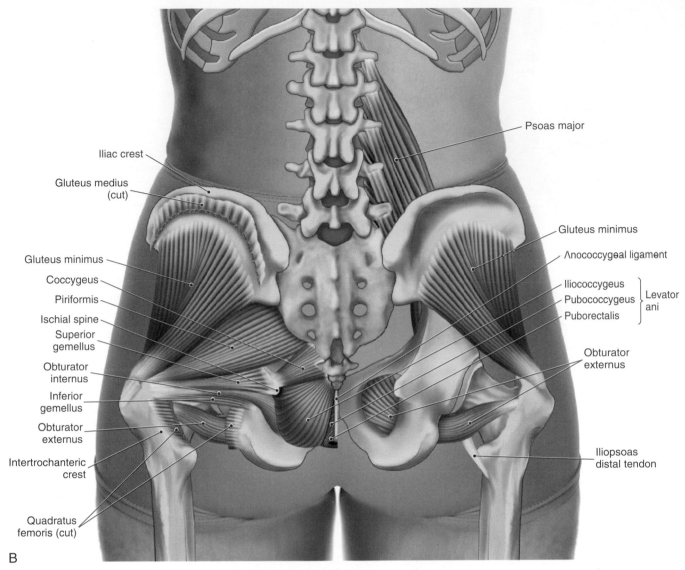

Iliac crest

Gluteus medius (cut)

Gluteus minimus

Coccygeus

Piriformis

Ischial spine

Superior gemellus

Obturator internus

Inferior gemellus

Obturator externus

Intertrochanteric crest

Quadratus femoris (cut)

B

Psoas major

Gluteus minimus

Anococcygeal ligament

Iliococcygeus
Pubococcygeus } Levator ani
Puborectalis

Obturator externus

Iliopsoas distal tendon

Figure 18-1, cont'd B, Deeper views.

18

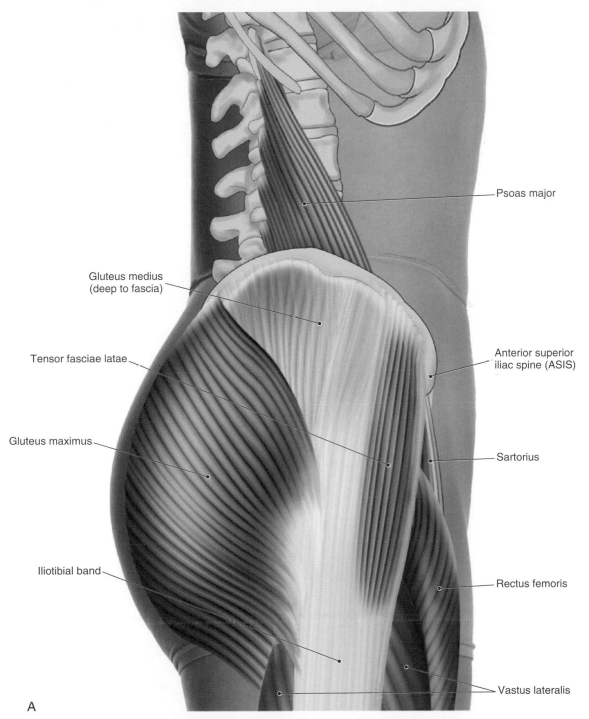

Figure 18-2 Right lateral views of the muscles of the pelvis. **A,** Superficial view.

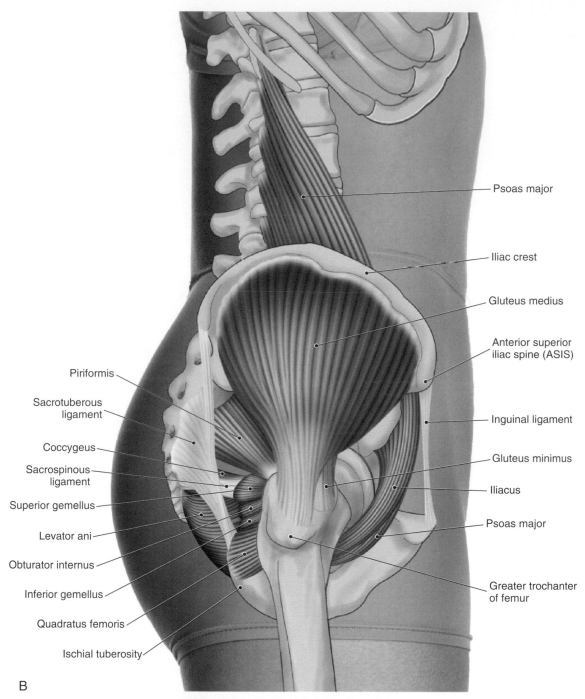

Psoas major

Iliac crest

Gluteus medius

Anterior superior
iliac spine (ASIS)

Inguinal ligament

Gluteus minimus

Iliacus

Psoas major

Greater trochanter
of femur

Piriformis

Sacrotuberous
ligament

Coccygeus

Sacrospinous
ligament

Superior gemellus

Levator ani

Obturator internus

Inferior gemellus

Quadratus femoris

Ischial tuberosity

B

Figure 18-2, cont'd B, Intermediate view.

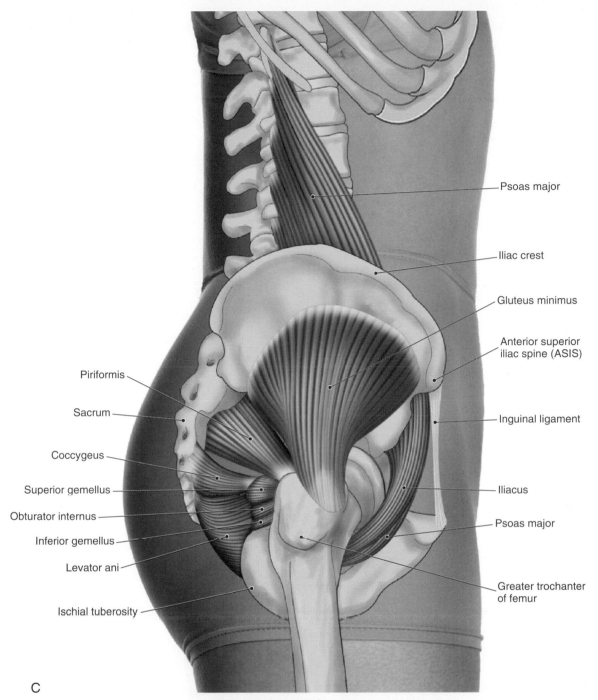

Psoas major

Iliac crest

Gluteus minimus

Anterior superior
iliac spine (ASIS)

Inguinal ligament

Piriformis

Sacrum

Coccygeus

Superior gemellus

Obturator internus

Inferior gemellus

Levator ani

Ischial tuberosity

Iliacus

Psoas major

Greater trochanter
of femur

C

Figure 18-2, cont'd C, Deep view.

18

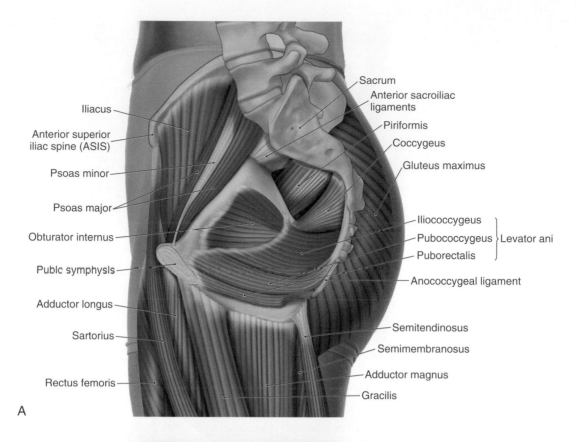

A

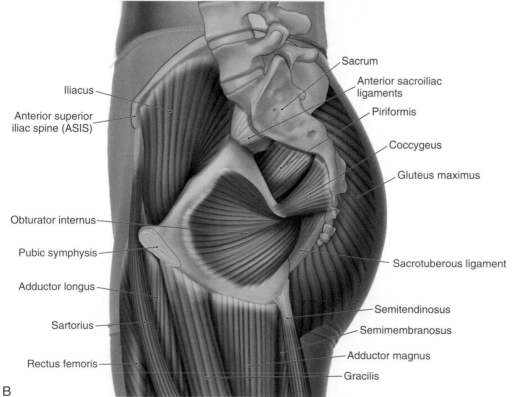

B

Figure 18-3 Medial views of the muscles of the right side of the pelvis. **A,** Superficial view. **B,** Deeper view.

18

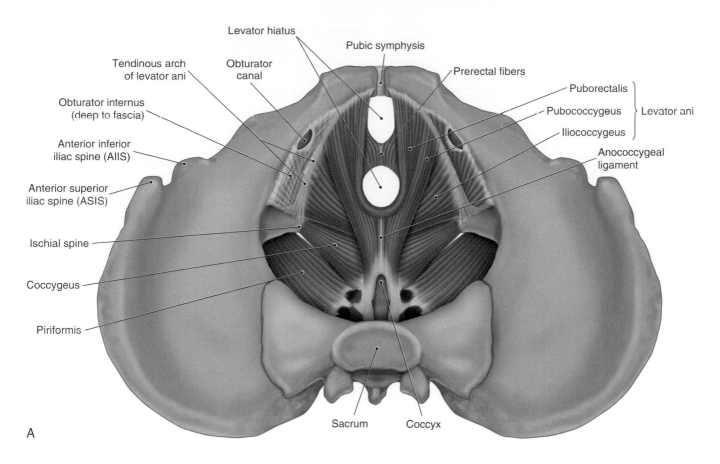

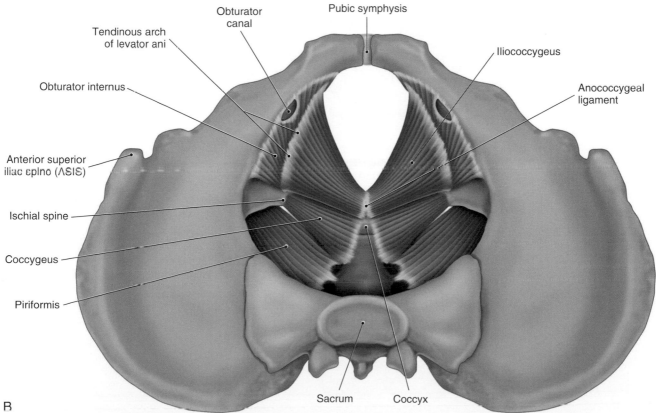

Figure 18-4 Superior views of the muscles of the pelvic floor; female pelvis. **A,** Superficial view. **B,** Deeper view.

18

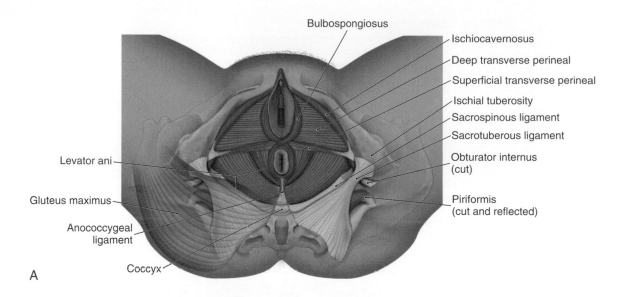

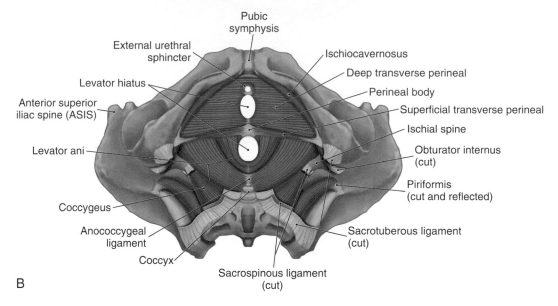

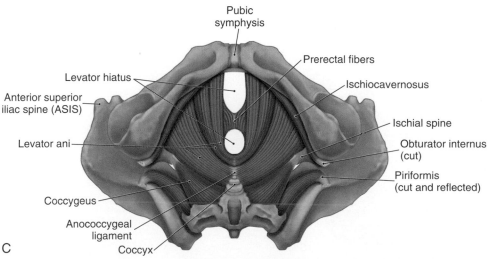

Figure 18-5 Inferior views of the muscles of the pelvic floor; female pelvis. **A,** Superficial view. **B,** Intermediate view. **C,** Deep view.

GLUTEUS MAXIMUS—PRONE

☑ATTACHMENTS

- ☐ Posterior iliac crest, posterolateral sacrum, and the coccyx

  to the

- ☐ gluteal tuberosity of the femur and the iliotibial band

☑ACTIONS

- ☐ Extends the thigh at the hip joint
- ☐ Laterally rotates the thigh at the hip joint
- ☐ The upper fibers abduct the thigh at the hip joint
- ☐ The lower fibers adduct the thigh at the hip joint
- ☐ Posteriorly tilts the pelvis at the hip joint

Starting Position (Figure 18-7)
- ■ Client prone
- ■ Therapist standing to the side of the client
- ■ Palpating hand placed lateral to the sacrum
- ■ Support hand placed on the distal posterior thigh if resistance is needed

Palpation Steps
1. Ask the client to extend and laterally rotate the thigh at the hip joint, and feel for the contraction of the gluteus maximus (Figure 18-8).
2. With the muscle contracted, strum perpendicular to the fibers to discern the borders of the muscle.
3. Continue palpating the gluteus maximus laterally and inferiorly (distally) to its distal attachments by strumming perpendicular to its fibers.

4. If desired, you may add resistance to the client's thigh extension to better engage the gluteus maximus.
5. Once the gluteus maximus has been located, have the client relax it, and palpate to assess its baseline tone.

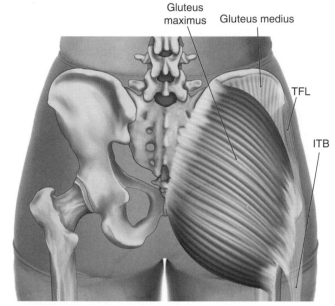

Figure 18-6 Posterior view of the right gluteus maximus. The tensor fasciae latae (TFL) and iliotibial band (ITB) have been ghosted in.

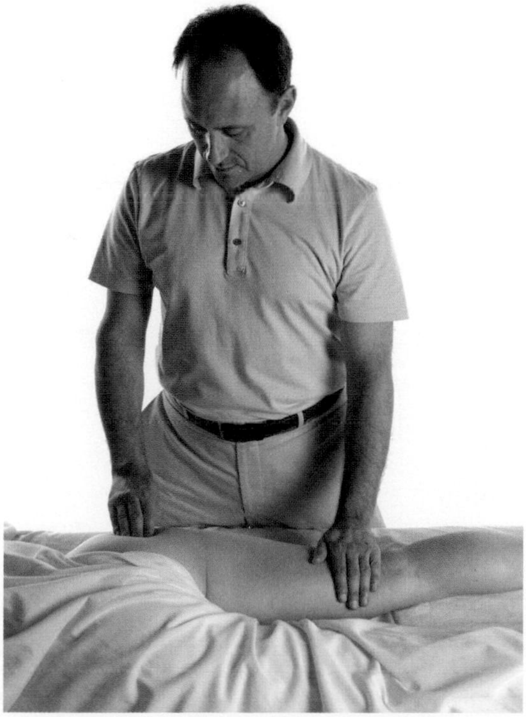

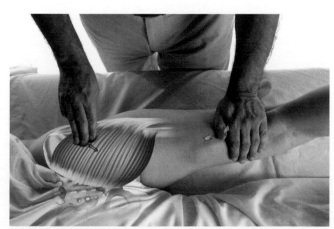

Figure 18-7 Starting position for prone palpation of the right gluteus maximus.

Figure 18-8 Palpation of the right gluteus maximus as the client extends and laterally rotates the thigh at the hip joint against resistance.

18

GLUTEUS MAXIMUS—PRONE—*cont'd*

PALPATION NOTES

1. The gluteus maximus is superficial and easy to palpate.
2. The gluteus maximus is known as the principle muscle of the posterior buttock. However, it does not cover the entire buttock. The gluteus medius is superficial supero-laterally. When following the gluteus maximus from the sacrum toward its distal attachment, be sure to follow it laterally and inferiorly (distally).

Alternate Palpation Position—Side Lying

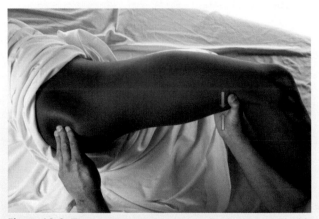

Figure 18-9 The gluteus maximus can also be palpated with the client side lying. Palpate the gluteus maximus on the side of the body away from the table while asking the client to actively extend and laterally rotate the thigh at the hip joint. However, because extension of the thigh is not against gravity when the client is side lying, the therapist must use the support hand to add resistance to extension to engage the gluteus maximus.

TRIGGER POINTS

1. Trigger points (TrPs) in the gluteus maximus often result from or are perpetuated by acute or chronic overuse (often with a strong eccentric contraction, such as walking uphill, especially if leaning over; or by concentric contraction, such as swimming the crawl stroke), prolonged lengthened position (e.g., sleeping with the hip joint flexed), prolonged sitting (especially if sitting on a thick wallet), direct trauma, irritation from injections, and Morton's foot. Deeper superior fibers have been discovered to attach from the sacrum directly to the pelvic bone. TrPs in this aspect of the muscle are often associated with sacroiliac joint dysfunction.
2. TrPs in the gluteus maximus may produce restlessness and pain with prolonged sitting, difficulty sleeping, pain walking uphill (especially if leaning over), pain when bending over, and restricted hip joint flexion.
3. The referral patterns of gluteus maximus TrPs must be distinguished from the referral patterns of TrPs in the gluteus medius, gluteus minimus, piriformis, tensor fasciae latae (TFL), vastus lateralis, semitendinosus, semimembranosus, quadratus lumborum, and pelvic floor muscles.
4. TrPs in the gluteus maximus are often incorrectly assessed as sacroiliac joint dysfunction, lumbar facet joint syndrome, trochanteric bursitis, coccygodynia, or disc compression upon a nerve.
5. Associated TrPs often occur in the gluteus medius, gluteus minimus, hamstrings, erector spinae group, rectus femoris, and iliopsoas.

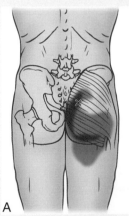
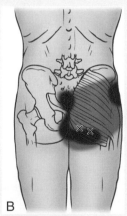

Figure 18-10 Posterior views of common gluteus maximus trigger points (TrPs) and their corresponding referral zones.

GLUTEUS MAXIMUS—PRONE—*cont'd*

STRETCHING THE GLUTEUS MAXIMUS

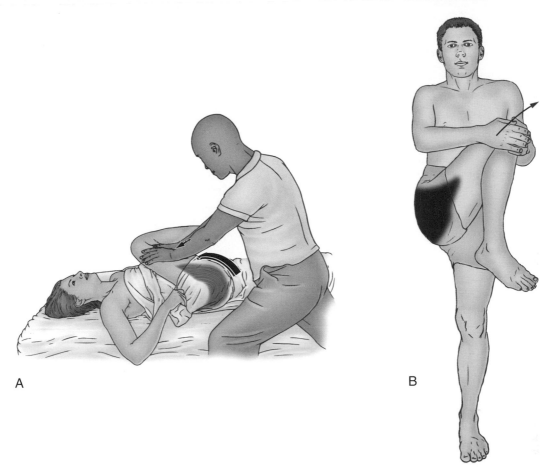

A

B

Figure 18-11 Stretching the right gluteus maximus. The client's thigh is flexed up toward the chest with the knee joint flexed. Bringing the thigh straight up toward the same-side shoulder (as seen in **A**) preferentially stretches the lower fibers. Bringing the thigh straight up toward the opposite-side shoulder (as seen in **B**) preferentially stretches the upper fibers. Note: If the client experiences a pinching sensation in the groin with this stretch, placing a small rolled up towel along the inguinal ligament often helps. **A,** Therapist-assisted stretch. The therapist contacts the client on the distal posterior thigh. Note: The client secures the draping by holding it with the hand. **B,** Self-care stretch.

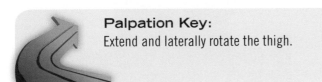

Palpation Key:
Extend and laterally rotate the thigh.

18

GLUTEUS MEDIUS—SIDE LYING

☑ ATTACHMENTS

☐ External surface of the ilium (from just inferior to the iliac crest)

to the

☐ lateral surface of the greater trochanter of the femur

☑ ACTIONS

Posterior Fibers
☐ Abduct the thigh at the hip joint
☐ Extend the thigh at the hip joint
☐ Laterally rotate the thigh at the hip joint
☐ Posteriorly tilt the same side of the pelvis at the hip joint
☐ Depress the same side of the pelvis at the hip joint

Middle Fibers
☐ Abduct the thigh at the hip joint
☐ Depress the same side of the pelvis at the hip joint

Anterior Fibers
☐ Abduct the thigh at the hip joint
☐ Flex the thigh at the hip joint
☐ Medially rotate the thigh at the hip joint
☐ Anteriorly tilt the same side of the pelvis at the hip joint
☐ Depress the same side of the pelvis at the hip joint

Starting Position (Figure 18-13)
■ Client side lying
■ Therapist standing behind the client
■ Palpating hand placed just distal to the middle of the iliac crest, between the iliac crest and the greater trochanter of the femur
■ Support hand placed on the lateral surface of the distal thigh

Palpation Steps
1. Palpating just distal to the middle of the iliac crest, ask the client to abduct the thigh at the hip joint, and feel for the contraction of the middle fibers of the gluteus medius (Figure 18-14). If desired, resistance can be added to the client's thigh abduction with the support hand.
2. Strum perpendicular to the fibers, palpating the middle fibers of the gluteus medius distally toward the greater trochanter.
3. To palpate the anterior fibers, place palpating hand immediately distal and posterior to the anterior superior iliac spine (ASIS), ask the client to flex and medially rotate the thigh at the hip joint, and feel for the contraction of the anterior fibers of the gluteus medius (Figure 18-15, *A*) (see Palpation Note #1). It may be necessary to add resistance.

4. To palpate the posterior fibers, place palpating hand over the posterosuperior portion of the gluteus medius, ask the client to extend and laterally rotate the thigh at the hip joint, and feel for the contraction of the posterior fibers of the gluteus medius (Figure 18-15, *B*) (see Palpation Note #1). It may be necessary to add resistance.
5. Once the gluteus medius has been located, have the client relax it, and palpate to assess its baseline tone.

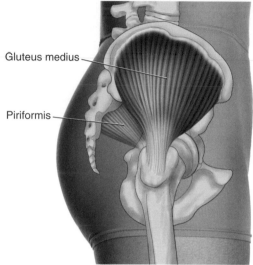

Gluteus medius

Piriformis

Figure 18-12 Lateral view of the right gluteus medius. The piriformis has been ghosted in.

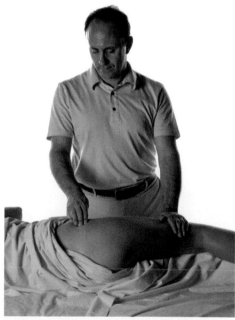

Figure 18-13 Starting position for side lying palpation of the right gluteus medius. Note: The therapist usually stands behind the client, but is shown standing in front of the client here so that the reader's view is not obstructed.

18

GLUTEUS MEDIUS—SIDE LYING—*cont'd*

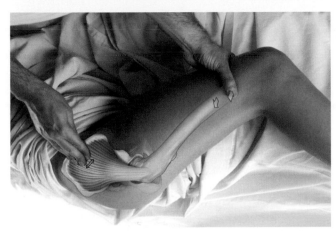

Figure 18-14 Palpation of the middle fibers of the right gluteus medius immediately distal to the center of the iliac crest as the client attempts to abduct the thigh at the hip joint against resistance.

PALPATION NOTES

1. The middle fibers of the gluteus medius are superficial and easy to palpate. The anterior fibers are next to and deep to the tensor fasciae latae (TFL) and are difficult to distinguish from the TFL. The posterior fibers are next to the piriformis and deep to the gluteus maximus, and are difficult to distinguish from these two muscles.
2. During walking, when one lower limb is off the ground and the body weight is being supported by the other lower limb, contraction of the gluteus medius on the weight-bearing side can be easily felt. Its role is to create a depression force on that side of the pelvis, which creates an elevation force on the other side of the pelvis, preventing the other side from falling (depressing) to the unsupported side of the body.

Palpation Key:
Palpate just distal to the middle of the iliac crest, and have the client abduct the thigh.

Alternate Palpation Position—Standing

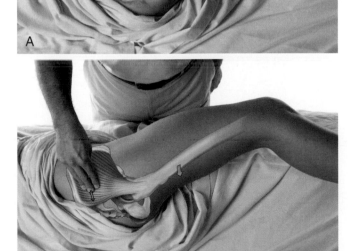

Figure 18-15 Side lying palpation of the anterior and posterior fibers of the right gluteus medius. **A,** Palpation of the anterior fibers of the gluteus medius as the client abducts and medially rotates the thigh. **B,** Palpation of the posterior fibers of the gluteus medius as the client abducts and laterally rotates the thigh.

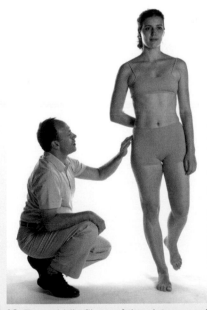

Figure 18-16 The middle fibers of the gluteus medius can be easily palpated with the client standing. Palpate just distal to the middle of the iliac crests, and ask the client to slowly walk in place or simply shift her body weight from one foot to the other. You will feel the contraction of the gluteus medius on the weight-bearing side.

18

GLUTEUS MEDIUS—SIDE LYING—*cont'd*

TRIGGER POINTS

1. Trigger points (TrPs) in the gluteus medius often result from or are perpetuated by acute or chronic overuse (e.g., excessive walking or running, walking on soft sand, prolonged standing on one lower extremity), prolonged immobility, sacroiliac joint dysfunction, sitting on a thick wallet, direct trauma, injections, and Morton foot.
2. TrPs in the gluteus medius may produce pain when sleeping on the involved side or walking, restricted hip joint adduction, hip joint pain, antalgic gait, sciatica-like pain referral, and a posturally depressed pelvis (with resultant scoliosis).
3. The referral patterns of gluteus medius TrPs must be distinguished from the referral patterns of TrPs in the gluteus maximus, gluteus minimus, and piriformis.
4. TrPs in the gluteus medius are often incorrectly assessed as low back pain, sacroiliac joint dysfunction, lumbar facet joint syndrome, or trochanteric bursitis.
5. Associated TrPs often occur in the gluteus maximus, gluteus minimus, piriformis, tensor fasciae latae (TFL), and quadratus lumborum.

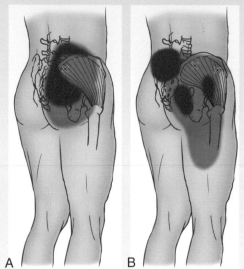

Figure 18-17 Posterolateral views of common gluteus medius trigger points (TrPs) and their corresponding referral zones.

STRETCHING THE GLUTEUS MEDIUS

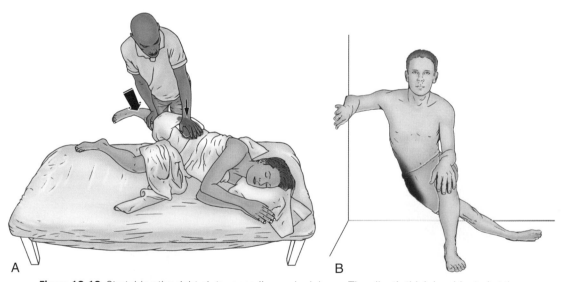

Figure 18-18 Stretching the right gluteus medius and minimus. The client's thigh is adducted at the hip joint. **A,** Therapist-assisted stretch. The therapist contacts the client's distal lateral thigh (not the leg). Note that the client's pelvis is stabilized from depressing by the therapist's left hand; a cushion is used for comfort. **B,** Self-care stretch. The client places the left foot in front of the right and then adducts the right thigh at the hip joint. See Figure 17-31 for another stretch of the gluteus medius.

18

GLUTEUS MEDIUS—SIDE LYING—*cont'd*

DETOUR

Gluteus Minimus:

The gluteus minimus attaches from the external ilium to the greater trochanter of the femur and is deep to the gluteus medius. It also has the same actions as the gluteus medius. Therefore it is extremely difficult to discern from the gluteus medius. Note: The most powerful action of the gluteus minimus is medial rotation.

Trigger Points:

1. Trigger points (TrPs) in the gluteus minimus often result from or are perpetuated by the same activities that create TrPs in the gluteus medius.
2. TrPs of the gluteus minimus generally produce the same symptoms as gluteus medius TrPs. However, the referral pain pattern for gluteus minimus TrPs often extends much farther distally (as far as the ankle joint) than the pattern of either the gluteus medius or maximus. Furthermore, the pain of gluteus minimus TrPs is often persistent and severe.
3. The referral patterns of gluteus minimus TrPs must be distinguished from the referral patterns of TrPs in the gluteus maximus, gluteus medius, piriformis, hamstrings, tensor fasciae latae (TFL), gastrocnemius, soleus, fibularis longus and brevis, popliteus, and tibialis posterior.
4. TrPs in the gluteus minimus are often incorrectly assessed as L5 or S1 nerve compression, or trochanteric bursitis.
5. Associated TrPs often occur in the gluteus medius, piriformis, vastus lateralis, fibularis longus, gluteus maximus, TFL, and quadratus lumborum.

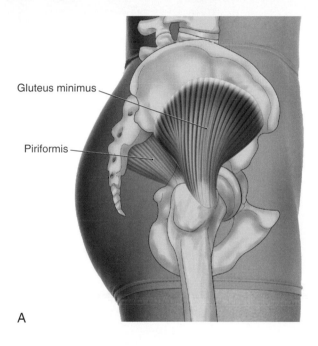

Gluteus minimus

Piriformis

A

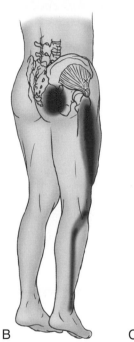

B

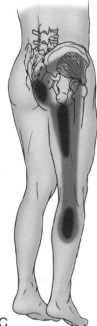

C

Figure 18-19 Views of the right gluteus minimus. **A,** Lateral view of the right gluteus minimus. The piriformis has been ghosted in. **B** and **C,** Posterolateral views of common gluteus minimus trigger points (TrPs) and their corresponding referral zones.

18

PIRIFORMIS—PRONE

✅ ATTACHMENTS

☐ Anterior surface of the sacrum

to the

☐ greater trochanter of the femur

✅ ACTIONS

☐ Laterally rotates the thigh at the hip joint
☐ If the thigh is first flexed approximately 60 degrees or more, the piriformis becomes a medial rotator of the thigh at the hip joint
☐ If the thigh is first flexed to 90 degrees, the piriformis horizontally abducts the thigh at the hip joint

Starting Position (Figure 18-21)

- Client prone with the leg flexed to 90 degrees at the knee joint
- Therapist standing to the side of the client
- Palpating hand placed just lateral to the sacrum, halfway between the posterior superior iliac spine (PSIS) and the apex of the sacrum
- Support hand placed on the medial surface of the distal leg, just proximal to the ankle joint

Palpation Steps

1. Begin by finding the point on the lateral sacrum that is halfway between the PSIS and the apex of the sacrum. Drop just off the sacrum laterally at this point, and you will be on the piriformis.
2. Resist the client from laterally rotating the thigh at the hip joint, and feel for the contraction of the piriformis (Figure 18-22). Note: Lateral rotation of the client's thigh involves the client's foot moving medially toward the midline (and opposite side) of the body.
3. Continue palpating the piriformis laterally toward the superior border of the greater trochanter of the femur while strumming perpendicular to the fibers as the client alternately contracts (against resistance) and relaxes the piriformis.
4. Once the piriformis has been located, have the client relax it, and palpate to assess its baseline tone.

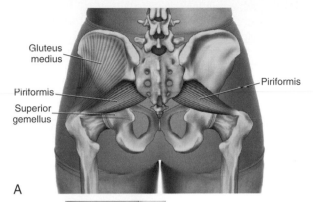

A

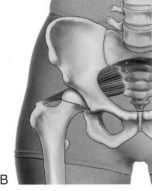

B

Figure 18-20 Views of the piriformis. **A,** Posterior view. The piriformis has been drawn on both sides. The gluteus medius and superior gemellus have been ghosted in on the left. **B,** Anterior view of the right piriformis, showing its attachment onto the anterior surface of the sacrum.

18

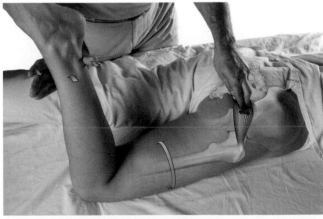

Figure 18-21 Starting position for prone palpation of the right piriformis.

Figure 18-22 Palpation of the right piriformis as the client attempts to laterally rotate the thigh at the hip joint against gentle to moderate resistance.

PIRIFORMIS—PRONE—*cont'd*

PALPATION NOTES

1. As soon as the midline of the sacrum is found, before beginning the palpation, it is helpful to find the greater trochanter of the femur and trace the course of the piriformis from the midline of the sacrum to the greater trochanter. This way, you do not have to interrupt the palpation protocol to find the greater trochanter.
2. When giving resistance to the client's lateral rotation of the thigh at the hip joint, do not let the client contract too forcefully, or the more superficial gluteus maximus (also a lateral rotator) may be engaged, blocking palpation of the deeper piriformis.
3. It can be challenging to discern the borders between the piriformis and the gluteus medius superiorly and superior gemellus inferiorly, because these muscles are also lateral rotators of the thigh at the hip joint and may be engaged when the client contracts the piriformis.

4. The sciatic nerve usually exits from the anterior pelvis into the buttock between the piriformis and the superior gemellus. Approximately 10% to 20% of the time, all or part of the sciatic nerve emerges through the belly of the piriformis itself. With either representation, be aware of the proximity of the sciatic nerve when palpating the piriformis.
5. The sacral attachment of the piriformis can be palpated on the anterior sacrum. To accomplish this, the therapist must use a gloved hand and access the piriformis through the rectum. However, local licensure laws may not allow this palpation.
6. If the thigh is first flexed at the hip joint approximately 60 degrees or more, the piriformis changes from being a lateral rotator to a medial rotator of the thigh at the hip joint. This change in action can change how the piriformis is stretched (Figure 18-23).

Palpation Key:
Find the midpoint of the lateral border of the sacrum. Then draw a line from there to the greater trochanter.

STRETCHING THE PIRIFORMIS

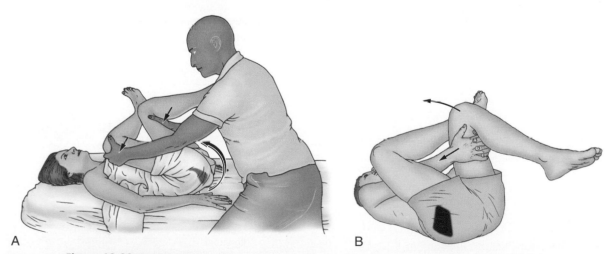

A   B

Figure 18-23 Stretching the right piriformis with the "figure 4 stretch." The client's thigh is flexed and laterally rotated at the hip joint. It is important to keep the pelvis down on the table. Note: Because the thigh is flexed so much, the piriformis being a medial rotator is stretched by lateral rotation. **A,** Therapist-assisted stretch. **B,** Self-care stretch. See Figure 18-29 for another stretch of the piriformis.

18

PIRIFORMIS—PRONE—*cont'd*

TRIGGER POINTS

1. Trigger points (TrPs) in the piriformis often result from or are perpetuated by acute or chronic overuse of the muscle, prolonged shortening of the muscle (e.g., driving with foot on the gas pedal, sleeping on one's side with the upper thigh flexed and adducted), sacroiliac joint sprain, hip joint arthritis, Morton foot, leg length discrepancy, and overpronation of the foot at the subtalar joint.

2. TrPs in the piriformis may produce restlessness and discomfort when sitting, lateral rotation of the thigh at the hip joint resulting in turn-out of the foot, restricted medial rotation of the thigh at the hip joint, and sacroiliac joint dysfunction.

3. The referral patterns of piriformis TrPs must be distinguished from the referral patterns of TrPs in the gluteus maximus, medius, and minimus; quadratus lumborum; and pelvic floor muscles.

4. TrPs in the piriformis are often incorrectly assessed as sacroiliac joint dysfunction, piriformis syndrome (compression of the sciatic nerve), herniated disc compression upon spinal nerves L5 or S1, or facet syndrome.

5. Associated TrPs often occur in the gluteus minimus, superior and inferior gemelli, obturator internus, coccygeus, and levator ani.

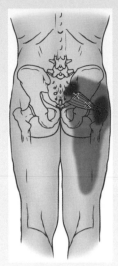

Figure 18-24 Posterior view of common piriformis trigger points (TrPs) and their corresponding referral zones.

DETOUR

Coccygeus and Levator Ani:

The coccygeus and levator ani are pelvic floor muscles and therefore not often thought of as muscles that can be palpated and worked by manual therapists. However, these muscles are quite accessible when working the posterior pelvic region of the client. In fact, the coccygeus is located directly inferior to the piriformis, and like the piriformis attaches to the sacrum (as well as the coccyx, as its name implies). The levator ani is found direcftly inferior to the coccygeus.

To palpate these muscles, begin by locating the piriformis, and then drop directly off it inferiorly, hugging along the lateral border of the sacrum. You will be over the coccygeus (deep to the sacrotuberous and sacrospinous ligaments). To access the levator ani, simply drop directly inferior to the coccygeus, hugging along the lateral border of the coccyx. The levator ani is superficial but often deep to subcutaneous connective tissue invested with fat. Once located, palpate these muscles while they are relaxed; it is usually not necessary to ask the client to engage them. If you would like the client to engage the coccygeus or levator ani to confirm your location, ask the client to perform a *Kegel exercise* (direct the client to contract and tighten the pelvic floor musculature as if to stop the flow of urine).

Given the location of these muscles, it is extremely important to appropriately drape the client. It might be best to palpate and work the levator ani from the opposite side of the body so that the direction of your force is away from the midline—in other words, oriented from medial to lateral.

The coccygeus and levator ani muscles are important to work because they help to stabilize the sacroiliac joint via their attachments to the sacrum and coccyx. As a part of the pelvic floor musculature, they also assist the multifidus and transversus abdominis to maintain the integrity of the abdominopelvic cavity and the core stabilization of the lumbar spine.

Trigger Points:

Trigger points (TrPs) in the coccygeus and levator ani generally refer pain to the sacrococcygeal region. In female clients, the levator ani may also refer pain to the vagina.

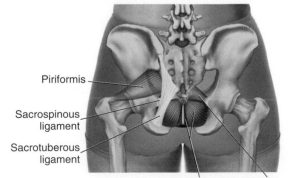

Figure 18-25 Posterior view of the coccygeus and levator ani. The piriformis has been ghosted in.

18

QUADRATUS FEMORIS—PRONE

✅ ATTACHMENTS
☐ Lateral border of the ischial tuberosity

to the

☐ intertrochanteric crest of the femur

✅ ACTIONS
☐ Laterally rotates the thigh at the hip joint

Starting Position (Figure 18-27)
■ Client prone with the leg flexed to 90 degrees at the knee joint
■ Therapist standing to the side of the client
■ Palpating hand placed just lateral to the lateral border of the ischial tuberosity
■ Support hand placed on the medial surface of the distal leg, just proximal to the ankle joint

Palpation Steps
1. Begin by finding the lateral border of the ischial tuberosity. This is usually best accomplished by first finding the inferior (distal) border and then palpating around to the lateral side. Once located, place palpating hand just lateral to the lateral border of the ischial tuberosity.
2. With gentle to moderate force, resist the client from laterally rotating the thigh at the hip joint, and feel for the contraction of the quadratus femoris (Figure 18-28).

Note: Lateral rotation of the client's thigh involves the client's foot moving medially toward the midline (and opposite side) of the body.
3. Continue palpating the quadratus femoris laterally toward the intertrochanteric crest by strumming perpendicular to the fibers as the client alternately contracts (against resistance) and relaxes the quadratus femoris.
4. Once the quadratus femoris has been located, have the client relax it, and palpate to assess its baseline tone.

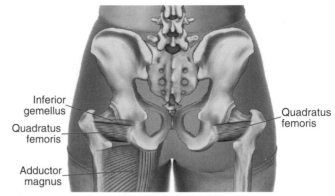

Figure 18-26 Posterior view of the quadratus femoris drawn on both sides. The inferior gemellus and adductor magnus have been ghosted in on the left side.

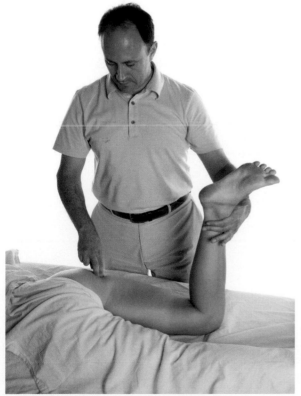

Figure 18-27 Starting position for prone palpation of the right quadratus femoris.

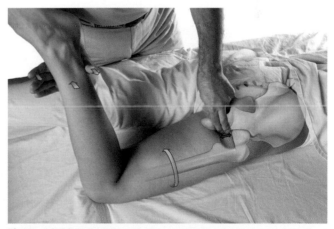

Figure 18-28 Palpation of the quadratus femoris as the client attempts to laterally rotate the thigh at the hip joint against gentle to moderate resistance.

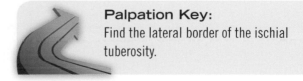

Palpation Key:
Find the lateral border of the ischial tuberosity.

18

QUADRATUS FEMORIS—PRONE—*cont'd*

PALPATION NOTES

1. When giving resistance to the client's lateral rotation of the thigh at the hip joint, do not let the client contract too forcefully, or the more superficial gluteus maximus (also a lateral rotator) may be engaged, blocking palpation of the deeper quadratus femoris.
2. Of all six "deep lateral rotators" of the thigh at the hip joint, the piriformis is the most well-known; however, the quadratus femoris is usually the largest.

3. If the thigh is first flexed at the hip joint 90 degrees, the quadratus femoris can horizontally abduct the thigh at the hip joint.
4. Proceed with caution when palpating the quadratus femoris, because the sciatic nerve courses directly over it.

STRETCHING THE QUADRATUS FEMORIS

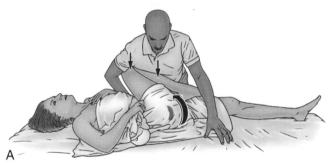
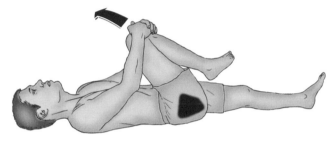

A   B

Figure 18-29 Stretching the right quadratus femoris. The client's thigh is horizontally flexed across the body toward the opposite shoulder. It is important to keep the pelvis down on the table. **A,** Therapist-assisted stretch. The therapist uses the axillary region to hold down the client's knee **B,** Self-care stretch. Note: If the client experiences a pinching sensation in the groin with this stretch, placing a small rolled up towel along the inguinal ligament often helps. See Figure 18-23 for another stretch of this region.

TRIGGER POINTS

Note: The patterns of trigger points (TrPs) and TrP referral zones for the quadratus femoris and the other deep lateral rotators (see Detour to Other Deep Lateral Rotators) have not been differentiated from the patterns for the piriformis.

Furthermore, factors that create or perpetuate TrPs in the quadratus femoris and other deep lateral rotators are likely to be the same as those for the piriformis.

QUADRATUS FEMORIS—PRONE—*cont'd*

DETOUR

Other Deep Lateral Rotators:
Of the six deep lateral rotators of the thigh at the hip joint (piriformis, superior gemellus, obturator internus, inferior gemellus, obturator externus, quadratus femoris), the piriformis is the most superior of the group and the quadratus femoris is the most inferior. The other deep lateral rotators are quite small and difficult to discern from each other, so it is best to palpate them as a group. To palpate these other deep lateral rotators, either find the piriformis and palpate inferior to it, or find the quadratus femoris and palpate superior to it. Follow the same procedure used to palpate the piriformis and quadratus femoris by giving gentle to moderate resistance to the client's lateral rotation of the thigh at the hip joint. Note: Given that the obturator externus is deeper than the rest, it is usually the most difficult of the group to palpate.

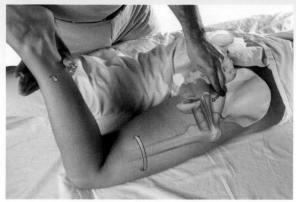

Figure 18-30 Palpation of the other deep lateral rotators by first locating the piriformis and then dropping inferiorly off it. This palpation is done as the client attempts to laterally rotate the thigh against gentle to moderate resistance.

18

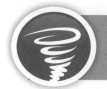

Muscles of the Pelvis

The following *Whirlwind Tour* is an abbreviated set of palpation protocols for the muscles of this chapter. Once you have read and become comfortable with each of the protocols presented thus far, this *Whirlwind Tour* allows you to quickly and efficiently run through the palpations protocols for all the muscles of the chapter.

Client Prone

1. **Gluteus maximus:** The client is prone; you are standing to the side of the client. Place your palpating hand just lateral to the sacrum, and feel for the contraction of the gluteus maximus as the client extends and laterally rotates the thigh at the hip joint (resistance can be added if desired). Once felt, continue to palpate the gluteus maximus toward its distal attachment while strumming perpendicular to its fibers as the client alternately contracts and relaxes the muscle.

Client Side Lying

2. **Gluteus medius:** The client is side lying; you are standing behind the client. Place palpating hand immediately distal to the middle of the iliac crest, and feel for the contraction of the middle fibers of the gluteus medius as the client abducts the thigh at the hip joint (resistance can be added if desired). Once felt, continue palpating the middle fibers distally to the greater trochanter of the femur while strumming perpendicular to the fibers as the client alternately contracts and relaxes the muscle. The anterior fibers and posterior fibers are mostly deep to other muscles and more difficult to palpate and discern. To palpate the anterior fibers, place your palpating hand immediately distal and posterior to the anterior superior iliac spine (ASIS), ask the client to flex and medially rotate the thigh at the hip joint, and feel for the contraction of the anterior fibers of the gluteus medius deep to the tensor fasciae latae (TFL). If felt, try to palpate the rest of the anterior fibers deep to the TFL. To palpate the posterior fibers, place your palpating hand over the posterosuperior portion of the gluteus maximus, ask the client to extend and laterally rotate the thigh at the hip joint, and feel for the contraction of the posterior fibers of the gluteus medius deep to the gluteus maximus. If felt, try to palpate the rest of the posterior fibers deep to the gluteus maximus. Note: The gluteus minimus is wholly deep to and has the

same actions as the gluteus medius. Therefore, although it can be palpated, it is extremely difficult to discern from the gluteus medius.

3. **Piriformis:** The client is prone with the leg flexed to 90 degrees at the knee joint; you are standing to the side of the client. Place your palpating fingers just lateral to the sacrum, halfway between the posterior superior iliac spine (PSIS) and the apex of the sacrum, and feel for the contraction of the piriformis as the client laterally rotates the thigh at the hip joint against gentle to moderate resistance. Note: Lateral rotation of the thigh in this position requires the client's foot to move medially toward the midline (i.e., the opposite side) of the body. Once felt, continue palpating the piriformis toward the greater trochanter attachment while strumming perpendicular to its fibers as the client alternately contracts and relaxes the muscle. Note: It can be difficult to discern the superior border between the piriformis and gluteus medius and the inferior border between the piriformis and superior gemellus.

4. **Quadratus femoris:** The client is prone with the leg flexed to 90 degrees at the knee joint; you are standing to the side of the client. Place your palpating fingers just lateral to the lateral border of the ischial tuberosity and feel for the contraction of the quadratus femoris as the client laterally rotates the thigh at the hip joint against gentle to moderate resistance. Note: Lateral rotation of the thigh in this position requires the client's foot to move medially toward the midline (i.e., the opposite side) of the body. Once felt, continue palpating the quadratus femoris toward its femoral attachment while strumming perpendicular to its fibers as the client alternately contracts and relaxes the muscle.

5. **Detour: Other deep lateral rotators (superior gemellus, obturator internus, inferior gemellus, obturator externus):** The client is prone with the leg flexed to 90 degrees at the knee joint; you are standing to the side of the client. These other deep lateral rotators located between the piriformis and quadratus femoris are small and deep, but they can usually be palpated. However, it is difficult to discern them from each other. (The obturator externus is deeper than the others and generally the most difficult to palpate.) To palpate these muscles, palpate between the piriformis and quadratus femoris and follow the same palpation procedure as for the piriformis and quadratus femoris by adding gentle to moderate resistance to the client's lateral rotation of the thigh at the hip joint.

Review Questions

1. List the attachments of the gluteus minimus.
2. List the attachments of the quadratus femoris.
3. What are the actions of the gluteus maximus?
4. What are the actions of the piriformis?
5. What change due to the effect of gravity, if any, is there when switching from a prone palpation of the gluteus maximus to a side lying palpation of the gluteus maximus?
6. Full palpation of the gluteus medius is difficult for what reasons?
7. What factors contribute to the extreme difficulty in discerning the gluteus minimus from the gluteus medius?
8. What is the first step in palpating the piriformis?
9. Why is caution advised when palpating the quadratus femoris?
10. By what means can the anterior sacral attachment of the piriformis be palpated?
11. What two muscles challenge proper discernment of the borders of the piriformis?
12. Which of the gluteal muscles has a TrP referral zone that extends as far distally as the ankle joint?
13. Pain when walking uphill and when bending over are hallmarks of TrPs in what muscle?
14. Describe the stretching protocol for the gluteus maximus, being sure to address both the lower and upper fibers.
15. A pinching sensation in the groin area during stretches for muscles like the quadratus femoris or the gluteus maximus can be minimized/alleviated by doing what first?
16. When walking, what is the reason for a depressive force on the pelvis on the weight bearing side?
17. What is the relationship between the action of lateral rotation of the thigh at the hip and the arch of the foot?

CASE STUDY

A 48-year-old male client comes in for his initial appointment to your office. His previous massage experience is limited to what he received from a physical therapist who treated him for a shoulder injury as a teenager. He now wishes to include regular massage as part of his care in his self-proclaimed "post-midlife crisis phase."

Previous medical history shows a left supraspinatus tear at age 16, a left inguinal hernia repair at age 25, and a fractured right radius at age 32. He plays on a recreational softball team and attends a martial arts class weekly. He reports having had high blood pressure for years as a result of his high-stress job as an accounts manager, which was only marginally helped by medication. One year ago he left that job for professional and health reasons, and now he works as a long-distance driver so that he can fulfill his wish of seeing more of the country.

His chief complaint is that of low back pain, but he also experiences intermittent pain that shoots down the back of his right thigh and occasionally feels pain in the lateral ankle. Onset began several weeks ago and has been getting progressively more intense. The pain is the least bothersome in the morning (2/10), but gets worse over the course of the day while working or during athletic activity (6-8/10). Over the counter pain medication has not helped. Both his dispatcher and his martial arts instructor suggested that massage therapy could be of help.

1. What muscles do you suspect are involved in this pain pattern?
2. Are there things that this client is doing, or can be doing, to aggravate or alleviate the condition? If so, what?
3. What other factor(s) should be considered in your assessment for this client?

18

CHAPTER 19

Tour #9 **Palpation of the Thigh Muscles**

Overview

This chapter is a palpation tour of the muscles of the thigh. The tour begins with the hamstring muscles in the posterior thigh, then addresses muscles primarily located in the anterior thigh, including the quadriceps femoris group, and then concludes with the muscles of the adductor group in the medial thigh. Except for the hamstring muscles, which are palpated prone, palpation for the rest of the muscles should be performed with the client supine with right thigh on the table and right leg hanging off the table (for palpation of the right side target muscles), and left hip and knee joints flexed with left foot flat on the table. This position of the client's left-side lower extremity stabilizes the pelvis and lumbar spine, allowing the client to be comfortable with the right leg hanging off the table. Please see the illustration below for this palpation position. (However, within the muscle layouts of this chapter, individuals are shown with both legs hanging off the table. This was done so as not to block the reader's view of the palpation protocol. Please be aware that having both legs hanging off the table can become uncomfortable for the client if maintained for any length of time.) Although the client is rarely placed in this position for treatment, it is an extremely effective position for palpation of the muscles of the thigh, because it affords the possibility of easily isolating contraction of each target muscle of the thigh. If desired, each of these palpations can be done with the client supine with the entire lower extremity on the table instead. Other alternate palpation positions are also described. The major muscles or muscle groups of the region are each given a separate layout. There are also a few detours to other muscles of the region. Trigger point (TrP) information and stretching, both therapist-assisted and self-care stretching, are given for each of the muscles covered in this chapter. The chapter closes with an advanced *Whirlwind Tour* that explains the sequential palpation of all the muscles of the chapter.

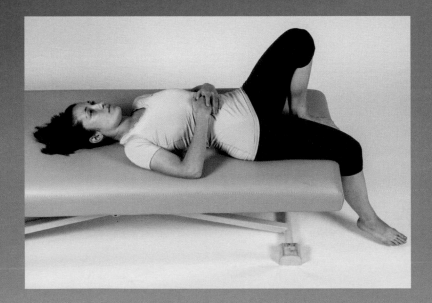

@ Go to http://evolve.elsevier.com/Muscolino/palpation for video demonstrations of the muscle palpations presented in this chapter.

Chapter Outline

Chapter Objectives

After completing this chapter, the student/therapist should be able to perform the following for each of the muscles covered in this chapter:

1. State the attachments.
2. State the actions.
3. Describe the starting position for palpation.
4. Describe and explain the purpose of each of the palpation steps.
5. Palpate each muscle.
6. State the "Palpation Key."
7. Describe alternate palpation positions.
8. State the locations of the most common TrP(s).
9. Describe the TrP referral zones.
10. State the most common factors that create and/or perpetuate TrPs.
11. State the symptoms most commonly caused by TrPs.
12. Describe and perform the therapist-assisted and self-care stretches.

19

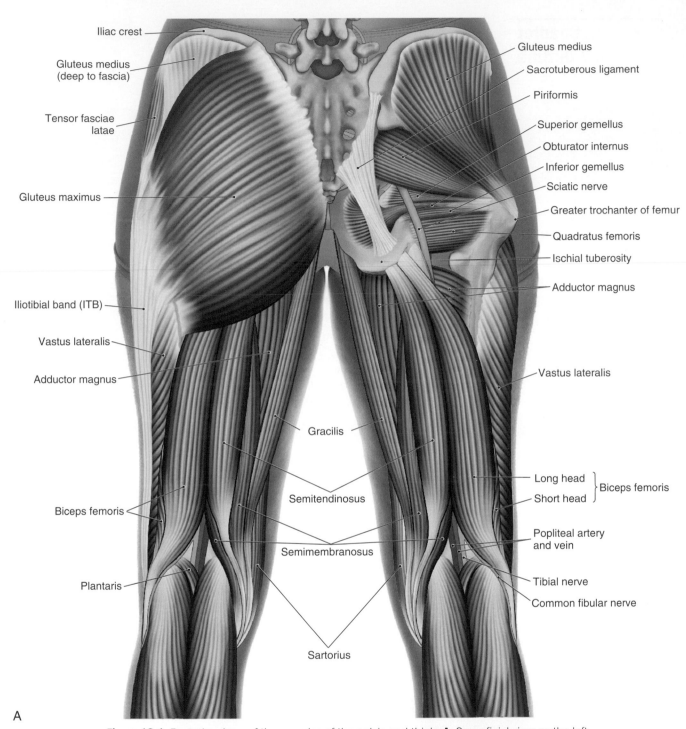

Figure 19-1 Posterior views of the muscles of the pelvis and thigh. **A,** Superficial view on the left and an intermediate view on the right.

A

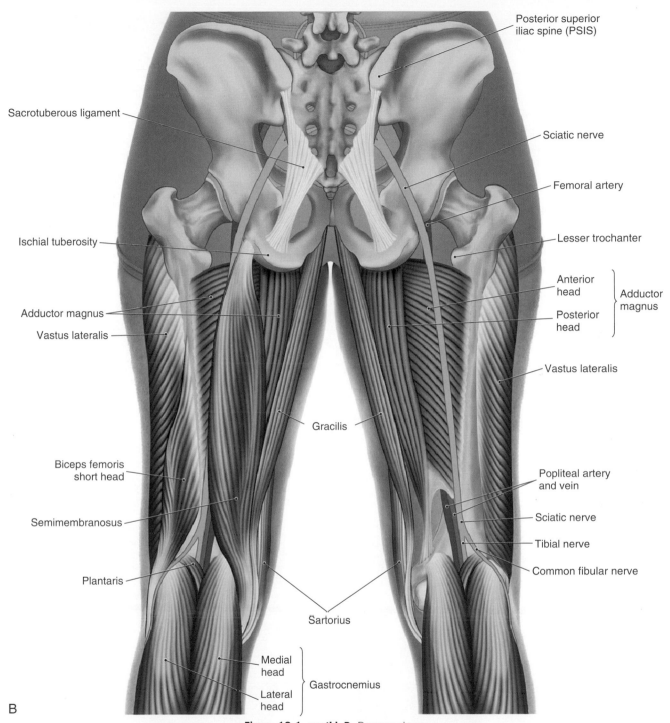

Posterior superior
iliac spine (PSIS)

Sacrotuberous ligament

Sciatic nerve

Femoral artery

Ischial tuberosity

Lesser trochanter

Anterior
head

Adductor
magnus

Adductor magnus

Posterior
head

Vastus lateralis

Vastus lateralis

Gracilis

Biceps femoris
short head

Popliteal artery
and vein

Semimembranosus

Sciatic nerve

Tibial nerve

Plantaris

Common fibular nerve

Sartorius

Medial
head

Gastrocnemius

Lateral
head

B

Figure 19-1, cont'd B, Deeper views.

19

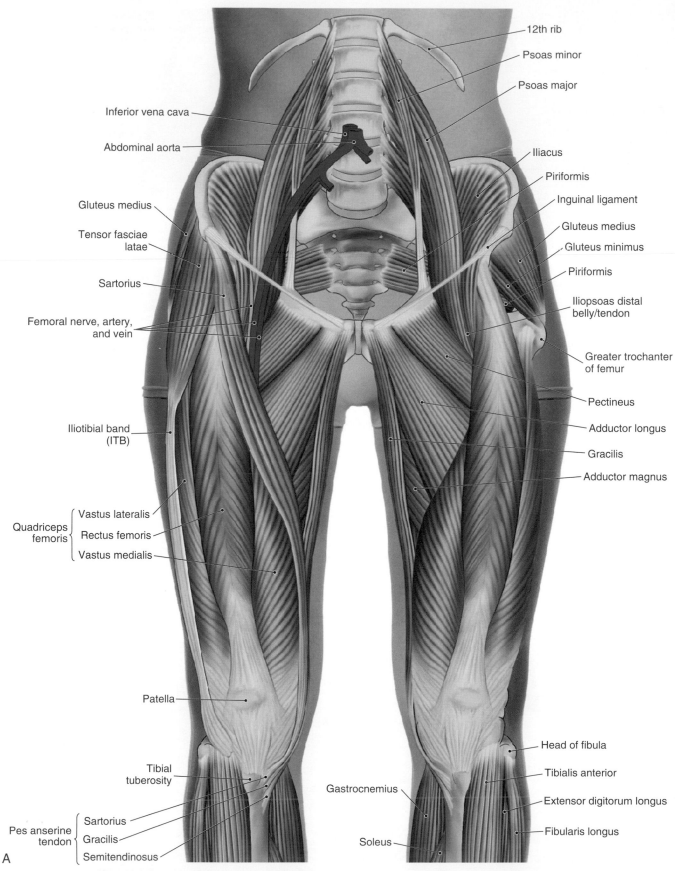

Figure 19-2 Views of the anterior thigh. **A,** Superficial view on the right and an intermediate view on the left.

19

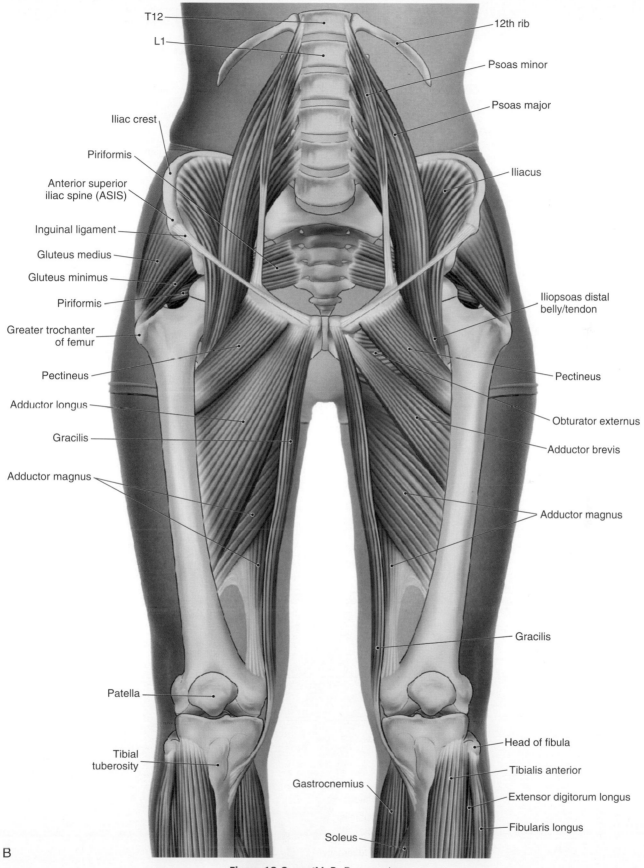

Figure 19-2, cont'd B, Deeper views.

B

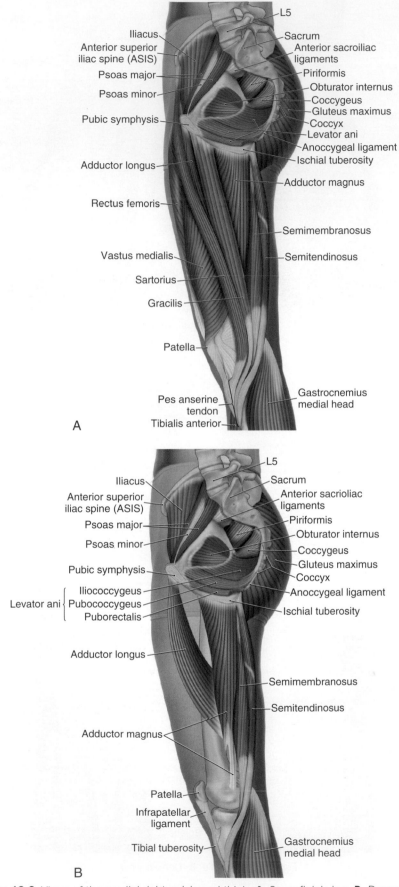

Figure 19-3 Views of the medial right pelvis and thigh. **A,** Superficial view. **B,** Deeper view.

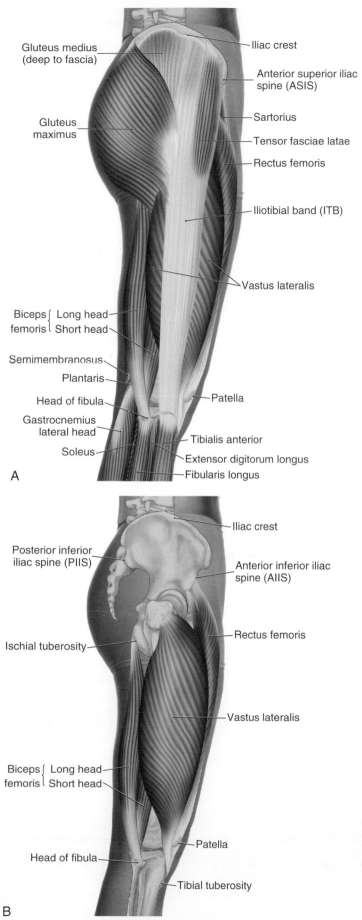

Gluteus medius
(deep to fascia)

Gluteus
maximus

Biceps { Long head
femoris { Short head

Semimembranosus

Plantaris

Head of fibula

Gastrocnemius
lateral head

Soleus

Iliac crest

Anterior superior iliac
spine (ASIS)

Sartorius

Tensor fasciae latae

Rectus femoris

Iliotibial band (ITB)

Vastus lateralis

Patella

Tibialis anterior

Extensor digitorum longus

Fibularis longus

A

Posterior inferior
iliac spine (PIIS)

Ischial tuberosity

Biceps { Long head
femoris { Short head

Head of fibula

Iliac crest

Anterior inferior iliac
spine (AIIS)

Rectus femoris

Vastus lateralis

Patella

Tibial tuberosity

B

Figure 19-4 Views of the right lateral thigh. **A,** Superficial view. **B,** Deep view (with only the quadriceps femoris group and biceps femoris of the hamstring group drawn in).

HAMSTRING GROUP—PRONE

Lateral hamstrings: Biceps femoris, long head and short head
Medial hamstrings: Semitendinosus and semimembranosus

☑ATTACHMENTS

Biceps Femoris

☐ Ischial tuberosity (long head) and the linea aspera of the femur (short head)

to the

☐ head of the fibula and the lateral tibial condyle

Semitendinosus

☐ Ischial tuberosity

to the

☐ pes anserine tendon at the proximal anteromedial tibia

Semimembranosus

☐ Ischial tuberosity

to the

☐ posterior surface of the medial tibial condyle

☑ACTIONS

All three hamstrings:
☐ Flex the leg at the knee joint
☐ Extend the thigh at the hip joint
☐ Posteriorly tilt the pelvis at the hip joint
Lateral hamstrings also:
☐ Laterally rotate the leg at the knee joint
Medial hamstrings also:
☐ Medially rotate the leg at the knee joint
Note: The short head of the biceps femoris does not cross the hip joint and therefore does not have an action at the hip joint.

Starting Position (Figure 19-6)

■ Client prone with leg partially flexed at the knee joint
■ Therapist standing to the side of the client
■ Palpating hand placed just distal to the ischial tuberosity
■ Support hand placed around the distal leg, just proximal to the ankle joint

Palpation Steps

1. Palpating just distal to the ischial tuberosity, resist the client from further flexion of the leg at the knee joint, and feel for the contraction of the hamstrings.
2. Strumming perpendicular to the fibers, follow the biceps femoris toward the head of the fibula. Repeat this procedure from the ischial tuberosity to follow the medial hamstrings toward the medial side of the leg (Figure 19-7).
3. Once each of the hamstrings has been located, have the client relax it, and palpate to assess its baseline tone.

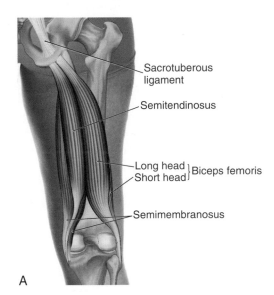

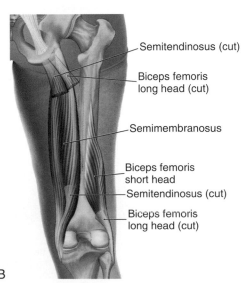

A

Sacrotuberous ligament
Semitendinosus
Long head ⎫ Biceps femoris
Short head ⎭
Semimembranosus

B

Semitendinosus (cut)
Biceps femoris long head (cut)
Semimembranosus
Biceps femoris short head
Semitendinosus (cut)
Biceps femoris long head (cut)

Figure 19-5 Posterior views of the right hamstring group. **A,** Superficial view of all three hamstring muscles. **B,** Deeper view. The proximal and distal tendons of the semitendinosus and the long head of the biceps femoris have been cut and ghosted in.

19

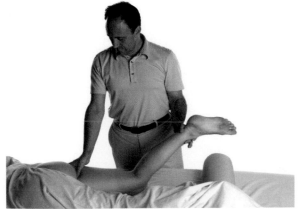

Figure 19-6 Starting position for prone palpation of the right hamstrings.

HAMSTRING GROUP—PRONE—*cont'd*

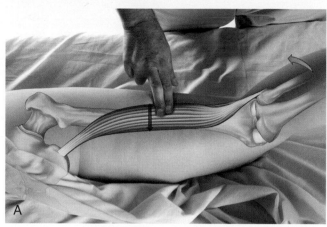 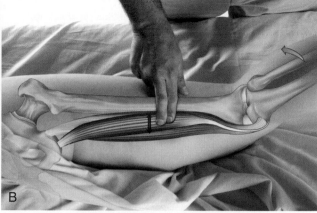

Figure 19-7 Palpation of the superficial hamstring muscles of the right thigh as the client attempts to flex the leg at the knee joint against resistance. **A,** Palpation of the long head of the biceps femoris on the lateral side. **B,** Palpation of the semitendinosus on the medial side.

PALPATION NOTES

1. Distally, the tendons of the medial and lateral hamstrings are quite far apart and easy to distinguish. Proximally, the muscles' bellies are closer to each other and more difficult to distinguish. Using rotation of the leg at the knee joint is an excellent way to discern between them. The medial hamstrings are medial rotators and the lateral hamstrings are lateral rotators. Keep in mind that the knee joint only allows rotations to occur if it is first flexed; the recommended flexion of the knee joint is 90 degrees.

2. When the client is not contracting the hamstrings to try to flex the leg at the knee joint against the resistance of your support hand, use your support hand to support the client's leg so that the hamstrings are allowed to fully relax. Otherwise, if the client has to hold the leg partially flexed in the air, the hamstrings will not relax between contractions. Full relaxation between contractions creates a greater change in muscle tone, making it easier to palpate and locate the target hamstring muscle.

3. It can be difficult to discern the bellies of the two medial hamstrings from each other. Note that the distal tendon of the semitendinosus is very prominent and easy to find. The semimembranosus can be palpated on either side of the distal semitendinosus, especially the medial side (Figure 19-8).

4. Directly anterior to the belly of the biceps femoris is the vastus lateralis muscle; use flexion versus extension of the leg at the knee joint to discern their border. Directly anterior to the medial hamstrings in the proximal thigh is the adductor magnus; use flexion of the leg to discern this border. The adductor magnus does not cross the knee joint and stays relaxed with leg flexion, whereas the hamstrings contract with leg flexion.

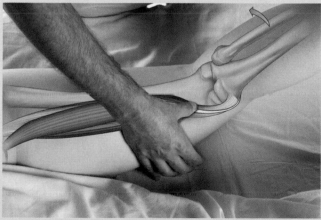

Figure 19-8 The distal semimembranosus can be palpated on either side of the distal tendon of the semitendinosus. Palpation on its lateral side is shown here.

19

HAMSTRING GROUP—PRONE—cont'd

Alternate Palpation Position—Seated

Having the client seated with the foot flat on the floor allows for easy use of rotations of the leg at the knee joint to locate the distal tendons of the biceps femoris, semitendinosus, and gracilis. With lateral rotation, the biceps femoris is easily palpable on the lateral side. With medial rotation, two tendons stand out on the medial side, the semitendinosus and gracilis. The semitendinosus is the larger of the two and more lateral (closer to the midline of the thigh).

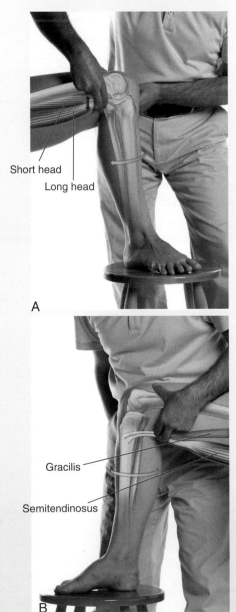

Figure 19-9 Palpation of the distal tendons of the biceps femoris, semitendinosus, and gracilis as the client rotates the leg at the knee joint. **A,** Palpation of the biceps femoris as the client laterally rotates the leg. **B,** Palpation of the semitendinosus and gracilis as the client medially rotates the leg. Note: For the purpose of these photos, the client is standing with the foot on a stool.

TRIGGER POINTS

1. Trigger points (TrPs) in the hamstrings often result from or are perpetuated by acute or chronic overuse of the muscle and ischemia caused by compression on the distal posterior thigh from sitting in an ill-fitting chair. They also commonly result from prolonged shortening of the muscle due to sleeping in the fetal position.
2. TrPs in the medial hamstrings tend to produce pain that is superficial and sharper in quality, whereas lateral hamstring TrPs tend to produce pain that is deeper and duller in quality. TrPs in the lateral hamstrings often wake clients at night, resulting in nonrestful sleep.
3. The referral patterns of hamstring TrPs must be distinguished from the referral patterns of TrPs in the piriformis, gluteus medius and minimus, obturator internus, vastus lateralis, popliteus, plantaris, and gastrocnemius.
4. TrPs in the hamstrings are often incorrectly assessed as sciatica or degenerative joint disease of the knee.
5. Associated TrPs often occur in the adductor magnus, vastus lateralis, gastrocnemius, iliopsoas, and quadriceps femoris muscles.

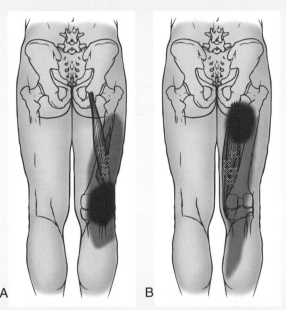

Figure 19-10 Posterior views of common lateral and medial hamstring trigger points (TrPs) with their corresponding referral zones. **A,** Lateral hamstring (biceps femoris). **B,** Medial hamstrings (semitendinosus and semimembranosus).

19

HAMSTRING GROUP—PRONE—*cont'd*

STRETCHING THE HAMSTRING GROUP

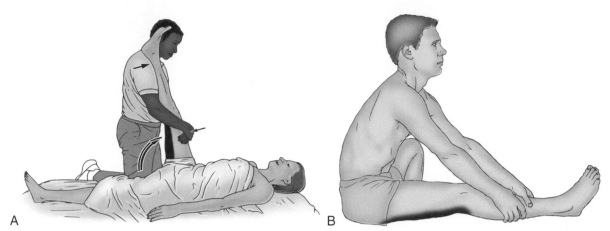

A   B

Figure 19-11 Stretching the right hamstring group. The client's hip joint is flexed while the knee joint is held in full extension. **A,** Therapist-assisted stretch. The hip joint is flexed by flexing the thigh at the hip joint. **B,** Self-care stretch. The hip joint is flexed by anteriorly tilting the pelvis at the hip joint. Note: The spine does not need to bend in this stretch.

Palpation Key:
Resist flexion of the leg at the knee joint.

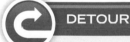 **DETOUR**

Adductor Magnus:
Once the medial hamstrings have been located in the proximal thigh, drop just medial (anterior) to their medial border and you will be on the adductor magnus. The adductor magnus is located between the medial hamstrings and the gracilis. To confirm your location, ask the client to flex the leg at the knee joint. This engages the hamstrings and the gracilis but not the adductor magnus between them. Resisted adduction of the thigh at the hip joint engages the adductor magnus (and the gracilis) (Figure 19-12).

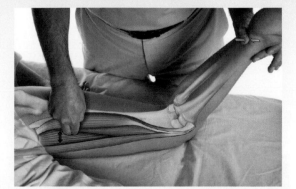

Figure 19-12 The adductor magnus can be palpated between the medial hamstrings and the gracilis. The medial hamstrings and the gracilis contract when the client flexes the leg at the knee joint, but the adductor magnus does not.

TENSOR FASCIAE LATAE (TFL)—SUPINE

☑ ATTACHMENTS

☐ Anterior superior iliac spine (ASIS) and the anterior iliac crest

to the

☐ iliotibial band (ITB), ⅓ of the way down the thigh

☑ ACTIONS

☐ Medially rotates the thigh at the hip joint
☐ Flexes the thigh at the hip joint
☐ Abducts the thigh at the hip joint
☐ Anteriorly tilts the pelvis at the hip joint
☐ Depresses the same-side pelvis at the hip joint

Starting Position (Figure 19-14)

■ Client supine with the right thigh on the table and right leg hanging off the table
■ Therapist standing to the side of the client
■ Palpating fingers placed just distal and lateral to the ASIS
■ If resistance is necessary, support hand placed on the distal anterolateral thigh

Palpation Steps

1. Ask the client to medially rotate and flex the thigh at the hip joint, and feel for the contraction of the tensor fasciae latae (TFL) immediately distal and slightly lateral to the ASIS (Figure 19-15).
2. Continue palpating the TFL distally to its ITB attachment by strumming perpendicular to the fibers.
3. Having the client contract to lift the medially rotated thigh up into flexion against gravity is usually sufficient resistance to bring out the TFL. However, if needed, additional resistance can be given with the support hand placed on the distal anterior thigh.
4. Once the TFL has been located, have the client relax it, and palpate to assess its baseline tone.

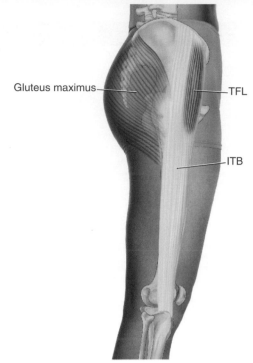

Figure 19-13 Lateral view of the right tensor fasciae latae (TFL). The gluteus maximus has been ghosted in. *ITB*, Iliotibial band.

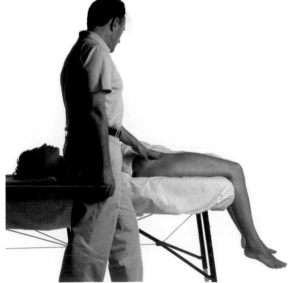

Figure 19-14 Starting position for supine palpation of the right tensor fasciae latae (TFL).

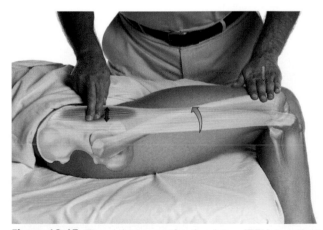

Figure 19-15 The right tensor fasciae latae (TFL) is palpated by asking the client to medially rotate and flex the thigh at the hip joint.

19

TENSOR FASCIAE LATAE (TFL)—SUPINE—*cont'd*

PALPATION NOTES

1. The TFL is superficial and easy to palpate.
2. It is interesting to compare the palpation procedures for the TFL and sartorius. Both muscles attach to the ASIS and are flexors of the thigh at the hip joint. However, the TFL is also a medial rotator of the thigh, and the sartorius is also a lateral rotator of the thigh. Therefore, to palpate the TFL, palpate immediately distal and lateral to the ASIS, and ask the client to medially rotate and flex the thigh at the hip joint. To palpate the sartorius, palpate immediately distal and medial to the ASIS, and ask the client to laterally rotate and flex the thigh at the hip joint.
3. Between the proximal attachments of the TFL and sartorius is the rectus femoris of the quadriceps femoris group.
4. The reason that the supine client is lying with the right leg off the table is that it allows for immediate and easy palpation and discernment of the rectus femoris by asking the client to straighten out (extend) the leg at the knee joint without contracting any flexors of the thigh at the hip joint. Locating the rectus femoris allows for better distinction between the TFL and the rectus femoris. This position also allows for easy palpation of other anterior and medial thigh muscles.

Alternate Palpation Position—Side Lying

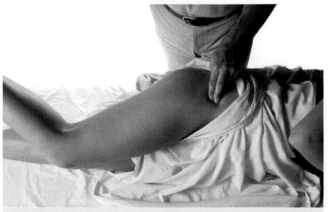

Figure 19-16 Because the tensor fasciae latae (TFL) is located in the anterolateral thigh, it can also be easily palpated with the client in side lying position. Ask the client to medially rotate and flex (slight abduction may also be added) the thigh at the hip joint, and feel for the contraction of the TFL.

TRIGGER POINTS

1. Trigger points (TrPs) in the TFL often result from or are perpetuated by acute or chronic overuse of the muscle, and prolonged shortening of the muscle due to sitting and sleeping in the fetal position.
2. The referral patterns of TFL TrPs must be distinguished from the referral patterns of TrPs in the anterior fibers of the gluteus medius and minimus, vastus lateralis, and quadratus lumborum.
3. TrPs in the TFL are often incorrectly assessed as trochanteric bursitis, sacroiliac joint syndrome, or meralgia paresthetica.
4. Associated TrPs often occur in the anterior gluteus minimus, rectus femoris, iliopsoas, and sartorius.

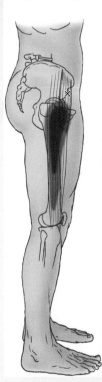

Figure 19-17 Lateral view of a common tensor fasciae latae (TFL) trigger point (TrP) with its corresponding referral zone.

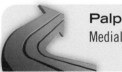

Palpation Key:
Medially rotate and flex the thigh.

19

TENSOR FASCIAE LATAE (TFL)—SUPINE—*cont'd*

STRETCHING THE TENSOR FASCIAE LATAE

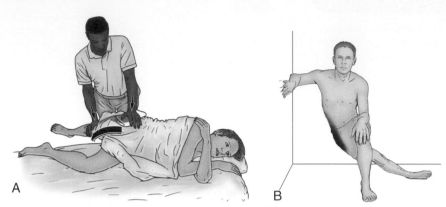

Figure 19-18 Stretching the right tensor fasciae latae (TFL). The client's thigh is extended and adducted. **A,** Therapist-assisted stretch. The therapist contacts the client's distal lateral thigh (not the leg). If the client's thigh is laterally rotated, it increases the stretch to the TFL. Note that the therapist's other hand stabilizes the client's pelvis from depressing; a cushion is used for comfort. **B,** Self-care stretch. The client can lean against a wall for stabilization and support. Note: It is important to not place too much weight on the ankle joint of the foot in back. See Figure 17-31 for another stretch of the TFL.

SARTORIUS—SUPINE

☑ ATTACHMENTS

☐ ASIS

to the

☐ pes anserine tendon at the proximal anteromedial tibia

☑ ACTIONS

☐ Laterally rotates the thigh at the hip joint
☐ Flexes the thigh at the hip joint
☐ Abducts the thigh at the hip joint
☐ Anteriorly tilts the pelvis at the hip joint
☐ Depresses the same-side pelvis at the hip joint
☐ Flexes the leg at the knee joint
☐ Medially rotates the leg at the knee joint

Starting Position (Figure 19-20)

■ Client supine with the right thigh on the table and right leg hanging off the table
■ Therapist standing to the side of the client
■ Palpating fingers placed just distal and medial to the ASIS
■ If resistance is necessary, support hand placed on the distal anteromedial thigh

Palpation Steps

1. Ask the client to laterally rotate and flex the thigh at the hip joint, and feel for the contraction of the sartorius immediately distal and slightly medial to the ASIS (Figure 19-21).
2. If necessary, use the support hand to add resistance when the client flexes the laterally rotated thigh.
3. Continue palpating the sartorius toward its distal attachment by strumming perpendicular to the fibers.
4. Once the sartorius has been located, have the client relax it, and palpate to assess its baseline tone.

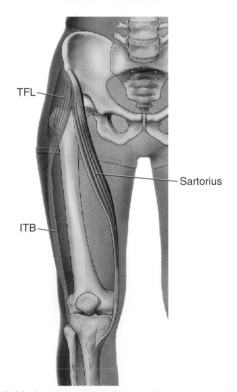

Figure 19-19 Anterior view of the right sartorius. The tensor fasciae latae (TFL) and iliotibial band (ITB) have been ghosted in.

19

SARTORIUS—SUPINE—*cont'd*

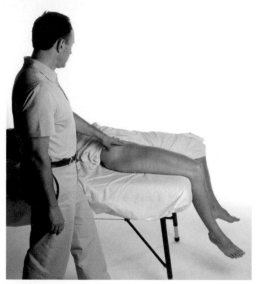

Figure 19-20 Starting position for supine palpation of the right sartorius.

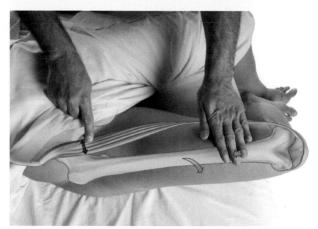

Figure 19-21 The proximal belly of the right sartorius engages and is easily palpable when the client laterally rotates and flexes the thigh at the hip joint. Note: The therapist usually palpates from the same side of the table but is shown here standing on the opposite side of the table for the purpose of this photo.

PALPATION NOTES

1. Even though it is superficial, the distal ½ of the sartorius is often challenging to palpate and discern from the adjacent musculature. One method to locate it is to first locate the vastus medialis in the distal thigh. (It is usually fairly prominent and often forms a bulge in well-developed individuals.) To engage the vastus medialis, have the client extend the leg at the knee joint. Once the vastus medialis has been found, move just medial (posterior) off it onto the sartorius. Then ask the client to flex the leg at the knee joint to engage the sartorius. In this position, this can be accomplished by asking the client to press the leg against the table (Figure 19-22).

2. In addition to asking the client to laterally rotate and flex the thigh at the hip joint, it can be helpful to ask the client to also abduct the thigh at the hip joint and flex the leg at the knee joint. These four actions are all the actions of the sartorius upon the thigh and leg.

3. The sartorius and TFL are palpated in a similar manner. To palpate the sartorius, palpate immediately distal and slightly medial to the ASIS, and ask the client to laterally rotate and flex the thigh at the hip joint. To palpate the TFL, palpate immediately distal and slightly lateral to the ASIS, and ask the client to medially rotate and flex the thigh at the hip joint. Note: Between the proximal attachments of the TFL and sartorius is the rectus femoris of the quadriceps femoris group.

4. Proximally, the medial border of the sartorius forms the lateral border of the femoral triangle. Located within the femoral triangle are the iliopsoas and pectineus muscles, and the femoral nerve, artery, and vein.

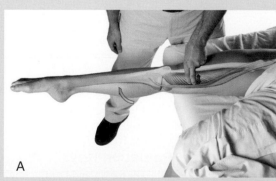
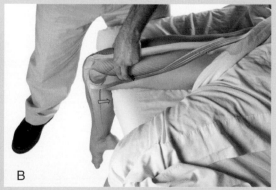

A   B

Figure 19-22 Palpation of the distal belly of the right sartorius by first locating the vastus medialis. **A,** Palpation of the engaged vastus medialis as the client extends the leg at the knee joint. **B,** Once the vastus medialis is located, the therapist palpates the distal belly of the sartorius immediately medial (posterior) to the vastus medialis as the client engages the sartorius by flexing the leg at the knee joint against the resistance of the table.

19

SARTORIUS—SUPINE—*cont'd*

Alternate Palpation Position—Supine with Entire Lower Extremity on the Table

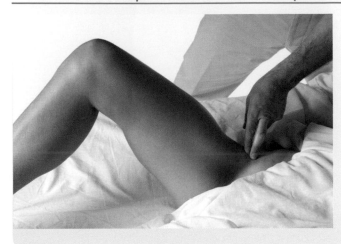

Figure 19-23 The sartorius can be palpated with the client supine with the thighs and legs on the table. The right sartorius is engaged and palpated here by asking the client to laterally rotate and flex the thigh at the hip joint.

TRIGGER POINTS

1. Trigger points (TrPs) in the sartorius often result from or are perpetuated by acute or chronic overuse of the muscle, or a prolonged shortening of the muscle due to sitting in the cross-legged lotus position or sleeping in the fetal position.
2. TrPs in the sartorius tend to produce superficial sharp pain or tingling compared with the usual deep dull pain typical of myofascial TrPs.
3. The referral patterns of sartorius TrPs must be distinguished from the referral patterns of TrPs in the vastus medialis, vastus intermedius, pectineus, iliopsoas, and the three "adductors" of the thigh.
4. TrPs in the sartorius are often incorrectly assessed as meralgia paresthetica or medial knee joint dysfunction.
5. Associated TrPs often occur in the quadriceps femoris and the three "adductor" muscles of the thigh.

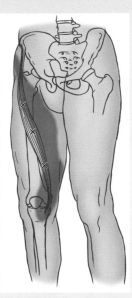

Figure 19-24 Anteromedial view of common sartorius trigger points (TrPs) with their corresponding referral zone.

Palpation Key:
Laterally rotate and flex the thigh.

SARTORIUS—SUPINE—cont'd

STRETCHING THE SARTORIUS

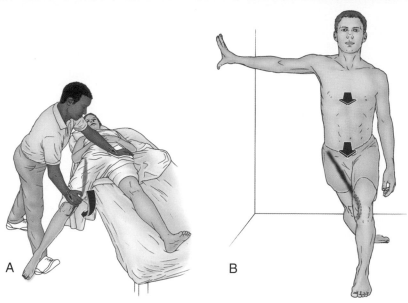

A   B

Figure 19-25 Stretching the right sartorius. The client's thigh is extended and medially rotated with the knee joint in full extension. **A,** Therapist-assisted stretch. It is important to abduct the client's thigh as little as possible. Note: The therapist's other hand stabilizes the client's pelvis from anteriorly tilted and rotating to the side of the stretch; a cushion is used for comfort. **B,** Self-care stretch. Adduction of the thigh is added to the extension and medial rotation. Note: It is important to make sure that excessive weight is not placed on the ankle joint of the foot in back.

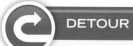

DETOUR

Iliopsoas Distal Belly and Tendon:

Slide medially off the proximal tendon of the sartorius, and you will be on the distal belly and tendon of the iliopsoas; confirm by asking the client to gently flex the trunk at the spinal joints (by doing a small abdominal curl-up) and feel for the tensing of the psoas major portion of the iliopsoas distal belly and tendon. (The psoas major portion is the more medial portion of the iliopsoas.) Be aware that a strong abdominal curl-up might cause other hip flexor muscles to contract to stabilize the pelvis, preventing it from posteriorly tilting (hip flexors are anterior tilters of the pelvis). Be aware of the presence of the femoral nerve, artery, and vein overlying the iliopsoas distal belly and tendon.

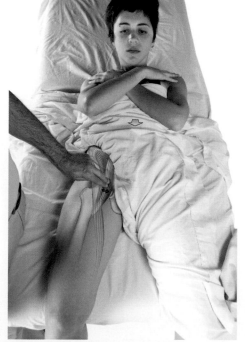

Figure 19-26 Palpation of the distal belly and tendon of the right psoas major portion of the iliopsoas medial to the sartorius as the client flexes the spine by doing a curl-up.

19

QUADRICEPS FEMORIS GROUP—SUPINE

The quadriceps femoris group is composed of the rectus femoris, vastus medialis, vastus lateralis, and vastus intermedius.

☑ ATTACHMENTS

Rectus femoris
☐ Anterior inferior iliac spine (AIIS)

to the

☐ tibial tuberosity

Vastus medialis, lateralis, and intermedius
☐ Linea aspera of the femur

to the

☐ tibial tuberosity

☑ ACTIONS

☐ All four quadriceps femoris muscles extend the leg at the knee joint

The rectus femoris also:
☐ Flexes the thigh at the hip joint
☐ Anteriorly tilts the pelvis at the hip joint

Starting Position (Figure 19-28)

■ Client supine with the right thigh on the table and right leg hanging off the table
■ Therapist standing to the side of the client
■ Palpating fingers placed on the proximal anterior thigh
■ If resistance is necessary, support hand placed on the distal leg, just proximal to the ankle joint

Palpation Steps

1. Proximally, the rectus femoris is located between the tensor fasciae latae (TFL) and sartorius. Either locate the proximal tendon of the TFL and drop off it medially, or locate the proximal tendon of the sartorius and drop off it laterally, and you will be on the rectus femoris.
2. Ask the client to extend the leg at the knee joint and feel for the contraction of the rectus femoris (Figure 19-29, *A*). If necessary, use the support hand to add resistance when the client extends the leg.
3. Continue palpating the rectus femoris distally to the tibial tuberosity by strumming perpendicular to its fibers.
4. For the vastus medialis, palpate in the anteromedial thigh, just proximal to the patella while the client extends the leg at the knee joint, and feel for its contraction. Then while strumming perpendicular to the fibers, palpate as much of the vastus medialis as possible (see Figure 19-29, *B*).
5. For the vastus lateralis, palpate in the anterolateral thigh, just proximal to the patella while the client extends the leg at the knee joint, and feel for its contraction. Then while strumming perpendicular to the fibers, palpate the vastus lateralis in the anterolateral thigh, in the lateral thigh deep to the iliotibial (ITB) and in the posterolateral thigh immediately posterior to the ITB (see Figure 19-29, *C*).
6. Once the quadriceps femoris muscles have been located, have the client relax them, and palpate to assess their baseline tone.

19

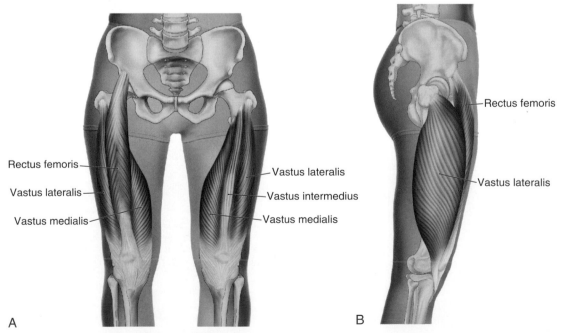

A   B

Figure 19-27 Views of the quadriceps femoris group. **A,** Superficial and deep anterior views. The right side is a superficial view. The rectus femoris has been removed on the left side to expose the vastus intermedius. **B,** Right lateral view.

QUADRICEPS FEMORIS GROUP—SUPINE—*cont'd*

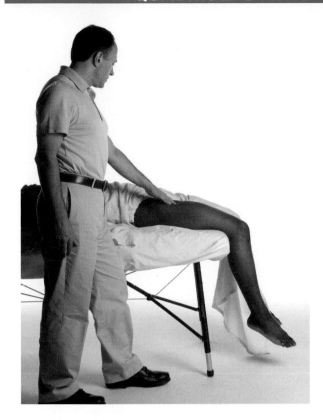

Figure 19-28 Starting position for supine palpation of the right quadriceps femoris group.

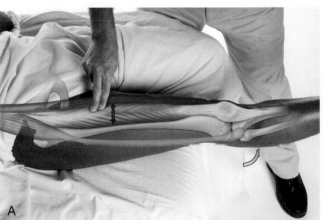

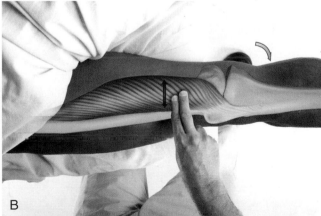

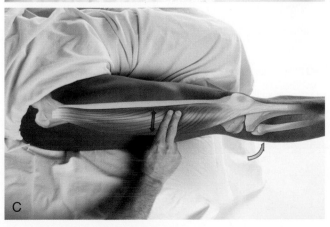

Figure 19-29 Palpation of the quadriceps femoris muscles as the client extends the leg at the knee joint. **A,** Anterolateral view showing palpation of the rectus femoris. **B,** Anterior view showing palpation of the vastus medialis. **C,** Anterior view showing palpation of the vastus lateralis.

19

QUADRICEPS FEMORIS GROUP—SUPINE—*cont'd*

PALPATION NOTES

1. When asking the client to extend the leg at the knee joint, make sure that the client does not also flex the thigh at the hip joint or all the hip flexor muscles will contract, making it difficult to discern the proximal rectus femoris.
2. Proximally, the rectus femoris is located between the TFL and the sartorius. Either of these two muscles can be used as a landmark to find the rectus femoris.
3. The rectus femoris can be palpated and followed all the way to the AIIS. Follow the rectus femoris proximally as far as possible with the client in the starting position (see Figure 19-28). Then passively flex the client's thigh at the hip joint as you continue palpating farther proximally toward the AIIS. Ask the client to alternately contract and relax the rectus femoris by extending the leg at the knee joint, and feel for the tensing of the proximal tendon. When you have reached the AIIS itself, make sure that the rectus femoris is relaxed and passively slackened so that the hard texture of the AIIS is discernable from the adjacent soft tissue texture of the proximal tendon of the rectus femoris (Figure 19-30).
4. In well-developed clients, it is usually possible to discern the borders between the rectus femoris and the vastus lateralis on the lateral side and rectus femoris and vastus medialis on the medial side. While the quadriceps femoris group is contracted, strum perpendicularly across the rectus femoris, feeling for the side-to-side width of the muscle. Then feel for a palpable indent/groove running vertically between the rectus femoris and the vastus muscles on either side.
5. The vastus medialis is superficial and easy to palpate in the distal thigh. However, proximally it is deeper and difficult to palpate and discern from adjacent musculature.
6. The vastus lateralis is superficial in the anterolateral thigh and deep only to the ITB in the lateral thigh. In these

locations, it is easy to palpate. It is also superficial and fairly easy to palpate immediately posterior to the ITB in the posterolateral thigh. However, the linea aspera attachment is quite deep and can be challenging to palpate and discern.
7. Because the vastus lateralis muscle is deep to the ITB, tension in this muscle is often incorrectly blamed on the ITB.
8. The vastus intermedius is extremely difficult to palpate and discern, because it is deep to the rectus femoris and vastus lateralis and has the same action as these other muscles.
9. The patella is a sesamoid bone that developed evolutionarily within the distal tendon of the quadriceps femoris tendon. Its major function is to increase the leverage force and therefore the strength of the quadriceps femoris muscles.

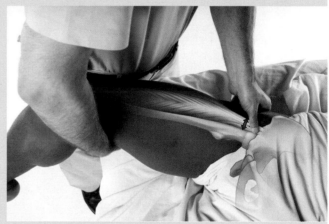

Figure 19-30 Palpation of the proximal tendon of the rectus femoris at the anterior inferior iliac spine (AIIS) (see Palpation Note #3).

Alternate Palpation Position—Side Lying

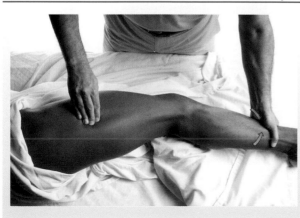

Figure 19-31 Because the vastus lateralis is located so far laterally, it is easily palpable with the client in side lying position. Palpate anterior, deep to, and posterior to the iliotibial band (ITB), and feel for the contraction of the vastus lateralis as the client extends the leg at the knee joint. Note: In this position, because extension of the leg is not against gravity, it is usually necessary to add resistance to leg extension with the support hand to increase the strength of the vastus lateralis contraction, thereby making it more easily palpable.

QUADRICEPS FEMORIS GROUP—SUPINE—cont'd

TRIGGER POINTS

1. Trigger points (TrPs) in the quadriceps femoris often result from or are perpetuated by acute or chronic overuse of the musculature (e.g., running, cycling), direct trauma, or a lack of stretching of the quadriceps femoris due to a lack of full knee flexion. (This may occur in sedentary individuals as well as those recovering from surgery or fracture of the hip or knee joints.) Other factors include placing a heavy weight on the lap when sitting (e.g., laptop computer, child) or receiving repeated intramuscular injections.

2. TrPs in the quadriceps femoris often produce knee joint pain (This is common in children and adults.); at times weakness of the knee joint occurs, sometimes resulting in a buckling of the knee joint when walking. Clients with vastus lateralis TrPs are often unable to sleep on the affected side.

3. The referral patterns of quadriceps femoris TrPs must be distinguished from the referral patterns of gluteus minimus, gluteus medius, sartorius, TFL, the three "adductors" of the thigh, gracilis, and possibly pectineus and iliopsoas.

4. TrPs in the quadriceps femoris are often incorrectly assessed as knee joint dysfunction, trochanteric bursitis, or meralgia paresthetica.

5. Associated TrPs often occur in the other quadriceps femoris muscles, hamstrings, iliopsoas, sartorius, the three "adductors" of the thigh, and gluteus minimus.

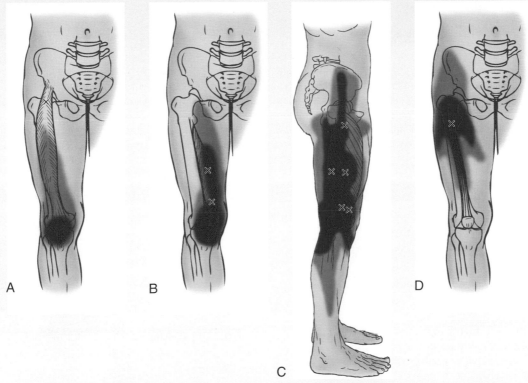

Figure 19-32 Views of the quadriceps femoris muscles' common trigger points (TrPs) with their referral zones. **A,** Anterior view of the rectus femoris. **B,** Anterior view of the vastus medialis. **C,** Lateral view of the vastus lateralis. **D,** Anterior view of the vastus intermedius.

19

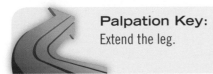

Palpation Key:
Extend the leg.

QUADRICEPS FEMORIS GROUP—SUPINE—*cont'd*

STRETCHING THE QUADRICEPS FEMORIS

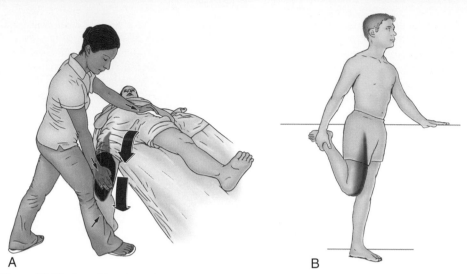

Figure 19-33 Stretching the right quadriceps femoris group. The client's knee joint is brought into flexion. If the hip joint is extended, the stretch is focused on the rectus femoris of the quadriceps. **A,** Therapist-assisted stretch. The therapist extends the client's hip joint by contacting the client's distal anterior thigh with her right hand and flexes the client's knee joint by contacting the client's anterior leg with her right leg. Note: The therapist's other hand stabilizes the client's pelvis from anteriorly tilted and rotating to the side of the stretch; a cushion is used for comfort. **B,** Self-care stretch. Note: It is important when doing this stretch to make sure that the knee joint is not rotated.

PECTINEUS—SUPINE

☑ ATTACHMENTS

☐ Superior pubic ramus

to the

☐ pectineal line on the proximal posterior shaft of the femur

☑ ACTIONS

☐ Adducts the thigh at the hip joint
☐ Flexes the thigh at the hip joint
☐ Anteriorly tilts the pelvis at the hip joint

Starting Position (Figure 19-35, *A*)

■ Client supine with the right thigh on the table and right leg hanging off the table
■ Therapist standing to the side of the client
■ Place palpating fingers on the proximal anteromedial thigh, and locate the proximal tendon of the adductor longus. To locate it, simply palpate along the pubic bone from lateral to medial until you encounter a prominent tendon (It is the most prominent tendon in the region.) (see Figure 19-35, *B*)
■ Support hand placed on the distal anteromedial thigh, just proximal to the knee joint

Palpation Steps

1. After locating the proximal tendon of the adductor longus, drop off it anteriorly (laterally), and you will be on the pectineus (see Figure 19-35, C).
2. To engage the pectineus, palpate against the pubic bone while asking the client to adduct the thigh at the hip

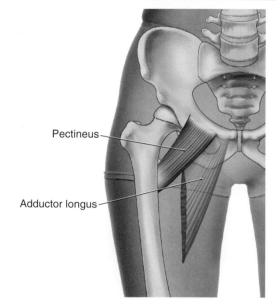

Figure 19-34 Anterior view of the right pectineus. The adductor longus has been cut and ghosted in.

joint. Using your support hand to add resistance is usually helpful (Figure 19-36).
3. Once located, strum perpendicular to the fibers and continue palpating the pectineus distally as far as possible.
4. Once the pectineus has been located, have the client relax it, and palpate to assess its baseline tone.

PECTINEUS—SUPINE—cont'd

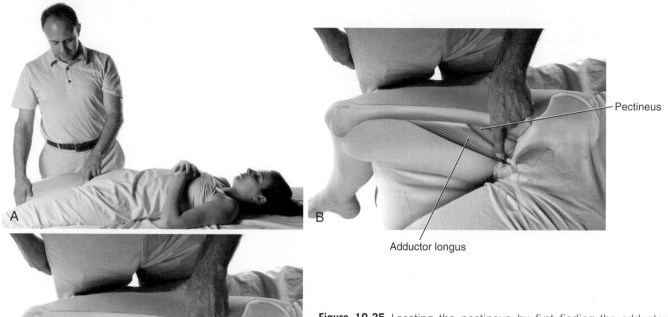

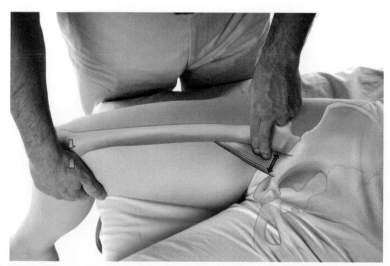

Figure 19-35 Locating the pectineus by first finding the adductor longus tendon. **A,** Starting position for supine palpation of the pectineus. **B,** The therapist first locates and palpates the proximal tendon of the adductor longus, which is the most prominent tendon in the region. **C,** The therapist drops anteriorly (laterally) immediately off the adductor longus tendon onto the pectineus.

Figure 19-36 This figure shows engagement and palpation of the pectineus as the client adducts the thigh against resistance.

PECTINEUS—SUPINE—*cont'd*

PALPATION NOTES

1. When locating the pectineus, the adductor longus tendon is an excellent landmark to use because it is the most prominent tendon in this region of the thigh. When locating it, it is necessary to palpate directly next to the pubic bone. If you are too far distal in the thigh, you will not be able to feel it.

2. Another way to find the pectineus is to first locate the distal tendon of the iliopsoas and then drop off it medially (posteriorly), and you will be on the pectineus. The border between the iliopsoas and pectineus can be distinguished by asking the client to perform a gentle to moderate curl-up of the trunk. This will tense the psoas major tendon but not the pectineus. If you are still on the iliopsoas, keep moving medially along the pubic bone; once you reach tissue that does not engage and tense with this trunk motion, you are on the pectineus.

3. Even though much of the pectineus is superficial, it is recessed compared with the adjacent muscles. When palpating for the pectineus, it often feels as though the palpating fingers drop into a depression or pocket. For this reason, it is sometimes slightly difficult to locate at first and may require either deeper pressure or greater resistance to adduction of the thigh at the hip joint.

4. Keep in mind that asking the client to actively adduct the thigh at the hip joint will cause the other adductors in the region to contract as well.

5. If asking the client to adduct the thigh at the hip joint does not engage the pectineus, you can try asking the client to flex the thigh instead, or to move in an oblique plane motion that combines flexion with adduction of the thigh. (Resistance can be added with your support hand.) However, keep in mind that all muscles in the anterior thigh will contract with thigh flexion.

6. Be careful when palpating the proximal anterior thigh, because the femoral nerve, artery, and vein are located over the iliopsoas and pectineus in this region. If you feel a pulse under your fingers, either gently move the artery out of the way or slightly move your palpating fingers off the artery. Similarly, if you are pressing on the femoral nerve and the client feels shooting pain, move your palpating fingers off the nerve.

TRIGGER POINTS

1. Trigger points (TrPs) in the pectineus often result from or are perpetuated by acute or chronic overuse of the muscle (during activities such as horseback riding, gymnastics, or sexual intercourse), or prolonged shortening of the muscle due to sitting cross-legged or sleeping in the fetal position. They may also occur secondary to degenerative joint disease of the hip.

2. TrPs in the pectineus tend to produce deep dull pain in the groin.

3. The referral patterns of pectineus TrPs must be distinguished from the referral patterns of TrPs in the iliopsoas, sartorius, gracilis, and the three "adductors" of the thigh.

4. TrPs in the pectineus are often incorrectly assessed as degenerative joint disease of the hip or obturator nerve entrapment.

5. Associated TrPs often occur in the iliopsoas, gracilis, and the three "adductors" of the thigh.

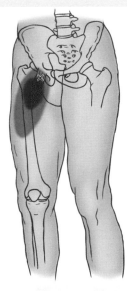

Figure 19-37 Anteromedial view showing a common pectineus trigger point (TrP) with its corresponding referral zone.

Palpation Key:
Drop anteriorly off the adductor longus tendon.

19

PECTINEUS—SUPINE—*cont'd*

STRETCHING THE PECTINEUS

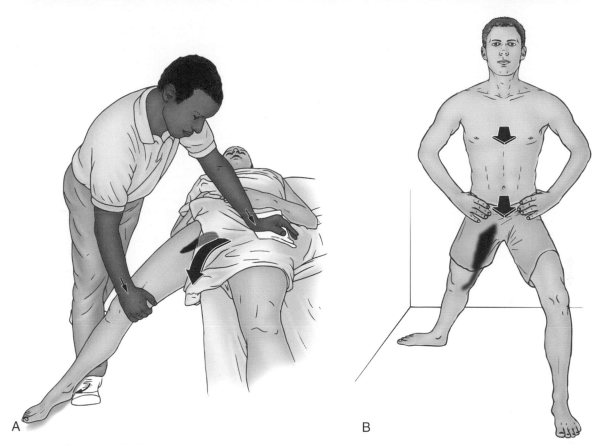

Figure 19-38 Stretching the right pectineus. The client's thigh is abducted, extended, and laterally rotated with the knee joint in full extension. **A,** Therapist-assisted stretch. The therapist moves the client's thigh with his right hand and maintains extension of the client's knee joint with his right foot and leg. Note: The therapist's other hand stabilizes the client's pelvis from anteriorly tilted and rotating to the side of the stretch; a cushion is used for comfort. **B,** Self-care stretch. Note: It is important to make sure that excessive weight is not placed on the ankle joint of the foot in back. See Figure 19-43 and Figure 19-57 for two other stretches of the pectineus.

19

ADDUCTOR LONGUS—SUPINE

☑ ATTACHMENTS

☐ Body of the pubic bone

to the

☐ linea aspera of the femur

☑ ACTIONS

☐ Adducts the thigh at the hip joint
☐ Flexes the thigh at the hip joint
☐ Anteriorly tilts the pelvis at the hip joint

Starting Position (Figure 19-40)

■ Client supine with the right thigh on the table and right leg hanging off the table
■ Therapist standing to the side of the client
■ Palpating fingers placed on the prominent tendon of the adductor longus in the proximal anterior thigh
■ Support hand placed on the distal anteromedial thigh, just proximal to the knee joint

Palpation Steps

1. The proximal tendon of the adductor longus is the most prominent tendon in the medial thigh and usually easily palpable. To locate it, simply palpate along the pubic bone from lateral to medial until you encounter a prominent tendon.
2. Once located, to confirm that you are on it, ask the client to adduct the thigh at the hip joint against resistance, and feel for it to tense (Figure 19-41).
3. Strum perpendicular to the tendon to palpate its width.
4. Continue to palpate it distally as far as possible toward its linea aspera attachment.
5. Once the adductor longus has been located, have the client relax it, and palpate to assess its baseline tone.

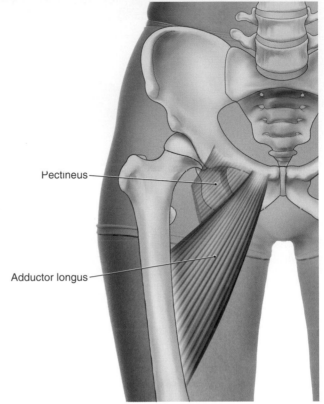

Figure 19-39 Anterior view of the right adductor longus. The pectineus has been cut and ghosted in.

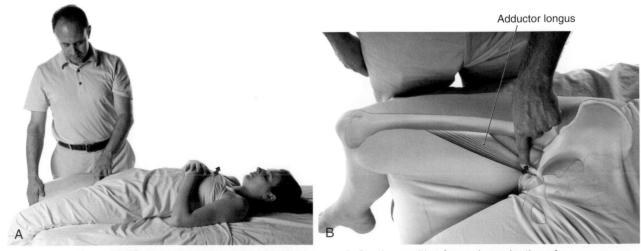

Figure 19-40 Palpation of the right adductor longus. **A,** Starting position for supine palpation of the adductor longus. **B,** Location of the proximal tendon of the adductor longus, which is the most prominent tendon of the region.

19

ADDUCTOR LONGUS—SUPINE—*cont'd*

Figure 19-41 Engagement and palpation of the right adductor longus as the client adducts the thigh at the hip joint against resistance.

PALPATION NOTES

1. The proximal tendon of the adductor longus is very prominent and easily palpable, even when the muscle is relaxed. It is also an excellent landmark to use to find the pectineus (located anterior to the adductor longus) and the gracilis (located posterior to the adductor longus). If you encounter difficulty locating the adductor longus' proximal tendon, then you are probably not palpating proximally enough. It is necessary to palpate directly along the pubic bone.
2. Proximally, the medial border of the adductor longus forms the medial border of the femoral triangle. Located within the femoral triangle are the iliopsoas and pectineus muscles, and the femoral nerve, artery, and vein.

Palpation Key:
Most prominent tendon in the groin region.

TRIGGER POINTS

1. Trigger points (TrPs) in the adductor longus often result from or are perpetuated by acute or chronic overuse of the muscle (during activities such as horseback riding), or prolonged shortening of the muscle due to sleeping on one's side with the thigh in adduction, or sitting for prolonged periods, especially with the legs crossed.
2. TrPs in the adductor longus may be the leading cause of groin pain, and often restrict abduction of the thigh at the hip joint.
3. The referral patterns of adductor longus TrPs must be distinguished from the referral patterns of TrPs in the other two "adductor" muscles, pectineus, sartorius, and the vastus medialis.
4. TrPs in the adductor longus are often incorrectly assessed as an adductor tendinitis/periostitis, degenerative joint disease of the hip, inguinal hernia, prostatitis, or nerve entrapment of the obturator or genitofemoral nerves.
5. Associated TrPs often occur in the other two "adductor" muscles, the gracilis, pectineus, and the vastus medialis.

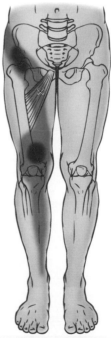

Figure 19-42 Anterior view showing a common adductor longus trigger point (TrP) with its corresponding referral zone.

19

ADDUCTOR LONGUS—SUPINE—*cont'd*

STRETCHING THE ADDUCTOR LONGUS AND BREVIS

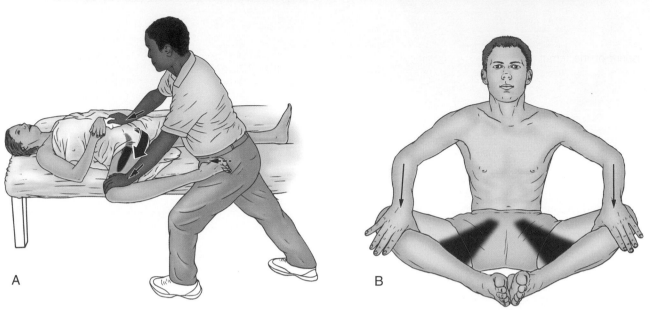

A   B

Figure 19-43 Stretching the adductors longus and brevis. The client's thigh is abducted and laterally rotated at the hip joint and the knee joint is flexed. **A,** Therapist-assisted stretch of the right adductors longus and brevis. The therapist pushes downward with the left hand on the client's distal thigh and forward against the client's foot placed on the anterior superior iliac spine (ASIS). Note: The therapist's right hand stabilizes the client's pelvis from rotating to the side of the stretch and stabilizes the opposite (left) side pelvis from depressing; a cushion is used for comfort. **B,** Self-care stretch for the adductors longus and brevis bilaterally. The client sits and lets gravity pull the thighs into abduction and extension; the client can then use his hands to increase the stretch. See Figure 19-38 and Figure 19-57 for two other stretches of the adductors longus and brevis.

ADDUCTOR LONGUS—SUPINE—*cont'd*

DETOUR

Adductor Brevis:

The adductor brevis attaches from the pubic bone to the linea aspera of the femur and is usually located entirely deep to other adductors of the hip joint, principally the adductor longus. It also has the same actions (adduction and flexion of the thigh at the hip joint) as the nearby adductors. For this reason, it is extremely difficult to palpate and discern the adductor brevis. However, a small part of it is sometimes accessible between the adductor longus and the gracilis. To palpate the adductor brevis, find the border between the adductor longus and gracilis, and try to press between these two muscles, palpating deeper for the adductor brevis (Figure 19-44, *B*). Alternatively, you can try palpating the adductor brevis through

the adductor longus. Keep in mind that if you ask the client to adduct the thigh, all adductors in the region will likely engage, obscuring discernment of the palpation of the adductor brevis.

Trigger Points:

1. Factors that create and/or perpetuate trigger points (TrPs) in the adductor brevis and symptoms caused by TrPs in the adductor brevis are the same as for the adductor longus.
2. TrP referral patterns for the adductor brevis have not been distinguished from the referral patterns for the adductor longus.
3. Note: Due to its depth, palpating and discerning TrPs in the adductor brevis can be difficult.

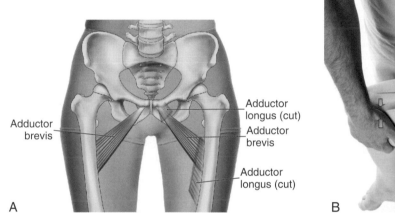

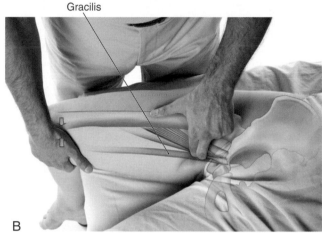

A   B

Figure 19-44 The adductor brevis. **A,** Anterior view. The adductor longus has been cut and ghosted in on the left. **B,** Palpation of the right adductor brevis proximally between the adductor longus (ghosted in) and gracilis as the client adducts the thigh against resistance.

Palpation Key:

Palpate between the adductor longus and gracilis.

19

GRACILIS—SUPINE

✅ ATTACHMENTS

☐ Body and inferior ramus of the pubic bone

to the

☐ pes anserine tendon at the proximal anteromedial tibia

✅ ACTIONS

☐ Adducts the thigh at the hip joint
☐ Flexes the thigh at the hip joint
☐ Flexes the leg at the knee joint
☐ Medially rotates the leg at the knee joint
☐ Anteriorly tilts the pelvis at the hip joint

Starting Position (Figure 19-46, *A*)

■ Client supine with the right thigh on the table and right leg hanging off the table
■ Therapist standing to the side of the client
■ Palpating fingers placed on the proximal medial thigh, on the proximal tendon of the adductor longus

Palpation Steps

1. First locate the proximal tendon of the adductor longus; it is the most prominent tendon in the region. To locate it, simply palpate along the pubic bone from lateral to medial until you encounter a prominent tendon (Figure 19-46, *B* and *C*). Then drop just off it posteriorly (medially), and you will be on the gracilis (Figure 19-47, *A*).
2. Ask the client to engage the gracilis by flexing the leg at the knee joint; this can be easily accomplished by asking the client to press the leg against the table. This engages the gracilis, but not the adductor longus and adductor

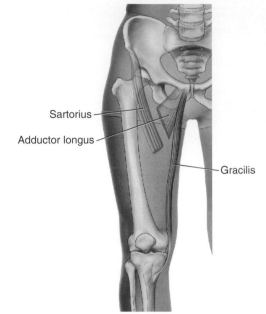

Figure 19-45 Anterior view of the right gracilis. The adductor longus and sartorius have been cut and ghosted in.

magnus on either side of it, making it easy to discern the gracilis in the proximal thigh (Figure 19-47, *B*).
3. Once located, strum perpendicular to the fibers and continue palpating the gracilis distally as far as possible.
4. Once the gracilis has been located, have the client relax it, and palpate to assess its baseline tone.

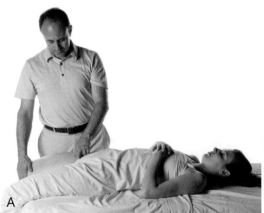

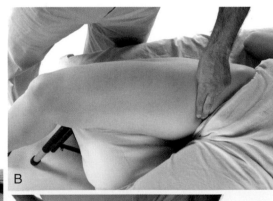

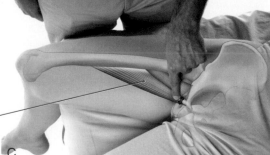

Figure 19-46 Locating the right proximal gracilis by first locating the adductor longus tendon. **A,** Starting position for supine palpation of the right gracilis. **B** and **C,** The therapist first locates and palpates the proximal tendon of the adductor longus, which is the most prominent tendon in the region.

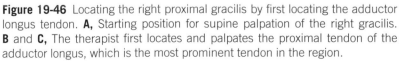
Adductor longus

GRACILIS—SUPINE—*cont'd*

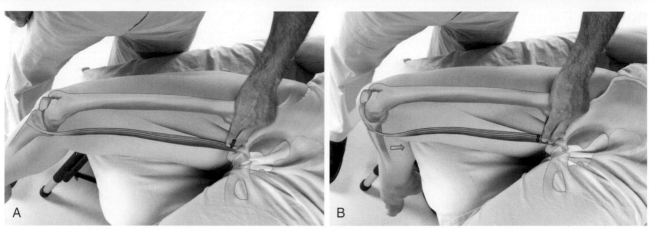

Figure 19-47 Palpation of the right proximal gracilis. **A,** The therapist locates the proximal tendon of the gracilis by dropping medially off the adductor longus tendon. **B,** Engagement and palpation of the gracilis as the client flexes the leg against the resistance of the table. Note: The adductor longus has been ghosted in.

PALPATION NOTES

1. In the proximal thigh, the gracilis is bordered by the adductor longus anteriorly and the adductor magnus posteriorly. Because neither of these other two muscles crosses the knee joint, having the client flex the leg at the knee joint against the table engages the gracilis but not these adjacent muscles. This allows for effective palpation and discernment of the gracilis proximally.
2. To distinguish the gracilis from the sartorius in the distal thigh, use abduction and adduction of the thigh at the hip joint. The sartorius engages with abduction; the gracilis engages with adduction.
3. The distal tendon of the gracilis can also be easily located. Palpate the distal posteromedial thigh while the client medially rotates the leg at the knee joint (The knee joint must be flexed to be able to rotate.), and feel for two tendons to noticeably tense (Figure 19-48). The gracilis is the smaller and more medial one of the two. (The semi-tendinosus is the other one and is larger and more lateral; in other words, closer to the midline of the thigh.) Once located, strum perpendicular and palpate the gracilis proximally toward the pubic bone.

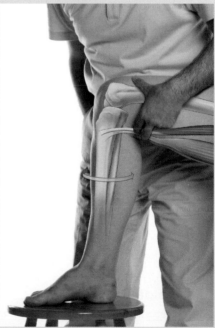

Figure 19-48 Seated palpation of the distal tendon of the right gracilis as the client medially rotates the leg at the knee joint. The semitendinosus has been ghosted in. Note: For the purpose of this photo, the client is standing with the foot on a stool.

19

Alternate Palpation Position—Seated, Prone, or Side Lying

The gracilis can be palpated with the client in a number of positions. Seated palpation is effective (see Palpation Note #3 and Figure 19-48). The gracilis can also be palpated with the client prone; from this perspective it is located beyond (anterior to) the adductor magnus. The gracilis can also be palpated with the client side lying. In this position, palpate the gracilis of the lower extremity that is against the table. Note: To access this gracilis, it is necessary to have the client's thigh of the lower extremity that is away from the table flexed at the hip and knee joints. Use resisted flexion of the leg at the knee joint to engage the gracilis and feel for its contraction (Figure 19-49).

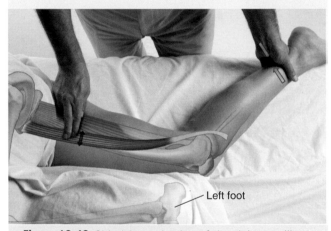

— Left foot

Figure 19-49 Side lying palpation of the right gracilis as the client flexes the leg at the knee joint against resistance. The adductor magnus has been ghosted in. Note: To access the right gracilis, the client's left lower extremity is flexed at the hip and knee joints.

Palpation Key:
Drop posteriorly off the adductor longus tendon.

TRIGGER POINTS

1. Trigger points (TrPs) in the gracilis often result from or are perpetuated by acute or chronic overuse of the muscle (during activities such as horseback riding), or prolonged shortening of the muscle due to sleeping on one's side with the thigh in adduction, or sitting for prolonged periods, especially with the legs crossed.
2. TrPs in the gracilis may produce either a hot stinging pain or a dull ache and may result in a decrease in range of the motion of abduction of the thigh at the hip joint. Clients with TrPs in the gracilis often have difficulty finding a position of comfort.
3. The referral patterns of gracilis TrPs must be distinguished from the referral patterns of TrPs in the three "adductors" of the thigh, pectineus, sartorius, and vastus medialis.
4. TrPs in the gracilis are often incorrectly assessed as an adductor tendinitis/periostitis, inguinal hernia, pes anserine bursitis, prostatitis, or nerve entrapment of the obturator or genitofemoral nerves.
5. Associated TrPs often occur in the distal sartorius.

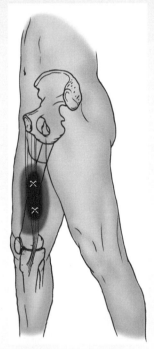

Figure 19-50 Medial view showing common gracilis trigger points (TrPs) with their corresponding referral zone.

GRACILIS—SUPINE—*cont'd*

STRETCHING THE GRACILIS

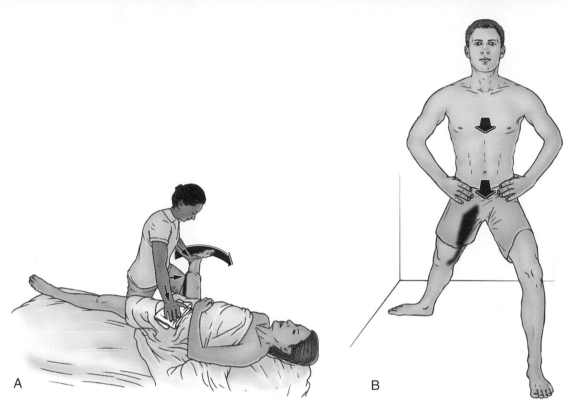

A   B

Figure 19-51 Stretching the right gracilis. The client's thigh is abducted, laterally rotated, and extended, while keeping the knee joint fully extended. **A,** Therapist-assisted stretch. The therapist contacts the client with her left hand and left thigh. Note: The therapist's right hand stabilizes the client's pelvis from rotating to the side of the stretch and stabilizes the opposite (left) side pelvis from depressing; a cushion is used for comfort. **B,** Self-care stretch. Note: It is important to not let the pelvis fall into anterior tilt and to make sure that excessive weight is not placed on the ankle joint of the foot in back. See Figure 19-57 for another stretch of the gracilis.

ADDUCTOR MAGNUS—SUPINE

☑ ATTACHMENTS

☐ Ischial tuberosity and the ischiopubic ramus

to the

☐ linea aspera and adductor tubercle of the femur

☑ ACTIONS

☐ Adducts the thigh at the hip joint
☐ Extends the thigh at the hip joint
☐ Posteriorly tilts the pelvis at the hip joint

Starting Position (Figure 19-53)

■ Client supine with the right thigh on the table and right leg hanging off the table
■ Therapist standing to the side of the client
■ Palpating fingers placed on the proximal medial thigh (between the gracilis and medial hamstrings)
■ Support hand placed on the distal medial thigh if resistance to adduction will be given

Palpation Steps

1. The adductor magnus is actually quite easily palpable in the proximal medial thigh between the gracilis and the medial hamstrings (semitendinosus and semimembranosus), where it is located in a depression between these muscles.
2. Locate the adductor magnus by first locating the gracilis and medial hamstrings, which contract with flexion of the leg at the knee joint, performed by asking the client to press the leg against the table. Once you feel these muscles palpably harden with leg flexion, feel for the adductor magnus between them (It will stay relaxed and soft during this joint action.) (Figure 19-54, *A*).
3. To engage the adductor magnus and confirm that you are on it, ask the client to either adduct the thigh against resistance supplied by your support hand, or to extend the thigh at the hip joint against the resistance of the table (as shown in Figure 19-54, *B*).

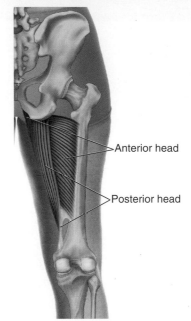

Figure 19-52 Posterior view of the right adductor magnus.

(labels: Anterior head, Posterior head)

4. Continue palpating the adductor magnus distally as far as possible while strumming perpendicular to the fibers as the client alternately contracts and relaxes it.
5. Once the adductor magnus has been located, have the client relax it, and palpate to assess its baseline tone.

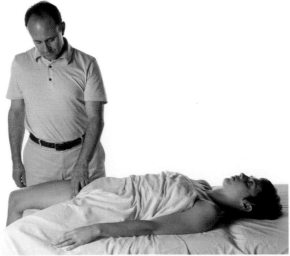

Figure 19-53 Starting position for supine palpation of the right adductor magnus.

19

ADDUCTOR MAGNUS—SUPINE—*cont'd*

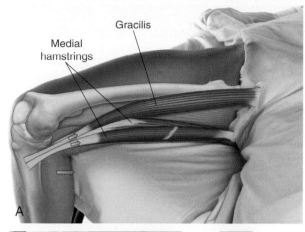

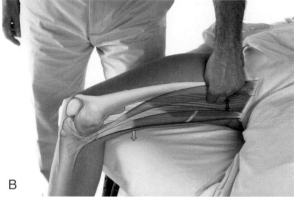

Figure 19-54 Palpation of the right adductor magnus in the medial thigh between the gracilis and medial hamstrings. **A,** The gracilis and medial hamstrings engage when the client flexes the leg at the knee joint by pressing the leg against the table. **B,** Engagement and palpation of the adductor magnus between these muscles as the client extends the thigh at the hip joint by pressing the thigh down against the table.

PALPATION NOTES

1. The easiest way to confirm that you are on the adductor magnus is to ask the client to flex the leg at the knee joint. The gracilis and medial hamstring musculature (semitendinosus and semimembranosus) located on either side of the adductor magnus contract with this joint action and become palpably hard, whereas the adductor magnus does not contract and remains relaxed and soft. If you are between these two other muscles, you are on the adductor magnus.
2. The adductor magnus itself can be engaged by asking the client to adduct or extend the thigh at the hip joint against resistance. Note that the gracilis also contracts with adduction, but not with extension. Also, the medial hamstrings contract with extension, but not with adduction. Therefore these actions can be used to distinguish the borders of the adductor magnus with these adjacent muscles.
3. The adductor magnus sits in a slightly recessed depression in the medial thigh between the gracilis and the medial hamstrings. Therefore it is usually necessary to gently but firmly press in to feel this muscle.
4. Other than the portion of the adductor magnus that is superficial in the proximal medial thigh, most of the rest of the muscle is deep and difficult to discern from adjacent musculature. From the anterior perspective, the adductor magnus can be looked at as a floor for the other more anterior adductor muscles of the thigh. From the posterior perspective, the adductor magnus can be looked at as a floor for the more posterior hamstring muscles of the thigh.
5. The attachment on the adductor tubercle of the femur at the medial side of the knee joint is often palpable.

Alternate Palpation Position—Prone or Side Lying

The adductor magnus can also be accessed with the client prone or side lying. In prone position, the adductor magnus is located directly anterior to the medial hamstring muscles (see Figure 19-1, *A*). In side lying position, the client's lower extremity that is away from the table must be flexed at the hip and knee joints so that the adductor magnus of the thigh that is against the table can be accessed.

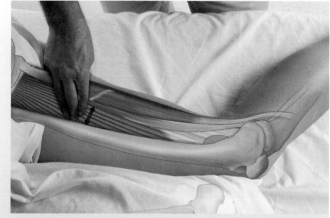

Figure 19-55 Side lying palpation of the right adductor magnus.

19

ADDUCTOR MAGNUS—SUPINE—*cont'd*

TRIGGER POINTS

1. Trigger points (TrPs) in the adductor magnus often result from or are perpetuated by acute or chronic overuse of the muscle (during activities such as skiing or horseback riding), or prolonged shortening of the muscle due to sleeping on one's side with the thigh in adduction, or sitting for prolonged periods, especially with the legs crossed.
2. Clients with adductor magnus TrPs often experience difficulty positioning their lower extremity at night. The more proximal TrP (Figure 19-56, *B*) of the adductor magnus can create pain that is felt within the pelvis; in some clients, this pain occurs during sexual intercourse.
3. The referral patterns of adductor magnus TrPs must be distinguished from the referral patterns of TrPs in the other two "adductors," pectineus, sartorius, vastus medialis, and perhaps the iliopsoas.
4. TrPs in the adductor magnus are often incorrectly assessed as an adductor tendinitis/periostitis, inguinal hernia, prostatitis, visceral or gynecologic disease, or nerve entrapment of the obturator or genitofemoral nerves.
5. Associated TrPs often occur in the other two "adductor" muscles, the pectineus, and the vastus medialis.
6. Note: Because much of the adductor magnus is deep, palpating TrPs in this muscle can be difficult.

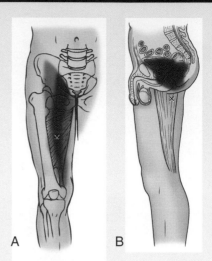

Figure 19-56 Views of the right adductor magnus with common trigger points (TrPs) and their corresponding referral zones. **A,** Anterior view. **B,** Medial view of a sagittal section through the pelvis showing another common adductor magnus TrP with its internal visceral referral zone.

STRETCHING THE ADDUCTOR MAGNUS

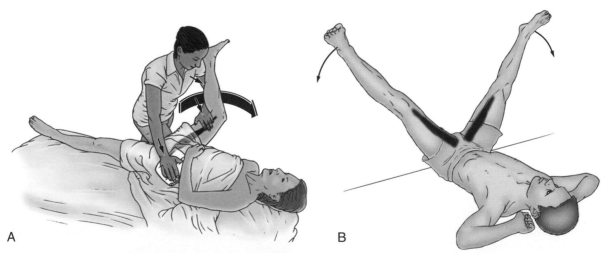

A   B

Figure 19-57 Stretching the adductor magnus. The client's thigh is abducted and flexed. **A,** Therapist-assisted stretch for the right adductor magnus. The therapist contacts the client with her left hand and left arm. Note: The therapist's right hand stabilizes the client's pelvis from rotating to the side of the stretch and stabilizes the opposite (left) side pelvis from depressing; a cushion is used for comfort. **B,** Self-care stretch for the adductor magnus bilaterally. The client lies against a wall and lets gravity pull his thighs into abduction. See Figure 19-43 for another stretch of the adductor magnus. Figure 19-51 shows a good stretch of the most proximal fibers of the anterior head of the adductor magnus.

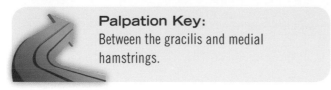

Palpation Key:
Between the gracilis and medial hamstrings.

19

WHIRLWIND TOUR

Muscles of the Thigh

The following *Whirlwind Tour* is an abbreviated set of palpation protocols for the muscles of this chapter. Once you have read and become comfortable with each of the protocols presented thus far, this *Whirlwind Tour* allows you to quickly and efficiently run through the palpations protocols for all the muscles of the chapter.

For all palpations of the muscles of the thigh, the therapist is standing to the side of the client.

Client Supine

For all palpations of the muscles of the thigh except the prone palpation of the hamstrings at the end, the client is supine with the right thigh on the table and right leg hanging off the table.

1. **Tensor fasciae latae (TFL):** Have the client first medially rotate the thigh at the hip joint and then flex the thigh into the air. Palpating just distal and lateral to the anterior superior iliac spine (ASIS), feel for the contraction of the TFL. Strum perpendicular, and palpate to the distal attachment.

2. **Sartorius:** Have the client first laterally rotate the thigh at the hip joint and then flex the thigh into the air. Palpating just distal and medial to the ASIS, feel for the contraction of the sartorius. Strum perpendicular, and palpate toward the distal attachment as far as possible. Distally, the sartorius is directly posterior to the vastus medialis; use extension of the leg at the knee joint to locate the vastus medialis. Confirm that you are on the distal sartorius by asking the client to flex the leg at the knee joint against the resistance of the table.

3. **Quadriceps femoris group:** Proximally, the rectus femoris is between the sartorius and the TFL. Find either one of these muscles and then drop onto the rectus femoris. Ask the client to extend the leg at the knee joint, and feel for the contraction of the rectus femoris. Strum perpendicular, and palpate to the distal attachment. Palpate in the distal anteromedial thigh for the vastus medialis and in the anterolateral, lateral, and posterolateral thigh for the vastus lateralis, always using leg extension to engage these muscles.

4. **Iliopsoas distal belly and tendon:** Find the proximal attachment of the sartorius and drop immediately medial onto the distal belly and tendon of the iliopsoas. Ask the client to do a gentle to moderate curl-up of the trunk and feel for the tensing of the belly and tendon of the psoas major. Be aware of the presence of the femoral nerve, artery, and vein in this region.

5. **Adductor longus:** Palpate along the pubic bone within the anteromedial thigh, feeling for the prominent tendon of the adductor longus. Once located, ask the client to adduct the thigh against gentle to moderate resistance, and feel for the contraction of the adductor longus. Strum perpendicular, and continue palpating distally as far as possible. Be aware that all adductors in this region will contract with resisted adduction of the thigh.

6. **Pectineus:** First locate the proximal tendon of the adductor longus, and then drop immediately off it laterally (anteriorly) onto the pectineus. Ask the client to adduct and/or flex the thigh at the hip joint, and feel for its contraction.

Pressing deeper and/or adding greater resistance may be necessary. Strum perpendicular, and continue palpating the pectineus distally as far as possible. Be aware of the presence of the femoral nerve, artery, and vein in this region.

7. **Gracilis:** First find the proximal tendon of the adductor longus, and then drop off it immediately medially (posteriorly) onto the gracilis. Ask the client to flex the leg at the knee joint by pressing the leg against the table, and feel for the contraction of the gracilis. Strum perpendicular to the fibers and follow distally to the pes anserine. Note: The distal tendon can also be located by palpating the distal posteromedial thigh and asking the client to medially rotate the leg at the knee joint, feeling for the gracilis and semitendinosus tendons to noticeably tense. The gracilis is the smaller and more medially located of the two tendons. Strum perpendicular, and palpate it proximally to the pubic bone.

8. **Adductor magnus:** Palpate immediately posterior from the gracilis onto the adductor magnus. You know you are on the adductor magnus when you do not feel a contraction when the client presses the leg against the table (flexion of the leg at the knee joint). Confirm you are on the adductor magnus by resisting the client from adducting the thigh at the hip joint (Be aware that all adductors in this region may engage with this action.) or by extending the thigh at the hip joint by pressing the thigh against the table. (Be aware that the hamstrings will likely engage with this action.) Palpate distally as far as possible while strumming perpendicular to the fibers. Note: The adductor magnus is located between the gracilis and medial hamstring musculature; these muscles can be felt to contract when the client presses the leg against the table (flexion of the leg at the knee joint). The adductor magnus does not cross the knee joint and stays relaxed when the leg flexes at the knee joint.

9. **Hamstrings (supine):** From the adductor magnus, palpate immediately posterior onto the medial hamstrings (semitendinosus and semimembranosus). Confirm that you are on the hamstrings by feeling their contraction when the client presses the leg against the table (flexion of the leg at the knee joint).

Client Prone with the Leg Partially Flexed at the Knee Joint

10. **Entire hamstring group:** Resist the client from further flexing the leg at the knee joint, and feel for the common proximal attachment of the hamstring group just distal to the ischial tuberosity. Strum perpendicular to the fibers, and continue palpating the biceps femoris distally toward the head of the fibula. Then strum perpendicularly and continue palpating the medial hamstrings distally toward the medial side of the leg. The medial and lateral hamstrings are side by side in the proximal thigh, but they diverge in the distal thigh. Note: The semitendinosus is generally superficial to the semimembranosus, and its distal tendon is very prominent. Palpate on either side of the distal semitendinosus for the semimembranosus.

19

Review Questions

1. List the attachments of the TFL.
2. List the attachments of the pectineus.
3. What are the actions of the sartorius?
4. What are the actions of the gracilis?
5. Palpation of the hamstring group generally utilizes flexion of the leg at the knee joint as all the muscles of this group share this action. Is there an alternate, shared action at another joint that can be used?
6. What advantage does placing the client supine with the leg hanging off the table give when palpating the TFL?
7. To what important anatomic feature does the medial border of the proximal sartorius contribute?
8. What type of bone is the patella, and what is its function in relation to the quadriceps femoris muscles?
9. Though the pectineus is a superficial muscle, what physical feature of it can present palpatory difficulty? Is there any other structure or feature of the muscle that suggests caution on the part of the therapist?
10. The adductor longus is used as a landmark for palpation of adjacent musculature for what reason?
11. What muscle is located between the gracilis and the medial hamstrings?
12. TrPs in what muscle might cause difficulty in positioning the lower extremity at night for sleeping, and pelvic pain that can manifest during sexual intercourse?
13. What differences, if any, are there in the pain intensity and location for TrPs in the hamstring group?
14. What is a proper stretch for the left TFL?
15. How would you instruct a client to stretch the left gracilis?
16. Describe how a therapist can be sure to distinguish the medial and lateral borders of the hamstring group from the surrounding musculature.
17. Describe a method by which a therapist may palpate and distinguish the gracilis from the adductor magnus.

CASE STUDY

A 45-year-old man comes in for a massage session complaining of pain and discomfort in the posterolateral right knee and posterior thigh. The issue began as a dull ache a few months ago and has become steadily worse over time. He now experiences periods of sharp pain and often wakes up from the discomfort when he is sleeping.

The client works both as database manager whose job consists mostly of desk work with an occasional call to leave the office to perform hardware repair and as an independent contractor troubleshooting software programs. Medical history reveals that he is being treated for high blood pressure, high cholesterol, and has been advised that he is at least 40 pounds overweight. After several visits to his primary care physician for knee pain, he received a magnetic resonance imaging (MRI) scan, which was negative for any injury. He tried a few weeks of physical therapy which consisted of resistance strengthening exercise, but he felt that the pain increased during that time, so he stopped treatment.

Physical exam and palpation shows decreased flexion of the right thigh at the hip joint, some muscle weakness in flexion of the right leg at the knee joint, and a bilaterally hypotonic gluteus maximus.

1. Do this client's symptoms fit any known TrP pain distribution patterns? What other muscular patterns are demonstrated here?
2. What factors in the client's life may have precipitated these symptoms, and how would that lead to his current situation?

CHAPTER 20

Tour #10

Palpation of the Leg Muscles

Overview

This chapter is a palpation tour of the muscles of the leg. The tour begins with the muscles of the anterior compartment, then covers the muscles of the lateral compartment, and concludes with the muscles of the superficial and deep posterior compartments. Palpation of the muscles of the anterior compartment is shown supine; palpation of the muscles of the lateral compartment is shown side lying; and palpation of the muscles of the posterior compartments is shown prone. Alternate palpation positions for most of the muscles are also described. The major muscles or muscle groups of the region are each given a separate layout. There are also a few detours to other muscles of the region. Trigger point (TrP) information and stretching, both therapist-assisted and self-care stretching, are given for each of the muscles covered in this chapter. The chapter closes with an advanced *Whirlwind Tour* that explains the sequential palpation of all of the muscles of the chapter.

Chapter Outline

Tibialis Anterior—Supine
Extensor Digitorum Longus (EDL)—Supine
    Detour to the Fibularis Tertius
Extensor Hallucis Longus (EHL)—Supine
Fibularis Longus and Fibularis Brevis—Side Lying
Gastrocnemius—Prone
    Detour to the Plantaris
Soleus—Prone
Popliteus—Prone
Tibialis Posterior (TP), Flexor Digitorum Longus (FDL), and Flexor Hallucis Longus (FHL)—Prone
Whirlwind Tour: Muscles of the Leg

Chapter Objectives

After completing this chapter, the student/therapist should be able to perform the following for each of the muscles covered in this chapter:
1. State the attachments.
2. State the actions.
3. Describe the starting position for palpation.
4. Describe and explain the purpose of each of the palpation steps.
5. Palpate each muscle.
6. State the "Palpation Key."
7. Describe alternate palpation positions.
8. State the locations of the most common TrP(s).
9. Describe the TrP referral zones.
10. State the most common factors that create and/or perpetuate TrPs.
11. State the symptoms most commonly caused by TrPs.
12. Describe and perform the therapist-assisted and self-care stretches.

e Go to http://evolve.elsevier.com/Muscolino/palpation for video demonstrations of the muscle palpations presented in this chapter.

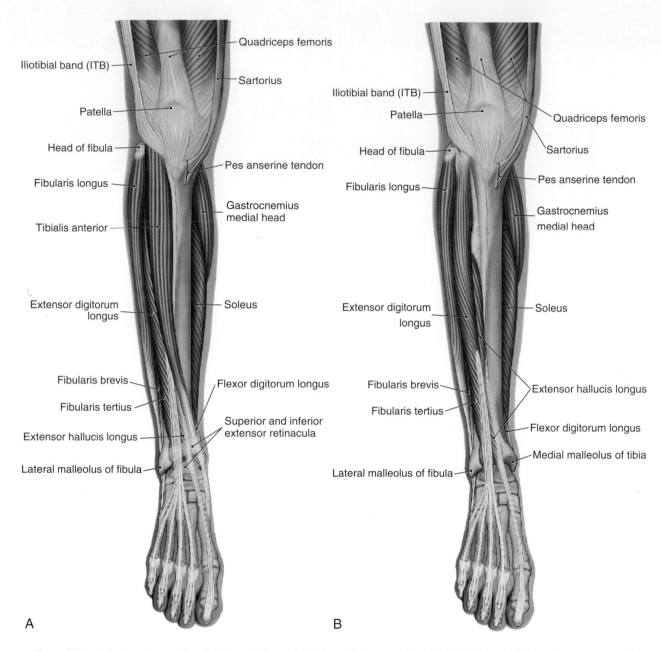

Iliotibial band (ITB)
Quadriceps femoris
Sartorius
Patella
Head of fibula
Pes anserine tendon
Fibularis longus
Gastrocnemius medial head
Tibialis anterior
Extensor digitorum longus
Soleus
Fibularis brevis
Flexor digitorum longus
Fibularis tertius
Superior and inferior extensor retinacula
Extensor hallucis longus
Lateral malleolus of fibula

Iliotibial band (ITB)
Quadriceps femoris
Patella
Sartorius
Head of fibula
Pes anserine tendon
Fibularis longus
Gastrocnemius medial head
Extensor digitorum longus
Soleus
Fibularis brevis
Extensor hallucis longus
Fibularis tertius
Flexor digitorum longus
Medial malleolus of tibia
Lateral malleolus of fibula

A   B

Figure 20-1 Anterior views of the right leg. **A,** Superficial view. **B,** Deeper view. (The tibialis anterior has been removed.)

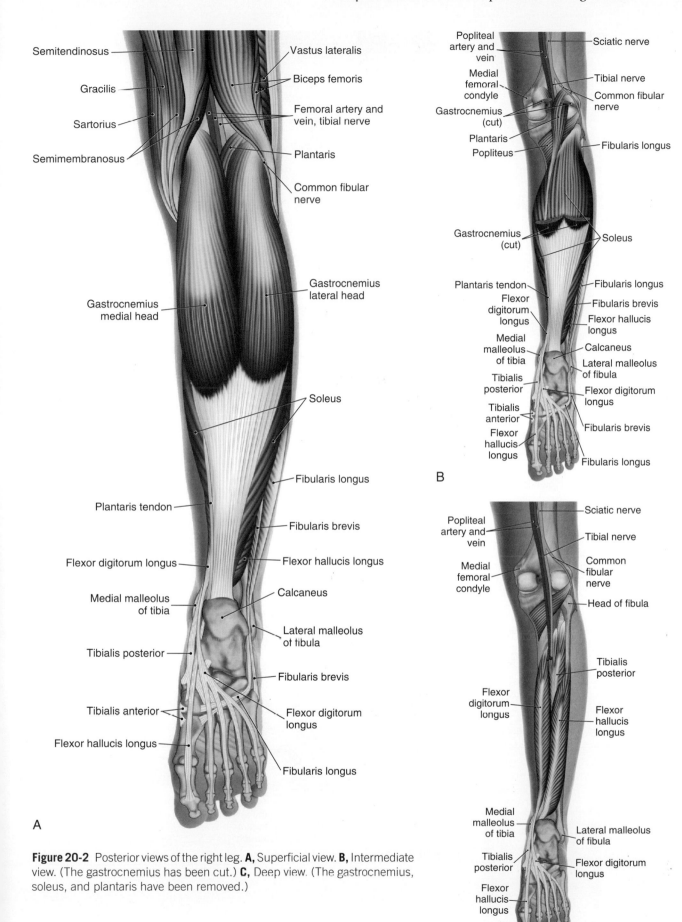

Figure 20-2 Posterior views of the right leg. **A,** Superficial view. **B,** Intermediate view. (The gastrocnemius has been cut.) **C,** Deep view. (The gastrocnemius, soleus, and plantaris have been removed.)

20

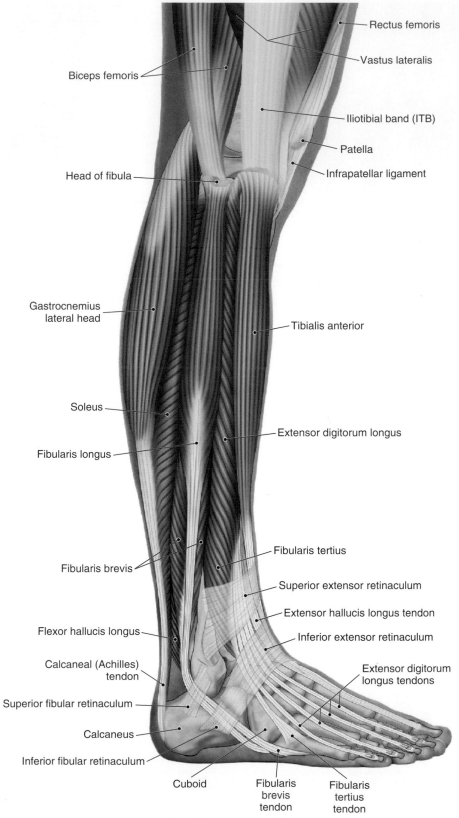

Rectus femoris

Vastus lateralis

Biceps femoris

Iliotibial band (ITB)

Patella

Infrapatellar ligament

Head of fibula

Gastrocnemius lateral head

Tibialis anterior

Soleus

Extensor digitorum longus

Fibularis longus

Fibularis tertius

Fibularis brevis

Superior extensor retinaculum

Extensor hallucis longus tendon

Inferior extensor retinaculum

Flexor hallucis longus

Extensor digitorum longus tendons

Calcaneal (Achilles) tendon

Superior fibular retinaculum

Calcaneus

Inferior fibular retinaculum

Cuboid

Fibularis brevis tendon

Fibularis tertius tendon

Figure 20-3 Lateral view of the right leg.

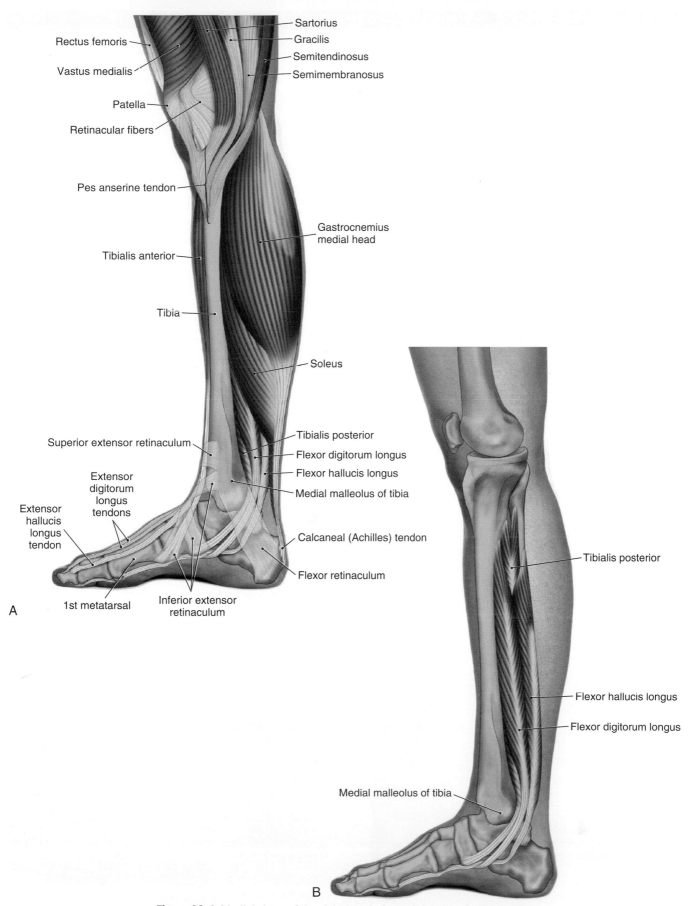

Rectus femoris
Vastus medialis
Patella
Retinacular fibers
Pes anserine tendon
Tibialis anterior
Tibia
Superior extensor retinaculum
Extensor digitorum longus tendons
Extensor hallucis longus tendon
1st metatarsal
Inferior extensor retinaculum

Sartorius
Gracilis
Semitendinosus
Semimembranosus

Gastrocnemius medial head

Soleus

Tibialis posterior
Flexor digitorum longus
Flexor hallucis longus
Medial malleolus of tibia

Calcaneal (Achilles) tendon

Flexor retinaculum

A

Tibialis posterior

Flexor hallucis longus

Flexor digitorum longus

Medial malleolus of tibia

B

Figure 20-4 Medial views of the right leg. **A,** Superficial view. **B,** Deep view.

20

TIBIALIS ANTERIOR—SUPINE

✅ATTACHMENTS

- ☐ Lateral tibial condyle and the proximal ⅔ of the anterior border of the tibia

  to the

- ☐ first cuneiform and the base of the first metatarsal

✅ACTIONS

- ☐ Dorsiflexes the foot at the ankle joint
- ☐ Inverts the foot at the tarsal joints

Starting Position (Figure 20-6)

- ◼ Client supine
- ◼ Therapist standing to the side of the client
- ◼ Palpating hand not yet placed on the client
- ◼ Support hand placed on the medial side of the distal foot

Palpation Steps

1. Resist the client from dorsiflexing and inverting the foot and look for the distal tendon of the tibialis anterior on the medial side of the ankle joint and foot; it is usually visible (Figure 20-7).
2. Palpate the distal tendon by strumming perpendicular across it. Continue palpating the tibialis anterior proximally to the lateral tibial condyle while strumming perpendicular to the fibers. Its belly is located directly lateral to the border of the tibia in the anterior leg (Figure 20-8).
3. Once the tibialis anterior has been located, have the client relax it and palpate to assess its baseline tone.

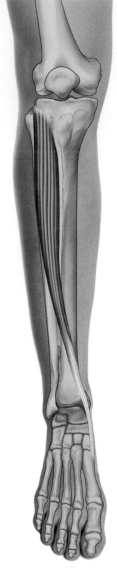

Figure 20-5 Anterior view of the right tibialis anterior.

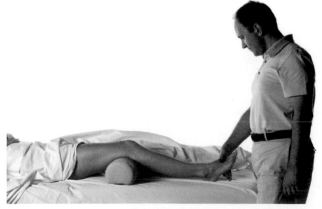

Figure 20-6 Starting position for supine palpation of the right tibialis anterior.

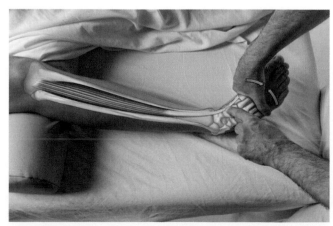

Figure 20-7 With resisted dorsiflexion and inversion of the foot, the distal tendon of the tibialis anterior is usually easily visible.

20

TIBIALIS ANTERIOR—SUPINE—cont'd

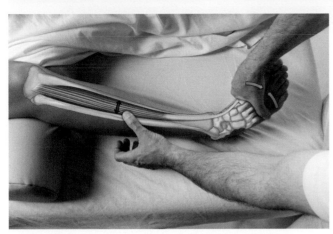

Figure 20-8 Palpation of the belly of the right tibialis anterior.

Alternate Palpation Position—Seated

The tibialis anterior can also be easily palpated with the client seated.

PALPATION NOTES

1. As with all superficial muscles, it is always best to look before placing your palpating hand over the muscle. Otherwise your hand may block your view, making it difficult to see and locate the muscle and its tendon.
2. The distal tendon of the tibialis anterior is usually very prominent and visible. The belly is also usually prominent and visible directly lateral to the shaft of the tibia in the anterior leg. If the tendon and belly are not visible, they can usually be easily palpated by strumming perpendicularly.
3. The distal attachment of the tibialis anterior can be discerned with careful palpation. Follow the tibialis anterior toward the first cuneiform and base of the first metatarsal while having the client alternately contract and relax the tibialis anterior against gentle resistance (see Figure 20-7).
4. To clearly discern the border between the tibialis anterior and the adjacent extensor digitorum longus (EDL), do not ask the client to dorsiflex the foot because it will engage both muscles. Instead use inversion and eversion. Inversion engages the tibialis anterior but not the EDL; eversion engages the EDL but not the tibialis anterior.
5. The belly and tendon of the extensor hallucis longus (EHL) are located directly next to the tibialis anterior, and this muscle also contracts with dorsiflexion and inversion of the foot. If the presence of this muscle makes it difficult to discern the tibialis anterior, ask the client to flex the big toe while you gently resist dorsiflexion and inversion of the foot. Flexion of the big toe will reciprocally inhibit the EHL. (Remember that strong resistance to foot dorsiflexion/inversion will likely override reciprocal inhibition of the EHL.)

TRIGGER POINTS

1. Trigger points (TrPs) in the tibialis anterior often result from or are perpetuated by acute or chronic overuse of the muscle, trauma, postures that result in chronic shortening of the muscle, and tight antagonistic ankle joint plantarflexor muscles.
2. TrPs in the tibialis anterior may produce weakness of dorsiflexion of the foot (which may result in foot drop or foot slap).
3. The referral patterns of tibialis anterior TrPs must be distinguished from the referral patterns of TrPs in the extensor hallucis longus (EHL), extensor digitorum longus (EDL), fibularis tertius, extensor digitorum brevis, extensor hallucis brevis, and first dorsal interosseus pedis.
4. TrPs in the tibialis anterior are often incorrectly assessed as anterior compartment syndrome, anterior shin splints, L5 nerve compression, or first metatarsophalangeal joint dysfunction.
5. Associated TrPs often occur in the fibularis longus, EHL, and EDL.

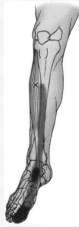

Figure 20-9 Anteromedial view showing a common tibialis anterior trigger point (TrP) and its corresponding referral zone.

Palpation Key:
First look for the distal tendon.

20

TIBIALIS ANTERIOR—SUPINE—*cont'd*

STRETCHING THE TIBIALIS ANTERIOR

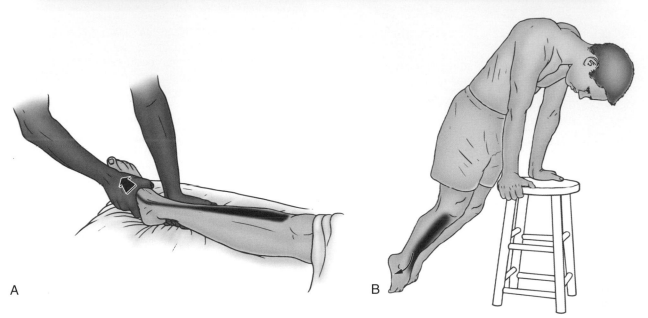

A

B

Figure 20-10 Stretching the tibialis anterior. The client's foot is plantarflexed and everted. **A,** Therapist-assisted stretch for the right tibialis anterior. Note that the therapist uses the other hand to stabilize the client's leg. **B,** Self-care stretch for the tibialis anterior bilaterally. The stool is used for support and to prevent the client from placing excessive weight upon the toes and feet.

EXTENSOR DIGITORUM LONGUS (EDL)—SUPINE

☑ ATTACHMENTS

☐ Proximal ⅔ of the anterior fibula and the lateral tibial condyle

to the

☐ dorsal surface of the middle and distal phalanges of toes two to five

☑ ACTIONS

☐ Extends toes two to five at the metatarsophalangeal (MTP) and interphalangeal (IP) joints
☐ Dorsiflexes the foot at the ankle joint
☐ Everts the foot at the tarsal joints

Starting Position (Figure 20-12)

■ Client supine
■ Therapist standing to the side of the client
■ Palpating hand not yet placed on the client
■ Fingers of the support hand placed on the dorsal surfaces of toes two to five

Palpation Steps

1. Resist the client from extending toes two to five at the MTP and IP joints and look for the tendons of the extensor digitorum longus (EDL) to become visible on the dorsum of the foot.
2. Palpate the distal tendons by strumming perpendicularly across them (Figure 20-13, *A*).
3. Continue palpating the EDL proximally while strumming perpendicular to the fibers (see Figure 20-13, *B*). Most of its belly is located between the tibialis anterior and the fibularis longus (see Figure 20-1, *A*).
4. Once the EDL has been located, have the client relax it, and palpate to assess its baseline tone.

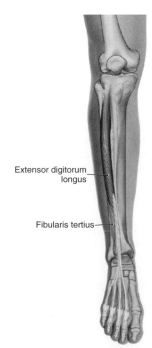

Figure 20-11 Anterior view of the right extensor digitorum longus (EDL). The fibularis tertius has been ghosted in.

Extensor digitorum longus

Fibularis tertius

20

EXTENSOR DIGITORUM LONGUS (EDL)—SUPINE—*cont'd*

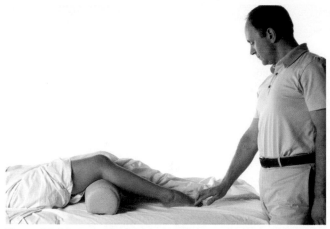

Figure 20-12 Starting position for supine palpation of the right extensor digitorum longus (EDL).

Alternate Palpation Position—Seated

The EDL can also be easily palpated with the client seated.

Palpation Key:
First look for the distal tendons going to toes two to five.

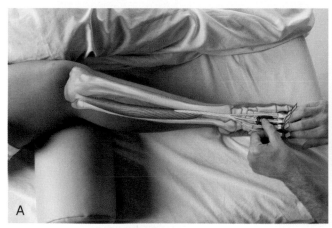
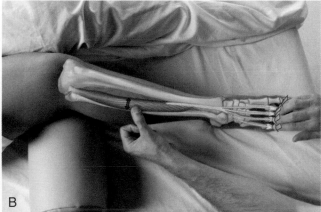

A

B

Figure 20-13 Anterior views of palpation of the right extensor digitorum longus (EDL) as the client extends toes two to five against resistance. **A,** Palpation of the distal tendons on the dorsum of the foot. **B,** Palpation of the belly in the anterolateral leg.

PALPATION NOTES

1. Many people have difficulty isolating motion of their toes. The client may be unable to extend toes two to five without also extending the big toe. If this occurs, do not restrain the big toe from extending. This may stop the big toe from moving but will not stop the extensor hallucis longus (EHL) muscle from isometrically contracting. It is the contraction of the belly of the EHL that is not wanted.

2. As with all superficial muscles, it is always best to look before placing your palpating hand over the muscle. Otherwise your hand may block your view, making it difficult to see and locate the muscle and its tendon. The distal tendons of the EDL are usually very prominent and visible and can be palpated by strumming perpendicularly.

3. To clearly discern the border between the EDL and the adjacent tibialis anterior, do not ask the client to dorsiflex the foot because it will engage both muscles. Instead use inversion and eversion. Eversion engages the EDL but not the tibialis anterior; inversion engages the tibialis anterior but not the EDL.

4. To clearly discern the border between the EDL and the adjacent fibularis longus, do not ask the client to evert the foot because it will engage both muscles. Instead use dorsiflexion and plantarflexion. Dorsiflexion engages the EDL but not the fibularis longus; plantarflexion engages the fibularis longus but not the EDL.

20

EXTENSOR DIGITORUM LONGUS (EDL)—SUPINE—*cont'd*

TRIGGER POINTS

1. Trigger points (TrPs) in the EDL often result from or are perpetuated by acute or chronic overuse of the muscle (especially because of a weak fibularis longus), postures that result in chronic shortening of the muscle (e.g., driving with a sharply angled gas pedal), chronic lengthening of the muscle (e.g., wearing high-heeled shoes or sleeping with foot in dorsiflexion), tight antagonistic ankle joint plantarflexor muscles, trauma, tripping (with ankle joint forced into plantarflexion), anterior compartment syndrome, and L4-L5 nerve compression.
2. TrPs in the EDL may produce ankle joint dorsiflexion weakness (which may result in foot drop or foot slap), entrapment of the deep fibular nerve (which may further dorsiflexion weakness), growing pains, and night cramps in the belly of the muscle.
3. The referral patterns of EDL TrPs must be distinguished from the referral patterns of TrPs in the fibularis longus, fibularis brevis, fibularis tertius, extensor digitorum brevis, dorsal interossei pedis, and extensor hallucis brevis.
4. TrPs in the EDL are often incorrectly assessed as tarsal joint dysfunction, MTP joint dysfunction, or L4 nerve compression.

5. Associated TrPs often occur in the fibularis longus, fibularis brevis, fibularis tertius, tibialis anterior, and extensor hallucis longus (EHL).

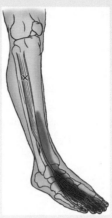

Figure 20-14 Anterolateral view showing a common extensor digitorum longus (EDL) trigger point (TrP) and its corresponding referral zone.

STRETCHING THE EXTENSOR DIGITORUM LONGUS

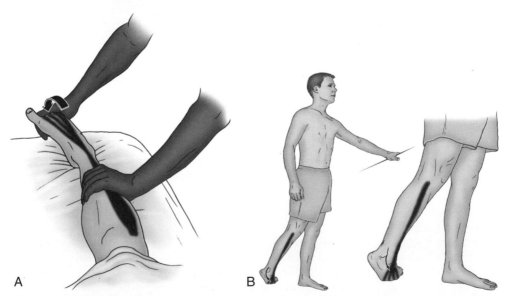

A   B

Figure 20-15 Stretching the right extensor digitorum longus (EDL). The client's toes (two to five) are flexed, and the foot is plantarflexed and inverted. **A,** Therapist-assisted stretch. Note that the therapist uses the other hand to stabilize the client's leg. **B** and **C,** Self-care stretch. The client should hold on to a stable object for support and to prevent placing excessive weight upon the foot in back.

20

EXTENSOR DIGITORUM LONGUS (EDL)—SUPINE—*cont'd*

DETOUR

Fibularis Tertius:

The fibularis tertius is actually the most distal and lateral aspect of the extensor digitorum longus (EDL) and attaches from the distal anterior fibula to the base of the fifth metatarsal. First find the distal tendon of the EDL that goes to the little toe on the dorsum of the foot; then palpate directly lateral to it, feeling for a tendon that goes to the fifth metatarsal. It may not be visible, so you may need to strum perpendicular to its fiber direction to feel for it; it may even be necessary to gently use a fingernail to feel it. If it is not readily palpable, then resist the client from everting and dorsiflexing the foot (actions of the fibularis tertius) and palpate again for its tendon (Figure 20-16, *B*). Once you have located the distal tendon of the fibularis tertius, resist the client once again from performing the actions of this muscle and palpate the fibularis tertius proximally into the leg (see Figure 20-16, *C*). Given its actions of dorsiflexion and eversion of the foot, the fibularis tertius would be stretched by plantarflexing and inverting the foot.

Note: The fibularis tertius is often missing, unilaterally or bilaterally.

Trigger Points:

1. Factors that create and/or perpetuate trigger points (TrPs) in the fibularis tertius and symptoms caused by TrPs in the fibularis tertius are the same as for the EDL.
2. TrPs in the fibularis tertius may cause pain with active dorsiflexion of the foot at the ankle joint or pain at the end range of motion of plantarflexion of the foot.
3. TrPs in the fibularis tertius are often associated with TrPs in the fibularis longus, fibularis brevis, and EDL.

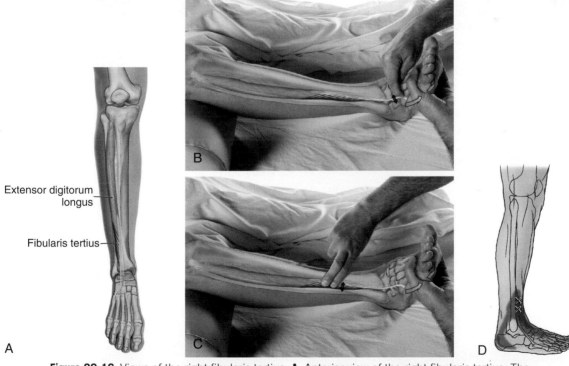

Extensor digitorum longus

Fibularis tertius

A

B

C

D

Figure 20-16 Views of the right fibularis tertius. **A,** Anterior view of the right fibularis tertius. The extensor digitorum longus (EDL) has been ghosted in. **B** and **C,** Anterolateral views showing palpation of the distal tendon and belly of the fibularis tertius respectively as the client everts and dorsiflexes the foot against resistance. The EDL has been ghosted in. **D,** Lateral view showing common fibularis tertius trigger points (TrPs) and their corresponding referral zone.

20

Palpation Key:

Palpate lateral to the EDL tendon to the little toe.

EXTENSOR HALLUCIS LONGUS (EHL)—SUPINE

☑ATTACHMENTS

☐ Middle ⅓ of the anterior fibula

to the

☐ dorsal surface of the distal phalanx of the big toe

☑ACTIONS

☐ Extends the big toe at the metatarsophalangeal (MTP) and interphalangeal (IP) joints
☐ Dorsiflexes the foot at the ankle joint
☐ Inverts the foot at the tarsal joints

Starting Position (Figure 20-18)

■ Client supine
■ Therapist standing to the side of the client
■ Palpating hand not yet placed on the client
■ Fingers of the support hand placed on the dorsal surface of the distal phalanx of the big toe

Palpation Steps

1. Resist the client from extending the big toe at the MTP and IP joints and look for the tendon of the extensor hallucis longus (EHL) to become visible.
2. Palpate the distal tendon by strumming perpendicular across it (Figure 20-19, *A*).
3. Continue palpating the EHL proximally by strumming perpendicular to the fibers. Once the EHL goes deep to the tibialis anterior and extensor digitorum longus (EDL); do not strum perpendicular to it. Instead feel for its contraction deep to these other muscles when the big toe extends (see Figure 20-19, *B*).
4. Once the EHL has been located, have the client relax it, and palpate to assess its baseline tone.

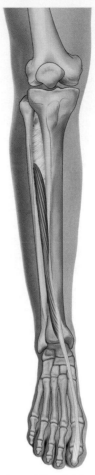

Figure 20-17 Anterior view of the right extensor hallucis longus (EHL).

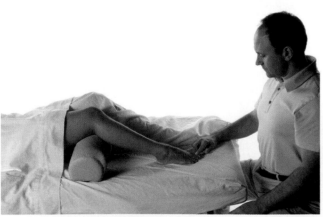

Figure 20-18 Starting position for supine palpation of the right extensor hallucis longus (EHL).

20

EXTENSOR HALLUCIS LONGUS (EHL)—SUPINE—*cont'd*

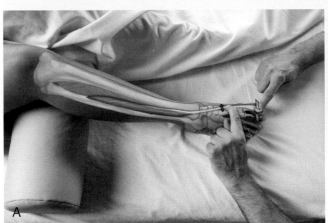
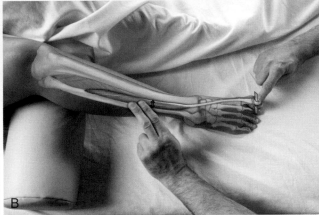

Figure 20-19 Palpation of the right extensor hallucis longus (EHL) as the client extends the big toe against resistance. **A,** Palpation of the distal tendon on the dorsum of the foot. **B,** Palpation of the belly in the anterolateral leg.

PALPATION NOTES

1. Many people have difficulty isolating motion of their toes. The client may be unable to extend the big toe without extending the other toes. If this occurs, do not restrain the other toes from extending. This may stop them from moving but will not stop the extensor digitorum longus (EDL) muscle from isometrically contracting; it is the contraction of the belly of the EDL that we do not want.

2. Most of the belly of the EHL is located between and deep to the tibialis anterior and EDL. As you palpate the EHL proximally, deep to these other muscles, it can be helpful to close your eyes to eliminate visual sensations from distracting you, and press very lightly with your palpating fingers, feeling for the subtle contraction deeper within the tissue of the EHL when the client extends the big toe, either with or without resistance (see Figure 20-19, *B*).

3. Do not allow the client to dorsiflex the foot at the ankle joint when palpating the EHL, because all muscles of the anterior leg will contract with dorsiflexion. Also, do not allow the client to invert the foot at the tarsal joints because that will engage the tibialis anterior; similarly do not allow the client to evert the foot, because that will engage the EDL. Any other muscles that contract when palpating the EHL will make it more difficult to palpate and discern it.

Alternate Palpation Position—Seated

The EHL can also be easily palpated with the client seated.

Palpation Key:
First look for the distal tendon to the big toe.

TRIGGER POINTS

1. Trigger points (TrPs) in the EHL often result from or are perpetuated by acute or chronic overuse of the muscle, postures that result in chronic shortening of the muscle (e.g., driving with a sharply angled gas pedal), chronic lengthening of the muscle (e.g., wearing high-heeled shoes, sleeping with foot in dorsiflexion), tight antagonistic ankle joint plantarflexor muscles, trauma, tripping (with ankle joint forced into plantarflexion), anterior compartment syndrome, and L4 nerve compression.

2. TrPs in the EHL may produce ankle joint dorsiflexion weakness (which may result in foot drop or foot slap), growing pains, and night cramps in the belly of the muscle.

3. The referral patterns of EHL TrPs must be distinguished from the referral patterns of TrPs in the tibialis anterior and extensor hallucis brevis.

4. TrPs in the EHL are often incorrectly assessed as MTP joint dysfunction or L4-L5 nerve compression.

5. Associated TrPs often occur in the tibialis anterior, extensor hallucis brevis, EDL, and fibularis tertius.

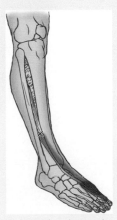

Figure 20-20 Anterolateral view showing a common extensor hallucis longus (EHL) trigger point (TrP) and its corresponding referral zone.

EXTENSOR HALLUCIS LONGUS (EHL)—SUPINE—*cont'd*

STRETCHING THE EXTENSOR HALLUCIS LONGUS

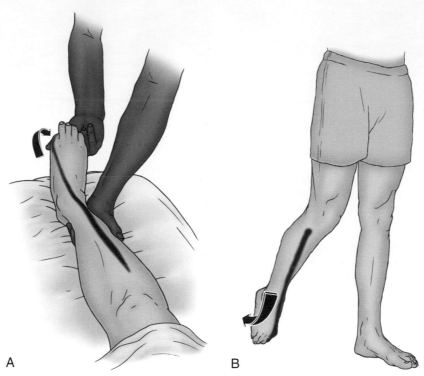

A   B

Figure 20-21 Stretching the right extensor hallucis longus (EHL). The client's big toe is flexed with the foot plantarflexed and everted. **A,** Therapist-assisted stretch. Note that the therapist uses the other hand to stabilize the client's leg. **B,** Self-care stretch. The client should hold on to a stable object for support and to prevent placing excessive weight upon the foot in back.

FIBULARIS LONGUS AND FIBULARIS BREVIS—SIDE LYING

☑ ATTACHMENTS

Fibularis longus
☐ Proximal ½ of the lateral fibula

to the

☐ first cuneiform and the base of the first metatarsal

Fibularis brevis
☐ Distal ½ of the lateral fibula

to the

☐ lateral side of the base of the fifth metatarsal

☑ ACTIONS

Fibularis longus and brevis:
☐ Evert the foot at the tarsal joints
☐ Plantarflex the foot at the ankle joint

Starting Position (Figure 20-23)

■ Client side lying
■ Therapist standing to the side of the client
■ Palpating hand placed on the lateral side of the fibula, just distal to the head of the fibula
■ Support hand placed on the lateral side of the foot

Palpation Steps:

1. Resist the client from everting the foot at the tarsal joints and feel for the contraction of the fibularis longus (Figure 20-24).
2. Continue palpating the fibularis longus distally while strumming perpendicular to the fibers. Note that the fibularis longus becomes tendon approximately halfway down the leg.
3. The distal tendon of the fibularis longus can usually be fairly easily palpated immediately posterior to the lateral malleolus of the fibula (Figure 20-25).
4. To palpate the fibularis brevis, palpate on either side of the fibularis longus in the distal half of the leg (Figure 20-26, *A*).
5. The distal tendon of the fibularis brevis is often visible and palpable in the proximal foot distal to the lateral malleolus of the fibula (see Figure 20-26, *B*).
6. Once the fibularis longus and brevis have been located, have the client relax them and palpate to assess their baseline tone.

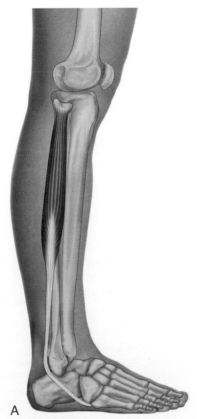
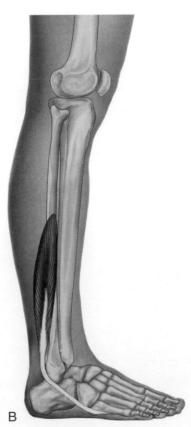

A   B

Figure 20-22 Lateral views of the right fibularis longus and brevis. **A,** Fibularis longus. **B,** Fibularis brevis.

20

FIBULARIS LONGUS AND FIBULARIS BREVIS—SIDE LYING—cont'd

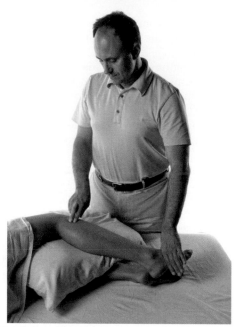

Figure 20-23 Starting position for side lying palpation of the right fibularis longus and brevis.

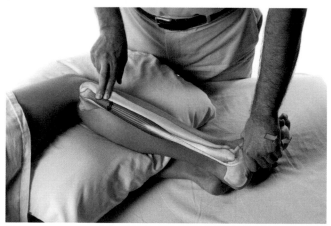

Figure 20-24 Palpation of the belly of the fibularis longus as the client everts the foot against resistance.

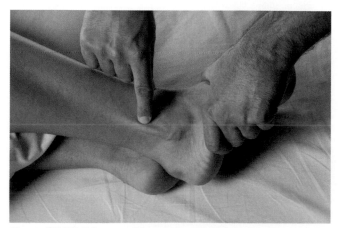

Figure 20-25 When resistance is applied to eversion of the foot, the distal tendon of the fibularis longus is often visible just proximal to the lateral malleolus of the fibula.

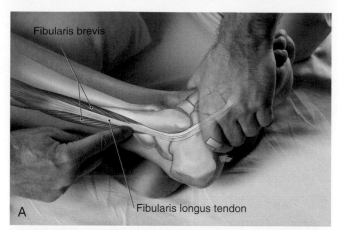

Fibularis brevis

A   Fibularis longus tendon

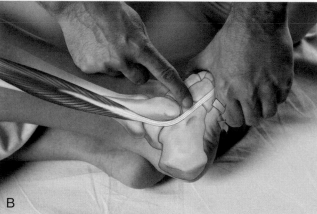

B

Figure 20-26 Palpation of the right fibularis brevis as the client everts the foot against resistance. **A,** Palpation of its belly immediately posterior to the fibularis longus tendon. **B,** Palpation of its distal tendon distal to the lateral malleolus.

PALPATION NOTES

1. The distal tendon of the fibularis longus is also often visible and palpable distal to the lateral malleolus of the fibula before it dives around the cuboid to enter the plantar surface of the foot to make its way to the medial side of the foot. Once the distal tendon of the fibularis longus enters the plantar side of the foot, it is located very deep and is not discernable except perhaps at the distal attachment on the first metatarsal and first cuneiform.

2. Having the client do eversion of the foot at the tarsal joints does not help discern the border between the extensor digitorum longus (EDL) and the fibularis longus and brevis. To discern this border, use dorsiflexion and plantarflexion of the foot at the ankle joint. The EDL engages with dorsiflexion, and the fibularis longus and brevis engage with plantarflexion. (Note: Eversion of the foot will discern the border between the fibularis longus and brevis muscles and the soleus because the soleus is an invertor of the foot.)

FIBULARIS LONGUS AND FIBULARIS BREVIS—SIDE LYING—*cont'd*

Alternate Palpation Position—Supine, Prone, or Seated

The fibularis longus and fibularis brevis can also be easily palpated with the client supine, prone, or seated.

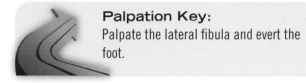

Palpation Key:
Palpate the lateral fibula and evert the foot.

TRIGGER POINTS

1. Trigger points (TrPs) in the fibularis longus and brevis often result from or are perpetuated by acute or chronic overuse of the muscle, prolonged shortening of the muscle (e.g., sleeping with the feet plantarflexed), prolonged immobilization (often due to wearing a cast), an ankle joint inversion sprain, chronic tension of the tibialis anterior and/or tibialis posterior (TP), wearing high-heeled shoes, flat feet, running on uneven (slanted side to side) surfaces, habitually sitting with one leg crossed over the other, TrPs in the gluteus minimus, Morton foot, or even socks with tight elastic bands that constrict circulation.

2. TrPs in the fibularis longus or brevis may produce weak ankles; pain with active eversion of the foot or with end range of motion of active or passive inversion of the foot; and entrapment of the common fibular nerve, deep fibular nerve (either of which may cause foot drop or foot slap), or the superficial fibular nerve.

3. The referral patterns of fibularis longus and brevis TrPs must be distinguished from the referral patterns of TrPs in the tibialis anterior, extensor digitorum longus (EDL), extensor hallucis longus (EHL), extensor digitorum brevis, extensor hallucis brevis, and gluteus minimus.

4. TrPs in the fibularis longus and brevis are often incorrectly assessed as lateral compartment syndrome or lumbar disc syndrome.

5. Associated TrPs often occur in the other fibularis muscles, EDL, TP, and gluteus minimus.

6. Note: The referral patterns of the fibularis longus and fibularis brevis muscles have not been distinguished from each other.

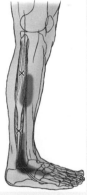

Figure 20-27 Lateral view showing common fibularis longus and brevis trigger points (TrPs) and their corresponding referral zones.

STRETCHING THE FIBULARIS LONGUS AND FIBULARIS BREVIS

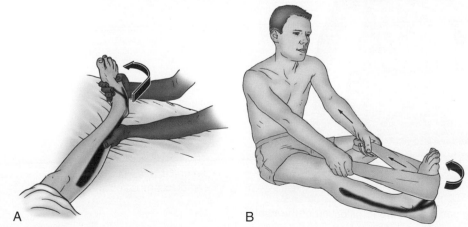

A

B

Figure 20-28 Stretching the right fibularis longus and brevis muscles. The client's foot is inverted and dorsiflexed. **A,** Therapist-assisted stretch. Note that the therapist uses the other hand to stabilize the client's leg. **B,** Self-care stretch. The client uses a towel to pull the foot into inversion and dorsiflexion.

GASTROCNEMIUS—PRONE

✔ ATTACHMENTS

☐ Posterior surfaces of the medial and lateral condyles of the femur

to the

☐ posterior surface of the calcaneus (via the calcaneal tendon)

✔ ACTIONS

☐ Plantarflexes the foot at the ankle joint
☐ Inverts the foot at the tarsal joints
☐ Flexes the leg at the knee joint

Starting Position (Figure 20-30)

■ Client prone with the knee joint fully or nearly fully extended
■ Therapist standing to the side of the client
■ Palpating hand placed on the proximal posterior leg
■ Support hand placed on the plantar surface of the foot

Palpation Steps

1. Ask the client to plantarflex the foot against your resistance and feel for the contraction of the gastrocnemius (Figure 20-31, *A*).
2. Palpate the medial and lateral bellies of the gastrocnemius in the proximal posterior leg.
3. Approximately halfway down the leg, the gastrocnemius becomes tendon. Palpate the tendon all the way to its attachment on the posterior surface of the calcaneus via the calcaneal (Achilles) tendon (see Figure 20-31, *B*).
4. Once the gastrocnemius has been located, have the client relax it, and palpate to assess its baseline tone.

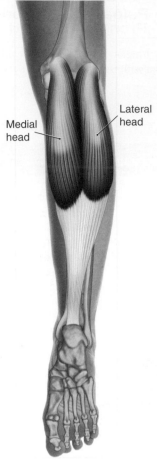

Medial head

Lateral head

Figure 20-29 Posterior view of the right gastrocnemius.

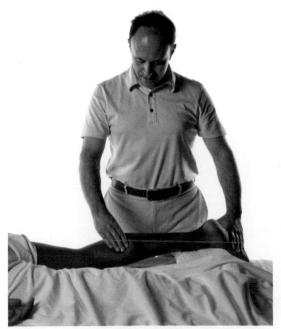

Figure 20-30 Starting position for prone palpation of the right gastrocnemius.

20

GASTROCNEMIUS—PRONE—cont'd

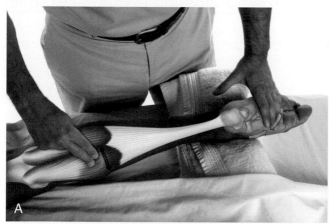
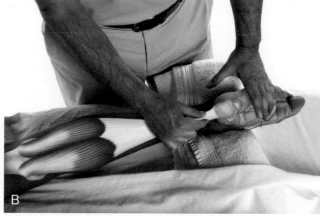

Figure 20-31 Palpation of the right gastrocnemius as the client plantarflexes the foot against resistance. **A,** Palpation of the medial belly. **B,** Palpation of the calcaneal (Achilles) tendon with a finger placed on each side of the tendon just proximal to the calcaneus.

PALPATION NOTES

1. The calcaneal tendon, also known as the *Achilles tendon,* is the common distal attachment of the gastrocnemius and soleus muscles.
2. The proximal attachments of the gastrocnemius on the posterior surfaces of the femoral condyles can be palpated. One at a time, follow a belly of the gastrocnemius proximally as the client alternately contracts and relaxes the muscle with resisted plantarflexion of the foot (with the knee joint extended). Be sure to stay medial to the biceps femoris distal tendon for the lateral head of the gastrocnemius and lateral to the semitendinosus and semimembranosus tendons for the medial head of the gastrocnemius (Figure 20-32). Once you

are in the popliteal region, passively flex the client's knee joint to approximately 90 degrees to slacken the hamstrings, and palpate for the femoral condyle attachments of the two heads of the gastrocnemius. Note: Be careful when palpating in the popliteal region because of the presence of the tibial and common fibular nerves and the popliteal artery and vein in the popliteal fossa (see Figure 20-2).
3. Discerning the proximal attachment of the lateral head of the gastrocnemius from the plantaris is challenging because these muscles are directly next to each other and have the same joint actions (see Figure 20-35, *B*).

Figure 20-32 Palpation of the proximal attachments of the gastrocnemius. **A,** Medial head. The semitendinosus and semimembranosus have been ghosted in. **B,** Lateral head. The plantaris is drawn in. The biceps femoris long and short heads are cut and ghosted in.

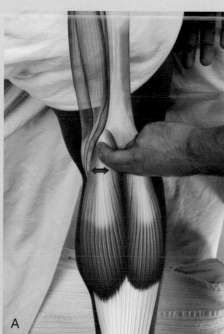
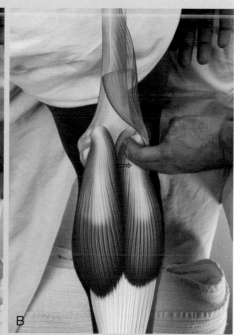

20

GASTROCNEMIUS—PRONE—*cont'd*

TRIGGER POINTS

1. Trigger points (TrPs) in the gastrocnemius often result from or are perpetuated by acute or chronic overuse of the muscle (e.g., walking/running uphill), prolonged shortening of the muscle (e.g., wearing high heels, sleeping with the feet in plantarflexion, driving with the foot plantarflexed on the gas pedal), riding a bicycle with a seat that is too low, chilling of the muscle, immobilization (e.g., wearing a cast), socks with tight elastic bands that constrict circulation, and S1 nerve compression.

2. TrPs in the gastrocnemius may produce calf cramps (including nocturnal cramps), intermittent claudication, and an inability to extend the knee joint when the ankle joint is dorsiflexed.

3. The referral patterns of gastrocnemius TrPs must be distinguished from the referral patterns of TrPs in the soleus, plantaris, popliteus, tibialis posterior (TP), flexor digitorum longus (FDL), hamstrings, and gluteus minimus.

4. TrPs in the gastrocnemius are often incorrectly assessed as posterior compartment syndrome, deep vein thrombosis, an S1 nerve compression, or growing pains.

5. Associated TrPs often occur in the soleus, hamstring muscles, tibialis anterior, extensor digitorum longus (EDL), extensor hallucis longus (EHL), and gluteus minimus.

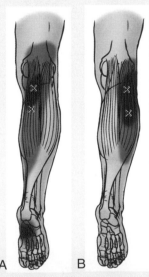

Figure 20-33 Posterior views showing common gastrocnemius trigger points (TrPs) and their corresponding referral zones. **A,** Medial head. **B,** Lateral head.

Alternate Palpation Position—Standing

The gastrocnemius can also be easily palpated with the client standing. Asking the client to go up on the toes engages the gastrocnemius, and its contours usually becomes visible.

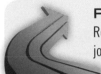

Palpation Key:
Resist foot plantarflexion with the knee joint extended.

GASTROCNEMIUS—PRONE—*cont'd*

STRETCHING THE GASTROCNEMIUS

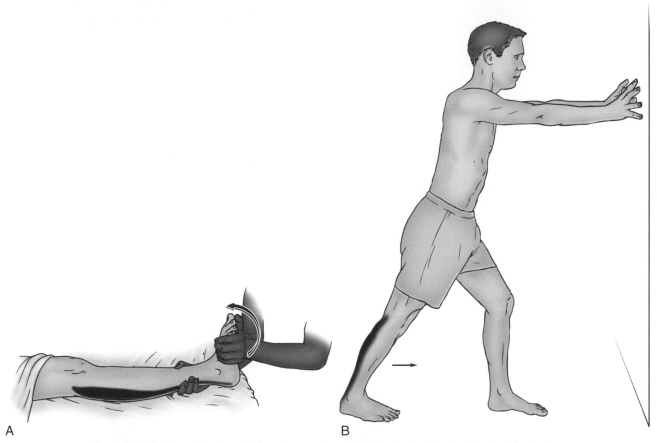

A   B

Figure 20-34 Stretching the right gastrocnemius. The client's foot is dorsiflexed with the knee joint extended. (If the knee joint is flexed, this becomes a soleus stretch.) **A,** Therapist-assisted stretch. Note that the therapist uses the other hand to stabilize the client's leg. **B,** Self-care stretch. It is important that the heel stays on the ground.

GASTROCNEMIUS—PRONE—*cont'd*

DETOUR

Plantaris:

The plantaris is a small muscle attaching from the lateral condyle of the femur to the calcaneus (Figure 20-35, *A*). It has a very short belly proximally, and an exceptionally long distal tendon. Its belly is located directly medial to the proximal attachment of the lateral head of the gastrocnemius (see Figure 20-32, *B*). To palpate the plantaris, begin with gentle palpation in the center of the popliteal fossa and gradually move laterally until you feel the presence of muscle tissue that contracts with plantarflexion of the foot at the ankle joint (see Figure 20-35, *B*). You are now on the plantaris. To discern the plantaris from the lateral head of the gastrocnemius can be challenging because these two muscles have identical

actions. Stretching the gastrocnemius would also stretch the plantaris.

Note: Trigger points (TrPs) in the plantaris may cause pain at the end range of motion of dorsiflexion of the foot. TrPs in the plantaris are often associated with TrPs in the gastrocnemius (see Figure 20-35, *C*).

Palpation Key:
Palpate medial to the attachment of the lateral head of the gastrocnemius.

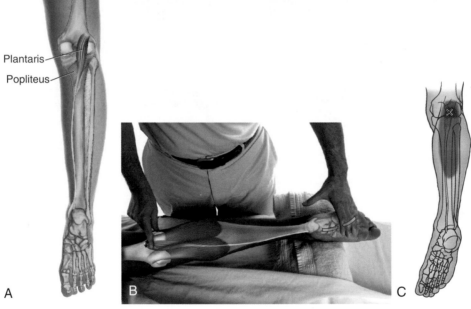

Plantaris

Popliteus

A   B   C

Figure 20-35 Views of the right plantaris. **A,** Posterior view of the plantaris. The popliteus has been ghosted in. **B,** Palpation of the plantaris. **C,** Posterior view showing a common plantaris trigger point (TrP) and its corresponding referral zone.

SOLEUS—PRONE

☑ ATTACHMENTS

☐ Head and proximal half of the posterior fibula and the soleal line of the posterior tibia

to the

☐ posterior surface of the calcaneus (via the calcaneal tendon)

☑ ACTIONS

☐ Plantarflexes the foot at the ankle joint
☐ Inverts the foot at the tarsal joints

Starting Position (Figure 20-37)

■ Client prone with the knee joint flexed to approximately 90 degrees
■ Therapist standing to the side of the client
■ Palpating hand placed on the proximal posterior leg
■ Support hand placed on the plantar surface of the foot

Palpation Steps

1. Ask the client to plantarflex the foot against gentle resistance and feel for the contraction of the soleus deep to the gastrocnemius (Figure 20-38, *A*).
2. Palpate the soleus to its proximal attachment, and palpate it distally to its distal attachment on the posterior calcaneus via the calcaneal (Achilles) tendon.
3. Although from the posterior perspective, the soleus is deep to the gastrocnemius; from the lateral perspective, the soleus is superficial and can be easily palpated (see Figure 20-38, *B*). Note: A portion of the soleus is also superficial on the medial side of the proximal leg and can be easily palpated (see Figure 20-4, *A*).
4. Once the soleus has been located, have the client relax it, and palpate to assess its baseline tone.

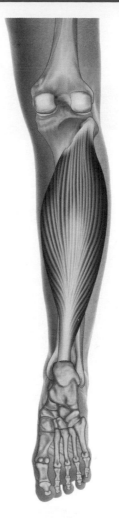

Figure 20-36 Posterior view of the right soleus.

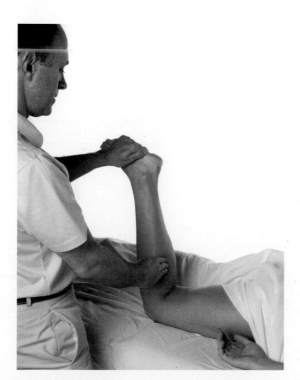

Figure 20-37 Starting position for prone palpation of the right soleus.

20

SOLEUS—PRONE—*cont'd*

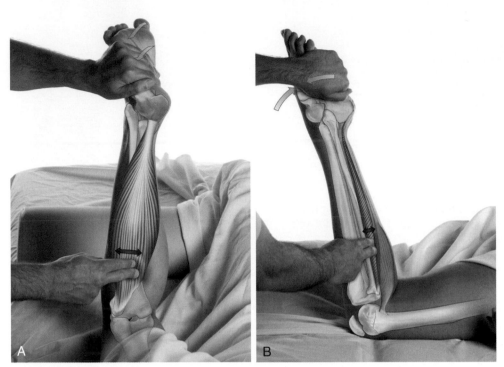

Figure 20-38 Palpation of the right soleus as the client plantarflexes the foot against gentle resistance with the knee joint flexed. **A,** Palpation of the posterior aspect through the gastrocnemius. **B,** Palpation of the lateral aspect where the soleus is superficial.

 PALPATION NOTES

1. The calcaneal tendon, also known as the *Achilles tendon,* is the common distal attachment of the soleus and gastrocnemius muscles.
2. The reason that the soleus is palpated with the client's leg flexed at the knee joint is that this position slackens and thereby inhibits the gastrocnemius from contracting (via the principle of shortened active insufficiency). If the gastrocnemius is inhibited, the soleus can be palpated through the gastrocnemius (in addition to where the soleus is superficial laterally as well as medially). Note: Do not provide too much resistance to the client's plantarflexion, or the inhibition of the gastrocnemius will be overridden, and it will contract, blocking the ability to palpate the soleus through it.

 Palpation Key:
Gently resist foot plantarflexion with the knee joint flexed.

SOLEUS—PRONE—*cont'd*

TRIGGER POINTS

1. Trigger points (TrPs) in the soleus often result from or are perpetuated by an acute or chronic overuse of the muscle (e.g., walking/running uphill), prolonged position of shortening of the muscle (e.g., wearing high heels, sleeping with the feet in plantarflexion, driving with the foot plantarflexed on the gas pedal), trauma, and chilling of the muscle.

2. TrPs in the soleus may produce restricted ankle joint dorsiflexion, pain when walking (especially uphill or upstairs), entrapment of the tibial nerve and associated vessels, heel pain upon weight bearing, and foot/ankle edema.

3. The referral patterns of soleus TrPs must be distinguished from the referral patterns of TrPs in the gastrocnemius, plantaris, tibialis posterior (TP), flexor digitorum longus (FDL), hamstrings, gluteus minimus, quadratus plantae, and abductor hallucis.

4. TrPs in the soleus are often incorrectly assessed as posterior compartment syndrome, posterior shin splints, growing pains, Achilles tendinitis, Baker cyst, deep vein thrombosis, S1 nerve compression, intermittent claudication, plantar fasciitis, or heel spur.

5. Associated TrPs often occur in the gastrocnemius, TP, FDL, flexor hallucis longus (FHL), and gluteus minimus.

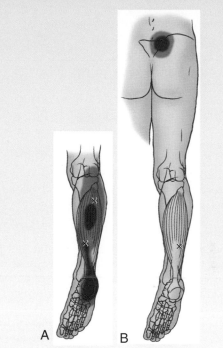

Figure 20-39 Posterior views of common soleus trigger points (TrPs) and their corresponding referral zones.

STRETCHING THE SOLEUS

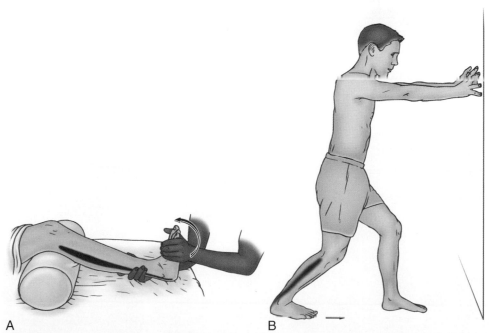

Figure 20-40 Stretching the right soleus. The client's foot is dorsiflexed with the knee joint flexed. (If the knee joint is extended, this becomes a gastrocnemius stretch.) **A,** Therapist-assisted stretch. A bolster is used to flex the knee. Note that the therapist uses the other hand to stabilize the client's leg. **B,** Self-care stretch. It is important that the heel stays on the ground.

20

POPLITEUS—PRONE

☑ ATTACHMENTS

☐ Lateral surface of the lateral condyle of the femur

to the

☐ medial side of the proximal posterior tibia

☑ ACTIONS

☐ Medially rotates the leg at the knee joint
☐ Flexes the leg at the knee joint

Starting Position (Figure 20-42)

■ Client prone with the leg flexed 90 degrees at the knee joint
■ Therapist standing to the side of the client
■ Palpating fingers curled around the posterior side of the medial border of the proximal tibia
■ If resistance will be given, support hand placed on the distal leg (just proximal to the ankle joint)

Palpation Steps

1. With your palpating fingers curled around and pressing against the tibia, ask the client to medially rotate the leg at the knee joint, and feel for the contraction of the popliteus. Resistance with the support hand can be given if desired (Figure 20-43).
2. Once the tibial attachment of the popliteus has been felt, try to continue palpating the popliteus through the gastrocnemius toward its proximal attachment while the client is alternately contracting and relaxing it by medially rotating the leg at the knee joint.
3. Once the popliteus has been located, have the client relax it, and palpate to assess its baseline tone.

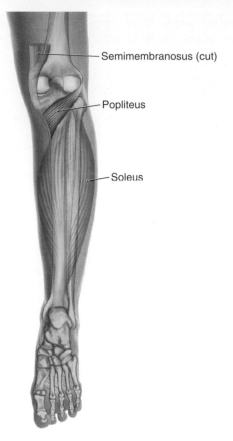

Figure 20-41 Posterior view of the right popliteus. The soleus and cut distal tendon of semimembranosus have been ghosted in.

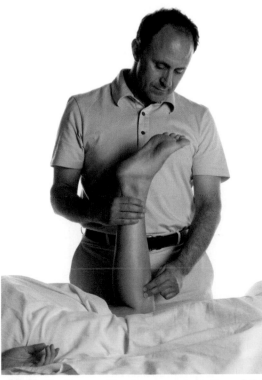

Figure 20-42 Starting position for prone palpation of the right popliteus.

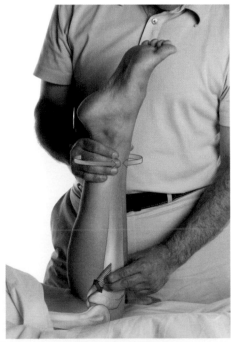

Figure 20-43 Palpation of the tibial attachment of the popliteus as the client medially rotates the leg against resistance.

20

POPLITEUS—PRONE—*cont'd*

 PALPATION NOTES

1. Many people have trouble isolating and performing medial rotation of the leg at the knee joint. To assist the client in doing this, before the actual palpation is done, move the client's leg into medial rotation so that the client can sense what this motion feels like; then ask the client to perform the motion once to practice it. This helps the client perform this joint action more easily when the palpation procedure is actually done. It is easier for the client to perform medial rotation of the leg at the knee joint when in the seated position (Figure 20-44).

2. Most of the belly of the popliteus is located deep to the gastrocnemius. As you palpate the belly of the popliteus through the gastrocnemius, it can be helpful to close your eyes to prevent visual sensations from distracting you, and press very lightly with your palpating fingers, feeling for the subtle contraction of the popliteus when the client medially rotates the leg at the knee joint, either with or without resistance. Continue palpating the popliteus toward its proximal attachment on the femur. At a certain point, its proximal attachment enters the joint cavity of the knee and is no longer palpable.

3. The proximal attachment of the popliteus on the lateral femoral condyle can be palpated. Palpate on the lateral surface of the lateral femoral condyle (just posterior to the lateral [fibular] collateral ligament) and resist the client from medially rotating the leg at the knee joint; feel for the tensing of the proximal tendon of the popliteus (Figure 20-45).

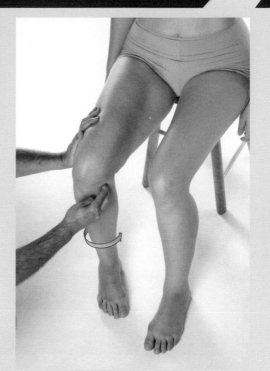

Figure 20-44 The advantage to palpating the popliteus with the client seated is that it is easier for the client to isolate medial rotation of the leg at the knee joint if the foot is flat on the floor. Palpate the popliteus with the client seated following the same steps used when the client is prone.

Alternate Palpation Position—Seated

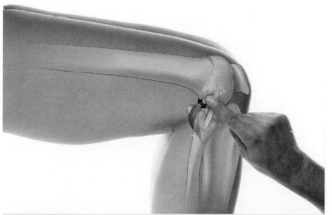

Figure 20-45 Palpation of the proximal attachment of the popliteus on the lateral femoral condyle.

 Palpation Key:
Curl your fingers around to the medial side of the proximal tibia.

POPLITEUS—PRONE—*cont'd*

TRIGGER POINTS

1. Trigger points (TrPs) in the popliteus often result from or are perpetuated by an acute or chronic overuse of the muscle (e.g., running or skiing downhill, planting and cutting on a semiflexed knee joint), excessive foot subtalar joint pronation, wearing high-heeled shoes, and a torn posterior cruciate ligament.

2. TrPs in the popliteus may produce posterior knee pain when crouching or walking/running downhill or downstairs, or decreased lateral rotation or extension of the leg at the knee joint.

3. The referral patterns of popliteus TrPs must be distinguished from the referral patterns of TrPs in the gastrocnemius, soleus, plantaris, hamstrings, and gluteus minimus.

4. TrPs in the popliteus are often incorrectly assessed as Baker cyst, instability of the knee joint, popliteus tendinitis/tenosynovitis, meniscal tear, or torn plantaris muscle.

5. Associated TrPs often occur in the gastrocnemius.

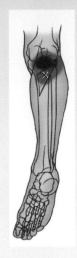

Figure 20-46 Posteromedial view showing a common popliteus trigger point (TrP) and its corresponding referral zone.

STRETCHING THE POPLITEUS

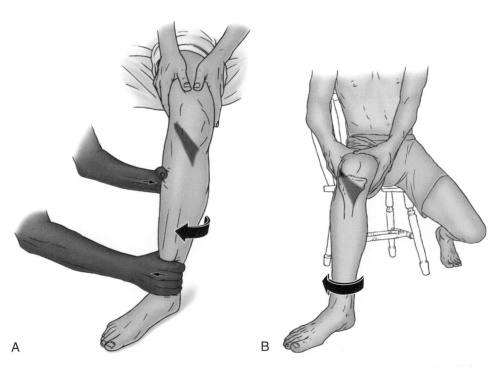

A   B

Figure 20-47 Stretching the right popliteus. The client's leg is laterally rotated at the knee joint. (The knee joint is flexed approximately 45 degrees from full extension.) The client stabilizes the thigh with his hands. **A,** Therapist-assisted stretch. The therapist uses both hands to laterally rotate the client's leg. **B,** Self-care stretch.

TIBIALIS POSTERIOR (TP), FLEXOR DIGITORUM LONGUS (FDL), AND FLEXOR HALLUCIS LONGUS (FHL)—PRONE

"Tom, Dick, and Harry Muscles" (Tibialis Posterior = Tom; Flexor Digitorum Longus = Dick; Flexor Hallucis Longus = Harry)

✅ ATTACHMENTS

Tibialis posterior (TP)
☐ Proximal ⅔ of the posterior tibia and fibula

to the

☐ plantar surface of the foot (metatarsals two to four and all tarsals except the talus)

Flexor digitorum longus (FDL)
☐ Middle ⅓ of the posterior tibia

to the

☐ plantar surfaces of the distal phalanges of toes two to five

Flexor hallucis longus (FHL)
☐ Distal ⅔ of the posterior fibula

to the

☐ plantar surface of the distal phalanx of the big toe

✅ ACTIONS

TP
☐ Inverts the foot at the tarsal joints
☐ Plantarflexes the foot at the ankle joint

FDL
☐ Flexes toes two to five at the metatarsophalangeal (MTP) and interphalangeal (IP) joints
☐ Inverts the foot at the tarsal joints
☐ Plantarflexes the foot at the ankle joint

FHL
☐ Flexes the big toe at the MTP and IP joints
☐ Inverts the foot at the tarsal joints
☐ Plantarflexes the foot at the ankle joint

Starting Position (Figure 20-49, *A*)
▪ Client prone with a roll under the ankles
▪ Therapist standing or seated on the other side of the client
▪ Palpating fingers placed just posterior and distal to the medial malleolus of the tibia, but not until after TP tendon has been visualized
▪ If resistance is needed, support hand placed on the foot

Palpation Steps
• Note: All three Tom, Dick, and Harry muscles are superficial and palpable in the distal medial leg; of the three, the FDL has the most exposure. The tendons of the TP and FDL are usually palpable and sometimes visible just posterior and distal to the medial malleolus of the tibia (see Figure 20-49, *B*).

TP

1. Ask the client to plantarflex the foot at the ankle joint and invert the foot at the tarsal joints, and look for the distal

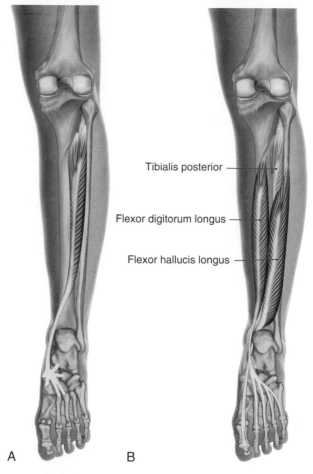

Figure 20-48 Posterior views of the right Tom, Dick, and Harry muscles. **A,** Tibialis posterior (TP; Tom). **B,** Flexor digitorum longus (FDL; Dick) and flexor hallucis longus (FHL; Harry). TP has been ghosted in.

tendon of the TP in the distal medial leg immediately posterior to the shaft of the distal tibia and immediately posterior and distal to the medial malleolus of the tibia. Resistance may be added with your support hand if needed to bring out the tendon (Figure 20-50, *A*).

2. Once located, palpate the distal tendon of the TP by strumming perpendicularly across it as the client alternately contracts and relaxes the muscle. Palpate proximally and distally as far as possible (see Figure 20-50, *B*). Note: The TP tendon is the closest of the three to the medial malleolus.

3. The belly of the TP is located very deep in the posterior compartment of the leg and can be very difficult to palpate and discern. To palpate its belly, press gently over it in the midline of the posterior leg, ask the client to invert the foot, and feel for its contraction (see Figure 20-50, *C*).

4. Once the TP muscle has been located, have the client relax it, and palpate to assess its baseline tone.

20

TIBIALIS POSTERIOR (TP), FLEXOR DIGITORUM LONGUS (FDL), AND FLEXOR HALLUCIS LONGUS (FHL)—PRONE—*cont'd*

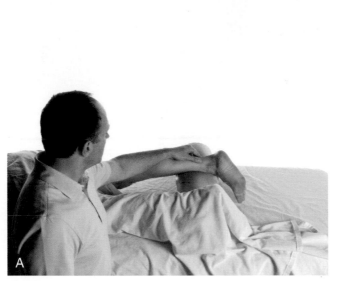

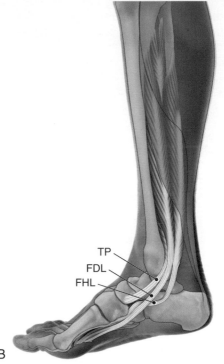

Figure 20-49 A, Starting position for prone palpation of the Tom, Dick, and Harry group. First try to visualize the tendons. **B,** All three Tom, Dick, and Harry muscles' distal tendons near the medial malleolus. The gastrocnemius and soleus have been ghosted in. Tom = tibialis posterior (TP); Dick = flexor digitorum longus (FDL); Harry = flexor hallucis longus (FHL).

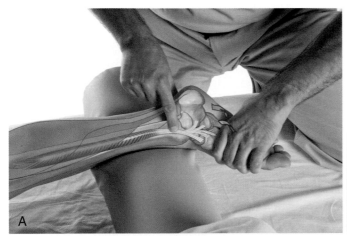

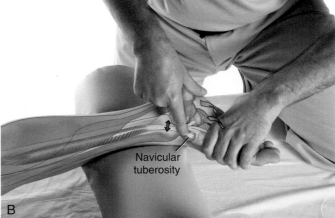

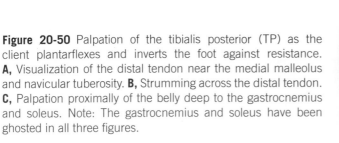

Figure 20-50 Palpation of the tibialis posterior (TP) as the client plantarflexes and inverts the foot against resistance. **A,** Visualization of the distal tendon near the medial malleolus and navicular tuberosity. **B,** Strumming across the distal tendon. **C,** Palpation proximally of the belly deep to the gastrocnemius and soleus. Note: The gastrocnemius and soleus have been ghosted in all three figures.

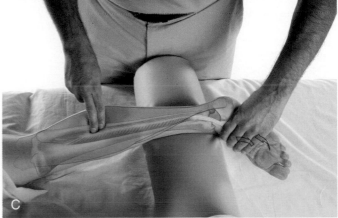

TIBIALIS POSTERIOR (TP), FLEXOR DIGITORUM LONGUS (FDL), AND FLEXOR HALLUCIS LONGUS (FHL)—PRONE—*cont'd*

FDL

5. Part of the belly of the FDL is superficial in the distal medial leg between the soleus and the shaft of the tibia. Ask the client to flex toes two to five, and feel for the contraction of the FDL (Figure 20-51, *A*). Resistance may be added with the fingers of your support hand if needed.
6. Once the FDL has been found, strum perpendicular to its fibers, and follow it proximally and distally as far as possible as the client contracts and relaxes the muscle.
7. At the level of the medial malleolus, the distal tendon of the FDL is usually palpable and sometimes visible posterior and distal to the medial malleolus (see Figure 20-51, *B*). It is located slightly farther from the medial malleolus than the distal tendon of the TP.
8. Within the plantar foot, the distal tendons of the FDL are fairly superficial and can usually be palpated if the client alternately contracts and relaxes the FDL by flexing toes two to five at the MTP and IP joints (see Figure 20-51, *C*). (Note: Some clients have a difficult time isolating flexion of toes two to five from flexion of the big toe.) However, precisely discerning the location of these tendons and their borders relative to adjacent musculature and soft tissue is sometimes difficult. Try to follow these tendons to the toes.
9. The belly of the FDL is located deep in the posterior compartment of the leg and can be challenging to palpate and discern. To palpate its belly, press gently over it in the posterior medial leg, ask the client to flex toes two to five, and feel for its contraction (see Figure 20-51, *D*).
10. Once the FDL muscle has been located, have the client relax it, and palpate to assess its baseline tone.

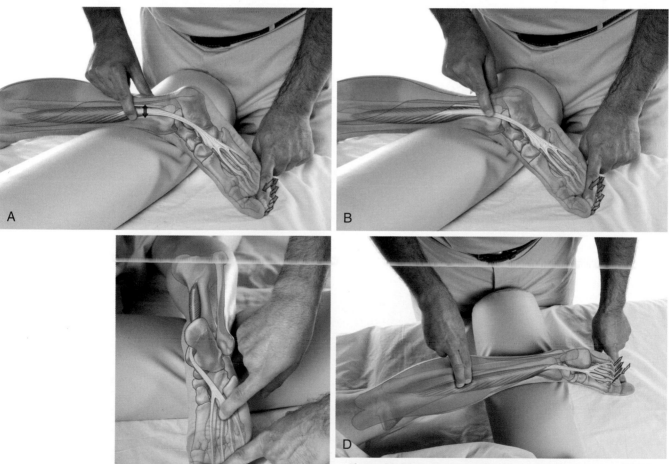

Figure 20-51 Palpation of the flexor digitorum longus (FDL) as the client flexes toes two to five against resistance. **A,** Palpation of the belly in the distal medial leg. **B,** Palpation of the distal tendon near the medial malleolus. **C,** Palpation of the distal tendons in the plantar foot. **D,** Palpation proximally of the belly deep in the posterior leg. Note: The gastrocnemius and soleus have been ghosted in **A, B,** and **D.**

20

TIBIALIS POSTERIOR (TP), FLEXOR DIGITORUM LONGUS (FDL), AND FLEXOR HALLUCIS LONGUS (FHL)—PRONE—cont'd

FHL

11. A small part of the distal belly of the FHL is superficial in the distal medial leg between the FDL and the calcaneal tendon. Ask the client to flex the big toe and feel for the contraction of the FHL (Figure 20-52, A). Resistance may be added with fingers of your support hand if needed.
12. Once the FHL has been found, strum perpendicular to its fibers, and try to follow it as far distally as possible. At the level of the medial malleolus, its distal tendon runs quite deep and is difficult to palpate.
13. Within the plantar foot, the distal tendon of the FHL is fairly superficial and can usually be palpated if the client alternately contracts and relaxes the FHL by flexing the big toe at the MTP and IP joints. (Note: Some clients have a difficult time isolating flexion of the big toe from flexion of the other toes.) However, precisely discerning the location of its tendon and its borders relative to adjacent musculature and soft tissue is sometimes difficult. Try to follow its tendon to the big toe (see Figure 20-52, B).

14. The belly of the FHL is located deep in the posterior compartment of the leg and can be challenging to palpate and discern. To palpate its belly, press gently over it in the posterior lateral leg, ask the client to flex the big toe, and feel for its contraction (see Figure 20-52, C).
15. Once the FHL muscle has been located, have the client relax it, and palpate to assess its baseline tone.

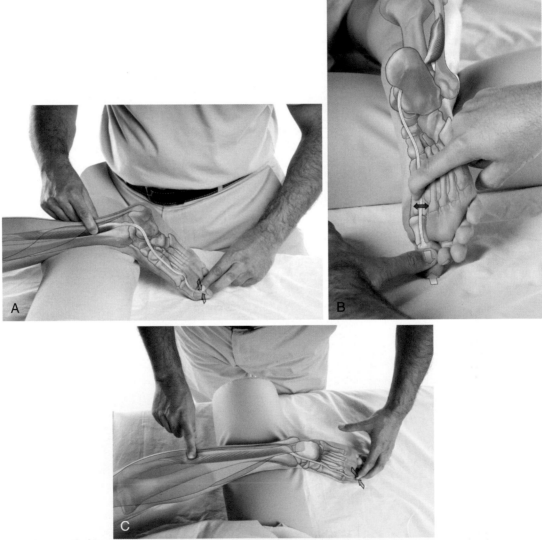

Figure 20-52 Palpation of the flexor hallucis longus (FHL) as the client flexes the big toe against resistance. **A,** Palpation of the belly in the distal medial leg. **B,** Palpation of the distal tendon in the plantar foot. **C,** Palpation proximally of the belly deep in the posterior leg. Note: The gastrocnemius and soleus have been ghosted in **A** and **C**.

20

TIBIALIS POSTERIOR (TP), FLEXOR DIGITORUM LONGUS (FDL), AND FLEXOR HALLUCIS LONGUS (FHL)—PRONE—*cont'd*

PALPATION NOTES

1. The "Tom, Dick, and Harry muscles" are so named because they all cross from the leg into the foot posterior and then distal to the medial malleolus of the tibia with the tibialis posterior (TP) closest to the medial malleolus, then the flexor digitorum longus (FDL), and then the flexor hallucis longus (FHL) farthest. Because they all cross the ankle joint posteriorly and the subtalar/tarsal joints medially, they all plantarflex the foot at the ankle joint and invert the foot at the tarsal joints.

2. When first palpating the Tom, Dick, and Harry muscles, look for the tendons of the TP and the FDL before placing the palpating hand on the client; otherwise your palpating hand will obstruct your view and visual identification.

3. When palpating for the TP, if you ask the client to extend all five toes, it will inhibit and relax the FDL and FHL from contracting, making it easier to palpate and discern the TP.

4. Do not use plantarflexion and/or inversion of the foot when palpating the FDL and FHL, because these actions will make all three Tom, Dick, and Harry muscles contract, making it difficult to discern the separate muscles.

5. The majority of fibers of the distal attachment of the TP attach into the navicular tuberosity; this attachment site can be easily palpated in the medial foot (see Figure 20-50, *B*). To do this, once the distal

tendon of TP is located near the medial malleolus, continue strumming it perpendicularly as the client contracts and relaxes the muscle until you reach the navicular tuberosity. The rest of the attachments of the TP distal tendon in the plantar surface of the foot are very deep and extremely difficult to palpate and discern from adjacent tissue.

6. When palpating the bellies of the Tom, Dick, and Harry muscles in the deep posterior compartment of the leg, it can be helpful to close your eyes (to eliminate distracting visual stimuli) and press very gently into the tissues, feeling for the vibration of the muscle's contraction when the client engages the muscle as described in the Palpation Steps for each muscle. Note that in the posterior leg, the FDL belly is medial, the FHL belly is lateral, and the TP belly is in the middle.

7. A small part of the FHL can often be palpated in the lateral leg between the soleus posteriorly and the fibularis longus and brevis muscles anteriorly (see Figure 20-3). Palpate for the FHL, while asking the client to flex the big toe against resistance. It is important that the client does not also plantarflex the foot at the ankle joint because this will cause the soleus and fibularis longus/brevis muscles to also contract.

Palpation Key for All Three Tom, Dick, and Harry Muscles:

Palpate in the distal medial leg and posterior and distal to the medial malleolus.

Alternate Palpation Position—Side Lying or Supine

The Tom, Dick, and Harry muscles can also be palpated with the client side lying or supine. If the client is side lying, the hip and knee joints of the lower extremity that is away from the table must be flexed to allow access to the medial side of the leg that is against the table.

TIBIALIS POSTERIOR (TP), FLEXOR DIGITORUM LONGUS (FDL), AND FLEXOR HALLUCIS LONGUS (FHL)—PRONE—cont'd

TRIGGER POINTS

1. Trigger points (TrPs) in the tibialis posterior (TP), flexor digitorum longus (FDL), and flexor hallucis longus (FHL) often result from or are perpetuated by an acute or chronic overuse of the muscle (e.g., walking on soft sand), walking/ running on uneven (slanted side to side) ground, excessive foot subtalar joint pronation, wearing high-heeled shoes, and Morton foot.

2. TrPs in the TP, FDL, and FHL may produce foot pain (plantar surface of the foot, especially the ball of the foot or the toes) when walking or running, spasm of the associated muscle, excessive foot subtalar joint pronation, and decreased extension range of motion of the associated toes.

3. The referral patterns of TP, FDL, and FHL TrPs must be distinguished from the referral patterns of TrPs in the other muscles of the deep posterior compartment; the gastrocnemius, soleus, and gluteus minimus (for TP); the adductor hallucis, plantar interossei, dorsal interossei pedis, and flexor digitorum brevis (for FDL and FHL); the abductor digiti minimi pedis (for FDL); and flexor hallucis brevis (for FHL).

4. TrPs in the TP, FDL, and FHL are often incorrectly assessed as shin splints, deep posterior compartment syndrome, tarsal tunnel syndrome, or tenosynovitis of the associated muscle's tendon.

5. Associated TrPs often occur in the other muscles of the deep posterior compartment; the fibularis longus, fibularis brevis, and fibularis tertius (for TP); the extensor digitorum longus (EDL), extensor digitorum brevis, and flexor digitorum brevis (for FDL); and the extensor hallucis longus (EHL), extensor hallucis brevis, and flexor hallucis brevis (for FHL).

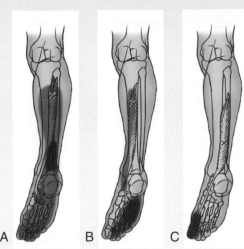

Figure 20-53 A to C, Posterior views showing common trigger points (TrPs) and their corresponding referral zones for the tibialis posterior (TP), flexor digitorum longus (FDL), and flexor hallucis longus (FHL) muscles, respectively.

TIBIALIS POSTERIOR (TP), FLEXOR DIGITORUM LONGUS (FDL), AND FLEXOR HALLUCIS LONGUS (FHL)—PRONE—*cont'd*

STRETCHING THE TIBIALIS POSTERIOR, FLEXOR DIGITORUM LONGUS, AND FLEXOR HALLUCIS LONGUS MUSCLES

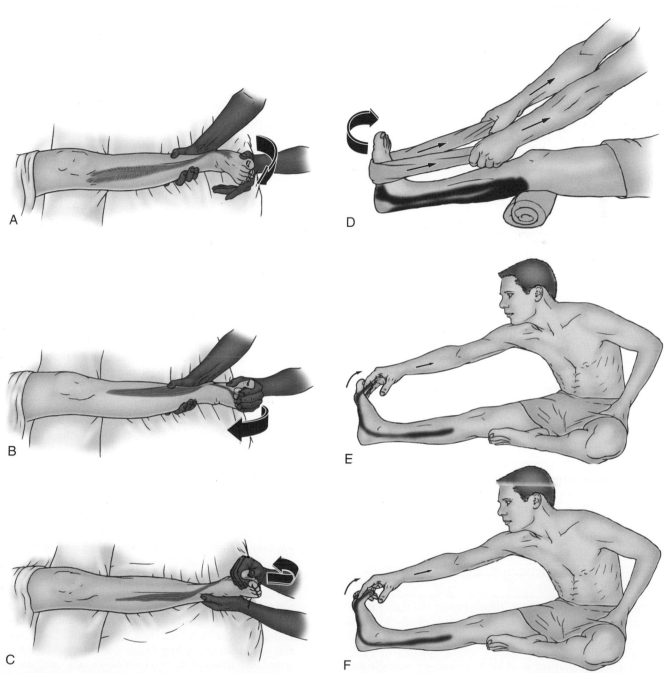

Figure 20-54 Stretching the right Tom, Dick, and Harry group. The tibialis posterior (TP) is stretched by dorsiflexing and everting the foot. The flexor digitorum longus (FDL) is stretched by extending toes two to five. (The stretch can be augmented by dorsiflexing and everting the foot.) The flexor hallucis longus (FHL) is stretched by extending the big toe. (The stretch can be augmented by dorsiflexing and everting the foot.) **A, B,** and **C,** Therapist-assisted stretches of the TP, FDL, and FHL respectively. In all cases, the therapist's other hand is used to stabilize the client's leg. **D, E,** and **F,** Self-care stretches of the TP, FDL, and FHL respectively. In **D,** a towel is used to dorsiflex and evert the foot.

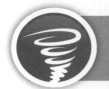

WHIRLWIND TOUR

Muscles of the Leg

The following *Whirlwind Tour* is an abbreviated set of palpation protocols for the muscles of this chapter. Once you have read and become comfortable with each of the protocols presented thus far, this *Whirlwind Tour* allows you to quickly and efficiently run through the palpations protocols for all the muscles of the chapter.

Anterior Compartment Muscles: Client Supine with the Knee Joint Extended

1. **Tibialis anterior:** Resist the client from dorsiflexing and inverting the foot, and look and feel for the tensing of the distal tendon of the tibialis anterior anteriorly and proximally on the dorsum of the foot. Continue palpating the tibialis anterior proximally along the lateral border of the tibia to its proximal attachment while strumming perpendicular to it.

2. **Extensor digitorum longus (EDL):** Resist the client from extending toes two to five and look and feel for the muscle's tendons on the dorsal surface of the foot. Continue palpating the EDL proximally to its proximal attachment by strumming perpendicular to it. Note: Proximally, the EDL is located between the tibialis anterior and the fibularis longus. Use eversion of the foot to engage and discern the EDL from the tibialis anterior; use dorsiflexion to engage and discern the EDL from the fibularis longus.

3. **Fibularis tertius:** Palpate just lateral to the tendon of the EDL that goes to the little toe, and ask the client to dorsiflex and/or evert the foot. Look and feel for the tendon of the fibularis tertius. Once located, follow the fibularis tertius proximally into the distal leg. Note: The fibularis tertius is often absent.

4. **Extensor hallucis longus (EHL):** Ask the client to extend the big toe against resistance, and look and feel for the distal tendon of the EHL on the medial side of the dorsum of the foot. Follow the EHL proximally by strumming perpendicular to it. When it is deep to the tibialis anterior and the EDL, press gently and feel for its contraction as the client extends the big toe.

Lateral Compartment Muscles: Client Side Lying

5. **Fibularis longus:** Ask the client to evert the foot against resistance, and feel for the contraction of the fibularis longus in the proximal lateral leg, just distal to the head of the fibula. Once located, continue palpating it distally to the lateral malleolus while strumming perpendicular. Note: The fibularis longus is located between the EDL and the soleus. Use plantarflexion of the foot to engage and discern the fibularis longus from the EDL; use eversion to engage and discern the fibularis longus from the soleus.

6. **Fibularis brevis:** Locate the tendon of the fibularis longus in the distal half of the leg. Then palpate on either side of it, and feel for the fibularis brevis as the client everts the foot (resistance may be added). The distal tendon of the fibularis brevis can often be visualized and palpated between the lateral malleolus and the fifth metatarsal.

Superficial Posterior Compartment Muscles: Client Prone

7. **Gastrocnemius:** With the client prone with the knee joints extended, ask the client to plantarflex the foot against resistance, and feel for the contraction of the gastrocnemius in the proximal posterior leg. Palpate both the medial and lateral heads, and then palpate to the attachment on the calcaneus.

8. **Plantaris:** Press gently into the center of the popliteal fossa as the client plantarflexes the foot. (Resistance can be added.) Gradually move laterally until you feel the presence of muscle tissue that contracts with plantarflexion of the foot. You are now on the plantaris. Strum across it perpendicularly. It can be challenging to discern the border between the plantaris and the lateral head of the gastrocnemius.

9. **Soleus:** With the client prone with the knee joint flexed to approximately 90 degrees, ask the client to plantarflex the foot (If resistance is given, offer only gentle resistance.) and feel for the contraction of the soleus through the gastrocnemius in the proximal posterior leg. Continue palpating the soleus distally to the calcaneal attachment. Note: The soleus is superficial and palpable in the lateral leg between the gastrocnemius and the fibularis longus, and it is superficial and palpable proximally in the medial leg between the gastrocnemius and the tibia (and flexor digitorum longus [FDL]).

Deep Posterior Compartment Muscles: Client Prone

For the popliteus palpation, you are standing to the same side of the client; for the rest of the palpations, you are seated or standing on the opposite side of the client.

10. **Popliteus:** With the client prone and the knee joint flexed to approximately 90 degrees, find the tibial tuberosity. Then curl your fingers around the tibia, and palpate against the posterior surface of the medial border of the tibia, feeling for the contraction of the popliteus as the client actively medially rotates the leg at the knee joint. (Resistance can be added if needed.) Once located, try to follow the popliteus deep to the gastrocnemius toward its femoral attachment as the client alternately contracts and relaxes the muscle.

11. **Tibialis posterior (TP):** The distal tendon of the TP is superficial in the distal medial leg directly posterior to the tibia. Ask the client to plantarflex and invert the foot and feel for the tendon of the TP to tense. Continue palpating the tendon to the navicular tuberosity by strumming perpendicularly across it. The distal tendon

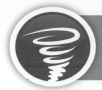

Muscles of the Leg—*cont'd*

of the TP is often visible and palpable directly posterior and then distal to the medial malleolus of the tibia. Palpate its belly proximally by pressing gently into the center of the posterior leg as the client plantarflexes and inverts the foot.

12. **Flexor digitorum longus (FDL):** Part of the FDL is superficial in the distal medial leg between the shaft of the tibia and the soleus. Ask the client to flex toes two to five (against resistance if needed) and feel for the contraction of the FDL. Continue palpating it distally as far as possible while strumming perpendicularly across it. Its tendon may be visible and palpable running posterior and then distal to the medial malleolus; its tendons may also be palpable in the plantar foot as the client contracts

the muscle. Palpate its belly proximally by pressing gently into the medial posterior leg as the client flexes toes two to five.

13. **Flexor hallucis longus (FHL):** A small part of the FHL is superficial in the distal medial leg between the FDL and the soleus. Ask the client to flex the big toe (against resistance if necessary) and feel for the contraction of the FHL. Continue palpating it as far distally as possible. It is usually not possible to palpate its distal tendon as it passes posteriorly and then distally to the medial malleolus; however, its distal tendon may be palpated in the plantar foot as the client contracts the muscle. Palpate its belly proximally by pressing gently into the lateral posterior leg as the client flexes the big toe.

20

Review Questions

1. List the attachments of the EDL.
2. List the attachments of the soleus.
3. What are the actions of the FDL?
4. What are the actions of the EHL?
5. Full assessment of the distal tendon of the tibialis anterior requires palpation along which two bones?
6. When palpating and assessing the EDL, what is it that needs to be remembered about the motions of the toes?
7. The distal tendon of what muscle can often be visualized and palpated distal to the lateral malleolus of the fibula?
8. Are there any positioning guidelines for palpation of the proximal attachments of the gastrocnemius?
9. What factors contribute to the ease or difficulty of palpating the soleus?
10. In what order are the tendons of the "Tom, Dick, and Harry" muscles from anterior to posterior?
11. What is the palpation key for the popliteus? In what position must the client be for proper muscle engagement during palpation and assessment?
12. Which muscle's TrPs may result in entrapment of the deep fibular nerve?
13. Compression of the S1 nerve, tight socks, and riding a bicycle with an improperly elevated seat may contribute to TrPs in what muscle?
14. What is the positioning for a stretch of the left EDL?
15. Describe an effective stretch for the fibularis longus and fibularis brevis.
16. Explain how a therapist can discern the border between the EDL and the tibialis anterior in the anterolateral leg.
17. Having found tightness in both the gastrocnemius and soleus, a client asks if she can be given a stretch that could help. How would you answer this client?

CASE STUDY

A 27-year-old male client is experiencing pain and muscle cramps in the posterior left leg and constant pain on the anterior side of his right leg. The pain in his left leg varies in intensity from four to seven on a scale of ten and the right leg pain intensity is at a five to six out of ten. The client is a long-time distance runner who has been training for the last 10 months to participate in an Ironman Triathlon (consisting of running, cycling, and swimming) later this year. His regular exercise routine has always included running and now includes weight lifting, cycling, and swimming.

History reveals no recent or past trauma to the legs and no other lifestyle changes other than training for a new type of sporting event. Evaluation by his medical doctor revealed nothing of significance, and it was recommended that he decrease his training for a couple of weeks and take over-the-counter pain medication as needed.

Physical examination shows moderate tenderness along the lateral border of the right tibia. Range of motion testing of the ankle produces pain (five out of ten) felt in the right anterior leg with active dorsiflexion of the foot. Manual resistance to dorsiflexion and inversion invoked a sharp, strong pain (seven out of ten) in the anterior leg. The left gastrocnemius is tight throughout its course with several active TrPs. It is also noted that the client's right medial longitudinal arch is slightly collapsed during weight bearing.

1. What about the client's lifestyle and activities may account for his complaints?
2. What is the effect of the collapsed right arch during weight bearing?
3. What would your treatment plan include?

CHAPTER 21

Tour #11 · Palpation of the Intrinsic Muscles of the Foot

Overview

This chapter is a palpation tour of the intrinsic muscles of the foot. The tour begins with the dorsal muscles and then addresses the plantar muscles. Palpation of the muscles on the dorsum of the foot is shown in the supine position; palpation of the plantar muscles is shown in the prone position. Alternate palpation positions are also described. The major muscles or muscle groups of the region are each given a separate layout. There are also a few detours to other muscles of the region. Many intrinsic muscles of the foot are relatively easy to palpate and discern. However, one difficult aspect to intrinsic foot musculature palpation is that clients are often unable to isolate the joint action necessary for isolated contraction of the target muscle. Trigger point (TrP) information and stretching, both therapist-assisted and self-care stretching, are given for each of the muscles covered in this chapter. The chapter closes with an advanced *Whirlwind Tour* that explains the sequential palpation of all of the muscles of the chapter.

Chapter Outline

Extensor Digitorum Brevis and Extensor Hallucis Brevis
Dorsal Interossei Pedis
Abductor Hallucis and Flexor Hallucis Brevis
    Detour to the Adductor Hallucis
Abductor Digiti Minimi Pedis and Flexor Digiti Minimi Pedis
    Detour to the Lumbricals Pedis and Plantar Interossei
Flexor Digitorum Brevis
    Detour to the Quadratus Plantae
Whirlwind Tour: Intrinsic Muscles of the Foot

Chapter Objectives

After completing this chapter, the student/therapist should be able to perform the following for each of the muscles covered in this chapter:

1. State the attachments.
2. State the actions.
3. Describe the starting position for palpation.
4. Describe and explain the purpose of each of the palpation steps.
5. Palpate each muscle.
6. State the "Palpation Key."
7. Describe alternate palpation positions.
8. State the locations of the most common TrP(s).
9. Describe the TrP referral zones.
10. State the most common factors that create and/or perpetuate TrPs.
11. State the symptoms most commonly caused by TrPs.
12. Describe and perform the therapist-assisted and self-care stretches.

e Go to http://evolve.elsevier.com/Muscolino/palpation for video demonstrations of the muscle palpations presented in this chapter.

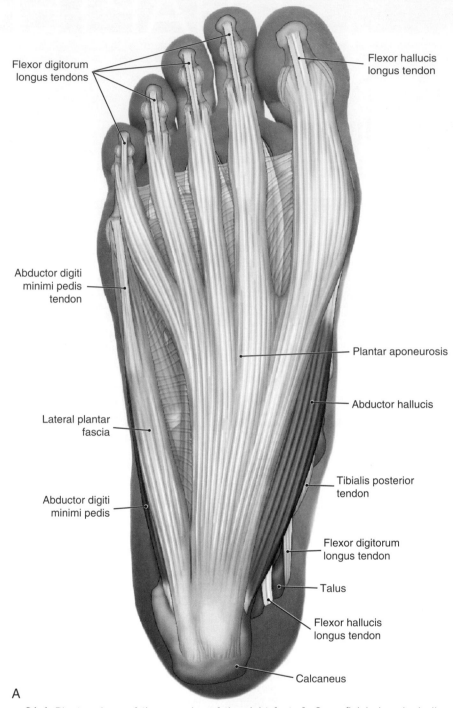

Flexor digitorum longus tendons

Flexor hallucis longus tendon

Abductor digiti minimi pedis tendon

Plantar aponeurosis

Abductor hallucis

Lateral plantar fascia

Tibialis posterior tendon

Abductor digiti minimi pedis

Flexor digitorum longus tendon

Talus

Flexor hallucis longus tendon

Calcaneus

A

Figure 21-1 Plantar views of the muscles of the right foot. **A,** Superficial view, including the fascia.

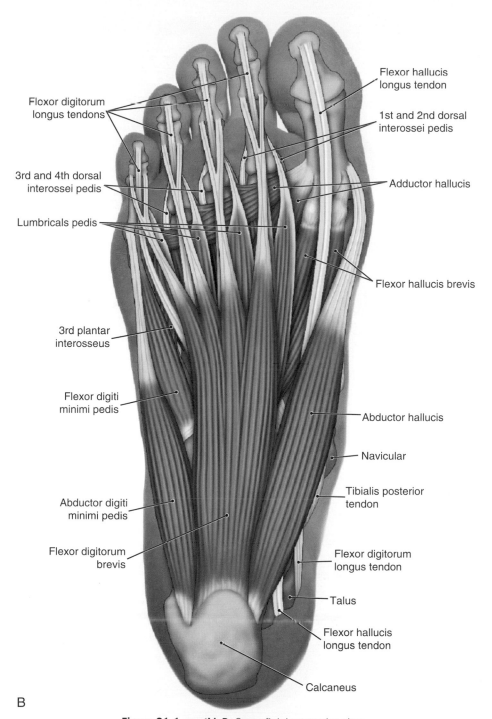

Flexor hallucis longus tendon

1st and 2nd dorsal interossei pedis

Flexor digitorum longus tendons

Adductor hallucis

3rd and 4th dorsal interossei pedis

Lumbricals pedis

Flexor hallucis brevis

3rd plantar interosseus

Flexor digiti minimi pedis

Abductor hallucis

Navicular

Tibialis posterior tendon

Abductor digiti minimi pedis

Flexor digitorum longus tendon

Flexor digitorum brevis

Talus

Flexor hallucis longus tendon

Calcaneus

B

Figure 21-1, cont'd B, Superficial muscular view.

21

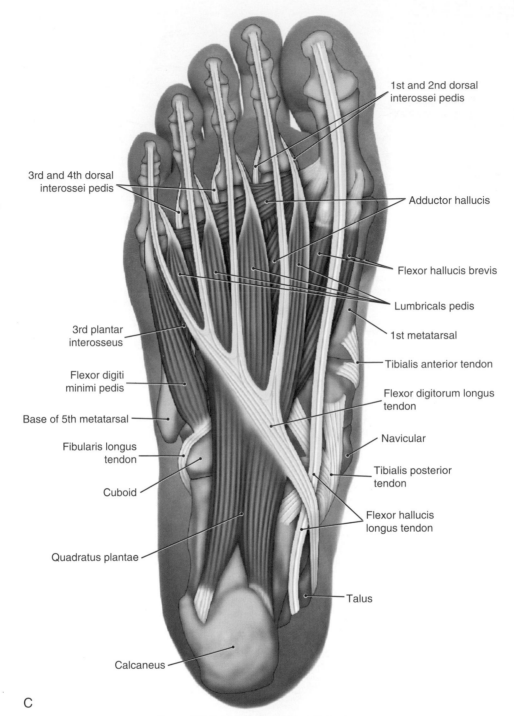

1st and 2nd dorsal interossei pedis

3rd and 4th dorsal interossei pedis

Adductor hallucis

Flexor hallucis brevis

Lumbricals pedis

3rd plantar interosseus

1st metatarsal

Flexor digiti minimi pedis

Tibialis anterior tendon

Base of 5th metatarsal

Flexor digitorum longus tendon

Fibularis longus tendon

Navicular

Cuboid

Tibialis posterior tendon

Quadratus plantae

Flexor hallucis longus tendon

Talus

Calcaneus

C

Figure 21-1, cont'd C, Intermediate view.

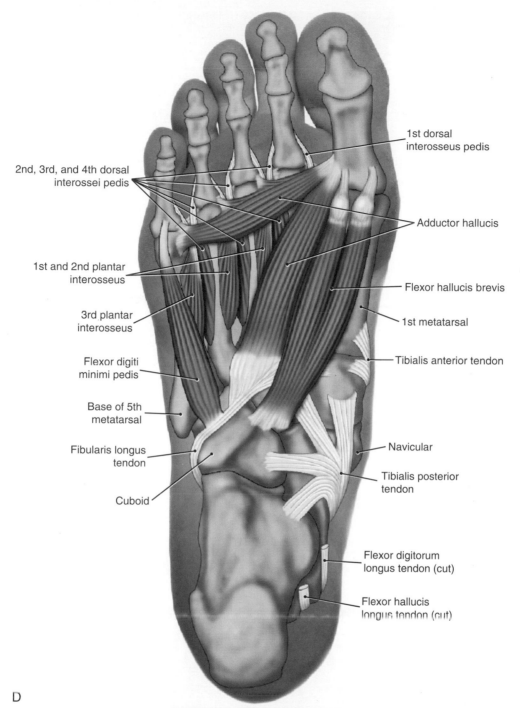

1st dorsal interosseus pedis

2nd, 3rd, and 4th dorsal interossei pedis

Adductor hallucis

1st and 2nd plantar interosseus

Flexor hallucis brevis

3rd plantar interosseus

1st metatarsal

Flexor digiti minimi pedis

Tibialis anterior tendon

Base of 5th metatarsal

Fibularis longus tendon

Navicular

Cuboid

Tibialis posterior tendon

Flexor digitorum longus tendon (cut)

Flexor hallucis longus tendon (cut)

D

Figure 21-1, cont'd D, Deep view.

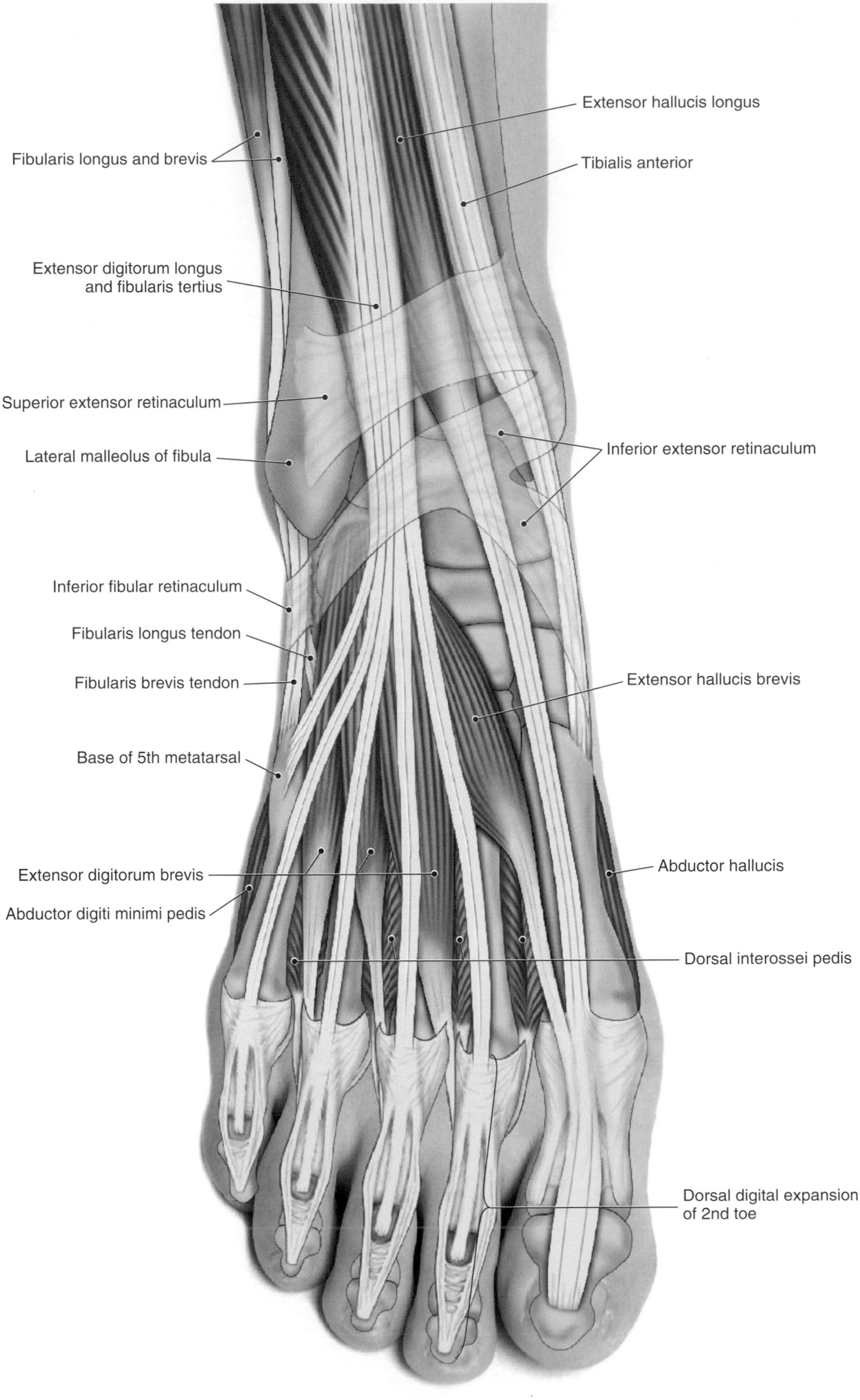

Fibularis longus and brevis

Extensor digitorum longus and fibularis tertius

Superior extensor retinaculum

Lateral malleolus of fibula

Inferior fibular retinaculum

Fibularis longus tendon

Fibularis brevis tendon

Base of 5th metatarsal

Extensor digitorum brevis

Abductor digiti minimi pedis

Extensor hallucis longus

Tibialis anterior

Inferior extensor retinaculum

Extensor hallucis brevis

Abductor hallucis

Dorsal interossei pedis

Dorsal digital expansion of 2nd toe

Figure 21-2 Dorsal view of the muscles of the right foot.

21

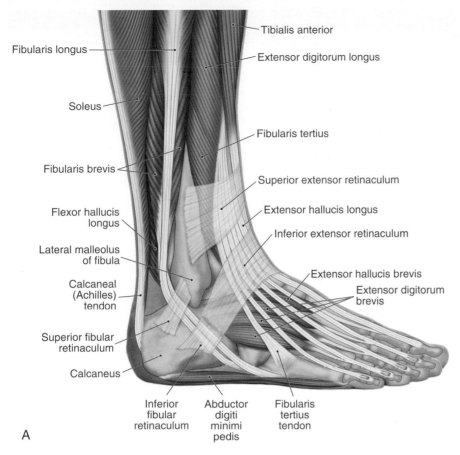

Tibialis anterior

Fibularis longus

Extensor digitorum longus

Soleus

Fibularis tertius

Fibularis brevis

Superior extensor retinaculum

Extensor hallucis longus

Flexor hallucis longus

Inferior extensor retinaculum

Lateral malleolus of fibula

Extensor hallucis brevis

Extensor digitorum brevis

Calcaneal (Achilles) tendon

Superior fibular retinaculum

Calcaneus

Inferior fibular retinaculum

Abductor digiti minimi pedis

Fibularis tertius tendon

A

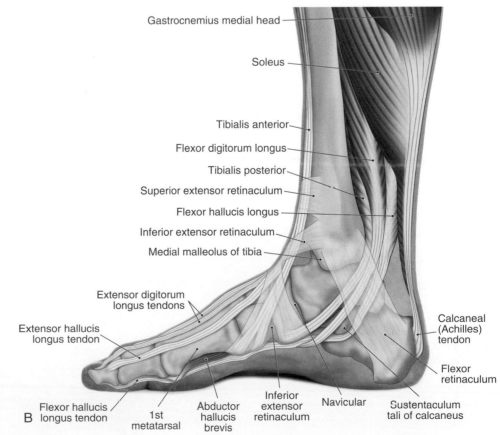

Gastrocnemius medial head

Soleus

Tibialis anterior

Flexor digitorum longus

Tibialis posterior

Superior extensor retinaculum

Flexor hallucis longus

Inferior extensor retinaculum

Medial malleolus of tibia

Extensor digitorum longus tendons

Calcaneal (Achilles) tendon

Extensor hallucis longus tendon

Flexor retinaculum

Flexor hallucis longus tendon

1st metatarsal

Abductor hallucis brevis

Inferior extensor retinaculum

Navicular

Sustentaculum tali of calcaneus

B

Figure 21-3 Lateral and medial views of the muscles of the right foot. **A,** Lateral view. **B,** Medial view.

21

EXTENSOR DIGITORUM BREVIS (EDB) AND EXTENSOR HALLUCIS BREVIS (EHB)—SUPINE

☑ ATTACHMENTS

☐ Proximally, both the extensor digitorum brevis (EDB) and extensor hallucis brevis (EHB) attach to the dorsal surface of the calcaneus.

☐ Distally, the EDB attaches to the lateral side of the distal tendons of the extensor digitorum longus of toes two through four.

☐ Distally, the EHB attaches to the dorsal surface of the base of the proximal phalanx of the big toe (toe one).

☑ ACTIONS

☐ The EDB extends toes two to four at the metatarsophalangeal (MTP) and proximal and distal interphalangeal joints.

☐ The EHB extends the big toe at the MTP joint.

Starting Position (Figure 21-5)

■ Client supine

■ Therapist is seated to the side of the client

■ After the common belly of the EDB and EHB is visualized, palpating fingers are placed on the belly of these muscles on the proximal dorsolateral surface of the foot (approximately 1 inch [2.5 cm] distal to the lateral malleolus of the fibula)

■ Fingers of the support hand placed on the proximal phalanges of toes two to four

Palpation Steps

1. Resist the client from extending toes two to four at the MTP joints by placing fingers of the support hand on the proximal phalanges of toes two to four, and look for the contraction of the belly of the EDB. After visualizing the contracted belly of the EDB, palpate it (Note: If the EDB cannot be visualized, then palpate for it on the proximal dorsolateral foot) (Figure 21-6, *A*).

2. To palpate the EHB, follow the same procedure used for the EDB except that the support hand is placed on the proximal phalanx of the big toe to provide resistance to extension of the big toe (see Figure 21-6, *B*).

3. Asking the client to alternately contract and relax the EDB or the EHB against resistance, try to follow the EDB distally toward toes two to four and the EHB toward the

big toe while strumming perpendicularly to the tendon(s) (Palpation Note #3).

4. Once the EDB and/or EHB have been located, have the client relax them, and palpate to assess their baseline tone.

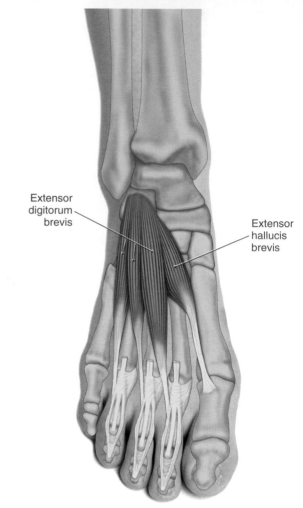

Figure 21-4 Dorsal view of the extensors digitorum and hallucis brevis (EDB and EHB).

Figure 21-5 Starting position for supine palpation of the right extensors digitorum and hallucis brevis (EDB and EHB).

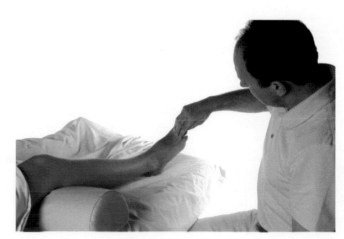

21

EXTENSOR DIGITORUM BREVIS (EDB) AND EXTENSOR HALLUCIS BREVIS (EHB)—SUPINE—*cont'd*

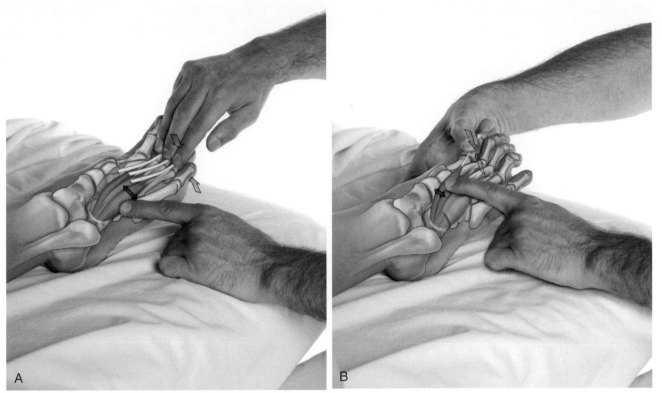

A   B

Figure 21-6 Palpation of the right extensor digitorum brevis (EDB) and extensor hallucis brevis (EHB). **A,** Palpation of the EDB as the client extends toes two to four against resistance. The EHB has been ghosted in. **B,** Palpation of the EHB as the client extends the big toe against resistance. The EDB has been ghosted in.

PALPATION NOTES

1. Structurally, the EDB and EHB are actually one muscle. They are functionally divided into two separate muscles based on their distal attachments. The fibers that attach distally to toes two to four are named the EDB, and the fibers that attach distally to the big toe are named the EHB.
2. Within the common belly of these two muscles, the fibers of the EDB are on the lateral side and the fibers of the EHB are on the medial side.
3. The distal aspects of the EDB and EHB can be difficult to palpate and discern because they are located deep to the distal tendons of the extensor digitorum longus, whose tendons (also) tense with extension of the proximal phalanges of toes two to four.

4. To discern the EDB from the EHB, it is necessary for the client to be able to isolate extension of the big toe from the other toes. Many people are unable to do this. It does not help to hold down whichever toe(s) that you want the client to not move, because even though the toe(s) might not move, the belly of the muscle that we want to be relaxed will be isometrically contracted, making it more difficult to discern these two muscles from each other. For example, if you are palpating the EDB and you want the EHB to stay relaxed, but the client cannot extend toes two to four without also extending the big toe at the same time, it does not help to restrain the big toe by holding it down, because the belly of the EHB will isometrically contract against the resistance of your finger.

Alternate Position—Seated

Both the EDB and EHB can also be easily accessed with the client seated.

EXTENSOR DIGITORUM BREVIS (EDB) AND EXTENSOR HALLUCIS BREVIS (EHB)—SUPINE—*cont'd*

TRIGGER POINTS

1. Trigger points (TrPs) in the EDB and EHB often result from or are perpetuated by acute or chronic overuse of the muscles, sustained postures that cause the muscles to lengthen (e.g., sleeping supine with tight sheets that hold the toes in flexion), sustained postures that allow the muscles to shorten (e.g., wearing high-heeled shoes), wearing shoes with an inflexible sole (not allowing motion of the MTP joints), wearing shoes that are too tight (or laced too tightly), trauma, or stress fractures of the metatarsals.
2. TrPs in the EDB and EHB may produce decreased flexion of the toes at the MTP joints, cramps in the foot, or an antalgic gait.
3. The referral patterns of EDB and EHB TrPs must be distinguished from the referral patterns of TrPs in the extensor digitorum longus, fibularis tertius, tibialis anterior, plantar and dorsal interossei pedis, and lumbricals pedis.
4. TrPs in the EDB and EHB may be incorrectly assessed as a metatarsal stress fracture or entrapment of a digital nerve between adjacent metatarsals.

5. Associated TrPs often occur in the extensor digitorum longus or extensor hallucis longus.
6. Note: The EDB and EHB share the same TrP pain referral pattern.

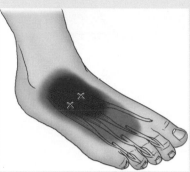

Figure 21-7 Anterolateral (dorsolateral) view showing common trigger points (TrPs) and their corresponding referral zone for the extensors digitorum and hallucis brevis (EDB and EHB).

Palpation Key:
Look for the bulge of the EDB and EHB laterally on the dorsum of the foot.

EXTENSOR DIGITORUM BREVIS (EDB) AND EXTENSOR HALLUCIS BREVIS (EHB)—SUPINE—*cont'd*

STRETCHING THE EXTENSOR DIGITORUM BREVIS AND EXTENSOR HALLUCIS BREVIS

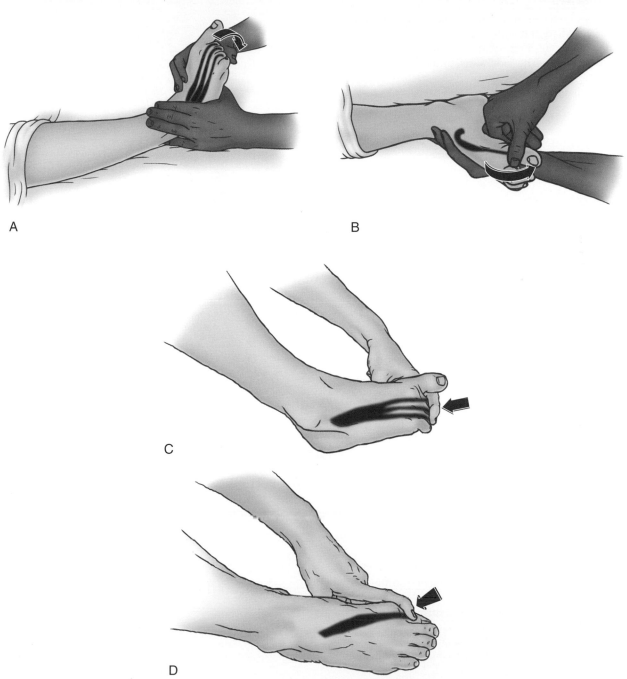

A

B

C

D

Figure 21-8 Stretching the right extensor digitorum brevis (EDB) and extensor hallucis brevis (EHB). For the EDB, the proximal, middle, and distal phalanges of toes two to four are flexed. For the EHB, the proximal phalanx of the big toe is flexed. **A** and **B,** Therapist-assisted stretches of the EDB and EHB respectively. Note: The therapist's other hand stabilizes the client's foot. **C** and **D,** Self-care stretches of the EDB and EHB, respectively.

21

DORSAL INTEROSSEI PEDIS—SUPINE

There are four dorsal interossei pedis muscles, numbered one to four from medial to lateral, respectively.

☑ ATTACHMENTS

☐ Proximally, each dorsal interosseus pedis attaches to both sides of the adjacent metatarsals.

☐ Distally, each one attaches to one side of the proximal phalanx of a toe (the side away from the center of the second toe), and to the tendon of the extensor digitorum longus to that toe.

☑ ACTIONS

☐ Abduct toes two to four at the metatarsophalangeal (MTP) joints

☐ Flex toes two to four at the MTP joints

☐ Extend toes two to four at the proximal and distal interphalangeal joints

Starting Position (Figure 21-10, *A*)

■ Client supine
■ Therapist is seated to the side of the client
■ Palpating fingers placed on the dorsal side of the foot between the fourth and fifth metatarsal bones
■ Fingers of support hand placed on the lateral side of the proximal phalanx of the fourth toe

Palpation Steps

1. Fourth dorsal interosseus pedis: Ask the client to abduct the fourth toe against your resistance, and feel for the contraction of the fourth dorsal interosseus pedis between the fourth and fifth metatarsals (see Figure 21-10, *A*).

2. Palpate the fourth dorsal interosseus pedis proximally and distally while the client alternately contracts against your resistance and relaxes the muscle.

3. Third dorsal interosseus pedis: Repeat this procedure for the third dorsal interosseus pedis by palpating on the dorsal surface of the foot between the third and fourth metatarsals and resisting the client from abducting the third toe (see Figure 21-10, *B*).

4. Second dorsal interosseus pedis: Repeat this procedure for the second dorsal interosseus pedis by palpating on the dorsal surface of the foot between the second and third metatarsals and resisting the client from performing fibular abduction of the second toe (see Figure 21-10, *C*).

5. First dorsal interosseus pedis: Repeat this procedure for the first dorsal interosseus pedis by palpating on the dorsal surface of the foot between the first and second metatarsals and resisting the client from performing tibial abduction of the second toe (see Figure 21-10, *D*).

6. Once each dorsal interosseus pedis has been located, have the client relax it and palpate to assess its baseline tone.

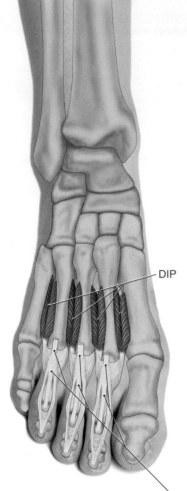

Figure 21-9 Dorsal view of the right dorsal interossei pedis (DIP).

21

DORSAL INTEROSSEI PEDIS—SUPINE—*cont'd*

Figure 21-10 Palpation of the dorsal interossei pedis. **A,** Palpation of the fourth dorsal interosseus pedis as the client abducts the fourth toe against resistance. **B,** Palpation of the third dorsal interosseus pedis as the client abducts the third toe against resistance. **C,** Palpation of the second dorsal interosseus pedis as the client does fibular abduction of the second toe against resistance. **D,** Palpation of the first dorsal interosseus pedis as the client does tibial abduction of the second toe against resistance.

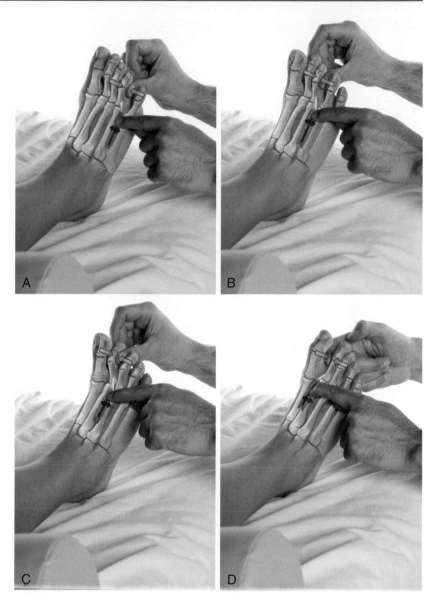

A   B

C   D

PALPATION NOTES

1. The second toe abducts in both directions. Fibular abduction is moving it laterally (i.e., toward the fibula); tibial abduction is moving it medially (i.e., toward the tibia).
2. Many clients cannot isolate abduction of the toes, especially fibular versus tibial abduction of the second toe. If a client cannot isolate a motion to engage one of the dorsal interossei pedis for palpation, then simply palpate the muscle in a relaxed state by its location.
3. Keep in mind that the extensor muscles of the toes (longus and brevis) lie superficial to the dorsal interossei pedis. For this reason, it is important that the client does not attempt to extend the toes, or these extensor muscles will contract, making palpation and discernment of the dorsal interossei pedis extremely difficult.

Alternate Position—Seated

The dorsal interossei pedis can also be easily accessed with the client seated.

Palpation Key:
Palpate between the metatarsals on the dorsum of the foot.

21

DORSAL INTEROSSEI PEDIS—SUPINE—*cont'd*

TRIGGER POINTS

1. Trigger points (TrPs) in the dorsal interossei pedis often result from or are perpetuated by acute or chronic overuse of the muscle (e.g., walking in soft sand), sustained postures that cause the muscles to lengthen (e.g., wearing high-heeled shoes), wearing ill-fitting shoes (that are either too tight or laced too tightly, or have a pointed toe), wearing shoes with an inflexible sole (not allowing motion of the MTP joints), immobilization due to a cast, excessive pronation of the foot (requiring greater stabilization by the intrinsic foot muscles), structural deformities of the foot, trauma, or stress fractures of the metatarsals.

2. TrPs in the dorsal interossei pedis tend to produce pain in a vertical pattern along the dorsal and plantar sides of the ray (metatarsal and phalanges) to which the dorsal interossei pedis attaches distally (Figure 21-11 shows the typical patterns for the first and fourth dorsal interossei pedis muscles). Dorsal interossei pedis TrPs also tend to produce tender and sore feet (especially when weight bearing), pain when walking, decreased or painful adduction or extension of toes two to five at the MTP joints, cramps in the foot, or an antalgic gait. Furthermore, TrPs in the first dorsal interosseus pedis may produce tingling in the big toe.

3. The referral patterns of dorsal interossei pedis TrPs must be distinguished from the referral patterns of TrPs in the flexor digitorum brevis (FDB), abductor digiti minimi pedis (ADMP), adductor hallucis, plantar interossei, lumbricals pedis, extensor digitorum longus, and flexor digitorum longus.

4. TrPs in the dorsal interossei pedis are often incorrectly assessed as plantar fasciitis, metatarsal stress fracture, entrapment of a digital nerve between adjacent metatarsals, or tarsal joint dysfunction.

5. Associated TrPs often occur in the plantar interossei and lumbricals pedis.

6. Note: The plantar interossei and lumbricals pedis share the same TrP pain referral patterns as the dorsal interossei pedis.

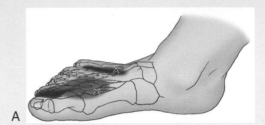

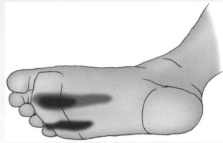

Figure 21-11 Views of common trigger points (TrPs) of the first and fourth dorsal interossei pedis muscles and their corresponding referral zones. **A,** Medial view showing common TrPs and their corresponding referral zones. **B,** Medial-plantar view that shows the remainder of the referral zones. Note: TrPs commonly occur in all four dorsal interossei pedis muscles.

21

DORSAL INTEROSSEI PEDIS—SUPINE—*cont'd*

STRETCHING THE DORSAL INTEROSSEI PEDIS

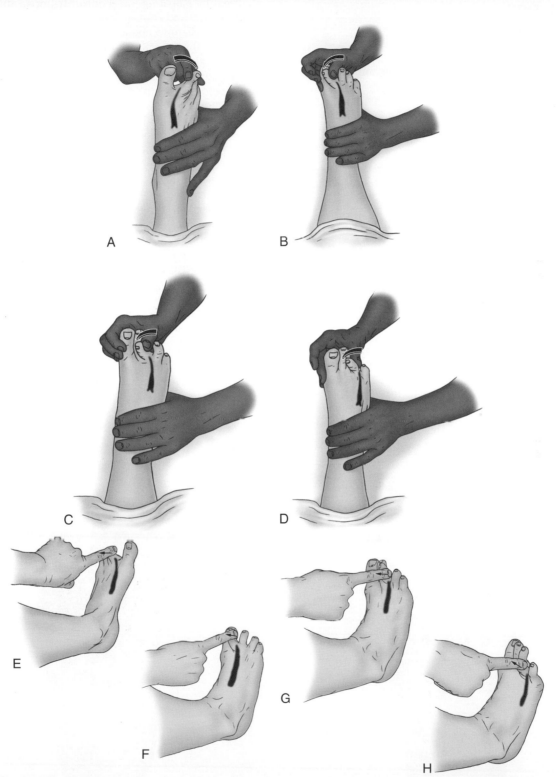

Figure 21-12 Stretching the right four dorsal interossei pedis muscles. Each dorsal interosseus pedis is stretched by moving the respective toe at the metatarsophalangeal (MTP) joint. To stretch the first dorsal interosseus pedis, the second toe is moved into fibular abduction. To stretch the second dorsal interosseus pedis, the second toe is moved into tibial abduction. To stretch the third dorsal interosseus pedis, the third toe is moved into adduction. To stretch the fourth dorsal interosseus pedis, the fourth toe is moved into adduction. **A, B, C,** and **D,** Therapist-assisted stretches of dorsal interossei pedis 1, 2, 3, and 4, respectively. Note: The therapist's other hand stabilizes the client's foot. **E, F, G,** and **H,** Self-care stretches of dorsal interossei pedis 1, 2, 3, and 4, respectively.

21

ABDUCTOR HALLUCIS (ABH) AND FLEXOR HALLUCIS BREVIS (FHB)—PRONE

Abductor Hallucis (AbH)

☑ATTACHMENTS

☐ Tuberosity of the calcaneus

to the

☐ medial plantar side of the base of the proximal phalanx of the big toe

☑ACTIONS

☐ Abducts the big toe at the metatarsophalangeal (MTP) joint
☐ Flexes the big toe at the MTP joint

Flexor Hallucis Brevis (FHB)

☑ATTACHMENTS

☐ Cuboid and third cuneiform

to the

☐ medial and lateral sides of the plantar surface of the base of the proximal phalanx of the big toe

☑ACTIONS

☐ Flexes the big toe at the MTP joint

Starting Position (Figure 21-15)
■ Client prone
■ Therapist seated at the end of the table
■ Palpating fingers placed on the medial side of the foot, close to the plantar surface

Palpation Steps

1. Begin by palpating the abductor hallucis (AbH), which is superficial and easily palpable.
2. Ask the client to abduct the big toe at the MTP joint, and feel for the contraction of the AbH. If desired, resistance can be given with the support hand on the medial side of the proximal phalanx of the big toe (Figure 21-16).
3. Once located, palpate it proximally and distally toward its attachments while strumming perpendicular to its fibers.
4. Once the AbH has been located, have the client relax it, and palpate to assess its baseline tone.
5. To now palpate the flexor hallucis brevis (FHB), which is also superficial and easily palpable, move your palpating fingers over the first metatarsal bone on the plantar side of the foot.
6. Ask the client to flex the big toe at the MTP joint, and feel for the contraction of the FHB. If desired, resistance can be given with the support hand on the plantar surface of the proximal phalanx of the big toe (Figure 21-17).
7. Once located, palpate it distally to the proximal phalanx of the big toe while strumming perpendicular to its fibers. Then palpate it proximally as far as possible.
8. Once the FHB has been located, have the client relax it, and palpate to assess its baseline tone.

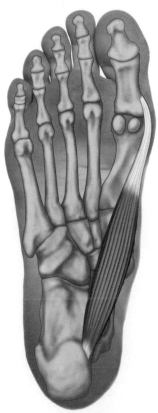

Figure 21-13 Plantar view of the right abductor hallucis (AbH).

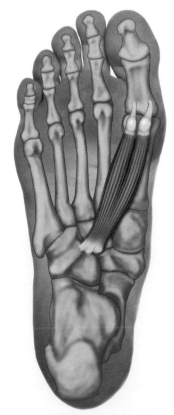

Figure 21-14 Plantar view of the right flexor hallucis brevis (FHB).

21

ABDUCTOR HALLUCIS (ABH) AND FLEXOR HALLUCIS BREVIS (FHB)—PRONE—*cont'd*

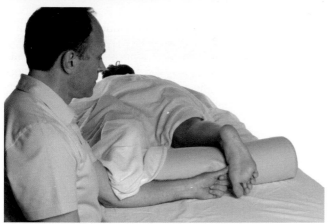

Figure 21-15 Starting position for prone palpation of the right abductor hallucis (AbH).

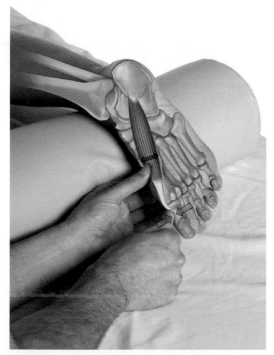

Figure 21-16 Palpation of the right abductor hallucis (AbH) as the client abducts the big toe against resistance.

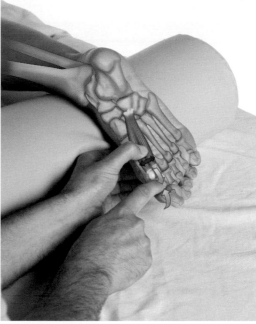

Figure 21-17 Palpation of the right flexor hallucis brevis (FHB) as the client flexes the big toe against resistance.

Alternate Position—Supine

Both the AbH and FHB can also be easily palpated with the client supine.

Palpation Key:
AbH: Palpate on the medial side of the foot, strumming up and down.
FHB: Palpate over the plantar surface of the first metatarsal while flexing the big toe.

ABDUCTOR HALLUCIS PALPATION NOTES

1. Abduction of the big toe at the MTP joint is a medial motion.
2. The entire abductor hallucis (AbH) can usually be palpated and discerned.
3. Many clients are unable to isolate big toe abduction. If this occurs, place a finger of your support hand against the medial side of the proximal phalanx of the big toe, and ask the client to press against it. Having the pressure of the resistance finger often helps the client create this motion.
4. If the client is still unable to perform abduction of the big toe against pressure (as in Palpation Note #3), then try resisting the client from flexing the proximal phalanx of the

big toe at the MTP joint, feeling for the AbH to contract on the medial side of the foot. Have the client keep the interphalangeal (IP) joint of the big toe extended; otherwise flexion of the proximal phalanx of the big toe will be carried out by the flexor hallucis longus and the AbH will not contract. Note: The flexor hallucis brevis (FHB) will also contract with flexion of the big toe at the MTP joint, so be sure that you are not palpating too far onto the plantar surface of the foot.

5. Another method to discern the AbH from the FHB is to ask the client to abduct and extend the big toe at the MTP joint. Extension will reciprocally inhibit and relax the FHB.

21

ABDUCTOR HALLUCIS (ABH) AND FLEXOR HALLUCIS BREVIS (FHB)—PRONE—*cont'd*

FLEXOR HALLUCIS BREVIS PALPATION NOTES

1. Even though the flexor hallucis brevis (FHB) is in the second plantar layer of the foot, the vast majority of it is fairly easily palpable. The most challenging aspect to palpate is the proximal attachment at the cuboid and third cuneiform. If the client is able to isolate flexion of the big toe without also flexing the other toes, even this proximal attachment can usually be well palpated and discerned from the more superficial flexor digitorum brevis (FDB). However, many clients cannot isolate this motion.

2. It does not help to stop toes two to five from flexing with the fingers of your support hand, because even though these other toes might not move, the belly of the FDB that we want to be relaxed will still contract (isometrically),

making it more difficult to palpate the proximal attachment of the FHB through it.

3. Directly superficial to the FHB is the distal tendon of the flexor hallucis longus. Given that both these muscles contract with flexion of the big toe, it can be difficult to discern them from each other.

4. To discern the FHB from the more superficial distal tendon of the flexor hallucis longus, try to have the client isolate flexion of the big toe at the MTP joint while keeping the IP joint of the big toe extended. This tends to engage the FHB more than the flexor hallucis longus. However, many clients are unable to do this.

TRIGGER POINTS

1. Trigger points (TrPs) in the AbH and FHB often result from or are perpetuated by acute or chronic overuse of the muscle (e.g., walking in soft sand), sustained postures that cause the muscles to lengthen (e.g., wearing high-heeled shoes), wearing ill-fitting shoes (that are either too tight or laced too tightly, or have a pointed toe), wearing shoes with an inflexible sole (not allowing motion of the MTP joint), immobilization due to a cast, excessive pronation of the foot (requiring greater stabilization by the intrinsic foot muscles), structural deformities of the foot, trauma, or stress fractures of the metatarsals.

2. TrPs in the AbH and FHB tend to produce tender and sore feet (especially when weight bearing), pain when walking, decreased or painful adduction (AbH) or extension (FHB or AbH) of the big toe at the MTP joint, cramps in the foot, or an antalgic gait. Furthermore, the AbH may produce entrapment of the posterior tibial nerve and/or its two branches, the medial and lateral plantar nerves (resulting in sensory symptoms on the plantar surface of the foot and/ or weakness of the intrinsic muscles of the sole of the foot).

3. The referral patterns of AbH TrPs must be distinguished from the referral patterns of TrPs in the plantar interossei, dorsal interossei pedis, and lumbricals pedis between the first and second toes, quadratus plantae, and medial head of the gastrocnemius. The referral patterns of FHB TrPs must be distinguished from the referral patterns of TrPs in the flexor hallucis longus, adductor hallucis, tibialis anterior, and extensor hallucis longus.

4. TrPs in the AbH are often incorrectly assessed as calcaneal (Achilles) tendinitis or tarsal joint dysfunction. TrPs in the FHB are often incorrectly assessed as gout, plantar fasciitis, metatarsal stress fracture, or tarsal joint dysfunction.

5. Associated TrPs for the AbH often occur in the FHB and flexor digitorum brevis (FDB). Associated TrPs for the FHB often occur in the AbH, quadratus plantae, and flexor digitorum longus.

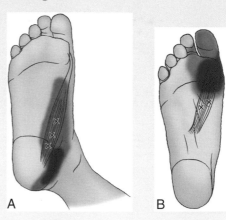

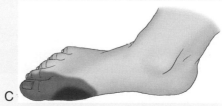

Figure 21-18 A, Medial-plantar view showing common abductor hallucis (AbH) trigger points (TrPs) and their corresponding referral zone. **B** and **C,** Plantar and medial views, respectively, of common flexor hallucis brevis (FHB) trigger points (TrPs) and their corresponding referral zones.

ABDUCTOR HALLUCIS (ABH) AND FLEXOR HALLUCIS BREVIS (FHB)—PRONE—cont'd

STRETCHING THE ABDUCTOR HALLUCIS AND FLEXOR HALLUCIS BREVIS

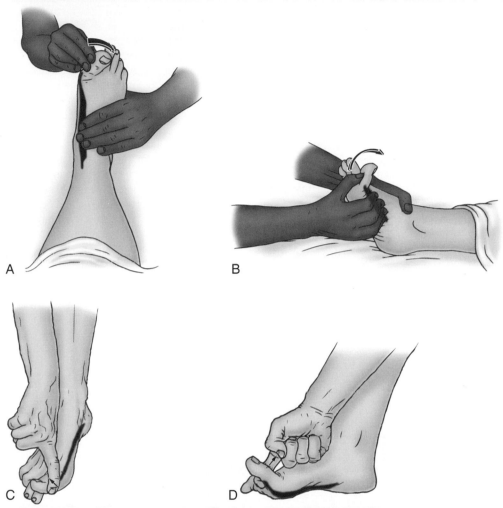

Figure 21-19 Stretching the right abductor hallucis (AbH) and flexor hallucis brevis (FHB) muscles. Each muscle is stretched by moving the big toe at the metatarsophalangeal (MTP) joint. For the AbH, the big toe is adducted and extended. For the FHB, the big toe is extended. **A** and **B,** Therapist-assisted stretches of the AbH and FHB muscles respectively. Note: The therapist's other hand is used to stabilize the client's foot. **C** and **D,** Self-care stretches of the AbH and FHB muscles, respectively.

21

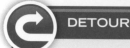

ABDUCTOR HALLUCIS (ABH) AND FLEXOR HALLUCIS BREVIS (FHB)—PRONE—*cont'd*

DETOUR

Adductor Hallucis:

The adductor hallucis has two heads, an oblique head and a transverse head, and attaches from metatarsals two to four, the tendon of the fibularis longus, and the plantar metatarsophalangeal (MTP) ligaments to the proximal phalanx of the big toe. Its actions are adduction and flexion of the big toe at the MTP joint. It is deep to the plantar fascia and the flexor digitorum brevis (FDB). Given its depth and the difficulty that most clients have isolating adduction of the big toe, this muscle can be challenging to palpate and discern. When palpating this muscle, palpate over the heads of the metatarsals of the second, third, and fourth toes while resisting the client from adducting the big toe and feel for the contraction of the transverse head. Try to palpate the oblique head in a similar manner.

Trigger Points:

1. Trigger points (TrPs) in the adductor hallucis usually result from the same factors that create or perpetuate TrPs in the abductor hallucis (AbH) and flexor hallucis brevis (FHB).
2. TrPs in the adductor hallucis often produce sore feet that cause pain when weight bearing and walking, antalgic gait, cramps, decreased abduction or extension of the big toe, or numbness in its TrP referral area.
3. The referral patterns of adductor hallucis TrPs must be distinguished from the referral patterns of TrPs in the FDB, flexor and abductor digiti minimi pedis (ADMP), FHB, plantar and dorsal interossei pedis, lumbricals pedis, flexor digitorum longus, and flexor hallucis longus.
4. TrPs in the adductor hallucis are often incorrectly assessed as plantar fasciitis, metatarsal stress fracture, or tarsal joint dysfunction.
5. Associated TrPs often occur in the FHB and AbH.

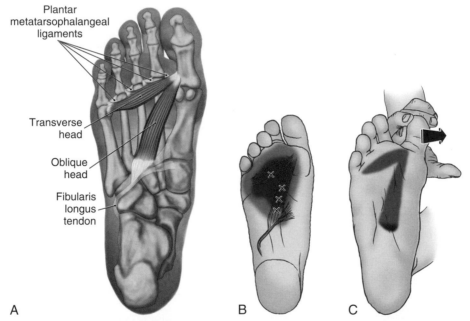

Figure 21-20 Views of the right adductor hallucis. **A,** Plantar view of the adductor hallucis (transverse and oblique heads). **B,** Plantar view showing common adductor hallucis trigger points (TrPs) and their corresponding referral zone. **C,** Stretch of the adductor hallucis in which the big toe is abducted away from the second toe and also slightly extended.

ABDUCTOR DIGITI MINIMI PEDIS (ADMP) AND FLEXOR DIGITI MINIMI PEDIS (FDMP)—PRONE

Abductor Digiti Minimi Pedis (ADMP)

☑ ATTACHMENTS

☐ Tuberosity of the calcaneus

to the

☐ lateral plantar side of the proximal phalanx of the little toe

☑ ACTIONS

☐ Abducts the little toe at the metatarsophalangeal (MTP) joint
☐ Flexes the little toe at the MTP joint

Flexor Digiti Minimi Pedis (FDMP)

☑ ATTACHMENTS

☐ The plantar surface of the base of the fifth metatarsal and the tendon of the fibularis longus

to the

☐ plantar surface of the base of the proximal phalanx of the little toe

☑ ACTIONS

☐ Flexes the little toe at the MTP joint

Starting Position (Figure 21-23)

■ Client prone
■ Therapist seated at the end of the table

■ Palpating fingers placed on the lateral side of the distal foot, close to the plantar surface

Palpation steps

1. Begin by palpating the abductor digiti minimi pedis (ADMP), which is superficial and easily palpable.
2. Ask the client to abduct the little toe at the MTP joint, and feel for the contraction of the ADMP. If desired, resistance can be given by placing fingers of the support hand on the lateral side of the proximal phalanx of the little toe (Figure 21-24).
3. Once located, palpate it proximally and distally toward its attachments while strumming perpendicular to its fibers.
4. Once the ADMP has been located, have the client relax it, and palpate to assess its baseline tone.
5. To now palpate the flexor digiti minimi pedis (FDMP), which is also superficial and easily palpable, move your palpating fingers over the fifth metatarsal bone on the plantar side of the foot.
6. Ask the client to flex the little toe at the MTP joint, and feel for the contraction of the FDMP. If desired, resistance can be given with the support hand on the plantar surface of the proximal phalanx of the little toe (Figure 21-25).
7. Once located, palpate it distally to the proximal phalanx of the little toe while strumming perpendicular to its fibers. Then palpate it proximally as far as possible.
8. Once the FDMP has been located, have the client relax it, and palpate to assess its baseline tone.

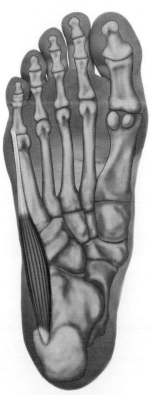

Figure 21-21 Plantar view of the right abductor digiti minimi pedis (ADMP).

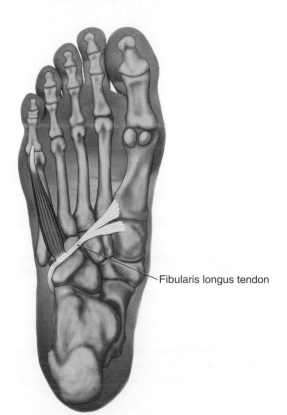

Fibularis longus tendon

Figure 21-22 Plantar view of the right flexor digiti minimi pedis (FDMP).

21

ABDUCTOR DIGITI MINIMI PEDIS (ADMP) AND FLEXOR DIGITI MINIMI PEDIS (FDMP)—PRONE—*cont'd*

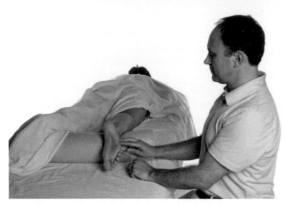

Figure 21-23 Starting position for prone palpation of the right abductor digiti minimi pedis (ADMP).

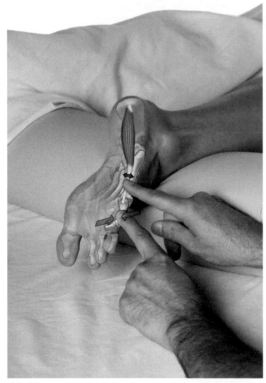

Figure 21-24 Palpation of the right abductor digiti minimi pedis (ADMP) as the client abducts the little toe against resistance.

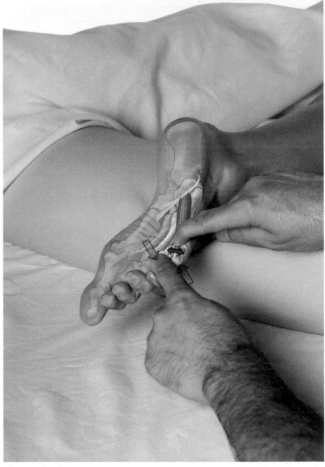

Figure 21-25 Palpation of the right flexor digiti minimi pedis (FDMP) as the client flexes the little toe against resistance.

ABDUCTOR DIGITI MINIMI PEDIS PALPATION NOTES

1. The abductor digiti minimi pedis (ADMP) is superficial and easily palpable.
2. Abduction of the little toe at the MTP joint is a lateral motion.
3. Although all of the ADMP can usually be palpated and discerned, it is easiest to palpate it in the distal half of the foot.
4. Many clients are unable to isolate the motion of abduction of the little toe. If this occurs, place a finger of your support hand against the lateral side of the proximal phalanx of the little toe, and ask the client to press against it. Having the pressure of the resistance finger often helps the client create this motion.
5. To discern the border of the ADMP from the flexor digiti minimi pedis (FDMP), make sure that the client is not flexing the little toe as abduction is done. If necessary, the client can be asked to abduct and extend the little toe at the MTP joint. Extension will reciprocally inhibit and relax the FDMP.

21

ABDUCTOR DIGITI MINIMI PEDIS (ADMP) AND FLEXOR DIGITI MINIMI PEDIS (FDMP)—PRONE—*cont'd*

FLEXOR DIGITI MINIMI PEDIS PALPATION NOTES

1. The flexor digitorum brevis and the tendon of the flexor digitorum longus to the little toe lie superficial to the flexor digiti minimi pedis (FDMP). For this reason, it can be difficult to discern the FDMP from these other muscles because they also contract when the little toe flexes.
2. To discern the FDMP from the more superficial flexors digitorum brevis and longus, try to have the client isolate flexion of the little toe at the MTP joint while keeping the interphalangeal (IP) joints of the little toe extended. This tends to engage the FDMP more than the flexors digitorum brevis and longus. Unfortunately, most clients are unable to do this.

TRIGGER POINTS

1. Trigger points (TrPs) in the abductor digiti minimi pedis (ADMP) and flexor digiti minimi pedis (FDMP) often result from or are perpetuated by acute or chronic overuse of the muscle (e.g., walking in soft sand), sustained postures that cause the muscles to lengthen (e.g., wearing high-heeled shoes), wearing ill-fitting shoes (that are either too tight or laced too tightly, or have a pointed toe), wearing shoes with an inflexible sole (not allowing motion of the MTP joint), immobilization due to a cast, excessive pronation of the foot (requiring greater stabilization by the intrinsic foot muscles), structural deformities of the foot, trauma, or stress fractures of the metatarsals.
2. TrPs in the ADMP and FDMP tend to produce tender and sore feet (especially when weight bearing), pain when walking, decreased or painful adduction (ADMP) or extension (FDMP or ADMP) of the little toe at the MTP joint, cramps in the foot, or an antalgic gait.
3. The referral patterns of ADMP and FDMP TrPs must be distinguished from the referral patterns of TrPs in the flexor digitorum brevis (FDB), plantar interossei, dorsal interossei pedis, and lumbricals pedis between the fourth and fifth toes, adductor hallucis, and flexor digitorum longus.
4. TrPs in the ADMP and FDMP are often incorrectly assessed as plantar fasciitis, metatarsal stress fracture, or tarsal joint dysfunction.

5. Associated TrPs often occur in the FDB.
6. Note: The ADMP and FDMP share the same TrP pain referral pattern.

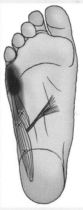

Figure 21-26 Plantar view showing common trigger points (TrPs) and their corresponding referral zone in the abductor and flexor digiti minimi pedis (FDMP) muscles.

Alternate Position—Supine

Both the ADMP and the FDMP can also be easily accessed with the client supine.

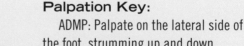

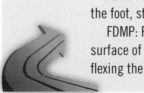

Palpation Key:

ADMP: Palpate on the lateral side of the foot, strumming up and down.

FDMP: Palpate over the plantar surface of the fifth metatarsal while flexing the little toe.

ABDUCTOR DIGITI MINIMI PEDIS (ADMP) AND FLEXOR DIGITI MINIMI PEDIS (FDMP)—PRONE—*cont'd*

STRETCHING THE ABDUCTOR DIGITI MINIMI PEDIS AND FLEXOR DIGITI MINIMI PEDIS

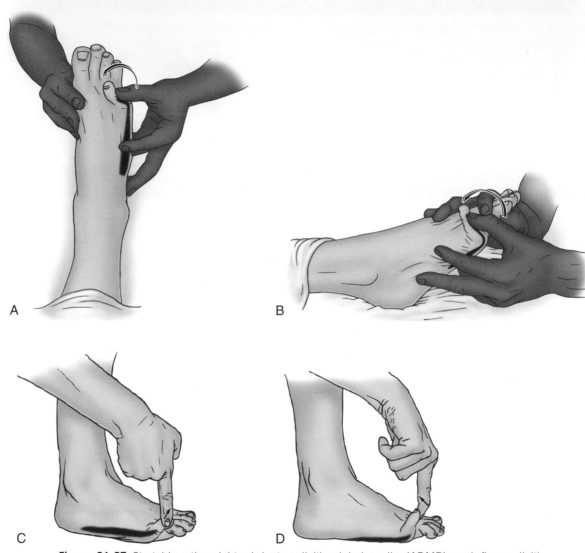

Figure 21-27 Stretching the right abductor digiti minimi pedis (ADMP) and flexor digiti minimi pedis (FDMP) muscles. Each muscle is stretched by moving the little toe at the metatarsophalangeal (MTP) joint. For the ADMP, the little toe is adducted and extended. For the FDMP, the little toe is extended. **A** and **B,** Therapist-assisted stretches of the ADMP and FDMP muscles, respectively. Note: The therapist's other hand is used to stabilize the client's foot. **C** and **D,** Self-care stretches of the ADMP and FDMP muscles, respectively.

21

ABDUCTOR DIGITI MINIMI PEDIS (ADMP) AND FLEXOR DIGITI MINIMI PEDIS (FDMP)—PRONE—*cont'd*

 DETOUR

Lumbricals Pedis:

There are four lumbricals pedis muscles, numbered one to four from medial to lateral. Even though they are located in the second plantar layer of the foot, they are fairly accessible to palpation. They attach from the distal tendons of the flexor digitorum longus to the distal tendons of the extensor digitorum longus (Figure 21-28, *A*). They flex toes two to five at the MTP joints and extend them at the IP joints. To palpate these muscles, palpate on the plantar side of the foot between the metatarsal bones. If the client is able to flex toes two to five at the MTP joints while keeping them extended at the IP joints, ask the client to do this and feel for their contraction. To stretch the lumbricals pedis, move toes two to five into extension at the MTP joints and flexion at the IP joints (see Figure 21-28, *B*).

Plantar Interossei:

There are three plantar interossei (PI) muscles, numbered one to three from medial to lateral. The plantar interossei (PI) attach from metatarsals three to five to the medial side of the proximal phalanges of toes three to five (see Figure 21-28, *C*) and are located deep to the lumbricals pedis; parts of them are also deep to the flexor digitorum brevis (FDB) as well as the plantar fascia. Their main action is to adduct toes three to five at the MTP joints; however, many clients are unable to isolate their action

of toe adduction. Given their depth and the difficulty of isolating their action, the plantar interossei are usually difficult to palpate and discern from adjacent soft tissues. To stretch them, move toes three to five into abduction (away from the second toe) at the MTP joints (see Figure 21-28, *D*).

Trigger Points:

1. Trigger points (TrPs) in the lumbricals pedis and plantar interossei usually result from the same factors that create or perpetuate TrPs in the abductor and flexor digiti minimi pedis (FDMP) muscles, and they produce approximately the same symptoms.
2. As with many intrinsic foot muscles of the plantar side, TrPs in the lumbricals pedis and plantar interossei tend to produce tender and sore feet (especially when weight bearing), pain when walking, decreased or painful extension of the affected toe at the MTP joint, cramps in the foot, or an antalgic gait.
3. Lumbricals pedis and plantar interossei TrP referral patterns are the same as for the dorsal interossei pedis and their TrPs are often incorrectly assessed as plantar fasciitis, metatarsal stress fracture, tarsal joint dysfunction, or entrapment of a digital nerve between adjacent metatarsals.
4. Associated TrPs often occur in the FDB, flexor hallucis brevis (FHB), and FDMP.

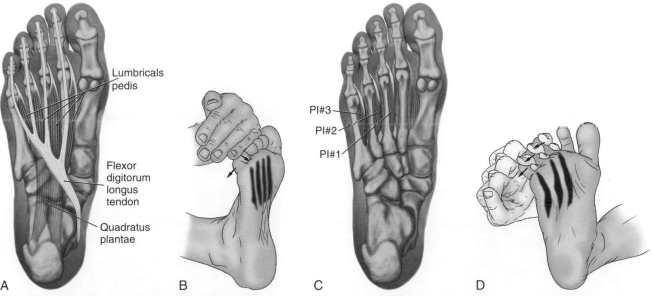

Figure 21-28 Views of the right lumbricals pedis and plantar interossei muscles. **A,** Plantar view of the lumbricals pedis; the quadratus plantae is ghosted in. **B,** Stretch of the lumbricals pedis. Toes two to five are extended at the metatarsophalangeal (MTP) joints and flexed at the interphalangeal (IP) joints. **C,** Plantar view of the plantar interossei (PI); the dorsal interossei pedis are ghosted in. **D,** Stretch of the plantar interossei. Toes three to five are abducted at the MTP joints.

21

FLEXOR DIGITORUM BREVIS (FDB)—PRONE

☑ ATTACHMENTS

☐ Tuberosity of the calcaneus

to the

☐ plantar surface of the middle phalanges of toes two to five

☑ ACTIONS

☐ Flexes toes two to five at the metatarsophalangeal (MTP) and proximal interphalangeal joints

Starting Position (Figure 21-30)

• Client prone
• Therapist seated at the end of the table
• Palpating fingers placed on the midline of the plantar surface of the proximal foot.
• If resistance is necessary, place fingers of the support hand on the plantar surface of the proximal or middle phalanges of toes two to five

Palpation Steps

1. Ask the client to flex toes two to five at the MTP joints, and feel for the contraction of the flexor digitorum brevis (FDB). If desired, resistance can be given with the support hand (Figure 21-31).
2. Once located, palpate it proximally to the calcaneus while strumming perpendicular to its fibers. Then palpate it distally as far as possible.
3. Once the FDB has been located, have the client relax it, and palpate to assess its baseline tone.

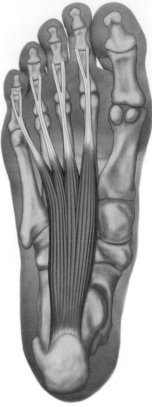

Figure 21-29 Plantar view of the right flexor digitorum brevis (FDB).

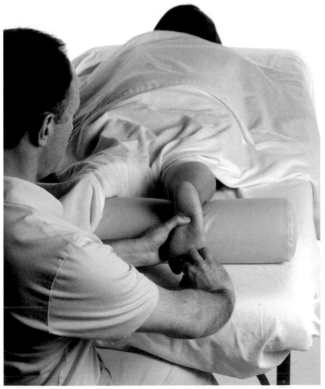

Figure 21-30 Starting position for prone palpation of the right flexor digitorum brevis (FDB).

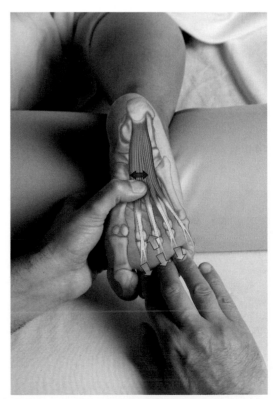

Figure 21-31 Palpation of the right flexor digitorum brevis (FDB) as the client flexes toes two to five against resistance.

21

FLEXOR DIGITORUM BREVIS (FDB)—PRONE—*cont'd*

PALPATION NOTES

1. Even though the flexor digitorum brevis (FDB) is deep to the plantar fascia, the contraction of its belly can usually be fairly easily palpated.
2. Directly deep to the FDB are the distal tendons of the flexor digitorum longus. Given that both these muscles contract with flexion of toes two to five, it can be difficult to discern them from each other. This is especially true in the distal end of the foot where the tendons of the FDB directly overlie the tendons of the flexor digitorum longus.
3. To discern the FDB from the deeper distal tendons of the flexor digitorum longus, try to have the client isolate flexion of the toes at the metatarsophalangeal (MTP) joints while keeping the interphalangeal (IP) joints extended. This tends to engage the FDB more than the flexor digitorum longus. Unfortunately, many clients are unable to isolate this action.
4. The quadratus plantae muscle is located directly deep to the FDB in the proximal foot and also flexes toes two to five. Therefore these two muscles can be difficult to discern from each other.

Alternate Position—Supine

The FDB can also be fairly easily palpated with the client supine.

Palpation Key:
Palpate in the center of the proximal plantar foot while flexing the toes.

TRIGGER POINTS

1. Trigger points (TrPs) in the FDB often result from or are perpetuated by acute or chronic overuse of the muscle (e.g., walking in soft sand), sustained postures that cause the muscles to lengthen (e.g., wearing high-heeled shoes), wearing ill-fitting shoes (that are either too tight or laced too tightly, or have a pointed toe), wearing shoes with an inflexible sole (not allowing motion of the MTP joints), immobilization due to a cast, excessive pronation of the foot (requiring greater stabilization by the intrinsic foot muscles), structural deformities of the foot, trauma, or stress fractures of the metatarsals.
2. TrPs in the FDB tend to produce tender and sore feet (especially when weight bearing), pain when walking, decreased or painful extension of toes two to five at the MTP joints, plantar fasciitis, cramps in the foot, or an antalgic gait.
3. The referral pattern of FDB TrPs must be distinguished from the referral patterns of TrPs in the adductor hallucis, flexor digitorum longus, flexor hallucis longus, abductor digiti minimi pedis (ADMP), flexor hallucis brevis (FHB), and plantar interossei, dorsal interossei pedis, and lumbricals pedis.
4. TrPs in the FDB are often incorrectly assessed as plantar fasciitis, metatarsal stress fracture, or tarsal joint dysfunction.
5. Associated TrPs often occur in the flexor digitorum longus, FHB, and flexor digiti minimi pedis (FDMP).

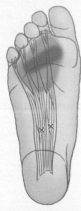

Figure 21-32 Plantar view showing common flexor digitorum brevis (FDB) trigger points (TrPs) and their corresponding referral zone.

21

FLEXOR DIGITORUM BREVIS (FDB)—PRONE—*cont'd*

STRETCHING THE FLEXOR DIGITORUM BREVIS

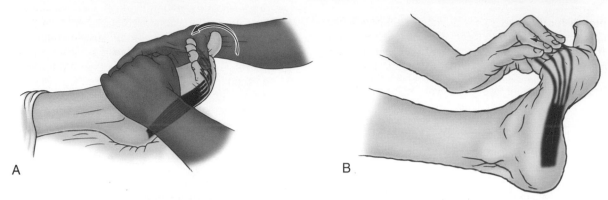

A   B

Figure 21-33 Stretching the right flexor digitorum brevis (FDB). The FDB is stretched by extending toes two through five at the metatarsophalangeal (MTP) and proximal interphalangeal joints. **A,** Therapist-assisted stretch. Note: The therapist's other hand is used to stabilize the client's foot. **B,** Self-care stretch.

DETOUR

Quadratus Plantae:

The quadratus plantae attaches from the calcaneus to the distal tendon of the flexor digitorum longus. To palpate this muscle, palpate on the midline of the plantar surface of the proximal foot, and ask the client to flex toes two to five. Because the quadratus plantae lies immediately deep to the flexor digitorum brevis (FDB), and both of these muscles flex toes two to five, it can be very difficult to palpate and discern the quadratus plantae from the FDB.

Trigger Points:

1. Trigger points (TrPs) in the quadratus plantae usually result from the same factors that create or perpetuate TrPs in the FDB. (However, their referral zones are quite different.)
2. The referral pattern for quadratus plantae TrPs must be distinguished from the referral patterns of TrPs in the soleus and abductor hallucis (AbH).
3. Associated TrPs often occur in the FDB and flexor digitorum longus.

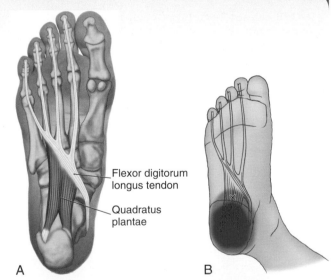

Flexor digitorum longus tendon

Quadratus plantae

A   B

Figure 21-34 Views of the right quadratus plantae. **A,** Planter view of the quadratus plantae. **B,** Medial-plantar view showing a common quadratus plantae trigger point (TrP) and its corresponding referral zone.

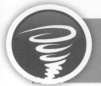

WHIRLWIND TOUR

Intrinsic Muscles of the Foot

The following *Whirlwind Tour* is an abbreviated set of palpation protocols for the muscles of this chapter. Once you have read and become comfortable with each of the protocols presented thus far, this *Whirlwind Tour* allows you to quickly and efficiently run through the palpations protocols for all the muscles of the chapter.

Client Supine

For the palpations of the following intrinsic muscles of the foot on the dorsal side, the client is supine with a roll under the knees and you are seated to the side of the client.

1. **Extensor digitorum brevis (EDB) and extensor hallucis brevis (EHB):** Visualize, locate, and palpate the belly of the EDB and EHB just distal to the lateral malleolus on the dorsal foot. Feel for its contraction as the client extends toes two to four at the metatarsophalangeal (MTP) and interphalangeal (IP) joints and the big toe at the MTP joint. The EDB fibers are located more laterally within the common belly, and the EHB fibers are located more medially within the common belly. Once the contraction is felt, continue palpating each of the tendons distally to its attachment on a toe while strumming perpendicular to it as the client alternately contracts and relaxes the muscle. Resistance can be added if needed.

2. **Dorsal interossei pedis:** Palpate between the metatarsals on the dorsal foot. To confirm that you are on a dorsal interosseus pedis muscle, ask the client to abduct the toe to which that muscle is attached. The fourth dorsal interosseus pedis between metatarsals four and five abducts the fourth toe; the third dorsal interosseus pedis between metatarsals three and four abducts the third toe; the second dorsal interosseus pedis between metatarsals two and three does fibular abduction of the second toe; and the first dorsal interosseus pedis between metatarsals one and two does tibial abduction of the second toe. Palpate proximally and distally as far as possible. Resistance can be added if needed.

Client Prone

For the palpations of the following intrinsic muscles of the foot on the plantar side, the client is prone with a bolster under the ankles and you are seated at the end of the table.

3. **Abductor hallucis (AbH):** Palpate on the medial side of the foot, close to the plantar surface, and feel for the contraction of the belly of the AbH as the client abducts the big toe at the MTP joint. Once located, palpate proximally and distally as far as possible while strumming perpendicular to its fibers. Resistance can be added if needed.

4. **Abductor digiti minimi pedis (ADMP):** Palpate on the lateral side of the foot, close to the plantar surface, and feel for the contraction of the belly of the ADMP as the client abducts the little toe at the MTP joint. Once located, palpate proximally and distally as far as possible while strumming perpendicular to its fibers. Resistance can be added if needed.

5. **Flexor digitorum brevis (FDB):** Palpate on the midline of the plantar surface of the proximal foot, and feel for the contraction of the belly of the FDB as the client flexes toes two to five at the MTP and proximal interphalangeal joints. Once located, palpate proximally to the calcaneus and distally as far as possible while strumming perpendicular to the fibers. Resistance can be added if needed. Detour: The quadratus plantae may be palpated in the midline of the proximal plantar foot as the client flexes toes two to five. However, it is deep to the FDB and difficult to discern from this muscle.

6. **Flexor hallucis brevis (FHB):** Palpate over the first metatarsal on the plantar side of the foot, and feel for the contraction of the FHB as the client flexes the big toe at the MTP joint. Once located, palpate as far proximally and distally as possible while strumming perpendicular to its fibers. Resistance can be added if needed.

7. **Flexor digiti minimi pedis (FDMP):** Palpate over the fifth metatarsal on the plantar side of the foot, and feel for the contraction of the FDMP as the client flexes the little toe at the MTP joint. Once located, palpate proximally and distally as far as possible while strumming perpendicular to its fibers. Resistance can be added if needed. Detour(s): (1) The lumbricals pedis can be palpated between the metatarsals in the plantar foot. If the client is able, ask the client to flex toes two to five at the MTP joints while keeping them extended at the IP joints. (2) The plantar interossei are extremely difficult to palpate and discern. To attempt to palpate them, ask the client to adduct toes three to five as you palpate between metatarsals two to five in the plantar foot.

Review Questions

1. List the attachments of the extensor hallucis brevis (EHB).
2. List the attachments of the abductor digiti minimi pedis (ADMP).
3. What are the actions of the lumbricals pedis?
4. What are the actions of the dorsal interossei pedis?
5. Where should a therapist add the resistance force when palpating the extensor digitorum brevis (EDB)?
6. What is the best way to deal with the situation where a client, who cannot separate individual motions of the toes, is extending toes other than the big toe during palpation of the extensor hallucis brevis (EHB)?
7. What extraneous joint motion can obscure palpation of the dorsal interossei pedis, and why?
8. If a client cannot isolate abduction of the big toe, how else can a therapist engage the abductor hallucis (AbH) for palpation?
9. In what plantar layer is the flexor hallucis brevis (FHB) located?
10. What muscle action or actions would you ask a client to perform to engage the plantar interossei?
11. The quadratus plantae is located directly deep to what muscle and shares what action?
12. What intrinsic foot muscle's TrP referral zone consists only of the heel of the foot?
13. Entrapment of the medial or lateral plantar nerves may be caused by TrPs in what muscle?
14. Explain how to stretch the dorsal interossei pedis.
15. Describe a stretch for the abductor digiti minimi pedis (ADMP)?
16. What can be said about both the structural and functional relationship of the extensor digitorum brevis (EDB) and the extensor hallucis brevis (EHB)?
17. Explain the procedure for discerning the border of the abductor digiti minimi pedis (ADMP) from the flexor digiti minimi pedis (FDMP).

CASE STUDY

A 38-year-old woman comes in for a massage complaining of foot pain. While walking her to the treatment room you notice that she has a limp and is limiting the time she spends weight-bearing on the right foot.

History reveals that she was an avid runner through her twenties and had occasional pain and discomfort in her feet and legs. At 30 she developed plantar fasciitis in both feet, but the left side resolved within 6 months, whereas the right side remained. At 35 and having had no relief from the pain in her right foot, she had fascia release surgery. After recovery and physical therapy, the pain decreased to only a mild, occasional discomfort. In the last 2 months, however, the pain in her right foot has returned. She indicates that the pain is on the medial side of the foot from the big toe to the heel and also occasionally spreads to the dorsum of the foot just anterior/distal to the calcaneus. There is also an occasional tingling/itching sensation that is felt on the plantar surface of her foot.

Physical exam of the right foot shows overpronation, tenderness to palpation along the path of the medial longitudinal arch, and decreased flexion of the toes. A recent x-ray report that the client provided indicates evidence of previous stress fractures of the second and third metatarsals and a bone spur on the calcaneus.

1. Based on the symptoms, what muscles might you expect to be tight on this client?
2. What effect may the plantar fascia release surgery have had on this client?
3. What might an initial treatment plan for this client include?

Index

Page numbers followed by b indicates boxes, f indicates illustrations, and t indicates tables.